11TH INTERNATIONAL CONGRESS OF THE WORLD CONFEDERATION FOR PHYSICAL THERAPY

The Barbican Centre, London, United Kingdom
28 July – 2 August 1991

PROCEEDINGS
BOOK II

Book I, II & III
ISBN 1 870905 27 X

Printed and bound in Great Britain

CONTENTS

Papers are printed under the same Subject Headings as in the Congress Programme, however please note that the paper titles may differ.

BOOK III

Clinical Practice

Resource Management

International Federation of Orthopaedic Manipulative Therapists

Authors Index

CLINICAL PRACTICE

KNEE DISORDERS MANAGEMENT

EFFICACY OF ELECTRICAL STIMULATION AS A FUNCTIONAL ORTHOSIS
FOR THE UNSTABLE KNEE

Authors: P.P. Tygiel, P.T. and S. Hardman, P.T.
Institution: Tygiel & Associates Physical Therapy
6606 E. Carondelet Dr. Tucson, Az. 85710, U.S.A.

While orthopedic surgical techniques for the
reconstruction and/or augmentation of torn knee
ligaments have advanced greatly over the past 50 years,
some patients still go on to be surgical failures and
developed chronically unstable knees. We have seen
several patients who eventually had multiple surgeries,
harvesting a variety of donor sites and even using
allographs and artificial augmentation devices, all to no
avail.

One can only speculate as to the reasons for the failures.
In some cases it might be that the initial damage was too
great to overcome. In others the ability of the body to
heal itself might have been compromised. Poor surgical
technique can always be suspected. In any case the
patient is left with a knee that gives out easily. Each
step can be an adventure. This presents a rather
difficult rehabilitation dilemma.

Strengthening of the lower extremity musculature proves
futile. Conventional bracing is not helpful. Most
conventional braces are designed for use in athletic
competition. They are to be worn for a few hours and then
taken off. Wearing them for a full day, day in and day
out, is extremely uncomfortable. Even with the brace on,
in certain positions the knee may give out anyway.
We have attempted an alternative stabilization technique
using functional electrical stimulation that has proven
quite successful. We have now used the technique on six
patients. There were three male and three females ranging
in age from 18 years to 42 years. Four had combined ACL,
PCL and MCL deficiencies. Of those, two had 3 surgeries,
one had 4 and one had 6.

Two patients had chronic PCL instability only.

The instability was sufficient to affect their ADL. They each failed two surgical attempts.

THE TECHNIQUE: A Medtronic Respond II unit was used to provide electrical stimulation to the hamstrings and quadriceps from heel strike through mid stance. Electrodes from one channel were placed on the hamstrings and from a second channel on the quadriceps.

The pulse rate was set for maximum tetany. The rise time was instantaneous for the hamstrings and set with a brief time delay for the quadriceps. This was done so that the hamstrings could decelerate the forward motion of the tibia under the femur before the quadriceps further stabilized the knee just as occurs in normal gait. The channels were set in synchrony rather than reciprocally. No fall time was set. The remote switch was set on reverse. Output percentage was 100% for both channels. (See Figure 1 for settings)

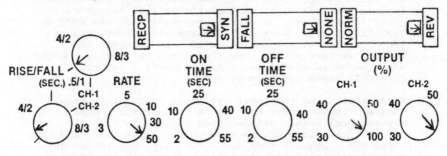

Figure 1

A foot plate was placed in the shoe of the involved leg. The switch in the foot plate made contact at heel strike and maintained contact through foot flat thus turning on the stimulation from heel strike through foot flat and turning it off upon heel off.

The patients were instructed to stand with the foot flat on the floor bearing full weight on that foot. They were then to turn on the two channels, one at a time, to the maximum they could comfortably tolerate. They would then begin walking with a normal gait pattern to see if they felt stable.

RESULTS: All six patients were totally, functionally stable during walking and general ADL activities. It was later found that the two PCL patients only needed the quadriceps stimulation for stability as tibial deceleration was not a problem. Surprisingly all of the patients were able to begin using the device full time immediately. No gradual accommodation phase was necessary.

Five of the patients continue to use the device as their main source of knee stabilization. One of them has now used it for seven years. One was unhappy that she would always require external stabilization and chose to seek further surgical consultation. She was the patient who had already under gone 6 surgeries to that knee and was probably being unrealistic about her future.

A few patients did have some problems with skin breakdown because of the electrodes. This was resolved with skin care and use of a variety of electrodes.

CONCLUSION: Electrical stimulation can be used as a functional orthosis for the chronically unstable knee. A more convenient unit than the Medcosonolator Respond II can probably be developed. The Respond II is rather cumbersome and provides for more adjustment than is needed for this technique.

The question really must be raised as to why it is possible for the knee to be stabilized electrically but not voluntarily. Further study of this phenomenon would certainly be in order.

It is also interesting to note that even though these people wore the unit daily for many hours a day, there was no significant functional strengthening that allowed them to ultimately be stable without the device. This would seem to raise serious questions about claims that one can increase strength with electrical stimulation alone or can get better strengthening with a combination of electrical stimulation and exercise.

NEUROPHYSIOLOGICAL APPROACH OF THE PHYSIOTHERAPEUTIC TREATMENT OF KNEE INJURIES

R.A.B. Oostendorp

National Institute of Research and Postgraduate Education in Physical Therapy, Amersfoort, The Netherlands; Free University Brussels, Faculty of Medicine and Pharmacology, Biomedical Sciences-Manual Therapy, Brussels, Belgium.

The conservative treatment of lesions of the ligaments of the knee and the postoperative treatment after reconstructive surgery of the ligaments of the knee often consists of a combination of immobilisation and physiotherapy. Many variations of this type of treatment have been discussed in the literature and are being used in actual practice. Whatever the choice of treatment may be, for a physiotherapist the underlying rationale for his treatment is always based on a number of functional impairments and disabilities of the patient, the appropriate treatment of which requires a good understanding not only of the biomechanical properties of collagen but of the (neuro)physiology of the knee joint as well. Over the past few years many in vivo and in vitro studies have been performed in the field of neurophysiology of joints in general. Impairments can, as a result of this research, be placed in a neurophysiological perspective:
* Partial immobilisation and limited joint motion in relation to the mechano-sensoric pattern and to the plasticity of the peripheral receptive field;
* Intra-articular swelling in relation to the inhibition of muscular function;
* Decompensated stability in relation to dyscoordination and protective muscular reflexes;
* Partial deafferentiation of the joint and joint stress in relation to the development of arthropathy and neurogenic inflammatory reaction (substance-P);
* Joint pain in relation to sensitization of free nerve endings (prostaglandine E2 and substance-P).
The implications of this approach will be discussed.

THE EFFECTS OF PAD PLACEMENT DURING ISOKINETICS ON ACL DEFICIENT KNEES

K E Wilk

Healthsouth Sports Medicine & Rehabilitation Ctr.,
Birmingham, Alabama, USA

Introduction: The purpose of this study was to compare the effects of proximal single pad placement (PSPP) vs distal single pad placement (DSPP) on tibial translation during isokinetic testing on anterior cruciate ligament (ACL) deficient knees.
Treatment: Twelve subjects participated in the study, each was randomized into 6 groups. Each subject exhibited greater than 10 mm of tibial translation determined by a computerized Lachman's Test performed on an Acufex Knee Signature System (KSS). Each subject was tested on the Biodex B-2000 isokinetic dynamometer at isokinetic speeds of 60, 180, and 300°/s with the KSS instrumented to determine tibial translation during testing. Pad placement consisted of PSPP just proximal to the medial malleoli and DSPP, 3" distal to tibial tuberosity.
Results: Results indicated PSPP rendered less tibial translation than the DSPP at all isokinetic speeds. The decrease in tibial translation ranged from 18%-28% with the greatest decrease at 60°/s. In addition, results indicated that higher speeds isokinetic 180 and 300°/s caused less tibial translation than 60°/s.
Conclusion: The clinical importance of this study indicates that when utilizing isokinetic exercise with an ACL client performing at 300°/s and/or 180°/s minimizes tibial translation compared to slow speed isokinetics at 60°/s. In addition, proximal single pad placement decreases tibial translation compared to the recommended distal pad placement for testing.

Isokinetic concentric and eccentric mode evaluation of suprapatellar plicae and patello-femoral disorders

J.E.Williams GradDipPhys MCSP SRP, L.Hall MCSP SRP, H.M.Porteous MCSP SRP
A.E.Strover FRCS,E.Rouholamin FRCS, S.Rao MD Orth and D.Bryson BSc.

There are three plicae or synovial folds commonly found within the knee joint :
The infrapatellar plica or ligamentum mucosum stretches from the top of the intercondylar notch fanning out distally to attach to the infrapatellar fat pad.
The mediopatellar plica or medial shelf originates at the distal end of the suprapatellar pouch or actually from a suprapatellar plica; it lies along the medial wall of the joint and runs obliquely down and attaches to the infrapatellar fat pad.
The suprapatellar plica is a synovial fold proximal to the superior pole of the patella, lying in a horizontal or tilted plane, when the knee is in extension (fig 1a). The anterior portion, which arises from the synovium deep to the quadriceps mechanism, moves as the patella descends into a vertical position on flexion. The plica can be anything from a small crescent to a complete septum.

The aim of this study was to evaluate the isokinetic findings of patients diagnosed as having a suprapatellar plica with or without other pathology, excluding those with a mediopatellar plica. We specifically aimed to determine if there was any correlation between the presence of a suprapatellar plica and the torque generated in concentric and eccentric modes and the graph shapes for quadriceps and hamstrings.

Materials and Methods
A group of 43 patients, 48 knees, 5 bilateral, were selected from their operative diagnosis as having a pathological suprapatellar plica and information about each patient including their pre-operative symptoms, isokinetic findings and per-operative video were analysed. Right leg 24, left 24; male 31, female 17. Average age 39 years, age range 14–82 years.

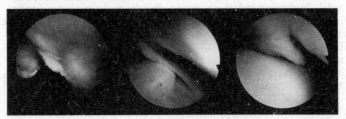

Figure1: Suprapatellar plica Type 2 viewed from a lateral suprapatellar portal a) knee in extension. b) Impingement or bowstrining, 36° flexion c) Trapped between quadriceps and femoral trochlea at 70° flexion

Patients were evaluated pre- and post-operatively using the Kincom Mk II[*] hydraulic computer controlled isokinetic machine. The normal and problem legs were assessed with the same set-up, ie. lever arm length, seat position and restraints (ref 1). The assessment was used to monitor the quadriceps and hamstrings at 30°/sec and 100°/sec in concentric and eccentric modes. A warm up period of 3 repetitions was used followed by the test of 3 repetitions.

For this study, readings were taken of the average and peak torque/weight for each patient and each graph shape described with reference to any changes from the normal. A normal concentric graph climbs from 90° flexion rapidly to its peak and then slowly fades towards 0°. The eccentric mode (fig 3a) climbs slowly from 0° to its peak at about 80° and fades. The continuous line on the graph is the mean value of the force readings and the dots above and below are the maximum and minimum values.

All patients underwent a diagnostic arthroscopy, followed by arthroscopic removal of the suprapatellar plica. The procedures were videotaped. In describing the types of suprapatellar plicae we have followed Deutsch's classification (ref 2) as shown in table 1.

Table 1 : Deutsch's Classification of Suprapatellar plicae

Type A –   An intact synovial septum completely dividing the suprapatellar pouch from the rest of the knee.

Type B –   A partially developed septum with a variably sized, centrally placed porta or opening.

Type C –   A variably sized crescent shaped fold.

An essential element in the arthroscopic method in these cases was the examination of the patello–femoral joint, via a lateral suprapatellar portal. This allows good visualization of the suprapatellar plica in its normal position (fig 1a) with the knee in extension and on flexion as it tightens, bowstrings then impinges on the medial femoral condyle (fig 1b) until at about 70° of flexion (fig 1c) it is trapped between the quadriceps mechanism and the femoral trochlea (ref 3).

Results

Analysis of Isokinetics

In our series of patients the peak torque in the quadriceps is consistently reduced compared with normal. This effect is more marked in the fast quadriceps test in the eccentric mode at 100°/sec.

The graph shape is altered with a plateau effect as indicated on figure 3b. The angle of flexion in this case was 36°, which was also the angle of initial impingement demonstrated at arthroscopy.

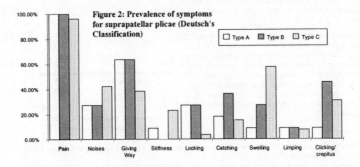

Figure 2: Prevalence of symptoms for suprapatellar plicae (Deutsch's Classification)

□ Type A   ▨ Type B   □ Type C

Clinical findings

The mean duration of symptoms was 19 months, range 2 weeks – 120 months. The prevalence of symptoms, expressed as percentages are given in figure 2 above for each of the different types of suprapatellar plicae. Operatively the plicae were classified as Type A 11 (%), Type B 11 (%) and Type C 26 (%) (Table 2).

The suprapatellar plica and associated pathology

In 18 patients, 22 knees, the only pathology found at arthroscopy was a suprapatellar plica.

The most common associated findings in our whole series were chondromalacia patellae in 19 (39.6%) and chondral softening of the medial femoral condyle in 11 (22.9%). The following operative procedures were also undertaken: lateral release 12 (25%), removal of chondral flaps 4 (8.3%), partial medial meniscectomy

6 (12.5%), partial lateral meniscectomy 9 (18.7%). Patello-femoral debridement for early osteoarthritis was necessary in 13 (27.1%) patients.

Discussion

The embryological origin of plicae has been described by Gray & Gardner (ref 1) and more recently by Ogata & Uhthoff (ref 2). The frequency of occurence in Ogata's study(ref 2) was suprapatellar 33.3%, mediopatellar 36.8% and infrapatellar 50%. The presence of a plica is not of itself pathological. Standard arthroscopic views may fail to demonstrate the presence or pathogenicity of a suprapatellar plica.

Our experience shows that a suprapatellar plica interfering with joint movements may slow recovery, prevent the knee returning to normal function, or it may mimic or mask patello-femoral or meniscal disorders.
The Isokinetic tests have been extremely valuable in pre- and post-operative monitoring, and can supplement the data a consultant has available prior to surgery and in assessing his patient at the end of the treatment.

The additional information that these tests provide mean that it is not always necessary to obtain MRI scans or contrast athrography views of the knee joint for the suprapatellar plica. In one patient an MRI failed to demonstrate a plica but the Kincom assessment pointed to the its presence, which was then confirmed by diagnostic arthroscopy.

The suprapatellar plica can act as a block to movement in the joint and give a false positive diagnosis of a meniscal lesion. A Kincom assessment showing abnormal shapes in the quadriceps graphs with "normal" hamstring graphs point to a patello-femoral problem which is commonly the direct result of a suprapatellar plica. Removal of the plica in our experience has always improved the shape of the graph, sometimes to normal or at least equivalent to the opposite side.

Figure 3: Graphs from Kincom MkII* Isokinetic machine

References

1. Gray D.J. and Gardner E. Prenatal development of the human knee and superior tibiofibular joints. Am.J.Anat. 1950;86:235–287.
2. Ogata S. and Uhthoff H.K. The development of synovial plicae in human knee joints : an embryologic study. Arthroscopy 1990;6(4):315–321.
3. Deutsch A.L., Resnick D., Dalinca M.K. et al. Synovial plicae of the knee. Diagnostic Radiol. 1981;141:627–634.
4. Hall L. and Williams J.E. The use of isokinetics in rehabilitation. Physiotherapy 1989;75(12):737–740.
5. Strover A.E., Rouholamin E., Guirguis N. and Behdad H. An arthroscopic technique of demonstrating the pathomechanics of the suprapatellar plica. Arthroscopy In Press.

* ® Chattex Corporation, Texas, USA.

MISCELLANEOUS

THE TOTAL CARE APPROACH TO THE MANAGEMENT OF PSORIASIS

Audrey Weiner
Physiotherapy Department, H.F. Verwoerd Hospital, Pretoria, South Africa

The relationship between the mind and the body was recognised by physicians and philosophers from the time of Socrates. He observed that "The reason why the cure of many diseases is unknown to the physicians of Hellas is because they disregard the whole, which ought to be studied, for the part can never be well unless the whole is well". (Plato c 390BC) (1). Today there is impressive evidence which demonstrates that the mind can affect the incidence, course and outcome of physical disease, and that physical disease can affect the mind, i.e. minds and bodies simply constitute different perspectives of an essentially unitary person (2). In this paradigm, Total Psoriasis Care encompasses the whole human being, attending to the physical, psychological and social aspects of the disease and incorporating humanistic concern for the patient.

Psoriasis is a common, chronic, non-contagious skin disease which affects 1-2% of the population. It can affect any part of the body and has several different forms. The effects of the disease can be devastating.

MANAGEMENT: The Physiotherapy Department at our Hospital has been designed so that the entire physical treatment of psoriatic patients takes place there. Both In- and Out-Patients are treated. The responsibility for administering the treatment rests on the physiotherapist. It has proved beneficial for one therapist to treat the patient, in that a strong physiotherapeutic relationship is established. It is of great importance that she understands the impact of the condition on the patient's life. An atmosphere of optimism, warmth, acceptance, trust, kindness, calmness and restfulness is created. The physiotherapist should be empathetic, tolerant, a skilled listener, supportive, non-judgemental, a competent counsellor, have good interpersonal skills and a sense of humour.

The patient is often bewildered, frightened, anxious and uninformed about his condition. Ingram (3) considers it a misdemeanour to emphasise the incurability of psoriasis and stated that patients should know that psoriasis can be cleared. Educating patients about their disease and encouraging them to take responsibility for self-care will lessen morbidity (4). They are taught to recognise triggering factors, which include streptococcal throat infection, injury, low humidity and emotional stress. The patients and their families are counselled and helped in coping with the condition as well as being informed of new developments and current research. The patients are treated with positive expectancy and are given an anticipated time for clearing.

A. Treatment: The aim of the treatment is to slow down the rapid cell division and to return the skin to normality. The physiotherapist assesses the history of photosensitivity, the use of photosensitising drugs, skin type, possibility of heat intolerance, percentage of body affected and the Psoriasis Area Severity Index Score. The condition should be cleared as soon as possible with the minimum intrusion into the patient's life. The type of treatment depends upon the patient's age and medical history, the type of psoriasis, its severity, extent and location.

1. Body: i) Ultraviolet light alone or with a thin film of liquid paraffin of white Vaseline.

   ii) Coal tar and Ultraviolet B - Goeckerman-type treatment.

   iii) Coal tar bath, Ultraviolet B and dithranol/anthralin - modified Ingram treatment. Dithranol is used either as short contact therapy or under occlusion. Thick plaques are steamed with moist hot packs.

   iv) DUVA - Dithranol and Ultraviolet A.

   v) Wolff's Helarium with or without dithranol.

   vi) PUVA - Psoralen and Ultraviolet A is used if there is no response to phototherapy and also for certain types of psoriasis.

2. Scalp: Thick scaly plaques are well lubricated with liquid paraffin and Ung Emulsificans Aquosum and steamed off with moist hot packs. Ultraviolet light is administered with a Psoracomb and a dithranol scalp cream applied.

3. Nails: The affected nails are soaked in a saline solution and then irradiated with a Dermalight Blue Point Light. With the use of a filter topical PUVA can be given.

4. Psoriatic Arthritis: Physiotherapeutic modalaties such as Curapulse, wax, Interferential and exercises are used as required.

Complete clearance with physical treatment is usually necessary to improve the prognosis. An even more lasting effect may follow early therapy, not only to the skin but also to the patient as a whole (5).

B. Stress Reduction: Ingram (3) considers emotional stress to be the most potent precipitating factor in psoriasis. Stressful events were found to be related to the onset and severity of psoriasis and Gaston et al (6) advocates that stress reduction be regarded as a part of the treatment offered for psoriasis. Patients with a clear insight into the possible relationship between stress and psoriasis had a better prognosis (5). Having psoriasis in itself can be stress producing. Patients need to cope with loss: of self-image, money, time and sometimes relationships and employment. Stress reduction is attended to according to the individual needs of the patient. It helps the patient maximise his own healing and recuperative potential.

1) Breathing: Diaphragmatic and Alternate Nostril Breathing are taught to help break the cycle of anxiety and tension.

2) Stretching exercises: These relax the back, neck, shoulders and face.

3) Massage: Used when there is a build up of tension in the neck, back and shoulders.

4) Music: The body posesses all the elements of music, namely sound, beat and rhythm. Music affects the body and mind. Slow movements from Baroque music lower the brain waves to Alpha, which help relieve stress and harmonise the body and mind. This music also provides a restful atmosphere.

5) Coping and basic life style skills: These are developed by means of discussions and hand-outs which include information on recognising sources and symptoms of stress, how to minimise worry, breaking stressful habits and quick and easy stress reducers.

C. Relaxation Techniques: According to Winchell et al (7), relaxation and other psychotherapeutic modalaties can be beneficial in the treatment of psoriasis, since psychological processes do affect the skin and have been found to be related to the onset and subsequent relapse in a high percentage of cases. Relaxation is a powerful self-help tool which encourages self-responsibility and provides an internal locus of control.

It also assists in gaining insight into one's potential inner resources for growth and self-regulation. Relaxation techniques are mainly taught within the treatment session, especially when using moist hot packs or when using short contact dithranol for a period of 20 minutes. Audio tapes are used with or without baroque music in the background. The techniques used are Tension/Release; Meditative relaxation; Guided and Self-Imagery of the healing process and Visualisation. Affirmations or self-talk are taught and used in the relaxed state when there is a greater access to the subconcious mind. These affirmations are for health, coping and living.
D. Nourishment: Although no dietary regimen has been of proven value, the patients are encouraged to partake of a healthy diet. Alcohol should be minimised, optimum weight should be maintained and any foodstuffs that affect the condition should be avoided.
E. Support: Patients receiving treatment have the opportunity to meet others with psoriasis. Group interaction is initiated by the physiotherapist; common problems are discussed, concerns are ventilated and some solutions shared. The support of families and friends should be mobilised. Social support helps keep the patients in treatment and promotes compliance with the prescribed regimens and may speed recovery. The patients are encouraged to join the Psoriasis Association which offers support, social interaction, meetings and journals.
RESULTS: The psoriatic lesions cleared within 2-4 weeks. Self-responsibility and a feeling of contributing to their own healing was established. The social isolation often induced by this condition was significantly reduced and self-image was improved. Longstanding cases went into remission for the first time. All patients reported feeling less stressed, more relaxed, more accepting of their condition and more in control of their lives.
CONCLUSION: The patients' quality of life improved and they were more equipped to cope with this chronic disease and its many implications. This Total Care approach assists in the return to wholeness of both body and mind, helping the patient to become a "Whole Human Being" again.

References
1. Plato (c 390 B.C.) Charmides dialogue. Sections 156-7. Princeton University Press 1978.
2. Schlebusch L. (1989). Mind-body synthesis. The interactive health-care equation. Pietermaritzburg : University of Natal Press.
3. Ingram J.T. (1954). The significance and management of psoriasis. British Medical Journal, ii, 823-828.
4. Faber E.M., Nall L. (1984). An appraisal of measures to prevent and control psoriasis. Journal of the American Academy of Dermatology 10:511-516.
5. Seville R.H. (1978). Psoriasis and Stress II. British Journal of Dermatology 98 : 151-153.
6. Gaston L, Lassonde M, Bernier-Buzzanga J, Hodgins S, Crombez J. (1987). Psoriasis and stress: A prospective study. Journal of the American Academy of Dermatology 17 : 82-86.
7. Winchell S.A., Watts R.A. (1988). Relaxation therapies in the treatment of psoriasis and possible pathophysiologic mechanisms. Journal of the American Academy of Dermatology 18 : 101-104.

Acknowlegements: To the late Professor G.H. Findlay, Professor of Dermatology and head of the Photobiology Research Unit for his support and encouragement; the Departments of Dermatology and Physiotherapy of the H.F. Verwoerd Hospital for support.

MUSCULOSKELETAL DEFICITS AND REHABILITATION INTERVENTION OF THE CANCER PATIENT

C.L. McGarvey and L.H. Gerber, M.D.
National Institutes of Health, Clinical Center, Department of Rehabilitation Medicine, 9000 Rockville Pike, Bldg. 10, Rm 6s235, Bethesda, MD 20892

Statistics from the National Cancer Institute's SEER Program, as published by the American Cancer society, indicate that approximately 500,000 Americans or 4 out of 10 patients with cancer will be alive 5 years following diagnosis.[1] This 4 in 10 ratio or 40% is referred to as the "observed" survival rate. When other factors such as normal, expected life processes are taken into account, a "relative" survival rate of 48% is calculated.

Musculosketal morbidity following primary cancer treatment may manifest in a variety of soft tissue, joint, cardiopulmonary, neurological or ambulation deficits.[2] Each of which, if not identified early and treated appropriately, could result in serious permanent physical disability. Disability which could effect the individuals potential to return to a functional vocation and meaningful life. Failure to achieve these goals would place personal and economic hardship on family, friends and medical support systems.

Table (1) again identifies some of the more common musculoskeletal problems but places them in a time frame identifying period during the treatment process in which the problem might occur. In addition, there are recommendations for specific treatment techniques, frequency of those treatments and their respective goals.

Table (2) identifies four current cancer treatment strategies employed in combinations to treat primary disease. Under each strategy one will note typical acute or chronic musculoskeletal sequalae. It is important to remember that although some columns identify a number of possible problems--the severity and functional disability from each is variable according to the type of neoplasm, the course of treatment and presence or absence of metastasis.

In summary, the information presented is an attempt to provide the reader with a general appreciation of the complexity involved in rehabilitation of the oncologic patient. Early referral and identification of responsible rehabilitation personnel could promote positive physical outcomes toward the goal of quality of life for the oncologic patient.

Table I

STAGE / COURSE of ACTION	POTENTIAL PROBLEM	REHABILITATION INTERVENTION TREATMENT	FREQUENCY of TREATMENT	GOAL
PRE-OPERATIVE	-delayed referral to rehabilitation medicine -delay in rehabilitation intervention	-initiate referral requesting: rehabilitation evaluation and treatment -educate in preliminary exercise program -identify risk factors of primary treatment	1-2 visits	Maintenance Prevention
Post-operative				
ACUTE STAGE -Bedrest -P.O.D. 1-4	Atrophy	-isometrics, active range of motion	1x/daily	Prevention Restoration
	Range of motion	-passive range of motion		
	Contracture	-static bracing, stretching		
	Pain	-electroanalgesia		
	Weakness	-isometrics		
	Decubiti	-functional bracing, body positioning		
	Neuropathy	-functional bracing		
INTERMEDIATE STAGE -Limited activity -P.O.D. 4-discharge	Weakness	-isokinetics, electrostimulation	2x/daily	Restoration
	Range of Motion	-active and active-assisted range of motion, mobilization		
	Gait deficits	-progressive ambulation and assistive devices		
	Joint instability	-temporary bracing with thermoplastic appliance		
	Neuropathy	-dynamic bracing, electrostimulation		
	ADL limitations	-assess ADL needs and provision of equipment		
POST-DISCHARGE STAGE -Unrestricted activity -Outpatient	Range of motion	-active and active-assisted range of motion	-dependent on musculoskeletal deficits and strategy of treatment, ie: chemotherapy and/or irradiation	-Restoration -Maintenance
	Weakness	-isotonic exercise		
	Edema	-pneumatic compression and pressure gradient sleeves		
	Neuropathy	-permanent bracing, electrostimulation		
	Gait deficits	-permanent prosthesis/orthesis		
	Role adjustment	-evaluation and referral to appropriate counseling service		

Table II

MUSCULOSKELETAL SEQUALAE
seen in
PRIMARY CANCER THERAPY

M-S PROBLEM / CANCER THERAPY	SURGERY	CHEMOTHERAPY	IRRADIATION	IMMUNOTHERAPY
ATROPHY	x			x
WEAKNESS	x			x
CONTRACTURE	x		x	
DECUBITI/wound development	x		x	x
EDEMA		x		x
GAIT DEFICITS	x	x	x	
JOINT INSTABILITY	x			
NEUROPATHY	x	x	x	x
PAIN	x		x	
RANGE OF MOTION DEFICITS	x		x	
CARDIOTOXICITY		x		x
CNS INVOLVEMENT (upper, lower)		x	x	

BIBLIOGRAPHY

1) 1991 Cancer Facts and Figures, American Cancer Society, Atlanta, Georgia.

2) Meyer W, and Leventhal B: Late Effects of Cancer Therapy. Complications of Cancer: Diagnosis and Management. Abeloff, M.D. John Hopkins Press, 1979,. p. 397.

3) Dietz JH: Rehabilitaiton Oncology. John Wiley & Sons, New York 1981.

4) Gunn AE: Cancer Rehabilitation. Raven Press. New York, 1984.

5) Hinterbuchner C: Rehabilitation of Physical Disability in Cancer. New York State Journal of Medicine, 78:106, 1978

6) Zislis JM: Rehabilitaiton of the Cancer Patient. Geriatrics, 25:150, 1970.

PHYSIOTHERAPY IN OPHTHALMOLOGY

A.T. Sterle
University Medical Centre, Dept. of Ophthalmology, Physiotherapy Unit,
61000 Ljubljana, Zaloška 2, Slovenia, Yugoslavia

The physiotherapeutic methods and techniques used in ophthalmology are highly specific and closely adapted to problems of the eye. We are concerned with patients who have different eye diseases and with patients who have undergone surgery or sustained an injury to the eye or adjacent parts of the face. The eye is a sensitive organ. The physiotherapist must take this into account when selecting the methods of work. These patients need primarily general physiotherapy. The physiotherapist must provide preventive care of the locomotor and respiratory systems and ensure that the rehabilitation is completed as soon as possible. The period of rest and strict confinement to bed, mandatory after some eye conditions and surgical interventions, should pass without cardiovascular and respiratory complications. General physical therapy is administered only to in-patients in hospital wards. Special physiotherapy is carried out at a suitably equipped physiotherapy clinic, attended by patients also after discharge from the hospital. A classical condition to illustrate the importance of general physiotherapy in ophthalmology is retinal detachment; the patient must lie in bed with precisely defined posture of the head. The duration of bed rest as well as the head posture and elevation before and after the operation are determined by the ophthalmologist, depending on the extent and site of detachment. The basic position is the horizontal supine position without a pillow, the posture and elevation of the head being precisely defined. Other operations require the prone position, which is expecially awkward for the patient. Each of these positions calls for a specific programme of exercises, which must not cause the patient to move his head or strain his eyes. Respiratory therapy is of great importance, especially in the preoperative period, but it must be non-aggressive. Coughing exercises, vibration massage and tapotement are not suitable.

Kinesitherapy: A basic problem for the physiotherapist working in an eye department is function of the eyelids. The main role of the lid is mechanical protection of the eye. In lagophthalmos the patient cannot close the eye. Drying of the lacrimal fluid leads to recurrent corneal inflammation, resulting in opacification of the cornea. Lagophthalmos develops as a result of abnormal function of the levator palpebrae muscle. The causes include post-traumatic scarring in the eyelid, neurologic deficits, such as paresis or paralysis of the facial nerve, and transient conditions following surgery. The opposite condition is ptosis, an inability to open the eye. Ptosis may be partial or complete. Before each therapeutic procedure, measurements of the lid function are carried out so that the effect of treatment can be evaluated. Exercises are performed by each patient individually and in a group, in front of a mirror. Exercises for paresis of the ocular muscles involve moving the eye in the direction of action of the paretic muscle. Detailed instructions are provided by the ophthalmologist on the basis of accurate diagnosis of the type of paresis. We must not forget that paresis of ocular muscles produces diplopia, which is very unpleasant for the patient. To improve his vision, the patient tends to tilt his head, and he soon acquires a faulty posture, frequently resulting in torticollis. Therefore the physiotherapist must remind the patient constantly of the proper posture to prevent additional complications.

Many problems and diseases in ophthalmology are related to impaired circulation. Therefore we have a special programme of exercises, aiming to improve blood supply to the head and motion of the cervical spine. Glaucoma patients receive in addition to the exercises also light massage to the eye globe. A basic item in this programme is the teaching of relaxation. Through breathing exercises patients are taught the correct breathing technique. The importance of proper and adequate oxygenation for the eye is well known.

Electrotherapy: Electrical stimulation is used in functional deficits of the ocular muscles. We have very good results in the treatment of post-traumatic and postoperative ptosis and lagophthalmos. Ocular muscle paresis is managed by indirect stimulation of the affected muscles and nerves; direct contraction cannot be elicited. Diadynamic currents are effective in reducing oedema, haematoma and paraesthesias and in providing relief of pain. In ophthalmology this is very important since even a minor swelling may cause serious problems by impairing function of the eyelid and facial muscles.

Thermotherapy: Infra-red light reduces pain by enhancing the circulation in the eye and its surroundings. A similar effect is obtained with dry and moist packs, which are also used as a preparation for other therapeutic procedures. A blue light filter is beneficial in neurogenic disorders, including different forms of neuritis, neuralgia and blepharospasm.

Micromassage: In traffic accidents, blows and other forms of trauma to the head the eyes, their surroundings and other parts of the face are often involved. Scarring in the eyelid, areas surrounding the eyes and the face interferes with normal function and causes emotional problems in the patient on account of unsightly appearance of the face. Frequently a reconstructive surgical intervention is required after primary surgical treatment. With the application of micromassage, packs, stretching and compression we try to soften the scars as much as possible and prevent the growth of keloid fibres.

Micromassage is often used in conjunction with kinesitherapy in an attempt to correct two opposite conditions of the lid: an ectropion, i.e. an outturned lid, and an entropion, i.e. an inturned lid margin.

Lymphatic drainage is used in refractory oedema of the lids, orbital tissues and face, such as occurs in allergies or endocrine disorders. Lymphatic drainage is especially valuable in cases where the location of oedema or a surgical procedure precludes the use of other techniques.

A group that deserves our special attention consists of patients whose eye has been removed because of disease or injury. The missing eye is substituted with an aesthetic prosthesis. Kinesitherapy and electrotherapy are used to prevent atrophy and functional muscle deficits. Exercises improve the function of the intraocular muscles and ensure good mobility of the prosthesis.

In my report I did not go into details of the various diagnostic and therapeutic procedures. My aim has been to describe briefly the physiotherapy programme maintained at our Department of Ophthalmology in Ljubljana, outline the use of individual techniques in ophthalmology and present our results. These include shortening of the rehabilitation period, restoration of function to the lids, ocular and facial muscles, and improved cosmetic appearance of the face. Undoubtedly, physiotherapy is a valuable adjunct to medical and surgical treatment.

REFERENCES
1. Medical encyclopaedia (in Croatian). Jugoslovenski leksikografski zavod, Zagreb.
2. Pavšič Z (1971) Ophthalmology (in Serbian). Medicinska knjiga, Beograd.
3. Čupak K (1990) Ophthalmology (in Croatian). Zagreb.
4. Leitman MW (1988) Manual for eye examination and diagnosis, 3rd edition.
5. Duke-Elder S (1971) System of ophthalmology: Neuroophthalmology. Henry Kimpton, London.
6. Duke-Elder S (1968) System of ophthalmology: the physiology of vision. Henry Kimpton, London.

TOTAL REHABILITATION OF A CHRONIC HEMODIALYSIS PATIENT

F. Endo, Y. Asakawa, M. Kameda, Y. Ando
Department of Rehabilitation, Hidaka Hospital, Nakao-cho 886,
Takasaki-shi, Gunma-ken, Japan

Key Word: Chronic hemodialysis patient - Total rehabilitation

1. Introduction

Progress in Hemodialysis (HD) technology in recent years has relieved several of the physical and mental restrictions which HD patients tend to develop over time. This has brought about increased opportunities for HD patients to return to society. However most previous reports have focused on exercise treatment or mental characteristics. We have worked for the return of HD patients to society under the concept of Total Rehabilitation and have organized a local society in which the hospital, sheltered workshop and company are connected. This net work was initially established in 1984. Based on this experience, we knew that "working" has an especially favorable effect. Even though there are many difficulties involved in "getting to work", these can be overcome with cooperation between medical treatment personnel and welfare.

Concrete suggests for facilitating the process of returning for HD patients to work are stated below.

2. Rehabilitation progress (Problems and methods/results)

(1) Because of the lack of medical data on working, adaptability and contraindications are unclear.

Firstly, Burger Exercise plus Straight Leg Raising and Cuff Pumping were done as exercises while in bed. The main purpose of this exercise regimen was to motivate patients to exercise and to promote mental well-being. However, consideration must be given to negative hemodynamic effects in HD patients. Exercise intensity was less 40 percent and the time was limited to 15 minutes. Group exercise instructions were given to 10 to 20 patients who got HD during the same period in one group, 3 times per week. One session was approximately 4 hours long.

And for subjects in whom we had developed an interest in aerobic power, we measured maximum oxygen intake. The method used was maximum exercise testing by bicycle ergometer. In addition, we measured heart rate and maximum oxygen intake individually by the primary revolution formula. The heart rate changes over a 24 hour period were recorded with portable heart rate gauges in time studies. From both records, we calculated working intensity and the intensities of several daily life activities based on heart rate. We then conductd individual interviews and gave them, and an instructor from their working places, advice pertaining to daily living activities.

We have found that the working intensity at a sheltered workshop is around 40 percent HR max and it is not recognised as being overly burdensome. Conversely, we were concerned about a drop in aerobic power as this level is the daily maximum heart rate.

(2) Patients have to undergo dialysis for 4 to 5 hous/day, 3 times/week on average. Under these conditions, they are unaccustomed to normal working conditions.

From the results of measuring working intensity, we considered the problem to be mainly one of duration of work. We therefore tried to overcome this difficulty by establishing sheltered workshops. The sheltered workshop is called the "GREEN PEER" for handicapped people. It opened in 1985, so 6 years have already passed since its establishment. At present, 16 HD patients and 30 others, including RA and CVA patients, are employed there assembling computor parts, planting carnations, and working in hospital shops. Furthermore, 6 of the instructors are also HD patients.

(3) Under the Japanese insurance system, the burden to employers is increased, therefore hemodialysis patients are not welcome in the workplace.

The problem is how to facilitate the transition from a sheltered workshop back to an ordinary company. We established "ABLE" and received 13 handicapped people. Among them, 3 are HD patients and one HD patient became President in 1990.

(4) Social Prejudice

Through this trial, HD patients became able to work continuously eventually finding solutions to the problem of working burden and working conditions. This brought financial independence by means of wages and promoted well-regulated life habits in these indivduals. Through human communication in the company setting, appropriate social positions were established. This allowed reliance on other people and made their social lives full.

3. Discussion

With the progress of HD technology, the number of patients of working age is increasing. The establishment of a physical activity standard for such patients is very important and the necessity for exercise treatment is very high. However, when we set social independence based on working as the target, the time limit becomes a problem.

We recognized, through this time trial, that it is necessary to follow HD patients through to the final stage of rehabilitation which is establishment of a working place for their return to society. Total Rehabilitation is necessary, which involves solving social problems by means of the cooperation of hospital staff, facilities and the government. In the future, we would like to examine the participation of HD patients in society with regards to the problems of physical activity standards and personal characteristics. Then we would like to work to overcome impediments in working and living conditions faced by handicapped people. We plan to develop substantial concepts and methods for Total Rehabilitation which embody a supporting program for independence.

4. Conclusion

   (1) We have established and managed a sheltered workshop and company for HD patients who hope to work so that they can return to society.

   (2) By managing the working conditions so as to limit aerobic output, patients are able to work continuously.

   (3) Continuous working has brought them getting wages and regulated their daily lives, leading to social independence.

   (4) Settlement of social problems is indispensable for total rehabilitation of HD patients. And supporting of a program for the independence to participate in local society, such as working opportunity, should also be examined.

References:
1) Carney RM, et al: Exercise Training Reduces Depression and Increases, The Performed of Pleasant Activities in Hemodialysis Patients. Nephron, 47(3): 194-198, 1987.

2) Gerver R.: Economic, Financial, and Social Sequelae of successful Kidney Transplantations. Schweiz Med Wocheschr, 119(33): 1113-1118, 1989.

3) Hase H. et al: A Comparison of Heart rate Methods for Predicting Exercise Intensity in Chronic Hemodaialysis Patients. J kidoney and dialysis. 6: 159-165, 1984.

4) Kobayashi T.: Social Rehabilitation of Patients. Sogo Rehabilitation, 18(7): 513-516, 1990

5) P. O. Astrand, K. Rodahl: Textbook of Work Physiology, 2nd ed. McGraw-Hill, New York, 1977.

REDEEMING EXPERT KNOWLEDGE: THE APPLICATION OF COMPUTERISED DECISION-SUPPORT SYSTEMS TO PHYSIOTHERAPY

Anne Parry, PhD MCSP DipTP and Sue Stone, MA MSc
Division of Health Sciences, School of Health and Community Studies,
Sheffield City Polytechnic, Collegiate Crescent, Sheffield S10 2BP, UK.

Computerised decision-support systems are more commonly known as "expert systems". A form of artificial intelligence (AI), they are a means of codifying the knowledge of human experts, emulating their reasoning, and making both accessible to novices and experienced practitioners. While AI itself is concerned with problem-solving in the abstract, expert systems capitalise on the knowledge of experts and computer technology to enhance the problem-solving ability of novices. For the experts themselves, they can provide a second opinion or a means of sharpening expertise.

Application of expert systems
Decision-making is often thought about in terms of the outcome although there are two discriminably different components: the decision itself and the process of making it. The implementation of expert systems is less to do with the decision than with the process and their support of clinical decision-making has been recommended for medicine[1] nursing[2] and both physiotherapy[3] and physical therapy[4].

Nearly twenty years ago, MYCIN[5] was found to be as reliable as, if slower than, medical experts diagnosing and prescribing treatment for infectious diseases. More efficient systems have been built since then for specific medical purposes: ONCOCIN selects therapies for cancer patients, CADIAG1 and CADIAG2 are applied to rheumatology and gastroenterology, and MEDCAT is a teaching and learning aid in diagnostic skills for medical students.

Nursing systems have been directed at identification of problems whose solution may lend them to expert systems[4]. Ozbolt[7] complains that two of them share a common flaw: the diagnosis, objectives and interventions proposed are fairly obvious and no nurse needs computer support for a problem that she or he can identify fairly quickly. While "diagnosis" is conventionally understood by its medical use of conferring a disease label to a set of signs and symptoms, diagnosis in physiotherapy has three parts: a dysfunction label (can't do this, can't do the other); an aetiology label (related to age, psychosocial status, etc); and a condition, or conventional diagnositic, label.

Physiotherapy diagnosis is the point at which the physiotherapist's decision-making starts: How shall I fulfil my aims? How shall I select from the repertoire of interventions at my disposal? Thus, the project was directed at aiding decision-making by codifying the experiential and intuitive "hidden" knowledge of expert physiotherapists and their reasoning. Although there was no evidence that physiotherapy would fit a rule-based computer system, there appeared to be an apriori case for assuming that electrotherapy would be a suitable domain.

Methodological issues

In an expert system, the general area of expertise, or the domain, is represented by symbols which are processed in a way similar to human reasoning and, therefore, how practitioners process conceptual knowledge qualitatively using IF-THEN-ELSE rules: *IF interferential is indicated AND there is no contraindication THEN apply interferential ELSE use a more appropriate modality.* Like all qualitative approaches, the symbolical approach appears less precise and thus less reliable than quantitative methods. The major advantage is that it represents the domain more validly and less arbitrarily.

What distinguishes expert systems from other automated knowledge-based systems is that in addition to rules, they require general and specific knowledge, tricks of the trade, exceptions, reasonable guesses, and reasoning from partial knowledge[8]. Knowledge is hidden in many ways and a substantial amount of tacit knowledge in physiotherapy is never stated in formal terms. Additionally, although knowledge engineers have a vast array of potential techniques at their disposal, knowledge elicitation is the acknowledged bottle-neck of AI because, not unlike physiotherapy, there are few objective results from research to guide selection of techniques, anticipation of problems or estimations of progress[9]. Consequently, eliciting from physiotherapists the knowledge and the combination of logic and heuristics of clinical decision-making in selecting treatments was the major challenge of the project.

System development

This is a repeating process involving structuring the elicited knowledge, developing preliminary sets of rules, evaluating them in the clinic, and using the feedback to make refinements which start the process again. Structuring the knowledge requires identification and examination of key constructs. Interferential therapy was singled out because it has entered the undergraduate curriculum relatively recently and established practitioners might be interested in whether knowledge about doses and contraindications could be presented in a structured and meaningful way.

Two concepts appear central to physiotherapists' clinical decision-making: the risk of harm and the assurance of benefit. The risk of harm concerns contraindications and dangers associated with application of a specific modality of treatment in specific circumstances, and this was the first module of the system modelled on the computer.

The simple prototype presented here concerns provision of benefit: or, in other words, fulfilment of aims. Although examination of therapuetic aims may enable general guidelines to be given, it requires more detailed scrutiny of physiological effect to begin to formulate more specific advice. Relief of pain is the obvious example. It is a complex phenomenon at the core of physiotherapy practice. There are different ideas about what mechanisms are involved in its production and perception and its relief. There is more than one mechanism for bringing it about and each of them might require application of a different treatment frequency. What many patients want is relief of pain. It is a subjective matter with a physiological basis. Therefore, it seemed essential to develop the system so that it encouraged practitioners to identify exactly

which physiological effect or effects would fulfil their therapeutic aim.
The module presented here shows how it is possible for a computer to
emulate clinical decision-making in selecting a treatment frequency to
fulfil a therapeutic aim. The algorithm has been presented in more detail
elsewhere[3].

Conclusion

Mayer[10] describes artificial intelligence programs as being able to think
and reason like a human being. Although no computer can simulate the
subtle interaction between practitioner and patient, expert systems might
liberate physiotherapists by processing complex information from
examinations and about therapy to aid clinical decision-making and to give
the novice access to the knowledge of an expert. As Ryan[11] says, by
capturing, replicating and distributing expertise, expert systems can
provide the competitive edge by fusing the knowledge of experts in
physiotherapy, especially those who are few and far between.

*This project was funded by the Physiotherapy Research Foundation of the
UK.*

1. Shortliffe EH, Buchanan BG, Geigenbaum E (1979) Knowledge engineering
   for medical decision making: A review of computer-based clinical
   decision aids. In, W J Clancy and E H Shortliffe (eds) Readings in
   Medical Artificial Intelligence; Reading, Mass: Addison-Wesley.
2. Laborde J (1984) Expert systems for nursing. Computers for Nursing,
   2: 130-135.
3. Parry A, Stone S (1991) Capturing the basics: the development of an
   expert system for physiotherapists. Physiotherapy, 77 3: 222-226.
4. Delitto A, Shulman AD, Rose SJ (1989) On developing expert-based
   decision-support systems in physical therapy; The NIOSH Low Back
   Atlas. Physical Therapy, 69 7: 554-558.
5. Waskell E (1984) Of MYCIN men. Medicine and Computers, Jul-Aug;
   28-35.
6. Change RL, Hirsch M (1988) An expert system for nursing diagnosis:
   Field testing of Phase 1, Assessment. Nursing and Computers:
   Proceeding of the Third International Symposium on Nursing Use of
   Computers and Information Science. St Louis: CV Mosby Company;
   152-164
7. Ozbolt JG (1987) Prologue: A practical language for decision-support
   systems in nursing. Proceedings of the Eleventh Annual Symposium on
   Computer Application in Medical Care. Nov 1-4, 1987: 79-84.
8. Peat FD (1988) Artificial Intelligence: How machines think. New
   York: Simon and Schuster; 81.
9. Fox J (1987) Dealing with uncertainty. In, O'Shea T, Self J and
   Thomas G, Intelligent knowledge-based systems: An introduction.
   London: Harper and Row: 73-74.
10. Mayer J (1987) AI on the threshold. Data Training, 6 3, February.
11. Ryan S (1985) An expert system for nursing practice. Computers in
    Nursing, March/April: 77-84.

SKIN TEMPERATURE CHANGES WITH DIFFERENT METHODS OF CRYOTHERAPY

G De Domenico, S Cotton, D Devereaux, H King, A McIntosh.
Electro-Physical Agents Laboratory, School of Physiotherapy
Dalhousie University, Halifax, Nova Scotia, Canada.

Introduction

Cryotherapy is a modality that has been in use as a therapeutic treatment since before the time of Hippocrates (460-370 B.C.). The uses, benefits and physiological effects of cryotherapy have been well documented, particularly in the treatment of soft tissue injuries, reduction of haemorrhage, facilitation of muscle contraction, and in the management of certain neurological disorders [1,2,3,4].

In physiotherapy, various methods of applying cryotherapy are currently in use. These include: ice in a wet towel (conventional ice packs), ice in a plastic bag with or without a wet towel, ice immersion, commercial cold packs, and ice massage [5,6]. However, some of these methods are more time consuming and less convenient for both patient and physiotherapist. In particular, conventional ice packs tend to leak once the ice melts and patients often report this method to be uncomfortable.

Comparatively few studies have been performed comparing the cooling effects of various methods of ice application [7,8,9]. In a similar study to that described here, Belitskyet al. (1987)[7] evaluated the effectiveness of ice in a wet towel (wet ice), ice in a plastic bag (dry ice), and cryogen packs in the reduction of skin temperature. Results revealed significant differences between the mean skin temperatures of wet and dry ice, and between wet ice and a cryogen pack after 15 minutes of cold application. Fifteen minutes following ice removal, no significant differences were found between the three methods.

The aim of the present study was therefore to compare skin temperature changes that occur with three different methods of cryotherapy. It was hypothesized that if no significant differences existed, then the most convenient and cost effective method should be used.

Methodology

Subjects: Ten, healthy, volunteers (5 males & 5 females), aged 19 to 27 (mean of 23 years), were recruited. Subjects had no known neurological, circulatory or orthopaedic disease, or consumption of stimulating / depressing agents.

Equipment: Skin temperature was measured using a Radiospares digital thermometer, air temperature by a Yellow Springs (Model 44TD) Telethermometer, and ice and water temperature by two Allied Fischer Scientific Dial thermometers. Other equipment included measuring scales, and standard plastic bags (34.5cm x 12.8cm) to enclose the ice. A 9.5 cm diameter rubber ring (70.9 cm^2) was used to standardize the area of skin in contact with the ice. The three methods of ice application were:- Method A (ice in a wet towel): Method B (ice in a plastic bag surrounded by a wet towel): Method C (ice in a plastic bag). Method A consisted of 400 grams of flaked ice in a terrycloth towel (58.0 cm x 37.5 cm). The towel had been previously immersed in water at 4°C. The towel was wrung so that a weight of 280 grams was obtained. Only one layer of towelling was between the ice and the skin. In method B, 400 grams of flaked ice were placed in a dry plastic bag and covered with a standardized wet towel. In Method C, 400 grams of flaked ice in a dry plastic bag, were applied to the skin.

Protocol: Each subject was tested once a week for three consecutive weeks, with random assignment of the three methods of ice application. Each subject was comfortably seated in a standard position on a plinth. All subjects spent 20 min. acclimatizing prior to testing. Room temperature was kept between 23.8 and 26.8°C.

The rubber ring was held securely in a standardized position, and the temperature probe fixed in the center of the ring. The probe-tip was insulated, such that only one side made direct contact with the skin. No other aspect of the probe-tip came into direct contact with the ice pack surrounding it. Ice temperature was monitored in all three methods and an insulated plastic sheet was placed over the pack to minimize heat transfer. The ice pack completely filled the rubber ring. Initial skin temperature was recorded before ice application, further readings being taken every 30 seconds during the 15 minutes of ice application. The ice pack was then removed and the waterproof towel replaced over the tested area. Skin temperature was monitored for an additional 10 minutes.

Results
The three methods produced similar cooling and re-warming trends (see Figure 1).
Data were normalized and expressed as a percentage of the initial temperature (100%)

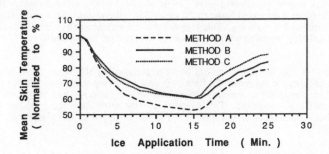

Figure 1. Mean, Normalized Skin Temperature Changes for Three Methods of Cryotherapy, during 15 min. of cooling and 10 min. of re-warming.

At ice removal (15 minutes), mean skin temperatures for Methods A, B and C were 6.7°C (± 1.9°C); 5.4°C (± 1.1°C) and 4.2°C (±2.2°C), respectively. Immediately following removal of the ice pack, mean skin temperature continued to decrease slightly before beginning to increase rapidly. Mean skin temperature readings at 10 minutes after ice removal were 14.7°C (± 2.3°C)for Method A; 12.5°C (± 1.5°C) for Method B, and 13.1°C (± 2.2°C) for Method C. A one factor, repeated measures ANOVA was performed on the raw data (data at the time of ice removal and at 10 minutes following ice removal). Results revealed no significant difference between the three methods at the time of ice removal. A significant difference in skin temperature means between method A and method C was found 10 minutes after ice removal (p =<0.01).

Discussion

Cooling curves from all three cryotherapy methods were very similar and no significant differences were apparent at ice removal. This suggests that as far as cooling efficiency is concerned, the three methods are interchangeable. Following ice removal skin temperature continued to drop in all three methods. This may be because the tissues require time to adapt to the new situation. It could also have been reinforced by evaporating moisture left on the skin with two of the methods (A & B).

The results obtained in this study both agreed and differed with those of similar studies [7,8,9]. This may be reflective of differences in experimental methodology between the various studies. In the present study, strenuous efforts were made to control the major variables. This was deemed to be essential if meaningful comparisons of different methods of cryotherapy were to be made. Despite the fact that the mass, temperature, site, area in contact with the skin and recording methodology were rigorously standardized; a significant difference between conventional ice pack and ice in a plastic bag, ten minutes after ice removal was seen. This may possibly be explained by the fact that a very wet towel was in contact with the skin in method A. Due to this, moisture remained on the skin after ice removal. This may have contributed to the slower temperature rise seen with this method. Water remaining on the skin evaporates when exposed to air, cooling the skin.

In an effort to resolve this issue, the entire experiment was repeated, using a similar protocol. In this case however, the re-warming phase was extended to 20 minutes and the skin was carefully dried following ice removal in all three methods. The cooling curves produced by this second experiment were almost identical to the present study. No significant differences were found between the mean skin temperature at ice removal, or following 20 minutes of re-warming. This suggests that the present results were due to the rather short period of re-warming and the presence of moisture on the skin surface.

Conclusion

Results indicate no significant differences between the cooling efficiency of all three methods of cryotherapy at ice removal. Results from a follow-up study indicate that no significant differences in the re-warming phases following cryotherapy treatments, when this phase is carefully controlled. This suggests that the most convenient method of applying ice should be advocated. In many cases, this will be flaked ice in a plastic bag.

References

1. **Knight KL (1987)** Cryotherapy: Theory, Technique and Physiology. Tennessee: Chattanooga Corporation.
2. **Olson JE, Stravino VD (1972)** A review of cryotherapy. Physical Therapy 52: 840-853
3. **Meeusen R, Lievens P (1986)**, The use of cryotherapy in sports injuries. Sports Medicine 3: 398-414
4. **Kowal MA (1983)** Review of the Physiological Effects of Cryotherapy. Journal of Orthopaedic and Sports Physical Therapy 5, 2: 66-73
5. **Wadsworth H, Chanmugan APP (1988)** Electrophysical Agents in Physiotherapy: Therapeutic and Diagnostic Use. (2nd ed.). Marrickville, NSW: Science Press
6. **Lee JM, Warren MP (1978)** Cold Therapy in Rehabilitation. Bell and Hymen : London
7. **Belitsky RB, Odam SJ, Hubley-Kozey C (1987)** Evaluation of the effectiveness of wet ice, dry ice and cryogen packs in reducing skin temperature. Physical Therapy 67: 1080-1084
8. **McMeeken, Lewis, and Cocks (1984)** Effects of cooling with simulated ice on skin temperature and nerve conduction velocity. Australian Journal of Physiotherapy 30:111-114
9. **McMaster WC, Liddle S, Waugh TR (1978)** Laboratory Evaluation of Various Cold Therapy Modalities. American Journal of Sports Medicine 6, 5: 291-294

No. 0173   CONSERVATIVE TREATMENT FOR
           INTRACTABLE FILARIAL LYMPHEDEMA.

Ms. A. A. ANDYAL
Department of Physiotherapy, Bombay Hospital Institute
of Medical Sciences and Research, Marine Lines, Bombay.

Introduction: It has been observed for many years in our Out Patient Clinic that patients with long standing inflammation of extremeties are seen. These patients come with great hope for curative treatment. To reduce this edema many medicines, several therapies and surgeries are tries. Surgery gave relief, but it was temporary. Many got recurrence often inflammation became more than at its earlier stage. They developed ulceration, secondary infection and several abnormalities of skin. Inspite of all the modern advances in medicine and surgery these patients remain untretable.

Filarial infection with Wuchereria bancrofti or Malayi is widely spread through out tropical and sub-tropical countries. It is common along the bank of rivers, except Indus and marshy lands. It is found in South China, West Indies, Pacific Islands, Western and Central Africa and South America. In India it is prevalent in coastal areas of Maharashtra, Goa, Kerala, parts of Andhra Pradesh, parts of Bengal and Assam.

Filaria is due to Nematode worn which is transmitted by Culex (Female mosquitoes). When in infected mosquito bites a human being at deposits third stage larvae on the skin. They are attracted by the warmth of the body through the functure of the bite into the lymphatics. They settle, grow, multiply and attain sexual maturity in 6-18 months. They produce millions of microfilariae and occupy the lymph nodes and lymphatics, then enter the blood stream. Microfilariae create mechanical insufficiency by reducing the lymphatic transport capacity and low lymph flow failure and stagnate the tissue proteins. This obstruction results into high protein edema or Lymphedema. Infection due to these parasites is known as an attack of Filariasis or Elephantisis. The attack of Erysipelas is accompanied by headache, bodyache, nausea, vomitting, pain, swelling, red hot and tender becomes the affected part, with high body temperature reaching 30-40 degree C or 103-104 degrees F. Lymph node and lymphatic get tender and hard like a cord. Microfilariae obstruct lymph flow, damage lymphatic wall and resulting into solid edema of the affected part. It may be an arm, one or both legs, brest, scrotum and some time kidneys. The periodic repeated attacks of Erysipelas weakens the patient bodily. If it is a child the education and future career is affected. Every attack goes on adding to the lymph edema size till it becomes big and heavy. It prevents mobility, if the leg is affected. The skin becomes rough, fissures, papillae are formed. The small papillae look like a bench of grapes and bigger hand like jack fruits. In these papillae lodge bacteria causing infection resulting in sores and ulcers. Maggots get into these infected spaces. They go on boring the skin and muscles underneath. This gives regularly high temperature every day, which damages the health.

Method: A specially made semi circular metal chamber is fitted with four rows of electric tungsten bulbs. Each row consisting of three bulbs of 100 watts. Each row has a separate switch to control the heat. It given 80 degree C temperature. Exercise programme includes simple full range of joint movements for legs, hips, knees, ankles and toes. Resistive Cycling, Simple Tread Mill for walking, Medicine balls of different weights and sizes for resistive exercises for ankles. For arms, shoulder scapular, elbows, wrists, fingers and thumb exercises are taught.

Compression banuage consists of thick elastic with veicro attached to both the ends. The length of the bandage varies from 3 to 17 meters, depending on the size of the lymphoedema/tous leg. A tubular cooton (like stocking) is used to avoid direct contact between skin and elastic to absorb perspiration.

Treatment: A few patients' lymphography is taken. The patients are examined and mostof them are found suffering for more than forty years. The size of the filarial leg is also huge. It is found that women are more vulnerable to the attack of Filariasis. The patients are examined. Metric and volumetric measurements of normal and abnormal limbs are taken for the sake of comparison. A photograph of the affected limb is taken. If a patient has oozing infected wound with foul smell then measurements are not possible. The infected wound is cleaned, a flow of ozone is administered to control tissue to bring about healing. If maggots are seen then they are removed with turpentine bath. The affected parts are in the heating chamer in supine and prone position for half an hour on eachside at 80 degree C constant temperature. The exercises are given to increase the mobility and endurance of the patient for forty to fifty minutes depending on the patient's condition. Compression bandage is applied, which is required to be kept for ten to twelve hours a day. Metric and volumetric measurements are taken every week for comparison.

Results: The lymphedema goes on reducing in size. The stretched skin changes its colour and texture. The patient feels lighter as time passes. The attacks of Erysipelas reduce in intensity and the period between two attacks is lengthened. This indicates recovery of the normal function of lymphatics to absorb the large serum albumin molecules. The lymph nodes of the affected side start functioning, the tenderness and hardness diminish. The heat increases the temperature tissues, which in turn increases the blood circulation and accelrate tissue metabolism, resulting into softing of the fibrous tissue and allowing lymphatics to be more efficient. The damaged walls and valves are bypassed by regeneration of collaterals to add to the efficacy of the lymphatic system, which has been proved by lymphography after treatment. After reducing the lymph edema the resulting loose skin of the limbs is treated with Accupunture to regain its normal elasticity and appearance. The patient recovers his health and confidence to stand, walk long distances and improves his endurance and is made fit for a job according to his ability. A partient can move freely as a useful and normal individual and thus he is rehabilitated.

Conclusion: The Conservative Treatment of Filarial Lymphedema requires long time for getting the desired results. More depends on the patient's determination and tenacity for following the instructions given to his such as continued exercises, bandaging of the affected limbs as directed. Periodically reporting for check up at the interval of three months is necessary. It is needless to state that success depends on the active cooperation of the patient in following the instructions religeously. From the year 1986 I have treated about 700 patients of varying degrees of abnormalities due to Filarial Lymphedema. Out of these 70% of the patients could regain normal size of their affected limbs.

References: (1) Temporary Relief with surgery - Ols zewski and Nielubowicz 1966, Kaye, Smith and Acland, 1980, Baumeisterd and Associates 1981.Mc Carthy, Plastic Surgery Lower Ex.Vol.6. (2) Geographical Distribution-Parasitology. By K.T.Chaterji. (3) Heat & Compression bandaging for Lymphedema-Prof Ti-Sheng Chang-International Plastic Surgery Conference, India 1986. (4) I visited 9th People's Hospital, Shanghai, China in response to the invitation of Prof. Ti-Sheng Chang. I observed their methods of treatment and modified with the addition of special heating chamber, bandage and exercises suitable to the climate and patient's condition of my country. (5) "Lymphography can damage the remaining lymphatic system." Bollinger, Partsch and Worlfe - 1985. (6) "Reconstructive Surgery can not produce reversal lymphoedematous tissue" M.C. Mc Carthy Plastic Surgery Vol.6 Lower Extremeties. (7) Heat and Bandage Treatment- Zang and Associates, 1984.

PHYSIOTHERAPY CARE OF LUMBAR SURGERY PATIENTS IN THREE COUNTRIES

Sheila C. Morrison, Physiotherapy Department, Victoria General Hospital, 1278 Tower Road, Halifax, Nova Scotia, B3H 2Y9, CANADA

Introduction: This investigation was directed towards answering two questions: (1) How do physiotherapists perceive their role in the peri-operative care of lumbar surgery patients, and (2) Are these patients receiving physiotherapeutic care? The study population included English, Canadian and American therapists. This is the first study that examines the physiotherapist's perceived and actual role in the care of lumbar surgery patients.

Literature Review: The literature is sparse. Physical therapist Sawyer (1983) describes a program that emphasizes reinforcing healthy behavior to maintain strength and reduce complications. He recommends a pre-operative biomechanical evaluation and attendance at a back school, the use of a TENS immediately in recovery room, early exercise and graduated activity, and a return to the back school for further progression. A surgeon, Mooney (1979), who also suggests education and progressive exercises, points out that certain patients face psychological barriers and require a more complicated rehabilitative approach. Neither author discusses outcome measurement. Damrel and Holloway (1981) describe a scheme for objectively assessing function in lumbo-sacral fusion patients. The test consists of standing, kneeling, sitting and cycling activities. While the concept is welcome, the validity and reliability have yet to be adequately established. A retrospective study by surgeon Lehmann et al. (1987) to quantify pain and disability indicates that more than half of arthrodesis patients have pain and use medication twenty years after surgery. He concludes, on a positive but surprising note, that they are "generally doing well".

Purpose: We intended to clarify how physiotherapists perceive their role in peri-operative care of lumbar discectomy and fusion patients; to see whether practice reflects beliefs; to determine whether differences exist among English, American and Canadian physiotherapists.

Population and Sample: The sample was drawn from a population of hospital based physiotherapists working in orthopaedics or neurology where discectomies, laminectomies or fusions are performed. Of the 134 hospitals, 32 were American, 49 Canadian and 53 English.

Method: Responses to a mail-out survey with a closed-end response format were analyzed using descriptive statistics on a Systat computer program. An open-end question on the role of the physiotherapist, occupational therapist and nurse was included. Respondents were also requested to send copies of education programs where possible so that content could be analyzed.

Results: The response rate was 61% (n=82). The majority (52%) worked in orthopaedics, 23% in neurology. In response to how essential they felt their role to be, "always" or "often" was selected from a Likert scale by 79% of respondents for discectomies, 74% for fusions, and 84% for laminectomies. Subjects from England had much stronger feelings regarding essentialness of role than their Canadian or American counterparts. For example, 88.9% of the English saw their role with laminectomies as "always essential" compared to Canadian (40%) or Americans (0%).

When asked to select from nine items which would reflect their ideal role relative to each surgery, "patient education" stood out for all three countries. "Post-operative assessment" and "exercise" were important; for fusions 73% chose "teaching exercises" compared to 85% for discectomies and 86% for laminectomies. Except for education, English physiotherapists tended to select all items more frequently than their North American counterparts. For example 88.9% - 92.6% of English respondents felt "pre-operative assessment" to be an essential component of care as compared to fewer than 50% of North American therapists. "Post-operative assessment" was selected more frequently by all, but the number of Canadians and Americans still fell 30% below the number of English who felt this item essential. A similar question asked respondents how often these care items were actually performed. In nearly all cases the number who were offering this care was less than the number who perceived they ought to be doing so. The most common reason for not doing so was failure to receive a medical consult. One third of respondents stated that they receive sporadic referrals from physicians, one third routinely, and one third see patients on standing orders.

Eighty-eight percent reported spending an average of 93 minutes educating an individual patient. Only 14 respondents reported educating in a group setting for an average of 91 minutes per group. Sixty-six percent of the sample stated that they use some form of written materials; half sent copies (see discussion section).

Of those who commented on the role of the physiotherapist, nurse and occupational therapist, they commonly stated that the nurse and physiotherapist complemented each other, while the occupational therapist generally was not involved.

Discussion: Physiotherapists do believe they have a unique function in regards to lumbar surgery patient and are providing that service, albeit less frequently than they would like. Reasons for this are unclear. It may be that not all surgeons regard such a service as essential and do not consult physiotherapists. The biggest discrepancy between role perception and practice is in regards to teaching exercises to patients who have undergone a fusion. One could postulate that the reason for this is that surgeons are reluctant to have their patients begin an exercise program believing that this may stress the site of the graft. On the other hand, it is difficult to conceive why these patients should not undergo a properly designed program that does not stress the graft. Clearly, physiotherapists and surgeons need to collaborate to ensure optimal rehabilitation of these patients.

While a large number of therapists, particularly the English, routinely refer their patients to outpatient physiotherapy, it is unclear from this study what the criteria might be for referral, and what the treatment goals would be. The most interesting and perhaps most distressing information from this study comes from the material that is less easy to analyze. While the statistics reported above suggest a fairly consistent philosophy toward lumbar surgery patients, the patient education materials sent to the investigator suggest great variability in the content of education program. Some handouts were clearly reflections of surgeons' protocols and ranged from very conservative to very aggressive. In one English hospital physiotherapists use auto-assisted pulleys for straight leg raises after fusion and the criteria for discharge is achievement of 90°. In contrast, in another hospital physiotherapists use a tilt-table to mobilize fusion patients post-operatively. Exercise programs produced by physiotherapists varied greatly, some in direct opposition to each other. While one hospital teaches full spinal extension, another absolutely prohibits the same exercise for discectomy patients.

Conclusion: Clearly despite the community feeling regarding our unique role, the referral patterns and the content of programming vary sufficiently that some very researchable questions arise. What is the outcome of surgery? Does physiotherapy have an impact? Should there be selection criteria (age, occupation, psychosocial status) for rehabilitation? What kind of program will benefit which patient? Current differences in approach may reflect cross cultural differences in physiotherapy education, variability in surgeons' views on rehabilitation, and a lack of research in the physiotherapy community.

References:
1.   Sawyer, M.W.(1983) the role of the physical therapist before and after lumbar spine surgery. Orthopaedic Clinics of North America 14(3): 649-659.
2.   Mooney, V. (1979) Surgery and post-surgical management of the patient with low back pain. Physical Therapy 56: 1000-1006.
3.   Damrel, D., Holloway, G., Quinnell, R., (1981) An objective assessment of operative fusions of the lumbo-sacral spine. Physiotherapy 67(6), 164-176.
4.   Lehmann, T., Spratt, M., Tozzi, J., Weinstein, J., Reinarz, S., El-khoury, G., Colby, H. (1987) Long-term follow-up of lower lumbar fusion patients. Spine 12(2), 97-104.

MODIFICATION OF MOTONEURON ACTIVITY IN VARIOUS VOLITIONAL TASKS IN MAN

T Fujiwara*, *N Nishimura**, *T Kimura***
*Shishu Univ., School of Allied Med. Sciences, Matsumoto, 390 JAPAN, ** Tokyo Koseinenkin Hosp., Tokyo

Introduction
In all of Physical Therapy practice for the patients with CNS disorder, the fluctuation of the muscle tone is one of the most frequently encountered clinical conditions. However, its etiology is diverse and quantitative evaluation is not provided. The purpose of this investigation is to prove an amount of the influence toward spinal motoneuron excitability due to various volitional tasks on a certain body segment[1],[2] and to be reflected the result for a treatment programme among the various kinds of central nervous disorders.

Method
Influences of the inter-limb interaction and of the antagonistic muscle contraction with visual feedback control were observed in a total of 10 healthy human subjects. Hoffmann waves(H-wave) were led out from the sural muscles by Ag/AgCl surface EMG electrodes. The evoked EMG was observed using biophysical high sensitivity amplifier, memory scope, averager and electric stimulator. H wave fluctuation by the antaganistic inhibition technique was observed with or without visual biofeedback procedure(see Fig. 1). All the data was stored in a data recorder. Amplitudes and latencies of H-wave were calculated using a micro computer system with an extraordinally bio-information multi task analyzing programme (BIMUTAS ver. 3.0E, Kissei Comtec Co. Ltd.). In addition, the investigation was conducted in a quiet sealed room with a room temperature of 23 degree C at 45 % humidity.

Fig. 1 Isometric volitional contraction values of unilateral biceps brachii are shown in terms of percentage of maximum volitional contraction, and the evoked EMG of the bilateral triceps surae under the 0 - 70% MVC loads are led out under the uniform stimulus condition standardized by the subliminal pair pulse method.

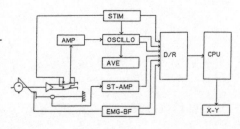

Result

1) Isometric volitional contraction of the right side elbow flexor muscles was subjected to randomized trials of 8 steps ranging at 0 to 70% maximum voluntary contraction. These tasks facilitated the amplitude of the H-wave from the ipsilateral leg with a positive correlation between wave amplitude and contracting force, and inhibited that of the contralateral side (see Fig. 2).

2) Antagonistic contraction inhibited the H-wave amplitude exponentially. Moreover, the phasic neuro-muscular component within the H-wave showed marked diminution by visual feedback control selectively (see Fig 3).

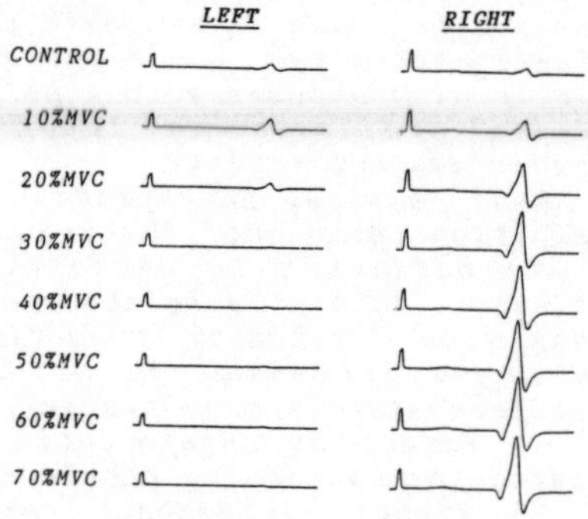

Fig. 2 This is an evoked EMG showing the triceps surae under the right side upper extremity volitional contraction. Eight trials from 0-70% MVC, including control without load, are averaged 8 times respectively. According as the conditioning load increased, the spinal reflex potential on the ipsilateral side shows a marked increase, and on the contralateral side, a decrease.

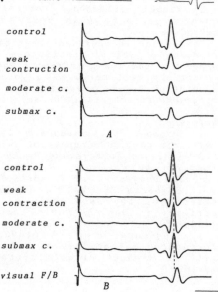

Fig. 3 H wave fluctuation by the antagonistic inhibition technique with or without visual biofeedback procedure
A: without biofeedback
B: with biofeedback in a poor responsive subject. (Note the latency delay.)

Discussion

The characteristics of this investigation are that observation were made on the inter-limb interaction between upper and lower extremities in man after the conditioning loads had been regulated in the strict sense. It was assumed that their modes of modification were in common with such physiological modes as inter-limb reflex and descending[5] propriospinal reflex in animal, and Jendrassik manoeuvre[3] in man. A spinal reflex are subjected to inhibition from the higher centre, and disinhibition is considered to take place when the descending volley of the cortico-spinal tract causing volitional contraction of upper extremity muscle temporarily increases. These apparent facilitatory phenomena cause to increase the H waves from the ipsilateral lower extremity. As is the case with above mentioned tasks, it is also necessary to consider the influences of such long spinal reflexes as inter-limb reflex and descending propriospinal reflex.

Many Physical Therapists have been used "Antagonistic inhibition technique" for reduction of spasticity. But it is very difficult to explain the physiological mechanisms cleary. According to the results of this study, patient who has some difficulty in motion due to spasticity, will be able to increase his or her voluntality by using EMG biofeedback exercise system with following precautions :

1) Effect of antagonistic inhibition technique is indicated for decreasing phasic conponent of muscular tone.

2) Visual biofeedback control method[4] are recommended when a patient shows poor sensitivity to the simple technique.

The auther is confident that the fact that in this investigation a part of muscle tone control system between the upper and the lower extremity was measured under controlled conditions will serve as a good foothold for urging consideration before preparing and executing related exercise programme for Physical Therapy in the future.

Reference

1. Gernandt BE, Shimamura M (1961) Mechanisms of interlimb reflex in cat. J Neurophysiol 24:665-676

2. Ishikawa T, Miyazawa T, Fujiwara T (1984) Characteristics of the spino-bulbo-spinal reflex with evoked EMGs in human subjects. Int J Sports Med 5:187-192

3. Hagbarth KE, Wallin G, Burke D, Lofstedt L (1975) Effects of the Jendrassik manoeuvre on muscle spindle activity in man. J Neurol Neurosurg Psychiat 38:1143-1153

4. Fujiwara T et al (1990) Modification of spinal motoneuron exitability by volitional task of antagonist with or without visual feedback control. J Jpn P T A 25:160

POSTER PRESENTATIONS

THE RESULTS OF THE REHABILITATION TREATMENT OF MOTOR
DYSFUNCTION

J.GROSSMAN and A.Ronikier
Metropolitan Rehabilitation Centre
Konstancin near Warsaw,Poland

In the Metropolitan Rehabilitation Centre in Konstancin near
Warsaw a search for a possibly objective method of assessment
of rehabilitation progress was conducted,for a rapid and
simple recording method,applicable in normal clinical
conditions,of changes in the functional state of our patients.
For this purpose investigation laboratories / electrophysiological,dynamometric,ergometric,locomotion and physical fitness/
were organized.The obtained objective data were found to be
useful in individual cases,but in view of time-consuming
methods of these investigations they could be used in some
cases only.
For this reason,a set of functional tests has been evolved
in our Centre,making possible assessment of all treated and
rehabilitated patients,independently of the disease,sex and
age.
After elimination it has been esteblished that the locomotor
fitness and adaptation to self-dependent life of subjects
with various disabilities are influenced essentially by such
physiological parameters as : pain,mobility of joints,muscle
strenght,general fitness,locomotion,self-care,gripping ability
of the upper extremities and socio-occupational situation.
Assuming that these parameters enable a strict determination
and characterization of motor self-dependence and fitness to
be made,and thus they were accepted as test parameters.
The main aim of the study was determination of the degree of
self-dependence in life and the degree to which the patients
could make themselves independent of the help of other
persons after rehabilitation treatment carried out in hospital

The results of rehabilitation treatment of 2500 patients who were treated and rehabilitated at the Center from 1988 to 1989 are analyzed.All the patients treated at that time were regarded as severe cases with poor locomotor efficiency, needing intensive nursing in the initial stage of treatment. The methods of movement rehabilitation were selected to suit individual needs of the patients.The selection was based on the evaluation of the patient´s : locomotor efficiency, general fitness,local disorders,concomitant diseases and the social situation.

The data were processed by computerized mathematical analysis The data obtained show that the duration of hospital stay necessary to achieve the pre-set rehabilitation results ranged from 6,2 to 10,6 weeks,depending on the diagnosed disease.Taking into account the age of the patients and the diagnosed disease the average duration of hospitalization should be regarded as very short,the more so that the movement rehabilitation was to a large extent dependent also on the fitting of prosthesis,braces,supplying with sticks, wheelchairs and other orthopaedic appliances contributing to the locomotor independence of the patients.

The mean numerical values for all tests were calculated on admission and discharge.On admission,as had been expected, the results of the tests were bad / high numerical values/. After rehabilitation treatment markedly better results of all the tests were recorded in all groups of patients / decreased numerical values /.High values for pain noted on admission were markedly diminished,so that pain was not a problem for the majority of patients on discharge.

The range of movement of the joints,muscle strength,general fitness,locomotion and independence in daily activities were all markedly improved and hence brought about significant improvement within the locomotor system and independence in daily activities of the whole group.Basing on the assumption that the general fitness of the patients to a large extent

determines their independence in daily living and that the
final evaluation of the effectiveness of rehabilitation is
the self-dependence of the patient,or in other words,the
patient´s independence of his/her environment,the
distribution of the self-service test results was
investigated.
The analysis shows that very few patients obtained score 1
at the initial testing.The improvement depended on the
severity of the disease.From 80 to 100% of patients were
independent at least at home conditions.
A comparison of the results obtained in the equation of
regression estimated for the data obtained on discharge from
the hospital,in which the studied variable was self-care,
with the results of an analogous equation estimated on
admission to hospital showed a considerable decrease of the
regression coefficients for the explaining variables,i.e.
pain and range of movements.The regression coefficients for
sex,age and locomotor activity were at a similar level.On
the other hand,there was an increase of the effect on the
self care of such factors as muscle strenght,general fitness
and prehensile ability of the hands.Similarly,in both
estimated self-care models the values of the parameters
reflecting the adjustment of the obtained equation to the
initial data / on which they were based / were of a similar
order.
Even in difficult cases of locomotor dysfunction in geriatric
patients comprehensive rehabilitation can give satisfactory
results of treatment and of social readaptation.To obtain
these aims,however,certain requirements must be met,namely :
rehabilitation programme must be started early,must be
parallel to the basic treatment and must be carefully
selected to suit individual needs and be continued after
discharge from hospital to home conditions.

EFFECTS OF ATHLETIC PROGRAM ON LAXITY AND TORQUE PRODUCTION OF THE KNEE

S. Henry, M. Moffroid, L. Fernandez, M. Emery

Department Physical Therapy, University of Vermont
Burlington, Vermont 05401
U.S.A.

The purpose of this study was to assess the effects of athletic participation on joint laxity and on maximal concentric and eccentric torque measures of the knee. Measurements were made with the Genucom and LIDO respectively, both devices having been shown to have high intra-rater reliability.

Muscle tightness and joint tightness have been reported to vary positively with torque production at the knee. However, strength testing, cyclic loading and short term exercise have all been shown to increase joint laxity in humans.

Fifteen female varisy soccer and field hockey players consented to be pretested at the start of the season for joint laxity of the knee and for maximum torque of the quadriceps and hamstring muscle groups. Following an introductory session, torque measures of maximum concentric contractions were made followed by eccentric measures. Joint laxity was measured on the next day in two positions: A/P at 30 deg flexion and V/V at 0 deg position. Subjects then began their training and competition, (2 hours/day, 7 days/week). All subjects were posttested at the end of the season.

Analysis indicated these 15 subjects increased significantly ($p < .05$) in joint laxity in the A/P direction, and also in eccentric torque of both muscle groups. Subjects also showed increased laxity in the V/V direction, and increased concentric torque measures, although these were not significant. The authors conclude that short term athletic participation may increase joint laxity as well as torque.

A PILOT STUDY TO EVALUATE THE EFFECTIVENESS OF CHRONIC LOW FREQUENCY ELECTRICAL STIMULATION IN IMPROVING PELVIC FLOOR MUSCLE FUNCTION.

J M Gardner, K R Davidge, M Polden, S A Hyde.

Departments of Physiotherapy, Hammersmith Hospital and Queen Charlotte's and Chelsea Hospital, London England, United Kingdom.

The purpose of the study was to evaluate the effectiveness of electrical stimulation in patients with pelvic floor dysfunction. 18 female subjects referred for pelvic floor exercises with ages varying from 34 to 68 years took part in this ethics approved study. All gave their informed consent. Baseline measurements were made of pelvic floor muscle function using digital assessment and the Bourne perineometer. A visual analogue scale was used to record discomfort or urinary symptoms. A frequency/volume chart was completed if there were symptoms of genuine stress or idiopathic urge incontinence. In order to evaluate the effects of electrical stimulation a blind controlled study was undertaken.

All patients referred were assessed and then received exercise. After three months, if on reassessment there was little improvement patients were randomly assigned to two groups for a further three months: Group I had electrical stimulation and Group II continued exercising, acting as a control group. All subjects were finally reassessed.

Analysis will be by standard statistical methods and completion of the study is projected for January, 1991.

PHYSIOTHERAPY TO TORTURE SURVIVORS

K. Christensen, L. Olsen, B. Carstensen

Rehabilitation Centre for Torture Victims
Copenhagen
Denmark

Torture takes place in more than 90 countries
throughout the world.
The majority of the refugees arriving in Western
Europe have been exposed to torture.
The body is the entrance to a person's mind and
identity. The torturers exploit this correlation.
The education and knowledge, which physiotherapists
have, make us qualified to help and rehabilitate
survivors of torture.
An overview of clinical management in physical
therapy to torture survivors.
In cooperation with the Danish National Organisation
of Physiotherapists (Danske Fysioterapeuter) a proposal for a convention against physiotherapists'
participation in torture will be presented.

ASSESSMENT OF DYNAMIC BALANCE IN INDEPENDENT LIVING NURSING HOME AND
RETIREMENT COMMUNITY RESIDENCE: A PILOT STUDY

T L Kauffman, W Gamber, B Anderl, M J Griffith
Timothy L. Kauffman, M.S., P.T.
719 North Duke Street, Lancaster, PA 17602   USA

Introduction

Balance and mobility problems are major concerns in the elderly
population. The loss of balance or the inability to recover from a
postural perturbation is associated with falls. Assessment of balance
dysfunction has become increasingly sophisticated and costly through
the use of computerized pressure footplates, which measure static
balance. But, the physiological systems that control static balance
are not identical to those that modulate dynamic balance and mobility.
Possibly, dysfunction of dynamic balance and mobility is of greater
clinical significance within the geriatric population than is static
balance. Several excellent assessment tools have been described in the
literature including the Get Up and Go Test,[1] the Tinetti Balance
Mobility Scale,[2] and the Gait Abnormality Rating Scale.[3] Based upon
our earlier work with static balance and the unilateral stance test, we
developed a balance beam (BB) test to assess dynamic balance.[4,5] The
purpose of this pilot study was to assess the possible use of a
modified BB, 6 1/2 feet x 8 inches x 1/4 inch as a screening device for
possible balance problems.

Methods

The subjects were instructed to walk across the BB with a normal gait
pattern. A heel-to-toe walk style of gait was discouraged. If the
subject fell off the BB, they were instructed to step back onto the
beam and to continue walking. After one or two trials for
familiarization, each subject traversed the BB 5 times. A stop watch
was used to time each of the 5 crossings. Cumulative and average times
were appropriately calculated. The time was stopped when the subject
reached the end of the BB. If the subject fell off (stepped off) the
BB, the time continued. The number of falls was recorded.

A fall was defined as anytime the subject's foot touched the floor or
whenever for safety reasons an imminent fall was prevented by an
evaluator.

Results

Five persons out of the 19 did not fall off the BB. The average
cumulative mean time for these non-fallers was 20.83 seconds compared

to the average mean of 36.62 seconds for the 14 persons who did fall.
It took an average of 4.16 seconds for the non-fallers to traverse the
beam each time compared to 7.32 seconds for the fallers.

As can be seen in Figure 1 there was a clear direct relationship
between the number of falls and length of time to traverse the BB.
Also it is apparent from Figure 1 that some subjects who fell had a
cumulative mean time that was less than some of the subjects who did
not fall.

Due to the nature of this pilot study these data were not subjected to
tests of statistical significance.

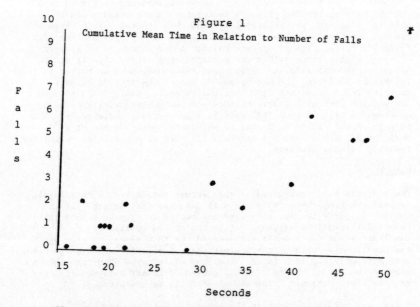

Figure 1
Cumulative Mean Time in Relation to Number of Falls

The number of falls is plotted for each subject in
relation to time. One Ss is not included in this figure
because he fell 12 times in 107 seconds.*

Conclusion

It was clear that the persons who fell traversed the BB with less speed which corresponds to reports that known fallers or persons with gait dysfunction have less velocity of gait and mobility.[1,2,3] With further study, the BB may be found to be a fast and inexpensive method to screen for balance and gait dysfunction.

References

1. Mathias S, Nayak and U, Isaacs B (1986) Balance and elderly patients: the "Get Up and Go" Test. Arch Phys Med Rehabil 67:387.

2. Tinetti M, Williams and T, Mayewski, R (1986) Fall risk index for elderly patients based on number of chronic disabilities. Am J Med 80:429.

3. Wolfson L, Whipple R et al (1990) Gait assessment in the elderly: a gait abnormality rating scale and its relation to falls. J Geron 45:M12.

4. Kauffman T (1990) Impact of age-related musculoskeletal and postural changes on falls. Top of Geriatr Rehabil 5:34.

5. Kauffman T (1987) Posture and age. Topics in Geriatric Rehabilitation 2:13.

INORGANIC PHOSPHATE AND INTRACELLULAR pH LEVELS IN YOUNG AND AGED SKELETAL MUSCLE STUDIED BY ^{31}P NUCLEAR MAGNETIC RESONANCE

J Ashmore 1, E B Cady 2, S Phillips 3, S A Rice 1.
1.Dept of Physiotherapy,The Middlesex Hospital,London,UK. 2.Dept of Medical Physics and Bio-engineering,University College,London,UK. 3.Dept of Physiology,University College,London,UK.

Introduction

Muscle weakness is a well documented feature of old age (1). Although atrophy accounts for some of the weakness associated with ageing it is not solely responsible (2,3). There appears to be a specific reduction in the ability of ageing muscle to produce force which results in a decrease in the maximal voluntary force per unit cross-sectional area (MVC/CSA). The cause of this has not yet been explained, but recent studies suggest that the deficit may be caused by an alteration in the behaviour of myosin, due either to high concentrations of inorganic phosphate (Pi) or a low intracellular pH (pHi)(3). It is believed that high Pi concentrations inhibit the power stroke of the cross bridge cycle (4) thus reducing the force that the muscle can produce (4,5,6). A low pHi also reduces isometric force development (7), but the mechanism is not known.

In this study, the hypothesis under investigation is that, in resting elderly muscle, the pHi is lower or the Pi level higher than that in young muscle.

An earlier study reported no difference between pHi or Pi levels in the resting flexor digitorum superficialis of young and elderly subjects (8). However, this muscle has not been shown to exhibit an age-related strength deficit and as the MVC/CSA of the muscle was not measured, it is not certain that these elderly subjects had a deficit. In the present study the adductor pollicis was investigated. This muscle has previously been found to demonstrate age-related weakness (2) and this study also includes a measurement of MVC/CSA.

Subjects

The study was performed on normal volunteers recruited from patients attending local physiotherapy departments and colleagues, parents and friends of the investigators. All subjects were right handed. The young subjects were 5 men and 7 women aged 21-39 years (mean age 29.7 years). The old group comprised 4 men and 8 women aged 74-83 years (mean age 80.3 years) who were healthy and leading active and independent lives. Subjects were excluded if they were taking any medication that could affect their motivation or muscle strength, as were those with any history of myelopathy, inflammatory joint, cardiovascular or neurological disease, diabetes, generalised osteoarthritis or metallic implants (9). Subjects were also excluded if they had pain, stiffness or weakness in their right arm and if their occupation or hobbies involved excessive use of the right thumb.

Methods

Pi and pHi were measured by ^{31}P nuclear magnetic resonance (NMR) spectroscopy, which provides a non-invasive method of investigating muscle metabolism. The palmar aspect of the subject's right adductor pollicis was placed over a 10mm radiofrequency coil which was positioned in the centre of a 1.9 Tesla, 26cm clear bore Oxford Instruments superconducting magnet interfaced to an Oxford Research Systems-Bruker TMR spectrometer. The arm was restrained with padded straps. To reduce external radiofrequency interference, the subjects were earthed using an aluminium strap around the upper part of the arm. ^{31}P spectra were collected for 20 minutes using a 90° flip angle at the core centre and a 2.256s repetition time.

Measurement of the MVC/CSA of the right adductor pollicis of all subjects was carried out as previously described (10).

Data Analysis

The Pi levels (expressed as a fraction of total mobile phosphorus) and pHi values were determined as previously described (11).

Results

The results for pHi and Pi levels are shown in table 1.

Table 1. Mean Pi and pHi values of the resting adductor policis. (Standard deviation in parenthesis)

	Young	Elderly
Age Range	21-39	74-83
Age Mean	29.7	80.3
pHi (SD)	7.133 (0.107)	7.118 (0.069)
Pi (SD)	0.083 (0.026)	0.078 (0.031)
Number of subjects	12	12

The results were analysed using a two-tailed unrelated t-test. The difference between the mean pHi for the elderly and young was not significant (t=0.43, p=0.671). The difference between the mean Pi levels was also not significant (t=0.43, p=0.674). The MVC/CSA was found to be lower in the elderly subjects, the results being significant (t=5.25, p<0.001) (Rice 1990 personal communication).

Discussion

The results show that there are no significant differences in pHi or Pi levels in the resting adductor pollicis of the two groups of subjects. However, the elderly group did show a significant reduction in the MVC/CSA and therefore had age-related muscle weakness. These results suggest that alterations in Pi and pHi are not responsible for age-related muscle weakness unless the myosin in elderly muscle is more sensitive to Pi or acidification than that in young muscle.

If this weakness is not due to changes in the intracellular environment of the contractile machinery then there must be a change to the contractile proteins themselves. Possible causes of this are inactivity (12) and hormonal factors, particularly in elderly women, where there is a link between a reduced ability to generate force and osteoporosis (13).

Conclusion

The results of the present study did not support the hypothesis that pHi is lower or Pi levels higher in elderly muscle. Therefore these factors are unlikely to be responsible for age-related muscle weakness. However, difficulties were experienced in obtaining good quality NMR spectra, problems being caused by radiofrequency interference and the size and location of the adductor pollicis. Therefore the results of this study should not be considered conclusive. The investigation of another muscle more suited to NMR may produce results of greater significance.

References

1. Larson L, Grimby G, & Karlsson J (1979). Muscle Strength and speed of movement in relation to age and muscle morphology. Journal of Applied Physiology 456: 451-456

2. Bruce SA, Newton D and Woledge RC (1989). Effect of age on voluntary force and cross-sectional area of human adductor pollicis muscle. Quarterly Journal of Experimental Physiology 74: 359-362.

3. Brooks SV & Faulkner JA (1988). Contractile properties of skeletal muscles from young adult and aged mice. Journal of Physiology 404: 71-82.

4. Hibberd MG & Danzig JA (1985). Phosphate release and force generation in skeletal muscle fibres. Science 228: 1317-1319.

5. Kentish JC (1986). The effects of inorganic phosphate and creatinine phosphate on force production in skinned muscle from the rat ventricle. Journal of Physiology 370: 585-604.

6. Elzinga G, Stienen GJM & Versteeg PGA (1989). Effect of inorganic phosphate on length responses to changes in load in skinned rabbit psoas. Journal of Physiology 415: 132.

7. Metzger JM & Moss RL (1987). Greater hydrogen ion-induced depression of tension in skinned single fibres of rat fast than slow muscles. Journal of Physiology 393: 727-742.

8. Taylor DJ, Crowe M, Bore PJ, Styles PO, Arnold DA & Radda GK (1984). Examination of the energetics of ageing skeletal muscle using nuclear magnetic resonance. Gerontology 30: 2-7.

9. Saunders R D & Smith H (1984). Safety Aspects of NMR Clinical Imaging. British Medical Bulletin 40: 148-154.

10. Bruce SA, Newton D & Woledge RC (1989). Effect of subnutrition on normalised muscle force and relaxation rate in human subjects using voluntary contractions. Clinical Science 76: 637-641.

11. Cady EB (1991). A reappraisal of the absolute concentration of phosphorylated metabolites in the human neonatal cerebral cortex obtained by fitting Lorentzian curves to the ^{31}P NMR spectrum. Journal of Magnetic Resonance (in press).

12. Klitgaard H, Mantoni M, Schiaffino S, Ausoni S, Gorza L, Lauren-Winter, Schnohr P & Saltin B (1990). Function, morphology and protein expression of ageing skeletal muscle: a cross-sectional study of elderly men with different training backgrounds. Acta Physiol Scand 140: 41-54.

13. Jones D A & Rutherford O M (1990). Effect of ageing and osteoporosis on the force generating capacity of the quadriceps muscle in women. Proceedings of the Phyisological Society (in the Press).

THE EFFECTS OF SPECIFIC TRAINING ON THE
BIOMECHANICS OF STANDING UP FOLLOWING TOTAL HIP
REPLACEMENT.

P. C. Westwood

School of Physiotherapy,
Cumberland College of Health Sciences,
The University of Sydney,
Sydney, Australia.

Introduction: The purpose of this study was to investigate the
effects on biomechanical variables of specific training of
standing up following total hip replacement (THR). Previous
studies have indicated that these patients continue to use
compensatory strategies when standing up even after discharge
from rehabilitation.
Method: Sixteen subjects following uncemented THR for
osteoarthritis of the hip were selected and randomly allocated
into either a control or a treatment group. Both groups of
subjects followed surgeon-prescribed activity of partial
weight-bearing for six weeks post surgery. Following this
period, all subjects were videotaped and forceplatform data
was collected as they stood up. The treatment group subjects
were then trained to stand up fully weight-bearing over a six
week period. Training comprised weekly supervised sessions
with daily practice of standing up according to guidelines set
by the physiotherapist. All subjects were retested six weeks
following the initial test.
Results: The results of this study will be presented in terms
of angular displacements and torques. Clinical implications
regarding the need to train activies specifically will be
discussed.

A SINGLE CASE STUDY TO INVESTIGATE THE EFFECTIVE-
NESS OF DIFFERENT PHYSIOTHERAPEUTIC METHODS IN
CONTROLLING UPPER LIMB LYMPHOEDEMA

W J Jefferson

Department of Physiotherapy, The Royal Free
Hospital, London, England

Introduction Previous work shows that lymphoedema can be
treated successfully by the skillful application of specific
physiotherapeutic measures. The results of this therapy can
be maintained if the patient is compliant. This case study
aims to identify the specific physiotherapeutic measures which
most effectively reduce and control lymphoedema of the arm in
women who have undergone surgery/radiotherapy for breast cancer
Method The study will evaluate the effectiveness of manual
lymphatic drainage and intermittent pneumatic compression combined with exercises, and multi-layer bandaging or containment
hosiery. The case selected is of severe lymphoedema, defined
as the affected limb measuring 4 cms. larger than the unaffected limb at defined points. Manual lymphatic drainage is the
manual stimulation of lymphatic flow by two techniques defined
as 'Call' and 'Absorb'. Intermittent pneumatic compression,
(using the LYMPHA PRESS) is the mechanical exertion of a pressure gradient through a multi-chambered sleeve. These two
techniques combined with exercises within bandaging or containment hosiery are used in accordance with a pre-set timetable.
Upper limb volume is measured, using a volumeter, at predetermined intervals of time.
Results Pilot studies indicate that these specific methods are
more effective in reducing and stabilising lymphoedema than
conventional techniques.
Conclusion This study identifies the specific physiotherapeutic
measures which are most effective. It therefore indicates the
need for further study and application of these techniques in
clinical practice.

AMPUTEES

ADVANCED METHODS OF PROSTHETIC GAIT TRAINING FOR HIGH TECH PROSTHETICS

R. Gailey, M.S.Éd., P.T.
University of Miami, Division of Physical Therapy
5915 Ponce de Leon Blvd, 5th Floor, Coral Gables, Florida 33146 USA

INTRODUCTION

The prosthetic field has made tremendous advances during the 1980's in fitting techniques, compent technology and improved function. With the onset of this new era in the prosthetic field, health professionals involved in amputee rehabilitation have a responsibility to keep current with options now available prosthetically, as well as to develop and promote rehabilitation techniques which take full advantage of the current prosthetic technology. The concept of this program is a systematic approach to amputee rehabilitation, which optimizes patient contact time in providing the skills necessary for maximum function with a minimum metabolic cost. A functional progression including: strengthening, stability training, weight shifting and balance activities provides the foundation for restoring pelvic, lower extremity and trunk mechanics. That is, the gait training process is taught in component parts, and once mastery of each splinter skill is achieved, greater success is experienced when ambulation is attempted.

The following is a four part comprehensive above-knee amputee rehabilitation program designed to progress the patient to independent ambulation in as short a time as possible. Part one is a pure isometric strengthening program. Part two is a pre-gait training program designed to orient the amputee to his center of gravity over his base of support, on either one or two limbs. Part three is the actual gait training where the components of gait biomechanics are practiced, and eventually drawn together for independent ambulation. Finally, part four develops advanced skills such as agility, balance and coordination that improve the amputee's confidence and level of skill with his prosthesis. As in all rehabilitation situtations, the results are partially dependent on the amputee's health status, motivation and level of skill.

An overview of the total rehabilitation program will be presented in the text of this article. The concept and rationale for each of the four segments of the functional progression program is the author's goal. Specific methods used to accomplish the desired therapeutic outcome may vary between therapists, naturally, as therapists must select rehabilitation techniques comfortable to them, which will in turn produce the best results for the patient.

PART ONE; AMPUTEE STRENGTHENING PROGRAM

Esiert (1954) first described dynamic exercise for lower extremity amputees. These exercises, with slight variations, have remained the most practical and productive residual limb strengthening exercises. Essentially, the hip is strengthened by placing a towel roll (for longer residual limbs, a small foot stool) under the limb and the amputee depresses the residual limb into the towel roll, raising the pelvis off the resting surface. This is technique is repeated for hip flexion, extension, abduction and adduction (illustration 1.0).

The knee extensors may be strengthened by placing the towel roll under the distal end of the residual limb, with the amputee prone, and a pillow under the distal thigh to prevent patellar compression. Knee flexors are best strengthened with the amputee supine or sitting, and attempting to flex the knee as the residual limb is depressed into the resting surface.

The trunk musculature must not be forgotten when teaching the amputee his strengthening program. The back extensors and abdominals play a significant role in gait, maintaining the trunk erect, and for amputees, preventing lateral leaning of the trunk. Traditional sit-ups, and back extension exercises in the prone position are two good ways to improve trunk strength. Additionally, bridging exercises assist with hip and low back extension, however, care must be taken not to let the amputated limb drop below horizontal. The sound limb internal rotators must contract to maintain equal height of the pelvis in the raised position. The strengthening of the sound side hip internal rotators will assist with transverse rotation of the pelvis, a movement necessary during gait training.

Although these exercises are dynamic by definition, the addition of an isometric component has proven clinically advantageous to the strengthening process. Amputees are instructed to follow a simple formula, the "Rule of Ten". The Rule of Ten is as follows: 10 second contraction, 10 second rest, 10 repetitions, 10 exercises, 10 times per day. The reason for a 10 second contraction is that a maximal contraction can be maintained for 6seconds. Additionally, there is a 2 second rise time and 2 second fall time in addition to the 6 second maximal contraction, thus equalling 10 seconds total contraction time. The rest is to permit adequate recovery. This time may be decreased depending on the level of fitness of each individual.

PART TWO; PRE-GAIT TRAINING EXERCISE PROGRAM

Once adequate strength has been developed, the next phase of this program is designed to reorient the amputees to the relationship between his center of gravity and his base of support. Visualization is a tool that has worked well in assisting patients to understand the concept of center of gravity. The patient is asked to visualize a small marble at his center of gravity (2 inches anterior to the second sacral level) and the therapist's hands can help the amputee locate and visualize this point. Next, the amputee imagines that the area under both feet is a square. Holding on to the P-bars with both hands, the amputee visualizes moving the small marble laterally to either edge of the imaginary square. In actuality, the amputee is displacing the center of gravity to either limit of the base of support. Once adequate displacement is achieved laterally, anterior and posterior displacement are practiced.

When the amputee is comfortable with these movements with bilateral upper extremity support, the sound side hand should be removed and the movements practiced in both directions again. By removing the sound side hand, increased weight-bearing through the prosthetic limb will be required. As single arm support movements become comfortable, both hands are removed from the P-bars for independent standing, as displacement of the center of gravity is practiced.

Obviously, the range of movement will decrease as upper extremity support is decreased. As the amputee concentrates on COG displacement, increased weight bearing, weight shifting and balance will be developed. Diagonal patterns may also be practiced in a similar fashion , to practice weight transfer from the rear foot to the forefoot as with walking.

One other exercise that has proven beneficial in promoting single limb balance on the prosthetic limb is the "stool stepping" exercise. A 6-8 inch step stool, or a thick phone book for lower heights, is placed in front of the amputee's sound limb while they are standing in the parallel bars. The amputee is asked to raise his sound limb onto the stool in a slow controlled manner, both hands remaining on the parallel bars. Once comfortable with this movement, the amputee is asked to free his sound side hand and again step onto the stool. In most cases, the foot moves extremely fast accompanied by lateral trunk leaning. At this time, visualization is employed again to help promote body and prosthetic awareness. The amputee should be asked to concentrate on three items; 1) muscular control of the hip on the prosthetic side, 2) controlling the prosthesis and receiving sensory input from the distal end of the residual limb within the socket, and 3) visualizing the movements about the prosthetic ankle, and between the sole of the prosthetic foot and ground. As mastery of these skills improves over time, both hands may be removed from the parallel bars. This one particular exercise will assist the amputee in developing adequate stance time during ambulation on the prosthetic limb, thus permitting equal stride length, stance time and decreasing lateral trunk lean.

PART THREE: GAIT TRAINING PROGRAM:

Gait training methods are intended to concentrate on the actual biomechanics of ambulation. To familiarize the amputee with his natural movement of lower extremity advancement, have the amputee stand in the parallel bars, taking a step forward and backward with his sound limb. As the patient continues the stepping movement, the therapist places his hands on the amputee's anterior superior iliac spines to feel for the forward pelvic rotation in the transverse plane. Once the motion of the pelvis and the step length of the sound limb are comfortable and appreciated by both the therapist and amputee, they are ready to begin to transfer this knowledge to the prosthetic limb. The amputee repeats the exercise of stepping forward and backward with the prosthetic limb the same way previously performed with the sound limb. Initially, what is commonly observed is a kicking motion of the prosthetic limb, accompanied by posterior rotation of the pelvis. As a result, the body's COG remains posterior, there is no smooth transition of the weight over the sound limb, and prosthetic knee flexion is severely compromised. To overcome these deviations, the prosthetic limb is placed posterior to the sound limb and the therapist passively rotates the pelvis in the desired transverse motion. When the amputee feels comfortable with the corrected motion, he begins to actively initiate the movement, progressing to taking a full step with the prosthetic limb. Stepping forward and backward with the prosthetic limb is practiced in the parallel bars concentrating on transfer of weight over the sound limb, maintenance of a straight line of progression with the prosthetic limb, and controlling stride length. The supporting hands may be released from the parallel bars, sound side hand first and then prosthetic side hand, as skill and confidence develop.

Returning to the sound limb stepping exercise, the amputee again practices with both hands on the parallel bars, concentrating on a slow sound limb step with an appropriate stride length. Releasing the sound side hand, the immediate response is usually a shorter, quicker step with a lateral leaning trunk over the prosthetic side. This response is the result of inadequate weight-bearing on the prosthesis and can be improved if the amputee utilizes the same skills learned when practicing the stool stepping exercise. Eventually, both hands should be removed from the parallel bars.

At this time, all the component parts of gait should be learned and well practiced. To tie the biomechanics together, resistive gait training in the parallel bars, progressing to resisted gait out of the parallel bars gives the amputee a sense of how to incorporate all the skills leaned into functional ambulation. Finally, trunk rotation must be taught to provide the additional balance, momentum, and symmetry necessary to increase stability and reduce metabolic cost. There are many ways to incorporate trunk rotation, including, rhythmic initiation, or passively moving the amputee's trunk via the shoulders to obtain the desired affect.

PART FOUR; ADVANCED TRAINING SKILLS:
There is a whole series of agility and balance exercises to help promote balance and improved coordination for a variety of patients. Any one of these would serve the amputee well to practice, and thereby help develop the relationship between his prosthesis and residual limb. A few examples are: toe and heel pivoting, tandem walking, braiding, walking in circles, and backward walking. Whatever the exercise chosen, it will help the amputee develop the skills necessary to improve prosthetic control, and overcome many barriers that might prohibit daily independent ambulation.

CONCLUSION:
Amputees today have many more options available to them than ever before, with newer socket designs and advanced prosthetic componentry. Rehabilitation techniques must keep up with this new technology, utilizing the advances to promote a higher level of skill and a more natural gait for amputees. The program presented in this article was designed to offer a few suggestions and stimulate further clinical experimentation by physical therapists for the enhancement of amputee rehabilitation.

PROSTHETIC REHABILITATION PROGRAM EXERCISES

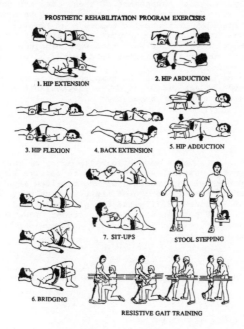

1. HIP EXTENSION
2. HIP ABDUCTION
3. HIP FLEXION
4. BACK EXTENSION
5. HIP ADDUCTION
7. SIT-UPS
STOOL STEPPING
6. BRIDGING
RESISTIVE GAIT TRAINING

REFERENCES

1. Brunnstrom S, Kerr D: The Training of the Lower Extremity Amputee. Springfield, IL. Charles C. Thomas Publishing, 1956.

2 . Eisert o, Tester O W: Dynamic exercises for lower extremity amputees. Arch Phys Med Rehabil 35:695-704, 1954.

FUNCTIONAL ASSESSMENT OF ONCOLOGIC AMPUTEES: A PROSPECTIVE STUDY

C.L. McGarvey, J. Hicks, M. Lampert, J. Danoff
National Institutes of Health, Clinical Center, Department of Rehabilitation Medicine, 9000 Rockville Pike, Bldg 10, Rm 6s235, Bethesda, MD 20892

INTRODUCTION:

Malignant neoplasms are responsible for approximately four percent of all amputations.[1] Melanomas and sarcomas represent two classifications of two such malignant neoplasms. Sarcomas, in particular, osteosarcoma (OS) and soft tissue sarcoma (STS) are among the most common neoplasms diagnosed.

Historically, surgical management of these patients has emphasized amputation of the involved extremity at levels higher than are usually accomplished for vascular or traumatic causes.[2,3,4] However recent advances in diagnostic technology and adjuvant therapies have fostered attempts toward more conservative surgeries which include limb sparing techniques such as wide local excisions (WLE) with and without prosthetic replacements.[5,6,7]

The purpose of this study was to compare the pre vs. postoperative effect of amputation on activities of daily living (ADL) for a group of oncology patients who underwent amputation.

METHODS:

SUBJECTS

Twenty-two (22) subjects were originally accepted into the study, two of these patients, however, were selected to receive limb sparing procedures. Of the ramaining twenty (20) who received amputation three (3) died prior to the administration of the post-test questionaire. In result, a total of seventeen (17) patients, nine males and eight females with a mean age of 22.6 participated in this study. Additional demographic information related to diagnosis and level of amputation is available from figures 1 and 2.

DESIGN:

Study was one group pretest-posttest design as described by Currier.[16]

DATA COLLECTION:

Data were collected by personal interview preoperative and one year post opertively using a twenty-two (22) item questionaire previously modified from a form described by Granger.[9] Included in the questionaire were assessment of the presence or absence of pain, phantom limb pain and phantom limb sensation. Also assessed were the levels of independence of activities of daily living such as: transfers, eating,

toileting, grooming, bathing, dressing, ambulation, vocational/
social/occupational issues and prosthetic application. Level of
function was rated in accordance with degree of independence per
activity. A sample of the questionaire is available for additional
review.

RESULTS:

No differences were found between (yes) and (no) responses for
"extremity pain" pre-amputation. Post amputation there were
significantly fewer (yes) responses and the number of (yes) responses
decreased significantly from pre to post amputation.

Significantly fewer (yes) responses were received for "pain
elsewhere" both pre and post amputation. For post-amputation only
responses, i.e., "phantom limb pain," "stump/residual pain," "phantom
limb sensation," and "pain elsewhere in body" (yes) and (no) responses
were approximately equal.

There were significantly more (yes) than (no) responses both pre
and post amputation for "transfer bed to chair," "feeds self," "on and
off toilet," "uses toilet," "grooms self," "in and out of shower,"
"bathes self," "dresses self," "prepares simple food," and "attends
school."

There were significantly more (yes) than (no) responses both pre-
amputation for "manipulates home appliances," "ambulates on level
surfaces," "ambulates on stairs," and "attends church."

There was a significant decrease in the number of (yes) responses
from pre-to-post amputation for "ambulates on level surfaces" and
"ambulates on stairs."

There were no other significant decreases comparing pre-to-post
amputation for any other of the questions.

CONCLUSION:

These results indicate that for oncology patients, in whom the
majority received high level amputations, very little difference is
noted in functional outcome when activities of daily living are compared
prior to and following amputation. Those significant changes detected
were in the patient ability to ambulate independently on level surfaces
and stairs. Obviously, the use of a prosthesis post-operatively
required additional assistance through the use of a cane, crutch or
handrail, however, did not appear to limit the amputee in participating
or performing other activities independently.

These data, although somewhat limited due to the small sample
population, appear to support Sugarbaker's[4] premise that the surgical
management of these lesions by amputation represent a reasonable
surgical choice in minimal deficits in functional outcome.

<u>REFERENCES</u>

1) Sanders GT: Lower Limb Amputations: A Guide to Rehabilitation. F.A. Davis, Philadelphia, pp. 35-37, 1986
2) Sugarbaker PH and Nicholson TH: Atlas of ExtremitY Sarcoma Surgery. J.B.Lippincott, Philadelphia, 1984.
3) Rosenberg SA, Suit HD, Baker LH and Rosen G: Sarcomas of the Soft Tissue and Bone. In: Devita VT, Hellman S and Rosenberg SA (eds) Cancer Principles and Practice of Oncology. J.B. Lippincott, Philadelphia, pp. 1037-1094, 1985.
4) Sugarbaker PH, Barofsky I, Rosenber SA and Gianola FJ: Quality of Life Assessment of Patients in Extremity Sarcoma Clinical Trials. Surgery 91: 17-23, 1982.
5) Arlen M and Marcove RC: Surgical Managemnet of Soft Tissue Sarcomas. W.B. Saunders Co. Philadelphia, 1987.
6) Morton DL, Eiber FR, Towsend CM et al.: Limb Salvage from a Multidisciplinary Treatment Approach for Skeletal and Soft Tissue Sarcomas of the Extremity. Ann Surg 184: pp. 268-278, 1976.
7) Rosenberg SA, Kent H and Costa J: Prospective Randomized Evaluation of the Role of Limb Sparing Surgery, Radiation Therapy and Adjuvant Chemoimmunotherapy in the Treatment of Adult Soft Tissue Sarcoma. Surger 84: pp. 62-69, 1978.
8) Granger,CV, Mcnamara MA: Funcitonal Assessment Utilitzation: The Long Range Evaluation System (LRES) In: Functional Assessment in Rehabilitation Medicine. Granger CV and Gresham GE (eds) Williams and Wilkins, Baltimore, 1984.
9) Granger CV: Health Accounting - Functional Assessment of the Long Term Patient. In: Krusen's Handbook of Physical Medicine and Rehabilitaiton. 3rd ed. Kottke FJ Stillwell GK and Lehmann JF (eds). W.B. Saunders Co., Phildelphia, 1982.
10) Lampert MH, Gerber LH, Glatstein R. Rosenberg SA and Danoff JV: Functional Outcome of Patients Undergoing Wide Local Excision and Radiation Tehrapy for Soft Tissue Sarcoma. Arch Phys Med Rehab 65: pp. 477-480, 1984
11) CAREY RG, Posavac EJ: Program Evaluation of Physical Medicine and Reahbilitaiton Unit: A New Approach. Arch Phys Med Rehab 59: pp. 330-337, 1978 (Level of Rehabilitaiton Scale (LORS).
12) Scranton J, Fogel ML, Erdman WJ: Evaluation of Functional Levels of Patients During and Following Rehabilitaiton. Arch Phys Med Rehab: pp. 1-21, Jan 1970 (Pielson Functional Evaluation Instrument).
13) Yates JW, Chalmer B, McKegkey FP. Evaluation of Patients with Advanced Cancer Using the Karnofsky Performance Status. Cancer 45: pp. 2220-2224, 1980 (Karnofsky Performance Status Scale (KPS).
14) Sarno JE, Sarno MT and Levita E: The Functional Life Scale. Arch Phys Med Rehab 54: pp. 214-220, May 19783 [Functional LIfe Scale (FLS)].
15) Kegal B, Carpenter ML, Burgess EM: Functional Capabilities of Lower Extremity Amputees. Arch Phys Med Rehab 59: pp.109-120, 1978 (Functional Capabilities Questionaire).

METABOLIC COST OF UNILATERAL ABOVE-KNEE AMPUTEES WALKING: A COMPARISON BETWEEN THE QUADRILATERAL
SOCKET AND THE CAT-CAM SOCKET

R. Gailey, MS Ed, PT, D. Lawrence, MS, PT, C. Burditt, MS, PT,
C. Newell, MS, PT, P. Spyropoulos, PhD, PT
University of Miami, Division of Physical Therapy
5915 Ponce de Leon Blvd, 5th Floor Coral Gables, Florida 33146 USA

INTRODUCTION

The energy expenditure of lower extremity above-knee amputees has consistently been reported as
being higher than non-amputee individuals. For example, James (1973) reported that above-knee
amputee's (AKA's) oxygen expenditure was 40% greater, while ambulating at a velocity 30% slower than
non-amputees. Traugh (1975) found AKAs to have a 65% increase in metabolic cost while ambulating at
a velocity 50% below non-amputees. Blessey (1976) noted a 37% increase in metabolic cost and a 13%
decease in ambulatory velocity as compared to non-amputees. Huang (1979) determined that AKAs had a
49% increase in metabolic cost compared to non-amputees while ambulating at a significantly slower
pace of 47 meters per minute (1.75 mph). All subjects who participated in the aforementioned
studies were assumed to be fitted with a quadrilateral socket.

The Contoured Adducted Trochanteric - Controlled Alignment Method (CAT-CAM) socket was introduced in
the early 1980's by John Sabolich. The CAT-CAM socket is designed to fit intimately with the
ischial ramus; thus, "locking" onto the pelvis encapsulating the ischial tuberosity as it is
considerably more narrow in the medial-lateral dimension than the quadrilateral socket .
Additionally, the CAT-CAM socket has been reported to improve muscular function, enhance pelvic
motion and maintain a more natural femoral adduction angle of the amputated limb. Consequently,
proponents of the CAT-CAM socket have suggested that there is a decrease in the energy required for
ambulation by above-knee amputees.

Limited research has been reported to substantiate the implied benefits of the CAT-CAM socket.
Beskin (1989) reported that five AKAs who formerly wore the quadrilateral socket, and who were
subsequently fitted with the CAT-CAM socket demonstrated reduced gait deviations, increased stride
length and ambulatory velocity, and significantly reduced oxygen consumption. Flandry (1989) noted
that AKAs wearing the CAT-CAM socket had improved efficiency as indicated by a reduction in oxygen
consumption and an increase in ambulatory velocity.

The purpose of this study was to determine whether or not the CAT-CAM socket is superior to the
quadrilateral socket with respect to metabolic cost during ambulation. Specifically, it was
hypothesized that (1) amputees fitted with the CAT-CAM socket would consume less O2 than amputees
fitted with the quadrilateral socket while ambulating at slow (1.25 mph) and fast speeds (2.5 mph);
and (2), heart rate values would be lower for CAT-CAM amputees than for quadrilateral amputees
during slow and fast ambulation.

METHODS

Subjects: Twenty unilateral above-knee amputees wearing either the CAT-CAM (n=10) or quadrilateral
QUAD (n=10) socket and ten non-amputee subjects (controls) participated in this study. The
following criteria served for the selection of our subjects: male gender between the ages of 18 -
55 years, amputation due to non-vascular pathology, absence of medical complications, unaffected
sound limb, at least six months experience with the tested prosthesis, and a minimum residual limb
length of six inches with the amputation site proximal to the femoral condyles.

Instrumentation: The MMC Horizon metabolic analyzer was used to collect expired air from our
subjects. This equipment was calibrated for gas, volume, and temperature prior to each testing
session and was corrected to standard volumes for temperature, pressure and humidity. Expired air
samples were collected every 15 seconds throughout the experimental procedure by means of a rubber
mouthpiece connected to a Hans-Rudolf non-rebreathing valve. Air exchange was prevented through the
nasal airway by way of a rubber nose clip. The Vantage Performance Transmitter was strapped around
each individual's chest at the point of maximal impulse to record heart rate (HR) values. Two
telemetry wristwatch/signal receivers were placed on the subject and were programmed to record HR
values at 15 second intervals throughout the experimental procedure.

Procedure: Subjects each walked at two different speeds, 1.25 mph and 2.5 mph, which were randomly assigned to each participant. Each subject was first connected to the Vantage Performance Monitor and simultaneously to the Metabolic Analyzer. Non-exercise VO2 and HR measurements were obtained during a one minute standing rest period. Subsequently, each subject walked at one of the two designated speeds for eight minutes around a 118-foot, L-shaped, industrial carpeted indoor track. A metronome and verbal cues were used as pacing devices. Following the eight minutes, each person remained standing for one minute to obtain post-exercise VO2 and HR values. Twenty minute rest periods were assigned between the two different speed testings.

Data Analysis: VO2 & HR mean values, obtained during steady state, were analyzed via a two-way ANOVA. Differences among means were further located through the Tukey and the simple effects tests.

RESULTS

Means and standard deviations for VO2 & HR are presented in Table 1. Significant differences were detected between the control group and CAT-CAM subjects regarding VO2 ($p < .05$) and HR ($p < .01$) values. The control and QUAD individuals were also different with respect to their VO2 ($p < .01$) and HR ($p < .01$) means. Faster speeds required more exercise energy expenditure ($p < .01$) and produced higher HR ($p < .01$) than slower speeds. In fast speeds, there was a significantly ($p < .01$) higher demand in energy expenditure in the QUAD than in the CAT-CAM group.

TABLE 1: MEANS AND STANDARD DEVIATIONS OF OXYGEN UPTAKE AND HEART RATE

	SLOW SPEED (1.25MPH)		FAST SPEED (2.5MPH)	
GROUP	**VO$_2$**	**HR**	**VO$_2$**	**HR**
CAT-CAM	10.37±1.34	101.42±13.27	15.12±1.89	116.42±14.48
QUAD	11.72±2.70	100.82±10.61	18.98±5.52	119.75±16.28
CONTROL	8.48±1.08	83.86±9.22	11.08±1.88	90.04±8.60

DISCUSSION

This study does support the suggestion that the CAT-CAM socket reduces the metabolic cost of ambulation by 20% for unilateral above-knee amputees at 2.5 mph or normal human locomotion velocity. For the amputee, the CAT-CAM socket not only has the clinical advantages described by prosthetists and consumers alike, but also provides a physiologically economical alternative to the quadrilateral socket design that has proved to be the standard for so many years.

As proponents of the CAT-CAM socket suggest, by "locking" on to the ischial ramus and containing the ischial tuberosity within the socket, the metabolic cost reduction may be a result of the restored pelvic motions that appear clinically to produce more normalized gait biomechanics. Additionally, there seems to be a more graphic difference in energy cost reduction with faster speeds. That is, as the amputee approaches normal walking speed, energy cost drastically increases with the quadrilateral socket, whereas the difference between slow and fast speed ambulation in CAT-CAM socket wearers is considerably less. This may indicate that amputees will find it less taxing and more comfortable to walk at normal speeds with the CAT-CAM socket.

One question that stands out is why there was a significant difference with VO2 and not with heart rate between, and within the groups. No suitable explanation can be rendered presently for this paradoxial result.

REFERENCES

1. James U (1973) Oxygen uptake and heart rate during prosthetic walking in healthy male unilateral above-knee amputees. Scand J Rehab Med 5:71-80

2. Traugh GH, Corcoran PJ, Rudolpho LR (1975) Energy expenditure of ambulation in patients with above-knee amputations. Phys Med Rehabil 56:67-71

3. Blessey RL, Hislop HJ, Waters RL (1976) Metabolic energy cost of unrestrained walking. Phys Ther 56:1019-1024

4. Huang CT, Jackson JR, Moore NB, et al (1979) Amputation: energy cost of ambulation. Arch Pys Med Rehabil 60:18-24

5. Sabolich J (1985) Contoured adducted trochanteric-controlled alignment method (CAT-CAM): introduction and basic principles. Orthotics and Prosthetics 9:15-26

6. Beskin J, Chambers R, Flandry F (1989) The effect of the CAT-CAM above-knee prosthesis on functional rehabilitation. Clinical Orthopaedics and Related Research 239:249-262

7. Flandry E, Beskin J, Chambers R, et al (1989) The effects of the CAT-CAM above-knee prosthesis on functional rehabilitation. Clin Orthop 239:249-262

DRAMATIC IMPROVEMENTS IN PROSTHETICS AND ORTHOTICS IN THE LEAST DEVELOPED WORLD.

Lawrence Golin L. P. T. (Michigan)
Memorial Christian Hospital,
P.O. Malumghat, Cox's Bazar Dist, BANGLADESH 4743

INTRODUCTION: The needs of the least developed world provide a great challlenge to the practice of physical therapy.[1] Disabling conditions are more prevalent there than in the developed world. Heavy manual labor, medical malpractice and minimal nutrition are only some of the factors that increase the incidence of disability. Poliomyelitis, cerebral malaria, bone tuberculosis, and leprosy are disabling ilnesses rarely seen in developed countries. In the past, the problems were so overwhelming that rehebilitation of disabled people was difficult or impossible. The problem was not a lack of compassion, but rather a dearth of inexpensive materials needed for making the necessary appliances. Western technologies were not suitable for countries where people squat rather than sit in chairs, where people walk barefoot instead of wearing shoes or boots, and where there are no insurance companies to pay for expensive calipers or dynamic splints.

Braces made from bamboo or steel rods with wooden clogs were previously used. They were not durable, too heavy, and were unattractive. Artificial limbs were either made from a western model or were modified peg legs. Both of these were either too expensive to make, or unsuitable for the needs of the people. The western type limb required a leather shoe with leather sole. This shoe could not withstand the insult of using it in a rural area where most people live. Therefore it wore out very quickly and the poor farmer, unable to purchase a new pair of shoes, hung the prosthesis on the wall and reverted back to his crutches or peg leg.[2]

In the past 20 years, materials have appeared in the market place that are cheap and suitable for making durable, functional appliances.

JAIPUR FOOT PROSTHESIS: In 1974 Drs. P.K. Sethi, M.P. Udowat, and Mr. R. Chandra of S.M.S. Hospital Rehabilitation Center in Jaipur, India published a paper entitled: "Lower Limb Prosthetics for Amputees in Rural Areas."[3] This paper described the fabrication of a foot piece using readily available vulcanized tire and microcellar rubber foam. The materials were fitted into a sand casted aluminum mold in such a way that the fabricated foot imitated the anatomy of the human foot. Ordinary village people accepted this Jaipur foot, for it allowed them to carry out their normal daily activities.

Another step forward, was using aluminum as a shank beaten into the shape of the stump and molded into a P.T.B. socket. With this prosthesis, an amputee could squat and sit cross legged, which was impossible with the conventional artifical limb. In addition, the aluminum shank made it possible to revise the socket after normal shrinkage of the amputee's stump. Expensive resin plastics, PVA sheeting, plaster of paris bandages, and complicated jigs are not needed to fabricate these sockets. Furthermore, the aluminum shanks are much lighter in weight and can be made by village tin workers

a western type prosthetic foot. This technology works well for village children and facilitates normal dorsiflexion at heel strike.

Keds type running shoes are more popular for children who come from the cities of the developing world. In such cases, a fitted-into-shoes-AFO would be the orthotic of choice. However, importing expensive plastic and plastic forming equipment is beyond the resources of most organizations in countries that have poor foreign exchange reserves. This problem has been overcome by the use of inexpensive soft plastic buckets now available in the market. The availability of these buckets has made it possible to fabricate a plastic AFO which can be molded with a heat gun over a plaster of paris mold of a childs' foot. The result is a plastic ankle-foot orthosis that is nearly equal in strength and appearance to that made elsewhere. The orthosis is especially effective for hemiplegic cerebral palsied children after serial casting. It maintains the range of motion achieved through this intervention better than any other methods.

SUMMARY: In spite of the many socio-economic problems affecting the burgeoning populations of the least developed countries, ingenious new technologies are emerging to meet the needs of the disabled population. Inventions like the Jaipur foot have demonstrated that a developing country can draw upon its own resources and skills to make appliances that can revolutionize the lives of their indigent people.

It is a delight to see farmers, laborers, rickshaw pullers, and seamstresses working as though they had no disability. They are now supporting their families and raising their standard of living. Children who had handicaps that prevented their social development are now able to go to school.

Let us, therefore, continue developing these indigenous orthotic and prosthetic appliances so that the disabled of the developing world will have an opportunity to be as independent as those in the developed world.

ENDNOTES

1. Golin, Lawrence D., Physical Therapy and Physical Rehabilitation in Bangladesh; Proceedings, IX International Congress of the World Confederation for Physical Therapy: Stockholm, Sweden, May 24, 1982, pp 658-663.

2. Prof's M. Upadhaya, S.R. Chandra Sharma, Dr. S. Sharma; "Modification of the Below Knee Prosthesis of Aluminum Shank with Jaipur Foot by High Density Polyethelene Shank"; Proceedings, VI North Zone Annual Conference of Orthopedic Surgeons, Patiala Punjab, India; April 1987, p 2.

3. Sethi P.K.; Udawat, M.P.; Chandra, R. (1974): "Lower limb Prosthesis for Amputees in Rural Areas"; in Surgical Rehabilitation in Leprosy; Edited by Mode-Well, F. and Enna, C. The Williams and Wilkins Co. Baltimore.

4. "The Triumph of the Jaipur Foot"; Asiaweek, October 2, 1981, p 29.

5. Prabhakar, Girija; "The Courage of Sudha Chandran:" Readers Digest; November, 1985; pp 90-95.

6. Prof's M. Upadhaya, S.R. Chandra Sharma, Dr. S. Sharma; Ibid p 3.

7. Ibid, p 4.

8. Ibid, pp 5-8.

9. Ibid, pp 12-16.

10. Alimed Rehab and Ortho Catalogue, 1989 Edition; 297 High St., Dedham Ma., 02026 U.S.A. p 63.

11. Fess, E.E.; Gettle K.S. Dr. Strickland J.W.; "Hand Splinting, Principles and Methods:" C.V. Mosby Co., St. Louis, Mo., 1981.

who require less remuneration than professional trained prosthetists. These artisians can measure an amputee for a new limb and complete the fitting in 45 minutes.[4]

The cost of the limb is sufficiently low, that with the help of local philanthropists, the limb can be given free of cost to all applicants. Jaipur foot wearers have achieved such independence in their daily activities, that some have even been able to climb date palm trees to obtain nectar or return to classical dancing.[5]

In 1985 Jaipur prostheses were introduced at Memorial Christian Hospital in southern Bangladesh. Presently we are the only center in Bangladesh producing this prosthesis. We hope to institute amputee camps in major centers for periods up to two weeks, so that this technology can be extended to people throughout Bangladesh.

More recently, in 1987, an improvement was made in the Jaipur foot technology which made its' weight and fit even more like that of a normal limb. Master Ram Chandra Sharma, who played a significant role in developing the Jaipur foot piece in 1974,[6] tried to replace the aluminum shank with high density propylene pipe used by farmers to irrigate their fields.[7] First a plaster of paris mold of the clients stump was formed. Next, a piece of HDPE pipe was cut according to the length of the positive mold. It was covered inside and outside with a stockinette; then a wooden rod was inserted in the pipe to prevent collapse of the pipe and adherence of its wall. This pipe, along with the wooden stick, was heated in a convection electric oven at a constant temperature of 300^0 C for half an hour. This made the pipe malleable enough to sleeve over the positive mold of the stump. After cooling, the plaster of paris mold filled into this HDPE pipe was hammered out. The original Jaipur foot piece was then attached to the shank by heating the lower end of the socket.[8]

The result proved to be a great improvement over the wooden or aluminum shank; it was much lighter and had a better grip and fit over the stump. This gave greater mobility to the amputee.[9] The only drawback is that HDPE pipe may not be available in every country of the developing world. An attempt was made to form a shank from more readily available PVC pipe with no success in our limb center at Malumghat Hospital.

ORTHOTICS: During the last 20 years, various forms of polyethelene plastics have been introduced as hand splinting material in the developed world. They are lightweight and easily formed to the hand and arm with low heat devices. They can be formed and shaped into a multitude of serial, static, and dynamic applications. However, in the less developed world the cost of such materials and import restrictions prohibit their use. One sheet of low temperature splinting material 1/8"X18"X24" costs US $35.[10] This is equivalent to one months salary for many workers in our part of the world. Consequently, the local craftsmen made crude splints from scrap metal which were still costly and poor fitting.

During the past 10 years, PVC pipe has become the low cost alternative to masonry pipe in the third world. A 10 ft. length of pipe 1/8" thick, and 6 inches in diameter, may cost only the equivalent of US $5.00. It is easily malleable at low temperatures.

We have used this material extensively in all our dynamic and static hand splinting with good results. A form is molded according to the model presented in the book; "Hand Splinting Principles and Methods," by Fess, Gettle and Strickland.[11] An ordinary hot plate, heat gun, or water cooker melts the PVC pipe into a form to fit a hand that is covered by a piece of felt. Some of the results will be shown at our poster display.

PLASTIC ANKLE FOOT ORTHOSIS: In our center we see may cerebral palsy and polio-affected children. We often fit these with adaptive AFO sandal, which have fixed ankle side bars made of aluminum window framing and a solid ankle cushion heel, much like

A SURVEY OF RECREATIONAL ACTIVITIES PARTICIPATED IN BY 1,214 LOWER EXTREMITY AMPUTEES

R. Gailey, M.S.Ed, P.T.,   R. Nickels, M.T., P.T., B. Ade, M.S., P.T., S. Swain, M.S., P.T.
University of Miami, Division of Physical Therapy
5915 Ponce de Leon Blvd, 5th Floor Coral Gables, Florida 33146 USA

INTRODUCTION

Rehabilitation for lower extremity amputees involves much more than learning how to walk with a prosthesis. Yet, most programs primarily focus on ambulation skills, often neglecting higher level functional skills necessary for a more active lifestyle. Recreational activities not only provide the potential to improve physical fitness, but may also improve the individual's social interaction and self confidence, as well as enhance the total restorative process.

Typically, the descriptive literature about amputees reports information centered on age, sex, level of amputation, mortality rates, and associated diagnoses. Kegel in 1978 and 1980 published two of the most the significant papers addressing amputees' attitudes toward the prosthetic rehabilitation team ,and their degree of participation in activities of daily living as well as in recreational activities, prior to and subsequent to their amputation.

The purpose of this study was to explore four topic areas: 1) the amputee profile, 2) prosthetic management, 3) degree of participation in recreational activities, and 4) the amputee's perception of their rehabilitative needs, and suggested improvements for the prosthetic rehabilitation management team. From the information gathered, valuable insight is gained into the physical, educational and psychosocial factors that influence participation in recreational activities, which will assist the rehabilitation professional to better serve the amputee population.

METHODS

The sample was composed of randomly chosen lower extremity amputees who received a 71 item questionnaire by mail. A total of 10,000 questionnaires were mailed to amputee organizations, support groups and prosthetic facilities over a three year period of time. Reminder cards were sent out when appropriate, and the deadline for all returns was December 31, 1990. A total of 1214 questionnaires were received, and the repsonses entered into a computer database system specifically designed for the study. The database system permits the user to identify unlimited, specific fixed variables such as level of amputation or medical status, and then provides responses for that entity to a specific question. The data was then computed for total number of responses for each category, within a question. Subsequently, percentages were calculated for each of the categories.

RESULTS

A total of 1214 questionnaires were received from: 41 hip disarticulation amputees, 592 above knee amputees, 492 below knee amputees, 23 symes amputees, 43 bilateral below knee amputees, and 23 bilateral above knee amputees. Demographical data showed that 27 per cent (%) of the sample reside in the Northeast, 23% in the Midwest, 21% in the Southwest, 19% in Southeast, and 7% in the Northwest. There were 971 males and 243 females between the ages of 4 to 91 years of age. The cause of amputation included 710 traumatic, 237 vascular, 160 tumorous and 54 congenital amputees. Veterans constituted 40 %of the sample population. The number of years since the participant's last amputation was reported by 8% as less than 2 years ago, by 37% as 2-10 years ago, by 21% as 11-20 years ago, and by 32% as greater than 20 years ago. Eighty five % reported experiencing phantom limb pain. When questioned about the unaffected limb, 60% stated they had no problems, and 11% reported vascular problems. Sixty per cent of participants reported that their amputaion had no influence on sexual activity, while 23% experienced changes in sexual activity.

Change of occupation after amputation occured in 26% of participants, no change occured in 28%, 27% retired, and 11% reported being unable to work due to amputation (figure 1). Prior to amputation, 23% of the respondents said they worked zero hours per week, 8% worked 1-39 hours, 35% worked 40 hours, and 27% worked > 40 hours. After amputation, 28% worked zero hours per week, 10% worked 1-39 hours, 33% worked 40 hours, and 22% worked > 40 hours (figure 2). Percentage of time standing at work prior to amputation was reported as 0 % by 267, 1-50% by 362, 51-100% by 499. Percentage of time standing at work since amputation was stated to be 0% by 355, 1-50% by 540, and 51-100% by 218 (figure 3). The reason for decreasing standing time at work after amputation was reportedly due to pain in 23% of participants, due to fatigue in 21%, and as a result of altered mobility in 12%.

EMPLOYMENT STATUS SINCE AMPUTATION

n=1,214	%	
NO ANSWER	5%	63
OTHER	7%	84
SAME OCCUPATION	28%	337
RETIRED	27%	328
CHANGED OCCUPATION	26%	311
UNABLE DUE TO AMPUTATION	11%	136
FULL-TIME STUDENT	4%	53
TOTAL	108%	1312

FIG. 1

HOURS WORKED PER WEEK BEFORE* AND AFTER** AMPUTATION

n=1,214	%	*	%	**
NO ANSWER	6%	77	7%	89
ZERO HOURS	23%	276	28%	342
1-8 HOURS	2%	23	1%	18
9-24 HOURS	3%	41	5%	57
25-39 HOURS	3%	34	4%	52
40 HOURS	35%	422	33%	401
41-50 HOURS	16%	197	14%	168
51- 60 HOURS	8%	102	6%	67
> 60 HOURS	3%	42	2%	20
TOTAL	100%	1214	36%	431

FIG. 2

The prosthesis is worn 0-9 hours per day by 19% of the amputees, 10-15 hours a day by 47%, and greater than 16 hours by 34% (figure 4). Reasons for limitation in wearing time include: skin irritation, 26%; fatigue, 24%; perspiration, 20%;prosthetic fit ,14%; soft tissue pain, 13%; and bone pain, 10%. Skin breakdown occured during daily activities 0-10% of the time in 893 persons, 11-50% of the time in 213 persons, and 51-100% of the time in 100 persons. Whereas, in strenuous activity, skin breakdown occured 0-10% of the time in 503 persons, 11-50% of the time in 245 persons, and 51-100% of the time in 205 persons (figure 5).

PERCENT OF DAY STANDING OR WALKING DURING EMPLOYMENT BEFORE* AND AFTER** AMPUTATION

n=1,214	%	*	%	**
NO ANSWER	7%	86	8%	101
ZERO %	22%	267	29%	355
1-10%	6%	76	11%	134
11-25%	7%	85	13%	155
26-50%	17%	201	21%	251
51-75%	10%	124	6%	74
76-90%	13%	158	6%	78
91-100%	18%	217	5%	66
TOTAL	100%	1214	100%	1214

FIG. 3

HOURS WEARING PROSTHESIS PER DAY

n=1,214	% ALL	ALL
NO ANSWER	0%	1
0 HOURS	6%	71
1-3 HOURS	3%	32
4-6 HOURS	3%	39
7-9 HOURS	7%	85
10-12 HOURS	22%	266
13-15 HOURS	25%	302
16-18 HOURS	33%	402
19 OR MORE	1%	16
TOTAL	100%	1214

FIG. 4

The type of assistive device used by the amputee includes: none by 55%, one cane by 20%, two crutches by 15%, walker by 5%, and wheelchair by 11%. The percentage of time using an assistive device involves 826 persons using a device 0-10% of the time, 95 using a device 11-50% of the time, and 188 using a device 51-100% of the time. Activities of daily living found difficult to do with a prosthesis include: running by 64%, jumping by 53%, squatting by 52%, kneeling by 42%, stair climbing by 35%, twisting by 21%, walking by 18%, sitting by 13%, and standing by 10% (figure 6).

PERCENT OF TIME EXPERIENCING SKIN BREAKDOWN OR IRRITATION DURING DAILY* AND STRENUOUS** ACTIVITIES WITH PRESENT SOCKET

n=1,214	%	*	%	**
NO ANSWER	1%	8	1%	11
0-%	38%	464	34%	413
1-10%	35%	429	24%	290
11-25%	10%	120	12%	143
26-50%	8%	93	13%	152
51-75%	2%	28	5%	64
76-90%	3%	34	5%	62
91-100%	3%	38	7%	79
TOTAL	100%	1214	100%	1214

FIG. 5

ACTIVITIES MADE DIFFICULT DUE TO PROSTHESIS

n=1,214	% ALL	ALL
NO ANSWER	7%	88
OTHER	0%	2
RUNNING	64%	781
JUMPING	53%	640
SQUATTING	52%	637
KNEELING	42%	513
STAIR CLIMBING	35%	423
TWISTING	21%	259
WALKING	18%	220
SITTING	13%	152
STANDING	10%	122
NOT APPLICABLE	8%	100
ALL	5%	58
TOTAL	329%	3995

FIG. 6

The five most frequently occuring recreational activities after amputation are: swimming, golf, fishing, walking, and dancing. The five most popular recreational activities cited prior to amputation include: swimming, dancing, bicycling, running and baseball. Running, baseball, football, basketball , and softball were the most frequently cited sports in which amputees were unable to participate (figure 7).

648

COMPARISON OF RECREATIONAL ACTIVITY PARTICIPATION

COLUMN 1			COLUMN 2			COLUMN 3			*COLUMN 4	
SWIMMING	51%	615	SWIMMING	40%	486	RUNNING	35%	425	SWIMMING	70.5
GOLF	48%	583	GOLF	25%	301	BASEBALL	24%	287	GOLF	23.2
FISHING	44%	537	FISHING	30%	360	FOOTBALL	23%	276	FISHING	46.5
WALKING	37%	450	WALKING	30%	367	BASKETBALL	22%	263	WALKING	66.6
DANCING	36%	441	DANCING	36%	437	SOFTBALL	19%	227	BICYCLING	56.9
BOATING	33%	401	BOATING	22%	273	BICYCLING	17%	207	MOTOR BOATING	29
BICYCLING	27%	331	BICYCLING	34%	414	TENNIS	16%	193	CAMPING	46.5
BOWLING	26%	313	BOWLING	31%	378	HIKING	15%	178	BOWLING	40.8
HUNTING	18%	223	RUNNING	32%	389	DANCING	13%	155	EXERCISE/EQUIP.	31.5
SNOW SKIING	14%	173	BASEBALL	32%	387	WATERSKIING	12%	151	BILLARDS	29.6
VOLLEYBALL	14%	166	SOFTBALL	27%	323	BOWLING	12%	146	VOLLEYBALL	25.1
HIKING	13%	161	HIKING	21%	256	VOLLEYBALL	12%	143	HIKING	23.5
HORSEBACK RIDING	13%	161	FOOTBALL	25%	309	WALKING	12%	142	AEROBIC EXERCISE	25.1
BASKETBALL	13%	154	BASKETBALL	30%	363	SOCCER	11%	131	BASKETBALL	26.2
RUNNING	5%	64	TENNIS	20%	239	HANDBALL	10%	121	RUNNING	24.8

COLUMN 1: ACTIVITIES CURRENTLY PARTICIPATED IN BY AMPUTEES; COLUMN 2: ACTIVITIES PARTICIPATED IN PRIOR TO
AMPUTATION; COLUMN 3: ACTIVITIES NOT ABLE TO PARTICIPATE IN DUE TO AMPUTATION; n=1214;
COLUMN 4: ABLE-BODIED ACTIVITIES PARTICIPATED IN BY MILLIONS.
*NATIONAL SPORTING GOODS ASSOCIATION BY THE NPD GROUP, INC., 1989.

FIG. 7

Regarding recreational activities, the amputees felt that their physical therapist was extremely informative 6% of the time, somewhat informative 14% of the time, uninformative 24% of the time. Forty two % answered not applicable. The prosthetist was said to be extremely informative 15% of the time, somewhat informative 32% of the time, uninformative 31% of the time. Thirteen % answered not applicable. The doctor was reported as extremely informative 6% of the time, somewhat informative 19%, uninformative 51% of the time. Sixteen % answered not applicable (figure 8). The most common suggestions for prosthetic modifications include: increased comfort 52%, decreased weight 43%, better foot mobility 39%, waterproofing 35%, and improved ventilation 33%. Most frequent requests to improve functional activity include: better prostheses (59%), amputee instructors (39%), "how to" literature (29%), organized sports (26%), and activity analysis research (20%).

DEGREE OF DOCTOR'S (MD), PROSTHETIST'S (PROS), AND
PHYSICAL THERAPIST'S (PT) INFORMATION CONCERNING
RECREATIONAL ACTIVITY

n=1,214	%	MD	%	PROS	%	PT
NO ANSWER	8%	99	9%	104	14%	165
UNINFORMATIVE	51%	623	31%	371	24%	289
SOMEWHAT	19%	226	32%	394	14%	172
EXTREMELY INFORMATIVE	6%	72	15%	182	6%	77
NOT APPLICABLE	16%	194	13%	163	42%	511
TOTAL RESPONSES	76%	921	100%	1214	58%	703

FIG. 8

DISCUSSION

Some of the most notable features of the survey results are the fact that the number of hours worked prior to, and after amputation are virtually unchanged. However, amputees stand and walk during working hours far less than prior to their amputation. Change of occupation occured in over one quarter of the population.

Not surprisingly, skin breakdown was far more prevolent during strenuous activity, than during activities of daily living. Some of the relatively strenuous activities of daily living are difficult for the amputee as seen in the survey results. As a result of amputation, amputees tend to participate in recreational activities which are less physically demanding, cause less impact on the residual limb, or do not require a prosthesis. However, when compared to the able-bodied population, there is little diffference in the most popular recreational activities.

Generally speaking , the amputee's perception of the rehabilitation team's knowledge regarding recreational activities suggests that either health professionals do not possess this knowledge, or that they are not adequately relaying this information to the amputee population. This survey provides insight into the needs and concerns of the amputee, which if attended to will facilitate a more complete rehabilitation for the amputee.

REFERENCES

1. Kegel B, Carpenter ML, Burgess EM (1978) Functional capabilities of lower extremity amputees. Arch Phys Med Rehabil 59:109-120

2. Kegel B, Webster JC, Burgess EM (1980) Recreational activities of lower extremity amputees: a survey. Arch Phys Med Rehabil 61:258-263

ENERGY EXPENDITURE OF BELOW-KNEE AMPUTEES DURING UNRESTRAINED AMBULATION

R. Gailey, MS Ed, PT, K. Erbs, MS, PT, M. Raya, MS, PT,
N. Kirk, MS, PT, M.A. Wenger, MS, PT, P. Spyropoulos, PhD, PT
University of Miami, Division of Physical Therapy, Coral Gables, Florida 33146 USA

INTRODUCTION

According to the National Center for Health Statistics, 161,425 below-knee amputations were performed in the United States from 1986-1988. Research repeatedly substantiates that below-knee amputees (BKA) expend significantly more energy than able-bodied individuals during normal ambulation.

However, these studies tended to employ non-representative samples of the total population, required designated walking velocities, did not consider whether the amputation was of a traumatic or vascular origin, and reported data only for gross levels of amputation. Collectively, these studies reported a wide range of 9-65% increase in energy expenditure over that of able-bodied ambulators. [2,3,4,5]

Currently, all studies save one have reported energy expenditure for BKAs without reference to stump length. Gonzalez (1976) considered level of amputation, and reported a statistically significant negative correlation between stump length and energy expenditure during ambulation in BKA subjects. However, this study grossly grouped levels of amputation into two categories of short and long, based on percentage of body height. [2]

Two previous studies imposed specific walking velocities on the subjects during ambulation. [2,4] Other research designs allowed individuals to use their comfortable walking speeds which varied from 1.99-3.00 mph. [3,5,6] Pagliarulo (1979) reported similar energy cost values for slow and fast velocity trials, which were approximately 13% higher than those observed during free walking. [5] Ganguli (1974), concluded that subjects use more energy when walking slower than their comfortable walking speed than when permitted to walk at their most comfortable pace. [4] It has been demonstrated, then, that individuals will expend the least amount of energy during unrestrained walking. Based on previous findings, this study design asked subjects to ambulate at their most comfortable walking speed.

In comparing vascular BKAs to traumatic BKAs, Waters et al reported that vascular amputees exhibited a 36% decrease in walking speed and a 30% increase in energy expenditure. [6] Pagliarulo et al also concluded that the amputee who has a vascular disease has a relatively higher physiological cost of walking. [5] Other studies did not consider this variable when assembling a sample group. This research design required that all subjects be non-vascular amputees.

The purpose of this study was to compare energy expenditure and speed of ambulation in BKAs to that of non-amputee ambulators, as well as to correlate percentage of residual limb length, and weight of prosthesis to energy expenditure in BKAs at their comfortable walking speeds. It was hypothesized that there is a correlation between residual limb length and energy expenditure, as well as between weight of the prosthesis and energy expenditure during unrestrained ambulation. It was also hypothesized that there is a difference in energy expenditure and in speed of ambulation between the experimental group of BKAs and the control group of non-amputee individuals.

METHODOLOGY

SUBJECTS: Thirty-nine healthy, male, BKAs between the ages of 22 and 75 ($\bar{x}$ = 47, +/- 16) who had been using a prosthesis for more than six months, and were independent of any assistive device volunteered to participate in this study. All amputations were performed due to non-vascular reasons (trauma, congenital, or tumor) with the residual limb free from skin breakdown, swelling, or restrictive pain. A control group of twenty-one healthy, male able-bodied ambulators, ranging in age from 24-47 ($\bar{x}$ = 31, +/-6), also agreed to participate in this investigation. All subjects were instructed in the procedure of the study and were asked not to eat or smoke for at least one hour prior to testing. A written statement of informed consent was obtained from each subject prior to their participation.

PROCEDURE: Each subject was instructed to ambulate at his most comfortable walking speed around a 118-foot L-shaped track. Heart rate (bpm) and oxygen consumption (ml O_2/kg/min) were monitored for one minute prior to ambulation to establish a non-exercise baseline, during eight minutes of ambulation, and for one minute after ambulation to record recovery. Speed of ambulation was determined according to distance traveled divided by the total time of ambulation. In addition, for all subjects in the amputee group, the prosthesis was weighed and both the residual limb length and the uninvolved limb length (distance from the medial tibial plateau to the distal end of the tibia) were documented using a measuring tape.

INSTRUMENTATION: Heart rate data were collected and recorded every 15 seconds using the Vantage Performance Monitor. Oxygen (VO2) consumption data was collected during ambulation by means of a rubber mouthpiece connected to a Hans-Rudolph non-rebreathing valve attached to a flexible tube connected to the breath port on the MMC Horizon metabolic cart.(b) The collected gas samples were analyzed for oxygen consumption and percent carbon dioxide according to standard values for weight, age, and sex. Collected values for VO2 (ml O_2/kg/min) and heart rate (bpm) during the sixth minute of testing were analyzed and used to represent each individual's ambulatory steady state.

STATISTICAL ANALYSIS: Means and standard deviations of speed, VO2, and HR before and during ambulation were calculated for both the BKA and the control group. In addition, means and standard deviations were calculated for VO2 and HR of BKA subjects wearing energy-storing or non-energy-storing feet. Pearson r correlation coefficients were calculated between the VO2, speed, HR, residual limb length, percent of residual limb length, resting VO2, and weight of the prosthesis. (Table 2)

RESULTS

Descriptive statistics for heart rate (HR), oxygen consumption (VO2), and walking speed for both the BKA group and the control group are shown in Table 1. In the BKA group, the mean HR was 102.5 $\pm$10.1 beats per minute (BPM), the mean steady state VO2 was 12.9 $\pm$2.3 ml O_2/kg/min, and the mean speed was 2.5 $\pm$0.3 mph. In the control group, the mean HR was 86.5 $\pm$14.1 BPM, the mean VO2 was 10.9 $\pm$3.0 ml O_2/kg/min, and the mean speed was 2.8 $\pm$0.5 mph. The mean HR and VO2 of the BKA group was 18% higher, and the mean BKA group walking speed was 10% slower than that of the control group.

Pearson r-values for each set of parameters in the BKA group are given in Table 2. None of the r-values show a significant correlation between any two parameters.

The mean VO2 value for BKA subjects wearing energy-storing feet was 12.6 $\pm$2.1, and the value for those wearing non-energy-storing feet was 13.1 $\pm$2.5. The mean resting VO2 of the BKA group was 4.5 $\pm$1.4, and that of the control group was 4.6 $\pm$1.5.

TABLE 1: MEANS AND STANDARD DEVIATIONS OF HR, VO$_2$, AND SPEED FOR BKA SAMPLE AND CONTROL GROUPS

	$\bar{X}$ HR (BPM)	$\bar{X}$ VO$_2$ (ml/O_2/kg/min)	$\bar{X}$ SPEED
CONTROLS	86.5±10.1	10.9±3.0	2.8±0.5
BKA SUBJECTS	102.5±10.1	12.9±2.3	2.5±0.3

TABLE 2: PEARSON R CORRELATION COEFFICIENT MATRIX FOR VARIABLES IN THE BKA SAMPLE

	VO$_2$/KG	SPEED	HR	RESID LIMB	% RESIDUAL	RESTINGVO$_2$	WEIGHT
VO$_2$/KG	1						
SPEED	.338	1					
HR	.171	-.445	1				
RESID LIMB	-.322	-.004	-.055	1			
% RESIDUAL	-.287	.049	-.106	.96	1		
RESTINGVO$_2$	.37	-.038	.108	-.084	-.071	1	
WEIGHT	.098	.253	-.128	.164	.179	-.224	1

DISCUSSION

The results of this study appear to be consistent with prior authors with respect to energy expenditure during unrestrained ambulation. BKA's tested in this study walked 10% slower than the control group, and showed an 18% increase in heart rate and oxygen uptake. If comfortable walking speed is considered to be the most energy efficient speed, then BKA patients should be encouraged to assume comfortable walking speeds that are comparable to what is considered normal walking velocity.

Another purpose of this study was to determine which parameters of the BKA population correlate with energy expenditure, and speed of ambulation. Commonly discussed parameters include length of residual limb and weight of prosthesis, neither of which correlated with either walking velocity or oxygen uptake in the BKA population. In addition, BKA's with energy storing feet or non-energy storing feet were examined with respect to oxygen uptake. Energy storing feet included the Flex-foot, Carbon-copy II, Quantum, and the Seattle foot (n=21), and non energy storing feet included the SACH foot, Greissenger foot, and Multiflex foot (n=18).[8] Oxygen uptake in subjects with energy-storing feet was only 4% lower than in subjects with non-energy storing feet. Additionally, the results of this study suggest that residual limb length and prosthetic weight have minimal effect on oxygen uptake during unrestrained ambulation.

REFERENCES

1. U.S. Department of Health & Human Services (1989) Vital and Health Statistics: Detailed Diagnoses and Procedures. National Hospital Discharge Survey Series 13, No. 100:196

2. Gonzalez EG, Corcoran PJ, Reyes RL (1974) Energy expenditure in below-knee amputees: Correlation with stump length. Arch Phys Med Rehabil 55:111-119

3. Huang CT, Jackson JR, Moore NB, et al (1979) Amputation: Energy cost of ambulation. Arch Phys Med Rehabil 60:18-24

4. Ganguli S, Datta SR, Chatterjee BB (1974) Metabolic cost of walking at different speeds with patellar tendon bearing prosthesis. J of Appl Physiol 36:440-443

5. Pagliarulo MA, Waters R, Hislop HJ (1979) Energy cost of walking of below-knee amputees having no vascular disease. Phys Ther 59:538-542

6. Waters RL, Perry J, Antonelli EE, et al (1976) Energy cost of walking of amputees: The influence of level of amputation. J Bone Joint Surg 58-A:42-46

7. Fisher SV, Gullickson G (1978) Energy cost of ambulation in health and disability: A literature review. Arch Phys Med Rehabil 59:121-132

8. Torburn L, Perry J, Ayyappa E, Shanfield SL (1990) Below-knee amputee gait with dynamic elastic response prosthetic feet: A pilot study. J Rehab Res and Develop 27(4):369-84

THE ROEHAMPTON APPROACH TO AMPUTEE REHABILITATION: A RETROSPECTIVE SURVEY OF PROSTHETIC
USE IN PRIMARY UNILATERAL LOWER LIMB AMPUTEES

P.J. Buttenshaw   J.E. Dolman
Physiotherapy Department, Roehampton Disablement Services Centre, Roehampton Lane,
London   SW15 5PR

This talk is divided into two parts; the first part is a brief explanation of the treatment regime for lower limb amputees at Queen Mary's University Hospital,
Roehampton, London.

The second part is a statistical analysis from a retrospective survey of
prosthetic use in primary unilateral amputees.

At Queen Mary's University Hospital a ward specifically designed for
amputees was built in 1974. This is a twelve bedded unit situated
adjacent to the limb fitting service at the Roehampton Disablement Service
Centre. The patient can be admitted and assessed pre operatively by all
members of the multidisciplinary team.

This team includes the surgeon, consultant in rehabilitation, prosthetist,
physiotherapist, occupational therapist, nursing staff, social worker
and counsellor.[1]

At most district general hospitals in England and Wales the prosthetist
and counsellor are not members of the multidisciplinary team.[2]

At this stage the rehabilitation programme is explained to the patient
and short term realistic goals are set. The relatives or carers must be
included at this early stage and involved throughout the amputees'
rehabilitation.[3]

Post operatively the patient is treated for the first three days on the
ward. After the drain is removed, the patient will continue physio
therapy in the main physiotherapy department, physiotherapy is only one
component of the patient's day programme of rehabilitation. A temporary
walking aid is used as an assessment tool and part of treatment
commencing between the 6th and 10th day post operatively.

If the patient is assessed to be a prosthetic user then measurement for a
prosthesis will take place at the appropriate time.

The prosthetic stage begins when the artificial limb is fitted by the
prosthetist. Gait training begins immediately.[4,5]

As the patient progresses, the prosthetist is able to monitor the fitting
of the prosthesis.[6]

Home visits for the amputee are arranged.
An early home visit immediately post-operatively ascertains major social problems. Before a patient is discharged a further visit must be accomplished to ensure the patient is managing with the hardware prescribed. Work visits and training using transport systems are necessary as well as coping with their local environment.[7,8]

Advice about hobbies and sporting activities should be included.[9]

A retrospective survey was carried out to include all patients admitted to the Limb Surgery Unit, Queen Mary's University Hospital who required unilateral amputation at a below or above knee level as a result of peripheral vascular disease.

Over a period of eighteen months, 32 patients were eligible for the survey.

Areas examined took into account age and sex of the patient, and looked into mobility and social service support at various stages of rehabilitation. I.e: pre operatively, at discharge and at follow up at six months.

REFERENCES

1. Engstrom B., Van de Ven C. 1985 Physiotherapy for Amputees: The Roehampton Approach. Ch.I. Published by Churchill Livingstone.

2. Bradway, J.K., Malone J.M., Racy, J., Poole, I. Psychological adaptation to amputation, an overview. 1984 Orthotics & Prosthetics Vol 38: (3) p45 50.

3. Ham R., Van de Ven C., 1986. The Management of the Lower Limb Amputee in England and Wales today. Physiotherapy Practice Vol 2 : 2.

4. Redhead R. G., Snowdon C. 1978. A New Approach to the Management of Wounds of the Extremities. Controlled environment treatment and its derivatives. Prosthetics & Orthotics International 2 : 148 156

5. Lein S., 1991. How are Physiotherapists Using the Pneumatic Post Amputation Mobility Aid?

6. Engstrom B., Van de Ven C., 1985. Physiotherapy for Amputees: The Roehampton Approach. Ch 14. Published by Churchill Livingstone.

7. Bolton P. Edited by banerjee S. N. 1982. Rehabilitation Management of Amputees. P.336 349. Published by Williams & Wilkings.

8. Van de Ven C., Edited by Downie P.A. 1990. Cash's Textbook of General medical and Surgical conditions for physiotherapists, 2nd Edition. Ch 17. Published by Faber and Faber.

9. Ellis P.M. Mensch G. 1987. Physical Therapy Management of Lower Extremity Amputations. Ch.4 Published by Heinemann Physiotherapy, London.

ANALYSIS OF ABOVE KNEE AMPUTEE RUNNING GAIT

R. Gailey, MS Ed, PT, J. Moore, MS, PT, D. Giaquinto, MS, PT,
D. Stinson, MS, PT, G. Hartley, MS, PT
University of Miami, Division of Physical Therapy, Coral Gables, Florida 33146 USA

INTRODUCTION

Studies have examined the kinematics of normal running gait. [1,2,3] Descriptions of "normal" running gait are usually categorized into three phases: stance phase, swing phase, and float phase. Due to an absence of descriptive/quantitative data regarding AKA running kinetics, this study proposes to examine and quantify AKA running gait through the use of two dimensional video gait analysis. Results will be reported and compared to a running gait model determined by the authors upon review of several established studies of gait analysis. [4,5]

METHODS

SAMPLE: Five healthy AKA males and one female volunteers with an age range of 17-40 years participated in this study. All amputations occurred at least five years prior to the time of data collection and were all a result of trauma or tumor. Residual limb length greater than or equal to five inches, and absence of skin irritation and breakdown were also criteria for participation in this study. Five subjects had Contoured Adducted Trochanteric-Controlled Alignment Mechanism (CAT-CAM) socket and the other subject had a quadrilateral socket. Other prosthetic components (i.e. knee, ankle and foot) varied with each amputee; 3 Mauch knees, 1 Endolite pneumatic knee, 3 Single axis Mach V knees, 3 Bouncy knees, 2 Seattle Lite feet, 1 Endolite foot, 3 Flex feet, 3 Endolite Multi-flex ankles.

PROCEDURE: Data was collected through a 60 Hertz NEC TI-23A CCD camera using a Cosmicar 8 millimeter lens. Films were then reviewed using a Panasonic AG 6300 video cassette recorder. Data from the films were digitized using a Motion Analysis MP 280, 386 and VP 110 computer system. Using the stick figure program available in Flex Trac software, phases of gait were determined. The computer generated joint angles, time, and distance for each frame identified as a phase of gait.

Reflective markers were placed on the subjects using the iliac crest, the greater trocanter, lateral knee joint, the lateral malleolus, the calcaneus, and the metatarsal breaks.

Video data was collected for the left and right sagittal views. Subjects were asked to run a distance of 30 feet on a
flat, carpeted surface, ten times for each of the two views.

DATA ANALYSIS: The software designed specifically for this study provided information on the sagittal view regarding hip, knee, and ankle joint angles, stance time and stride length. By referring to the phases of gait described by Slocum and James (running), the Rancho Los Amigos Medical Center (walking), and reviewing animated stick figure diagrams of each trial, the authors determined six different phases of running gait. The phases are described as follows:

1. Initial Contact (IC):   initial contact with the ground (foot strike)
2. Midstance (MSt):   foot is flat, before heel off (mid-support)
3. Take-off (TOFF):   before toes leave the ground
4. Initial Swing (ISw):   when the femur begins to swing forward (follow through)
5. Mid-swing (MSw):   maximum hip flexion (forward swing)
6. Terminal Swing (TSw):   full knee extension (foot descent)

Raw data was collected from six subjects for five trials each of their prosthetic and sound limbs. Frame by frame stick figure analysis yielded joint angles for the hip, knee, and ankle during the six phases of running gait previously identified.

Stride length and stance times were computed for each trial. Stride length was computed using the distance values taken from one IC to the next IC of the same leg. Stance phase was computed as a percentage of the gait cycle (IC to IC of the same leg). Velocity was computed using time values from IC to IC.

Further analysis of the group was performed producing means and standard deviations of stride length, stance time, velocity and joint angles at hip, knee, and ankle for each six gait phases for both limbs.

RESULTS

Table 1. summarizes mean and standard deviation statistics for both prosthetic and sound limb joint angles of the hip, knee and ankle. Means of the stride lengths of the prosthetic limb versus the sound limb are essentially identical. The mean value for the prosthetic limb was 198.5 cm (s = 41.45), and the sound limb mean was 197.39 cm (s = 41.73). Stance phase was described as a percent of the total gait cycle and reported values of 34.5% (s = 6.05%) and 31.4% (s = 4.77%) for the prosthetic and sound limb respectively. The remaining 65.5-68% is the swing or float phase. Mean velocity was recorded as 176.94 m/min (s = 39.75).

TABLE 1: ABOVE-KNEE AMPUTEE RUNNING DATA

JOINT	INITIAL CONTACT		MID-STANCE		TAKE-OFF	
	PROSTHETIC	SOUND	PROSTHETIC	SOUND	PROSTHETIC	SOUND
HIP	20.72 ± 7.60	28.13 ± 9.08	18.49 ± 6.23	27.00±11.33	-2.03 ± 7.14	-8.49 ± 1.85
KNEE	.34 ±5.81	21.43 ± 6.70	.61 ± 8.37	40.32± 8.16	24.94 ± 13.39	21.09 ± 6.79
ANKLE	4.12 ± 7.58	6.88 ± 7.23	-.73 ±3.82	12.14± 7.03	3.92 ± 5.99	-5.51 ±16.57

JOINT	INITIAL CONTACT		MID-STANCE		TAKE-OFF	
	PROSTHETIC	SOUND	PROSTHETIC	SOUND	PROSTHETIC	SOUND
HIP	3.24±10.26	-3.67± 8.47	27.64±13.07	20.77± 7.75	24.62 ±8.91	24.28±11.22
KNEE	54.46±16.32	35.30±10.95	98.51±11.34	72.26±18.92	-.13 6±6.30	14.26± 6.25
ANKLE	6.12± 6.10	-19.87±23.00	6.72± 7.21	.10±10.19	2.15 ±3.91	8.27 ±13.70

DISCUSSION

The authors found that prosthetic hip joint angles differed from sound hip joint angles in that there was less flexion of the prosthetic hip during initial contact and midstance. During take-off, midswing and terminal swing, the prosthetic hip displays more flexion than the sound hip.

The prosthetic knee was in full extension at initial contact, whereas the sound limb demonstrated knee flexion for shock absorption. If the prosthetic knee were allowed to flex significantly, collapse of the knee would occur due to a lack of eccentric quadriceps control. At take-off, the prosthetic knee was seen to passively flex, whereas the sound knee moves toward extension. An explanation for knee flexion is again due to lack of muscle control. The vertical displacement normally seen at take-off is created by control of the quadriceps and plantarflexors and as expected, is seen only on the sound side.

Excessive heel rise in the prosthetic limb occurs in the beginning of the swing phase. Factors contributing to this event include momentum, lack of muscular control of the prosthetic limb, and current cadence control devices. Cadence control devices currently on the market are not specifically designed for various running speeds.

Both ankles displayed approximately five degrees of dorsiflexion at initial contact which was in agreement with normal values found in the literature. At take-off, the sound ankle began to plantarflex and the prosthetic ankle increased its dorsiflexion. The suggested reason for the increase in dorsiflexion is that the prosthetic knee flexes forward over the foot, the ankle is passively dorsiflexed.

Stride length and stance phases are basically in agreement between prosthetic and sound limbs. Stance phase values found in this study were comparable with Mann's findings of thirty-one percent in normal runners.

Each runner self-selected a comfortable pace. Velocities of the runners in this study are in a range considered to be normal.

REFERENCES

1. Cavanaugh PR (1987) The biomechanics of the lower extremity action in distance running. Foot and Ankle 7:197-217

2. Mann RA (1982) Biomechanics of running. AAOS Symposium of the Foot and Leg in Running Sports 30-40

3. Vaughan CL (1984) Biomechanics of running gait. Critical Reviews in Biomedical Engineering 12(1):1-48

4. Slocum DB, James SL (1968) Biomechanics of running. JAMA 205(11):97-104

5. Rancho Los Amigos Medical Center (1989) Normal gait summary. Physical Therapy Department

PATTERNS OF RECOVERY FOR LOWER LIMB AMPUTATION IN THE UK

R. O. Ham, *C. Van de Ven, J. de Trafford
King's College School of Medicine and Dentistry, Dulwich
Hospital SE22. *Queen Mary's Hospital, Roehampton SW15

Introduction

A study has been carried out to evaluate the recovery patterns
in patients with residual hemiplegia after stroke (Partridge et
al. 1987). Functional activities of the patients were recorded
at referral and at weeks 1, 2, 4, 6 and 8. The results
obtained suggested that recovery follows a predictable pattern
producing useful baseline data for comparing scores, the
setting of goals and the examination of factors that influence
recovery. A similar study has now been carried out looking at
patients following lower limb amputation.

Method

Initially a group of specialist physiotherapists identified
suitable functional activities which were regarded as
rehabilitation "landmarks". A form was designed using these 9
activities over a 10-week period. A pilot study was then
carried out by a number of therapists with 37 patients.

Following the pilot study, the form was amended slightly and
all physiotherapists in the UK that treat amputees post-
operatively were contacted through their District or Area
Physiotherapist for their co-operation in the study. Over the
12-month period 1987-88, physiotherapists were asked to
complete these activity charts over a 12-week period. The
activities included; moving about the bed, lying to sitting,
sitting balance, transfers, dressings, use of an early mobility
and the use of a prosthesis.

Results

Four hundred and fifty nine completed forms were received of
which 391 were suitable for analysis (85%). It has been
estimated that there are approximately 10,000 amputations
performed annually in the UK (Dormandy & Thomas 1988) so the
return number responds to <1% of the estimated UK total.

The major medical reason for amputation was as expected, vascular disease and diabetes but the transtibial or below-knee level of amputation was higher than recent national figures (Ham et al. 1989). This perhaps reflects the fact that interested centres with good practice were carrying out the study.

The mean age of the group was 69.5 years and the male:female ratio was 2:1.

Returns were received from 13 of the 14 health regions in England and the mean number of returns was 22 (SD18). One health region returned 90 forms and perhaps reflects the good network of communication that the therapists in South West Thames Region have.

Basic functional activities such as; moving about the bed, lying to sitting, and sitting balance were achieved by most patients by week 2 post-operatively (87%). Transferring and dressing the upper part of the body took 3 to 4 weeks (76%). Dressing the lower half of the body was generally achieved in weeks 3 to 5 (65%). The use of an early walking aid (EWA) was started by some in the 2nd week (27%) but used by more by week 4 (43%). Ten percent were not allowed to use an EWA.

Prosthetic activities were achieved by only about $1/_3$ of the group and in weeks 6 onwards, milestones. Almost 40% were discharged or transferred before prosthetic rehabilitation was achieved and these patients were not monitored for the full 12 weeks.

Conclusion

The return numbers for the length of time of the study were poor and this perhaps reflects the lack of interest in treating this group of patients and in data collection and audit by physiotherapists at this time. The numbers are however large enough to give conclusive recovery patterns for this group which provides useful baseline data for rehabilitation for comparing scores, the setting of goals and the examination of factors that influence recovery.

References

Partridge C J, Johnson M, Edwards S (1987) Recovery from physical disability after stroke: normal patterns as a basis for evaluation. Lancet February 14th 373-375.

Dormancy J A, Thomas P R S (1988) What is the natural history of a critical ischaemic patient with and without his leg? In: Limb salvage and amputation for vascular disease ed. Greenhalgh R M, Jamieson C W, Nicolaides A N. W.B. Saunders Co.

Ham R O, Luff R, Roberts V C (1989) A 5-year review of referrals for prosthetic treatment in England, Wales and Northern Ireland. 1981-1985. Health Trends 21: 3-6.

INSTRUMENT TO EVALUATE THE FACTORS RELATED TO LOWER EXTREMITY AMPUTEES'
PROSTHETIC USE

C. Gauthier-Gagnon & M.-C. Grisé
Ecole de réadaptation, Université de Montréal, C.P. 6128, succursale A,
Montréal (Québec) H3C 3J7

The purpose of this study was to develop and validate a
questionnaire (mail and telephone versions) to evaluate the
frequency and extent of prosthetic use of Quebec's (Canada)
lower limb amputees (LLA) and identify the factors related to
prosthetic use.

The already existing instruments used to assess the locomotor
functional capabilities of LLA have proven to be inappropriate
to evaluate this problem. Some are non-specific to the
amputee population, they have been designed for a neurological
population.[1,2] Others, including the step-counter and the
activity score, evaluate prosthetic use but do not investigate
the factors related to it.[3,4] The already existing
questionnaires used with LLA give some superficial information
on factors related to prosthetic use but present
methodological limitations thus giving rise to important
biases.[5,6]

The present questionnaire was developed in three phases: the
planning, construction and validation phases.[7] The planning
phase consisted mainly in identifying the factors potentially
related to prosthetic use. Using the PRECEDE (Predisposing,
Reinforcant and Enabling causes in Educational Diagnosis and
Evaluation)[8] theoretical model, the factors considered most
likely to influence prosthetic use were identified and
classified in order of priority by a multidisciplinary group
of health professionals (n=13) from different medical centers
in Montreal, using the verbal brainstorming and the nominal
group techniques. A group of LLA (n=8) were also interviewed.
The factors identified include predisposing factors (level of
amputation, physical condition ...), facilitating factors
(physical capacities, physical environment ...) and
reinforcing factors (social environment, satisfaction with the
prosthesis ...).

Construction: the operationalization, format, measurement and
sequence of the questions in the questionnaire follow the
recommendations of Dillman and Sudman.[9,10] The questionnaire
contains 39 close-ended questions based on the predetermined
factors. The different measurement scales are primarily
qualitative and include nominal scales with dichotomous or

multiple choice answers, ordinal and ordinal additive scales and a few quantitative ratio scales of measurement. It can be filled out in 25 minutes. The mail and telephone versions of the questionnaire were translated from French to English using the Del Greco's back translation technique.[11]

The content validity of the questionnaire was first determined by the group of health professionals who verified the relevancy of the questions. The role of the group was to determine whether the questions were measuring what they intended to measure and reflected the specific objectives of the instrument. Then the instrument was pretested with a random sample of the adult unilateral above and below-knee amputee population (n=26), who had completed a prosthetic training program at the Montreal Rehabilitation Institute. This sample of LLA (French and English speaking) were asked to complete and comment the questionnaire with regard to the clarity and easy understanding of instructions, questions, format, wording and typography.

To evaluate the psychometric properties of the instrument, reliability tests (test-retest, internal consistency) and validity tests (construct and concurrent) are actually being conducted with a sample of 95 French and English speaking LLA who have undergone a prosthetic training. To determine the reliability of the intrument, the questionnaire will be completed twice, in a short time frame, by the LLA. The second questionnaire includes the Reintegration to Normal Living index developped by Wood Dauphinee et al..[12] This index will serve to determine construct validity (convergent and discriminant) of the questionnaire. The statistical analyses will include correlation tests (Kappa, Pearsons), coefficient alpha (Cronback), principal components and factor analyses. Preliminary results which are not available at the present time, will be presented and discussed at the WCPT Congress.

Upon completion of the validation process, the revised questionnaire will be sent to a stratified random sample of the LLA population following discharge from the various prosthetic rehabilitation centers of the province of Quebec (n=600). Eventually, the results of the latter study could help adapt the prosthetic training and follow-up programs to the needs of LLA.

This project is supported by the Fonds de la recherche en santé du Québec and the National Health Research and Development Program Canada.

REFERENCES

1. Granger CV (1982) Health accounting - Functional assessment of the long-term patient, 12, Krusen's Handbook of Physical Medecine and Rehabilitation. Third edition, Kohke Fj & al, WB Saunders Company

2. O'Toole DM, Goldbert RT, Ryan B (1985) Functional changes in vascular amputee patients : evaluation by Barthel index, Pulses profile and Escrow scale, Arch Phys Med Rehabil 66(8):508-511

3. Holden JM, Fernie GR (1987) Extent of artificial limb use following rehabilitation. J Orthop Res 5:562-568

4. Day HJB (1981) The assessment and description of amputee activity. Prosthet Orthot Int 5(1):23-28

5. Lam VT, Nieto J (1981) Réadaptation des amputés fémoraux unilatéraux, de plus de 55 ans, d'origine vasculaire. Union Med Can 110(9):774-779

6. Kegel B, Carpenter ML, Burgess EM (1978) Functional capabilities of lower extremity amputees. Arch Phys Med Rehabil 59(3):109-120

7. Benson J, Clark F (1982) A guide for instruments development and validation. Am J Occ T 36(12):789-800

8. Green LW, Kreuter MW, Deeds SG et al (1980) Health education planning. A diagnostic approach. Mayfiels Publishing Company, Palo Alto, California

9. Dillman DA (1978) Mail and Telephone surveys, the total design method. John Wiley and sons, New-York

10. Sudman S, Bradburn NM (1982) Asking questions, a practical guide to questionnaire design. Jossey-Bass, San Francisco

11. Del Greco L, Walop W, Eastbridge L (1987) Questionnaire development: 3. Translation, CMAJ 136:817-818

12. Wood-Dauphinée SL, Opzoomer MA, Williams JI, Marchand B, Spitzer WO (1988) Assessment of global function : The reintegration to normal living index. Arch Phys Med Rehabil 69:583-590

PROLONGED IMMOBILITY PROBLEMS

FACTORS INFLUENCING MUSCLE WEAKNESS DUE TO BED REST

T Sakamoto
Department of Physical Therapy, Kobe University Hospital, Chuo-ku, Kobe 650, Japan

INTRODUCTION

It is well known that inactivity causes changes in several aspects of the human body and often results in secondary problems. Some of previous investigations showed the loss of muscle strength as one of the effects of inactivity by designing bed rest or immobilization of limbs in casts. However, except for muscle length during a immobilized period, the experimental studies that noticed factors influencing muscle weakness induced by inactivity have not well established, though in a few review articles it was described that several factors, including age of subjects, duration of inactivity, pre-treatment conditions and others, influenced the effects of inactivity. The purpose of this study was to investigate how age of subjects, duration of bed rest, and the pathology of the joint influenced muscle weakness due to bed rest.

METHODS

1. Subjects

Subjects were 32 patients(3 men and 29 women) with unilateral or bilateral osteoarthritis of the hip joint between the ages of 25 and 82 years(mean=48.7, SD=±14.9), who were confined to bed between 9 and 60 days (mean=29.0, SD=± 13.0) after operations for the unilateral hip. The operations performed were osteotomy for the pelvis or femur, or hip arthroplasty. During a bed rest period, the subjects were allowed to only sit up with back support and no lower extremity weightbearing was allowed. Nutrition during bed rest was mainly taken from a standard hospital diet. There were no problems such as infection and mental deterioration during bed rest. No subjects performed special exercise for the nonoperated limb before and during bed rest. Informed consent had been obtained from all subjects before the start of the study.

2. Measurements

The muscle group tested was the hip abductors on the nonoperated limb. The voluntary isometric torque was measured using a REHAMATE kinetic evaluation and training machine(Kawasaki heavy industries, Ltd., Japan) within the week before the surgery and 48 hours after the subjects bore weight on the nonoperated limb to transfer to a wheelchair. In the supine position with the neutral positions of the hips and knees, the subjects performed ten repetitions of hip abduction for six seconds with maximal efforts. No subjects complained of pain and apprehension in the measurements. The maximal torque in the ten repetitions(MT) and the average of peak torque in each repetition(APT) were recorded as the measures of hip abductor muscle strength.

The anatomical and osteoarthritic changes of the tested hip were evaluated on roentgenograms. The anatomical changes were evaluated by measuring Sharp angle(1) and Center-Edge(CE) angle(2).

3. Data Analysis

Weakness index (WI: $\{1-($post-bed rest torque$/$pre-bed rest torque$)\} \times 100$) and WID (WI$/$days of bed rest) were calculated for each subject for both MT and APT.

Statistical analysis was performed using a multiple regression analysis. The dependent variable was WI or WID and the independent variables were age of the subjects, duration of bed rest, Sharp angle, and CE angle. An unpaired t-test was used to test significant differences in WI and WID between subjects with(n=15) and without(n=17) osteoarthritis of the hip (No significant differences between the two groups were found in both age and duration of bed rest). Statistical significance was accepted at $p<0.05$.

RESULTS

The matrix of correlations among variables for MT is presented in the table.
In both MT and APT, major findings were as follows :

1. Bed rest caused the loss of torque in the hip abductor muscles in 31 subjects(mean $\pm$SD of WI for MT = 23.6$\pm$12.2 ; for APT = 24.6$\pm$12.7).
2. WI was not correlated with duration of bed rest.
3. Age was the only significant explanatory variable of WI($p<0.05$).
4. Both age($p<0.01$) and duration of bed rest($p<0.05$) were the significant explanatory variables of WID.
5. No significant differences between the subjects with and without osteoarthritis of the hip were found in both WI and WID.

Matrix of Correlations(r) Among Variables for MT (N=31[a])

	WI	WID	Age	DBR[b]	Sharp	CE
WI	1.0	0.66**	0.39*	0.09	-0.22	0.17
WID		1.0	0.68**	-0.58**	-0.29	0.29
Age			1.0	-0.42*	-0.04	0.12
DBR				1.0	0.26	-0.23
Sharp					1.0	-0.77**
CE						1.0

[a]One outlying value was omitted ; [b]DBR = Duration of bed rest
*$p<0.05$; **$p<0.01$

DISCUSSION

Gogia et al.(3) reported that bed rest caused a proportionately higher percentage loss of torque in the antigravity muscles such as soleus, gastrocnemius-soleus, and knee extensors in healthy men. In the present study, the loss of torque in the hip abductors, which act as the "antigravity muscles in the frontal plane" when we walk, was found in 31 of the 32 subjects after bed rest. Weightbearing stimulus on the lower extremities would play an important role in maintaining the muscle strength.

The strength of the hip abductors was not always further decreased when duration of bed rest was prolonged. On the contrary, as duration of bed rest became shorter, the strength loss per day(WID) tended to become larger. Müller(4) showed that the strength loss in the upper extremity with immobilization of one arm in a plaster cast occurred mostly in the first seven days of immobilization. This previous report and the present findings might suggest that most of the strength loss induced by inactivity occur in the early phase of an inactivated period.

Tomonaga(5) showed that type II fast twitch muscle fibers atrophied selectively in elderly persons. Meanwhile, many investigators have reported that type I slow twitch fibers atrophied predominantly with inactivity. These findings might explain the present findings that subjects' age largely influenced WI and WID.

Sirca et al.(6) found the selective atrophy of the type II fibers in the gluteal muscles in patients with osteoarthritis of the hip. In the present study, however, in spite of the subjects experienced the inactivated condition such as bed rest, which might result in the predominant atrophy of the type I fibers, no significant differences between subjects with and without osteoarthritis of the hip were found in both WI and WID. No significant correlations between the anatomical changes(Sharp and CE angle) and the strength loss(WI and WID) were also found.

CONCLUSION

It is postulated that age is one of the major factors that affect muscle weakness induced by bed rest. In addition, it is suggested that the loss of muscle strength occur largely in the early phase of a bed rest period. In elderly patients, even if duration of bed rest is short,exercise should be more carefully programed to prevent a decrease in muscle strength.

REFERENCES

1.Sharp IK (1961) Acetabular Dysplasia. J Bone Joint Surg 43-B:268-272
2.Wiberg G (1939) Studies on dysplastic acetabula and congenital subluxation of the hip joint. Acta Chir Scand 83, Suppl 58
3.Gogia PP, Schneider VS, LeBlanc AD, Krebs J, Kasson C, Pientok C(1988)Bed rest effect on extremity muscle torque in healthy men. Arch Phys Med Rehabil 69:1030-1032
4.Müller EA (1970) Influence of training and of inactivity on muscle strength. Arch Phys Med Rehabil 51:449-462
5.Tomonaga M (1977) Histochemical and ultrastructural changes in senile human skeletal muscle. J Am Geriatr Soc XXV:125-131
6.Sirca A, Susec-Michieli M (1980) Selective type II fibre muscular atrophy in patients with osteoarthritis of the hip. J Neurol Sci 44:149-159

FREQUENCY-SPECIFICITY THEORY: ITS APPLICATION IN RETARDING DISUSE ATROPHY.

Chan PKL, Evans JH, Chow YN
Department of Rehabilitation Sciences, Hong Kong Polytechnic, Hung Hom
Hong Kong

INTRODUCTION
Disuse atrophy is commonly associated with joint immobilization, leading to degenerative changes and weakening of the muscle fibres. Various electrical stimulation protocols have been suggested for retardation of the disuse atrophy and results have been inconclusive [1]. The main reasons appeared to be related to the short duration of the stimulation session and the stimulation parameter:pulse frequency. Is this conventional stimulation frequency of 50-100Hz, the optimal one for all types of muscle fibres, slow and fast alike? A study has been conducted to examine the effects of treatment duration and the frequency parameter of an electrical stimulation programme in the retardation of disuse atrophy [2] and in this paper, the issue of frequency-specificity will be addressed.

Studies on muscle plasticity demonstrated clearly the importance of the neurotrophic influence of nerve on maintaining the physical characteristics of muscles. Muscle will be transformed when its nerve supply is changed[3]. Applying a pattern of stimulation which is foreign to the natural discharge frequency of the nerve will also produce a change in the muscle characteristic[4]. A low frequency (10Hz) for slow muscle and a high frequency (50-100Hz) have been advocated by previous researchers [5]. In disused quadriceps, it has been shown that fast type II fibres atrophy more than the slow type I fibres [6], thus in this study, a frequency of 50Hz was selected for investigation. It was hypothesized that this particular frequency range would retard disuse atrophy of type II more than type I fibres.

METHODS AND MATERIALS
Six patients with knee disorder (anterior cruciate ligament repair or fractured patella) requiring an extended period of 6 weeks immobilization were randomly allocated into the stimulation group who received 4 hour daily stimulation for 6 weeks or the control group who carried out daily isometric quadriceps exercise. A needle biopsy was first taken from vastus medialis muscle during the surgical repair procedure at the beginning of immobilization. The biopsy specimen was then frozen and cross-sections made. ATPase histochemical staining was used to map out the fast and slow fibres. The type I slow fibres were stained by ATPase at pH4.3 and type II fast fibres at pH9.4.Photomicrographs were then taken and later used for the morphometric analysis of the changes in fibre area, maximum and minimum diameter by the use of an image-analyzer system. The second biopsy was taken just before the immobilization unit was removed in close proximity to the that of the first biopsy site at the standardized depth.

Neurotech NT-4 portable units, pre-programmed with the following stimulation parameters: Frequency:50Hz; Pulse width:250μs; train on 2 sec and train off:8 sec were loaned to the ES subjects for the home programme. The stimulator usage time could be checked by an infra-red optical communication port of the main unit such that patients' compliances to the stimulation programme could be validated.

RESULTS
Over 100 fibres for each types of muscle were being assayed and their mean

fibre area, maximum and minimum diameter were computed for the pre-test and post-test measurement of each subject and the mean percentage changes in these morphometric measurement were being analysed. 2-tailed independent t-test comparison of data between the control group and ES group was conducted. Results showed that reduction in fibre area and minimum diameter were significantly less ($p \leq 0.05$) in the stimulated subjects when compared to the control subjects; change in maximum diameter was also consistently less in ES subjects though not statistically significant at 0.05level(see table 1,2 & 3).

Table 1: Comparison of mean percentage change in fibre area between control group and ES group.

Type	Mean % decrease in fibre area		Significance
	control gp	ES gp	
I	32.9↓ ± 5.4	7.7↓ ± 4.3	S* p=0.003
II	33.7↓ ± 4.3	11.98↓ ± 5.9	S* p=0.007

Table 2: Comparison of mean percentage changes in the minimum diameter of type I and II fibre between control and ES subjects.

	Mean % decrease in Dmin		Significance
	control gp	ES gp	
type I	25.69± 6.21	6.87 ± 0.39	S* p=0.006
type II	29.67± 13.72	7.19 ± 1.62	S* p=0.048

Table 3: Comparison of mean % changes of maximum diameter of type I and type II fibre between control and ES subjects.

	Mean % decrease in Dmax		Significance
	control gp	ES gp	
type I	19.81 ± 6.6	10.17 ± 5.3	NS p=0.122
type II	22.25 ± 7.97	9.78 ± 4.67	NS p=0.079

Table 4: Comparison of reduction of fibre area between type I and type II fibres.

	Mean % reduction in fibre area		Significance
	type I	type II	
control gp	32.89 ± 5.36	33.68 ± 4.34	NS p=0.853
CES gp	7.71 ± 4.38	11.98 ± 5.89	NS p=0.537

S = significant at 0.05 level

DISCUSSION

In the control subjects where effects of immobilization were profound, both type I and type II fibres showed a dramatic reduction in their area, (32.9 and 33.7% respectively). There were no significant differences between the diminution in size in the two types of fibres (see table 4 and fig.1). Selective atrophy of fast fibres of quadriceps was not found in this study. There were also no statistical differences in the percentage of reduction in fibre area and diameter between the fast and slow fibres in the ES subjects. In fact, the stimulated subjects showed a greater mean percentage

671

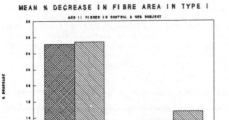

Fig.1: Bar chart illustration of mean % changes in type I & II fibre area in conrol and ES subjects.

reduction in their type II fast fibre which was contrary to the researcher's hypothesis.This finding was in agreement with previous work on animal and human studies [7,8]. However, caution must be exercised in the interpretation of results and in making clinical inference from this study because of its small sample size. To mimic the natural discharge frequency of a fast motoneurone supplying a fast muscle, a fixed frequency of 50-100Hz may not be able to represent the activity pattern completely. "Eutrophic stimulation" [9] may be a better alternative. Future work in this area is warranted, e.g. comparative study using different frequency range.

CONCLUSION

Although the present ES programme cannot conteract disuse atrophy completely, its beneficial effect on retarding disuse atrophy was supported. However, findings of the present study were unable to confirm the "frequency-specificity" hypothesis under such experimental conditions, suggesting that if the duration of stimulation session is long enough to compensate for the loss of activity associated with immobilization, the programme will retard disuse atrophy, both type I and type II fibres to similar extent.

REFERENCE:

1. St.-Pierre D, Gardiner P(1987) The effect of immobilization & exercise on muscle function: a review.Physio Can 39:24-36
2. Chan P (1991) The therapeutic value of a chronic electrical stimulation programme in disuse atrophy. MPhil Thesis, Hong Kong Polytechnic
3. Buller JA, Eccles JC (1960) Interaction between motorneurones and muscles in respect of the characteristic speed of their response. J. Physiol (London) 150:417-439
4. Vrbov'a G (1963) The effect of motoneurone activity on the speed of contraction of striated muscle. J Physiol 169:513-526
5. Hennig R, Lomo T (1987) Effect of chronic stimulation on the size and speed of long term denervated and innervated rat fast and slow skeletal muscle. Acta Physiol Scand 130:115-131
6. Baugher WH et al (1984) Quadriceps atrophy in the anterior cruciate insufficient knee. Am J of Sports Med 12:192-1957
7. Halkjer J, Ingemann T (1985) Wasting of the Human Quadriceps muscle after knee ligament injuries, I: Anthropometric consequences. Scand J Med Suppl 13:5-11
8. Eerbeek O et al (1984) Effects of fast & slow pattern of tonic long term stimulation on contractile properties of fast muscles in cat. J Physiol (London) 352:73-90
9. Faargher D et al (1987) Eutrophic electrical stimulation for Bell's Palsy. Clin Rehab 1:265-271

THE EFFECTS OF PROLONGED CAST IMMOBILIZATION ON TENDONS

Chukuka S. Enwemeka, Ph.D., P.T.

Division of Physical Therapy, Department of Orthopaedics & Rehabilitation, University of Miami School of Medicine, & Veterans Affairs Medical Center, 5915 Ponce de Leon Blvd, 5th Fl., Miami, FL 33146, U.S.A.

Introduction

Prolonged cast immobilization is well-known to produce muscle atrophy; but its effect on tendons remains poorly understood. Studies on primates indicate that cast immobilization reduces the tensile strength and energy absorption capacity of the anterior cruciate ligament, a dense connective tissue similar to tendons.[1,2] Additionally, it has been shown that immobilization induces joint stiffness, and that the induced stiffness is accompanied by corresponding biochemical changes in periarticular connective tissues.[3] These findings suggest that the biomechanical changes induced by immobilization may be accompanied by changes in the structure of dense connective tissues. Therefore, the purpose of this study was to determine the effects of prolonged cast immobilization on the ultrastructure and morphometry of rabbit calcaneal tendons.

Methods

Subjects: Fifteen rabbits were used for this study. The animals were kept under veterinary care, housed one per cage in a light-controlled environment maintained at $23 \pm 1°C$, and fed rabbit chow *ad libitum*.

Cast Immobilization: Under adequate anaesthesia, the right hind-limbs of 12 rabbits, assigned randomly to 4 equal groups, were immobilized in plaster. The immobilization casts were applied to maintain 90° of knee flexion and full plantar flexion of the ankle. The non-casted right hind-limbs of a fifth group of 3 rabbits served as controls. At each of 3, 4, 6 and 8 weeks post-immobilization, 3 rabbits were weighed, anaesthetized and their immobilized right calcaneal tendons surgically exposed to permit *in situ* fixation. Following satisfactory fixation, the tendon was excised, then processed for electron microscopy.

Tissue Processing & Electron Microscopy: The specimens obtained were first sliced into thin filaments, fixed for 6-8 hours in 2% paraformaldehyde/2.5% glutaraldehyde (pH 7.4), buffer washed, then post-fixed for another two hours in a 1% aqueous solution of osmium tetroxide (pH 7.4). Thereafter, each specimen was washed and dehydrated in graded alcohol before final dehydration in propylene oxide. After gradual infiltration with a mixture of propylene oxide and EMBED 812 resin (Electron Microscopy Sciences, Fort Washington, PA), each specimen was embedded in 100% resin and cured at 60°C for 65-70 hours. Each specimen was then trimmed and sectioned. Sections obtained were stained with both uranyl acetate and lead citrate for 10 minutes each, then visualized and photographed with a JEOL 100CX electron microscope.

Computer Morphometry: To objectively compare the ultrastructural morphometry of the collagen fibrils of the five groups of tendons, the high magnification electron micrographs obtained were placed on a Jandel Scientific digitizing tablet (Jandel Scientific, Corte Madera, CA) interfaced to a computer that has SIGMA-scan (Jandel Scientific, Corte Madera, CA), a software designed to facilitate computation of morphometric measurements. After calibrating the system, the electronic pen of the digitizer was used to carefully trace the outline of each fibril. Simultaneously, the cross-sectional area of each fibril was computed and stored in the computer. Then, the mean diameter of each fibril was obtained by mathematical transformation. A total of 15,804 collagen fibrils representing 2,390 to 3,711 fibrils per group were measured.

Data Analysis: Because the diameter of collagen fibrils exhibit a bi- or trimodal distribution, the normality of the data was first determined by Kolmogorov-Smirnov D statistic. This test revealed that the distribution of each group of fibrils differed significantly from a normal distribution, therefore, non-parametric ANOVA was used to compare the cross-sectional area and diameter of the five groups of rabbits. Thereafter, Mann-Whitney U tests were performed to distinguish groups that differ in diameter and cross-sectional area.

Results

Collagen Fibril Ultrastructure & Morphometry: The non-immobilized normal control tendons consisted of densely packed collagen fibrils with relatively few cells. Sections of these tendons revealed an array of

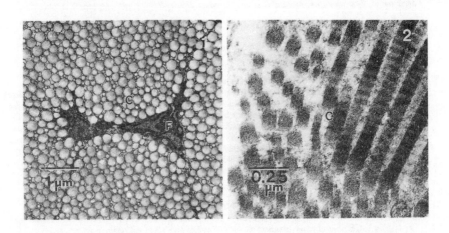

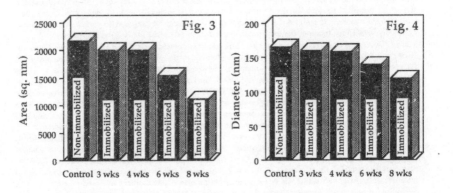

Figure Legends

Fig. 1: Electron micrograph of a cross-section of collagen fibrils in a normal control tendon (15,000X).

Fig. 2: A cross-section of collagen fibrils in a 6-week immobilized tendon; Note disorganization of collagen fibrils in this representative electron micrograph (62,600X). Figs. 1 & 2 differ in magnification.

Fig. 3: Mean cross-sectional area of control and immobilized tendons.

Fig. 4: Mean diameter of control and immobilized tendons.

longitudinally arranged collagen fibrils throughout the field (Fig. 1). In contrast however, the collagen fibrils of cast immobilized tendons were profoundly disorganized. In several of the sections, randomly distributed areas that were totally devoid of collagen were frequently seen. Although these changes were progressive with the duration of cast immobilization, notwithstanding, there were areas of relatively well-organized fibrils (Figs 2). The morphometric measurements revealed a statistically significant decrease in the mean cross-sectional area and mean diameter of the collagen fibrils after three weeks of cast immobilization ($P < .05$). This decrease in collagen fibril sizes progressed with the duration of immobilization. Thus, by the 8th week, both the cross-sectional area and the diameter of the collagen fibrils of immobilized tendons had declined to approximately 50% of control values (Figs. 3 & 4).

Tendon Fibroblasts: Within the matrix of cast-immobilized tendons that remained relatively well-organized, the fibroblasts had the same morphological characteristics as those of non-immobilized controls. Specifically, these cells had thin layers of cytoplasm around prominent nuclei that had dense clumps of heterochromatin along the inner surface of their nuclear membranes. The synthetic organelles of the rER and Golgi complex were not seen in these cells. In contrast, areas of disorganized matrix had fibroblasts that were always large, with massive cytoplasms, well-developed rER, and prominent nuclei that were rich in euchromatin.

Discussion & Conclusions

These findings demonstrate that cast immobilization of three weeks or more induces (1) progressive disorganization of tendon collagen, and (2) a gradual but steady decline in the sizes of collagen fibrils. Thus, the deleterious effects of prolonged cast immobilization are not limited to muscle atrophy and degenerative articular changes. Since the strength of tendons is directly related to the orderly arrangement and sizes of the collagen fibrils,[4] the present study suggests that prolonged cast immobilization may weaken tendons, as it has been shown to weaken anterior cruciate ligaments.[1,2] *Ipso facto*, rehabilitation strategies should be directed at restoring the structural integrity of both muscles and tendons; not muscles alone.

The presence of clusters of collagen fibrils that were relatively spared and apparently intact in casted tendons indicates that not all collagen fibrils are adversely affected by immobilization. Fibroblasts are well-known to collaborate with macrophages in collagen degradation.[5] Thus, it is plausible that the metabolically active fibroblasts visualized in areas of disorganized collagen were involved in active degradation of the collagen matrix. Besides collagen synthesis, fibroblasts are known to monitor and possibly adapt the matrix to environmental stresses.[6] Thus, it is possible that cast immobilization triggers a signal that either induces tendon fibroblasts to degrade rather than synthesize collagen, or hinder their ability to maintain the structure of existing matrix. Further studies are necessary to understand the biochemical processes associated with these changes.

References

1. Noyes FR, *et al.* (1974) Biomechanics of Ligament failure II: An analysis of immobilization, exercise and reconditioning effects in primates. J Bone Joint Surg 56A:1406-1418
2. Noyes FR (1977) Functional properties of knee ligaments and alterations induced by immobilization. A correlative biomechanical and histological study in primates. Clin Orthop Rel Res 123:210-253
3. Woo SL-Y, *et al.* (1975) Connective tissue response to immobility. Correlative biochemical measurements of normal and immobilized rabbit knees. Arthritis and Rheumatism 18:257-264
4. Parry DAD, Barnes GRG, Craig AS (1978) A comparison of the size distribution of collagen fibrils in connective tissue as a function of age and a possible relation between fibril size distribution and mechanical properties. Proc R Soc Lond [Biol] 203:305-321
5. Laub R, *et al.* (1982) Degradation of collagen and proteoglycan by macrophages and fibroblasts: Individual potentialities of each cell type and cooperative effects through the activation of fibroblasts by macrophages. Biochim Biophys Acta 721:425-433
6. Ten Cate AR (1989) The Fibroblast and its Products. In: AR Ten Cate (ed), *Oral Histology* 3rd edition, Mosby Publishers, St. Louis. pp 90-105

Supported in part by Veterans Affairs Rehabilitation Research & Development Grant.

A MODEL FOR THE IDENTIFICATION, ASSESSMENT, AND TREATMENT OF
ALGODYSTROPHY

M.R. Gersh
Department of Physical Therapy, Eastern Washington University,
Cheney, WA. 99004 USA

Algodystrophy is a symptomatology characterized by pain, tenderness,
and sympathetic nervous system hyperarousal. Symptoms often appear
following minor trauma or immobilization, and progress to complete
autonomic disregulation and limb atrophy. The early identification of the
physiological and behavioral correlates associated with the potential
development of algodystrophy permits the physical therapist to provide
early intervention critical to the arrest of the disease process prior to
complete limb dysfunction and disability.

Algodystrophy was first documented as causalgia by Mitchell in 1864,
in Civil War soldiers with peripheral nerve injuries following gunshot
wounds. Clinical variants of algodystrophy include Sudeck's atrophy of
bone, shoulder-hand syndrome, and reflex sympathetic or neurovascular
dystrophy (1). Algodystrophy has been associated with peripheral
phenomena including soft tissue trauma, arthritis, fracture, infection,
nerve injury, surgery, malignancy, vasculitis, amputation, and
immobilization, central disorders including cerebrovascular accident,
poliomyelitis, and spinal cord injury, and systemic conditions such as
herpes zoster, pregnancy, myocardial infarction, renal tubular
osteomalacia, and pneumonia (1,2). A precipitating event is not
identified in 50% of cases (2).

Symptoms may appear immediately following trauma, or may be delayed by
weeks, months, or years. While symptoms are often localized or regional,
they can extend to adjacent joints, throughout the extremity, or to
homolateral or contralateral limbs (2). The course of algodystrophy is
progressive and symptoms are grouped into stages of varying duration and
severity. Stage I (acute) is characterized by a sudden onset of severe,
persistent, burning pain, which is aggravated by dependency, movement,
cutaneous stimulation, or emotional stress. Edema and vasomotor
instability are present, the skin appears taut, shiny, and reddened, and
the limb may be hyperthermic. Hair and nail growth may be increased or
decreased, and the patient shields tha limb from all sensory and motor
functions. Stage II (dystrophic) is characterized by resolving edema,
dystrophic changes, hyperhidrosis, cyanosis, localized hypothermia, hair
loss and nail ridging.Spontaneous pain abates but pain is triggered by
any sensory stimulus or motor activity. Diffuse osteoporosis may be seen
radiologically. During Stage III (atrophic) pain spreads proximally and
limb dysfunction becomes disuse. Irreversible tissue damage, including
thin, shiny skin, thickened fascia, contracture, muscle atrophy, bone
demineralization, and joint ankylosis render the limb functionless, and
amputation may be necessary (1,2). Movement disorders, including weakness,
inability to initiate movement, tremor, spasm, hypertonus, hyperreflexia,
and dystonia have been described during all stages (3,4). These movement

disorders differ from those of peripheral or central nervous system origin, in that they are temporarily eliminated by regional sympathetic blockade.

Clinical symptomatology may be objectively measured by volumetry (edema), dolorimetry (hyperestesia), goniometry (mobility), and stress loading (pain) (5). Pain inventories are useful in quantifying the patient's response to treatment. A questionnaire has recently been developed to address the patient's perception of vasomotor involvement(5).

Maladaptive behaviors are often apparent in patients with algodystrophy, and may predispose some patients to development of the syndrome. Hyperarousal of the sympathetic nervous system may manifest in the patient's hyperemotional temperament and overtly anxious responses to stress (6). Patients with algodystrophy display elevated scores on scales for hysteria, hypochondriasis, and depression on the Minnesota Multiphasic Personality Inventory, when compared to a matched group of patients with brachial plexus injury without algodystrophic signs or symptoms. Patients share qualities common to patients with chronic pain, including high pain behavior, passivity, dependency, and poor compliance. In adolescents with algodystrophy poor self-concept, unstable home environment, substance or sexual abuse, or passivity are often identified. Psychopathology warrants a multidisciplinary approach to the management of algodystrophy, which includes supportive psychotherapy and behavior modification.

The confirmation of a clinical diagnosis of algodystrophy may be made by radiography, scintigraphy, thermography, or response to sympathetic blockade (1,2). No specific laboratory or electrophysiologic findings confirm a diagnosis of algodystrophy. However, these tests are useful to rule out diseases such as rheumatoid arthritis, scleroderma, or nerve trauma, whose symptoms may mimic those of algodystrophy. The prompt, accurate diagnosis of algodystrophy, as well as the identification and treatment of any underlying disease process, are critical to the successful treatment of the syndrome, and full restoration of function.

The most effective treatment of algodystrophy is prevention. Immobilization, either self-imposed or applied, is the hallmark on the development of this syndrome. Early identification of patients predisposed to algodystrophy, and prompt, consistent mobilization of traumatized regions can prevent the escalation of sympathetic hyperactivity. This principle is applicable regardless of the precipitating event, and particularly evident in the management of children and adolescents (7). The earlier a diagnosis of algodystrophy is established, the more immediate and complete the patient's response is to conservative, non-invasive treatment measures. Physical therapy interventions which reduce pain and hyperesthesia, control edema, inhibit sympathetic tone, and facilitate active movement are often sufficient to reverse the pathological process and restore function. Treatment may include thermal agents, retrograde massage, compression and elevation to reduce edema, assistive, active,and resistive exercises to restore motion, strength, and function, and desensitization techniques (8). Static splinting is contraindicated. Stress loading of the affected limb via weight bearing is effective in diminishing pain and resolving vasomotor instability. Transcutaneous electrical nerve stimulation (TENS) has been applied successfully to reduce burning pain and restore autonomic homeostasis, most notably in children (7). Normalization of peripheral circulation via autogenic relaxation training and electromyographic or thermal biofeedback have also been documented (9).

Once the patient exhibits significant dystrophic or atrophic changes, pharmacologic or surgical interruption of sympathetic activity is required in addition to those interventions previously described to reverse the pathology. Ultimately, treatment emphasizes the restoration of active, functional mobility. If pain is relieved and normal autonomic balance is restored without strict attention to mobilization of the affected body region, symptoms of algodystrophy can recur.

In summary, early identification of algodystrophy is established by patient history of a precipitating event, trauma, illness, or stress. A psychosocial history will often reveal predisposing risk factors. Signs and symptoms including persistent, burning pain, vasomotor and sudomotor instability, edema, hyperesthesia, and immobility, often unrelated to specific dermatomal or peripheral nerve distribution, are observed and measured. Confirmation of the clinical diagnosis is established via radiographic, scintigraphic, thermographic, or sympathetic evidence (4). The early recognition of the potential for a patient to develop algodystrophy enables prompt treatment directed at facilitating normal active motion in the affected region, and adjacent joints. Once clinical evidence of algodystrophy is present, treatment is directed towards pain control, and normalization of autonomic activity, with emphasis on facilitating patient participation in and compliance with active movement and restoration of functional mobility.

1. Schwartzman RJ, McClellan TL (1987) Reflex sympathetic dystrophy: A review. Arch Neurol 44:555-561
2. Doury P (1988) Algodystrophy: Reflex sympathetic dystrophy syndrome. Clinical Rheumatology 7:173-180
3. Schwartzman RJ, Kerrigan J (1990) The movement disorder of reflex sympathetic dystrophy. Neurology 40:57-61
4. Doury P, Dirheimer Y, Pattin S (1981) Algodystrophy: Diagnosis, and therapy of a frequent disease of the locomotor apparatus. Springer Verlag, Berlin
5. Atkins RM, Duckworth T, Kanis JA (1990) Features of algodystrophy after Colles' fracture. J of Bone and Joint Surgery 72B:105-110
6. Zucchini M, Alberti G, Moretti MP (1989) Algodystrophy and related psychological features. Functional Neurology 4:153-156
7. Kesler RW, Saulsbury FT, Miller LT, Rowlingson JC (1988) Reflex sympathetic dystrophy in children: Treatment with transcutaneous electric nerve stimulation. Pediatrics 82:728-732
8. Waylett-Rendall J (1990) Therapist's management of reflex sympathetic dystrophy. In Hunter JM, Schneider LH, Mackin E, Callaghan A: Rehabilitation of the Hand, third edition, CV Mosby Co., St. Louis, pp. 787-792
9. Grunert BK, Devine CA, Sanger JR, Matloub HS, Green D (1990) Thermal self-regulation for pain control in reflex sympathetic dystrophy syndrome. J of Hand Surgery 15A:615-618

ALTERNATIVE THERAPIES

BODY AWARENESS THERAPY AND THE BODY AWARENESS SCALE, BAS

Gertrud Roxendal, D M Sc
Lund University, Department of Physical Therapy
LUND, Sweden

Body Awareness Therapy is based on the bearing idea that physiotherapy can focus upon the patient´s body ego to reestablish motor ability as far as possible.

The body ego is mainly understood as:
Non verbal experience
and functions of the body
for an autonomic life
of a grown up person
who can do what he/she wants to.

The body ego thus contains experience and knowledge of the body as well as behaviour and actions with the body.

The overall goal of Body Awareness Therapy is to re-establish the body ego and to get the body integrated in the total experience of identity.

Functions of the body ego which are possible to observe and train are for instance:
Relation to the centre line (postural functions)
Relation to the ground in different positions
Ability to performe movements from the centre of the body
Breathing and integration of breathing and movements.

Body Awareness Therapy is applied in different areas of physiotherapy in Sweden, primary health care, preventive care, psychosomatic problems and psychiatry.

The Body Awareness Scale, BAS, is constructed to measure body ego functions in psychiatry and for psychosomatic patients. The BAS is based on a psychiatric rating scale, CPRS, (Comprehensive Psychopathological Rating Scale) with new constructed body items. The BAS contains items for the patient´s experience as well as those for the rater´s observation.
Information for the patient´s report is gathered in a structured interview and for the observation there is a structured movement test.

The scale steps are based on common principles, 0 represents the healthy dimension and 3 the extreme pathological dimension.

I will now present some studies performed with the BAS.

1. The first study was descriptive, its aim was to test the reliability of the BAS and to give a symptom pattern for the patients included in the study. This could give a first idea of the construct validy of the scale. 53 patients with chronic schizophrenia were included. Three psychologists and two physiotherapists took part in the study.

The reliability between raters was satisfactory. Four pairs of raters had a coefficient correlation of 0.96 and 0.98 for the whole scale. Seen item for item the reliability also was satisfactory. The lowest coefficient correlation was 0.65 for Personal space, all the other items had 0.77 or more. This is seen as satisfactory both for clinical use and for effect evaluation.

The mean scores in the study showed a high degree of symptoms concerning body-directed functions. This is a new and valuable information in psychiatric physiotherapy.

Some items concern the same symptoms for the patient´s report and for the rater´s observation. For these items the patient´s report had higher means than the rater´s observation in Inability to feel (Lack of appropriate emotion), Hostile feelings (Hostility), Autonomic disturbances and Hygiene. The rater´s observation gave higher mean than the patient´s report in Muscular tension.

2. A factor analytic study with 292 ratings gave clinically useful factors ruch as:

The Movement factor
General feeling of illness factor
Body image factor and
Anxiety factor
Of special interest in psychiatric care is the Limitation factor.

3. A discriminative study had the aim to compare two groups, one given Body Awareness Therapy and one given traditional treatment for schizophrenia. 32 patients took part, 20 in the therapy group and 12 in the control group. The therapy group showed significant improvement in The Movement factor, Body image factor, Anxiety factor and The Gaze & sexual interest factor. This must be seen as a strong result since the factors represent a big part of the BAS.

4. A Study with 100 non-psychotic patients with chronic pain in combination with other symptoms showed a significantly higher degree of symptoms in 17 out of 47 items of the BAS than did the schizophrenic patients. All these items had a non-psychotic character. The schizophrenic patients had a significantly higher degree of symptoms in 5 items, all of which had a psychotic character. This may indicate that the BAS can be used for a diagnostic purpose. (Vivianne Nordwall and Gertrud Roxendal)

5. One study with 12 patients with chronic pain and alexitymia showed that the reliability of the BAS was not satisfactory if used by not experienced raters. When the raters were experienced the reliability again was satisfactory. The author also found a congruity between high symptoms with the BAS and a high degree of alexithymia assessed with Schalling Sifneos rating scale (Anders Schiöler).

6. In another degree project the authors studied possible connection between body posture assessed with the BAS and life satisfaction assessed with psychological rating scales. The total scores of these assessments showed congruity for 18 patients out of 20; patients with low satisfaction of life also had a high degree of symptoms in their body posture. (Liselott Jönsson et al).

7. In a study in progress patients with fibromyalgia are treated with Body Awareness Therapy and measured with the BAS and other instruments. One preliminary result is that all of the patients in the study have a high degree of anxiety. They also show a low degree of centering measured in a BAS-item. Both chronic pain and low centering might be signs of a low self esteem. The findings give support to the possibility that one important problem might be a low self esteem at the patients in the study.

The BAS is a rating scale for symptoms and functions. To get a high score the patient must show extreemely pathological patterns of symptoms. Now there has occured an interest to apply the BAS with other groups of patients and healthy people. For that purpose I have changed the scale steps. I exluded the pathological dimension and developed a new system of scoring from the health dimension. I call the new scale BAS-H (Health). Preliminary results in studies in progress show satisfactory reliability between raters even for BAS-H.

Finally I would like to mention a study by a physiotherapist working especially with psychosomatic problems. Kerstin Ullberg Pettersson has developed a combination of group treatment including education, group talks and Body Awareness Therapy. She performed a retrospective study with 55 patients given the therapy combination. Initially the author had gathered enough data for a coming study. The results show, among other things, a significant decrease of medicine doses, of experienced pains and of increased working time. The patients expressed increased self confidence, body awareness and ability to influence on satisfaction of life. A great deal of the improvements remained even after a follow up time of two years. This indicates that the treatment has not only lead to a symptom reduction but also has supported a personal growth at the patients.

LITERATURE

1. Roxendal G, Ett helhetsperspektiv, Sjukgymnastik inför framtiden, Lund, Studentlitteratur, 1987

2. Hegna T, Sveram M, Psychological and Psychosomatic Problems, Roxendal G, Physiotherapy as an approach in psychiatric care with emphasis on Body Awareness Therapy, Edinburgh, Churchill Livingstone, 1990, 75-101

3. Åsberg et al, The CPRS - Development and Applications of a Psychiatric Rating Scale, Act psych Scand 1978: Suppl 216

4. Roxendal G, Body Awareness Therapy and the Body Awareness Scale, Treatment and Evaluation in Psychiatric Physiotherapy, (thesis), Göteborg University 1985

5. Roxendal G, Body Awareness Scale, Instruction, Manual, Movement Test and Factors for Subscales, in progress

PSYCHOMOTOR PHYSIOTHERAPY DEPARTS FROM TRADITIONAL PRINCIPLES

BH Bunkan.
Fysioterapihøgskolen i Oslo,
Pilestredet 56, 0167 Oslo 1, Norway

The method was developed in Norway during the 1940s by the psychiatrist Trygve Braatøy and the physiotherapist Aadel Bülow-Hansen. It is the first method in physiotherapy known to be based on clearly holistic principles. Although the method represents a departure from traditional concepts in physiotherapy and medicine it has its roots in these two disciplines.

In what way is this a departure from traditional physiotherapy?

The differences may be summarized as follows (1):
- The treatment is not symptom-oriented.
- The treatment includes the whole body.
- Respiration is the guiding factor in the treatment.
- The treatment is carried out undisturbed.
The treatment normally takes place once a week.
The therapeutic attitude is characterized by empathy.
There is an opportunity for trust and confidence.
The patient is given the opportunity to show his feelings.

What does the psychomotor theory involve?

The interplay between body and feelings is one of the pillars of the theory. People have different bodily reactions to emotional stress. Some react specifically by means of motor responses and tend to develop symptoms related to muscular movement. Others react primarily with the autonomic, endocrine, or immune system, and tend to develop symptoms in internal organs. We have all noticed how our body stretches upwards and our breathing becomes freer when we are feeling relaxed and optimistic, and how our shoulders become bowed and our bodily functions become more sluggish when we are depressed. Hunching of the back and shoulders (flexion) is a common reaction to excessive stress, and straightening the back (extension) is often an instinctive response in people who are pulling themselves together. Such physical expressions are especially noticeable in people wishing to hide their feelings. Another physical reaction is trembling legs caused by fear or anxiety. In psychomotor theory respiration is considered the most important means of regulating the expression of emotion. When emotions are held in check over a long period, respiration often becomes inhibited. The diaphragm then becomes tense, and natural spontaneous basal respiration at rest may become inhibited, even though the person may be able to breathe basally on request. When the spontaneous functioning of the diaphragm is restricted, this inhibits circulation to the internal organs, which predisposes to the development of disease. Peripheral circulation may also be weakened in certain areas, often the legs. When the basal respiration movements are restricted, increased use is often made of the auxiliary respiration muscles, which predisposes over time to thoracic outlet ailments and symptoms of muscular tension in the head, jaw, throat and cervical region. A tense diaphragm, resulting in the risk of increased compression around the 10th thoracic vertebrae. Hypomobile segments in this area, with hypermobility in surrounding areas, are a well-known finding.

What is the aim of psychomotor physiotherapy?
Psychomotor physiotherapy aims to change the person's entire way of functioning. This cannot be done by correcting isolated elements, but has to be achieved by an inner transformation. The objectives of psychomotor therapy are:
- freedom from symptoms,
- a posture in which the segments are able to move freely in relation to each other,
- a body with good flexibility and stability,
- free and adaptable respiration
- good body awareness and coordination,
- an increased awareness of one's own feelings,
- ability to resolve one's own conflicts.

What kind of patients can benefit from psychomotor therapy?
The indicatons are the same as those ordinarily treated with physiotherapy. Examples are: problems caused by muscular tension, musculoskeletal ailments, circulation-related symptoms, and certain psychiatric conditions.

Selection criteria are based on personal resources
The patient's physical resources are assessed by a special physical examination, which allows investigation of the interaction between posture, respiration, function, musculature, and autonomic reactions. Findings close to the optimal norms in physiotherapy are defined as good. They indicate the presence of the psychoemotional resources necessary to tolerate such a deep-reaching form of treatment. Supportive physiotherapy is suggested in the case of clini- cal findings that indicate excessive stress. The physical resources indicate the person's susceptibility to treatment, the prognosis, and the required dosage level of treatment.

The therapeutic approach in psychomotor therapy

The method aims to regulate tension primarily by means of massage and exercises related to respiration. Courses of treatment start with the legs, back, and arms before going on to the thorax, and face. Patients in a difficult emotional phase are given stabilizing bodily exercises. Primitive reactions like yawning, sighing, and so on are used as guidelines in treatment, and the respiratory check on such reactions is dessolved by a short, sharp pain stimulus to the muscles. The patient is asked to express respiratory, motor, and emotional responses to the pain. The stimulus provides a real situation against which to react, which helps to alter previously learned responses like the use of breathing to hold back feelings, and stiffening or deadening parts of the body. The patient's true reaction is thus given a chance to develop. This process aims to help patients release their breath passively during the expiraton phase. Yawning and sighing are gradually stimulated. A complete yawn provokes a strong stretching impulse involving the whole body from head to toe, including the respiratory organs and especially the diaphragm. Stretching and yawning cumulate in a profound release of tension, and when this is successful it releases the respiratory inhibitions. This allows for a better circulation in the internal organs. Evidence shows that a number of ailments affecting internal organs may improve of disappear when respiratory function improves. A reduction in respiratory control often releases suppressed or forgotten emotions, but this form of therapy does not aim at a strong acting out of such emotions but at less violent forms of reaction, within the therapist's control.

The therapeutic attitude in psychomotor physiotherapy

Common questions used to help feelings rise to the surface are "How do you feel"? "What do you feel"? The patient is encouraged to remain with the feelings that he becomes conscious of. Questions and remarks that encourage the patient to find his own solutions to his problems are part of the approach.

Psychomotor physiotherapy and psychotherapy

More serious types of conflicts may call for a combination of physiotherapy and psychotherapy. Psychomotor physiotherapy activates deep levels of the psyche and sometimes causes preverbal material to surface, which may be difficult to reach by means of verbal therapy. It may thus be a useful supplement to verbal psychotherapy.

Literature:
1. Bunkan BH, Thornquist E. (1990) Psychomotor therapy. International Perspectives in Physiotherapy. 5 Ed. Hegna T. Sveram M. Churchill Livingstone ISBN 0-443-03347-1.

THE INTEROBSERVER RELIABILITY OF A PHYSIOTHERAPEUTIC ASSESSMENT OF BODILY RESOURCES

R. Keskinen-Rosenqvist
Crisis Dept. Huddinge Hospital
S-141 86 Huddinge

G. Biguet
Dept. of Physical Therapy
Karolinska Hosp.S-104 01 Stockholm

Psychomotor Physiotherapy (PMP) is a physiotherapeutic method of examination and treatment which is based on the assumption that the human body is affected by psychological as well as physical causes.It was developed in Norway and is spreading throughout Scandinavia. The tradition is based on Reich´s theory that the individual´s defensive behavior manifests itself parallelly on the psychological and physical levels (1).

This examination method is used to assess a person´s bodily resources, and it stresses the connection between muscular tension, restrained breathing and emotions. It is based on solid, clinical physiotherapy, and it emphasizes that

- psychological factors play an important role in the formation of the individual´s body pattern;
- the entire body is always examined regardless of the local symtom;
- all findings are interpreted as parts of the whole. The breathing is of
  fundamental significance to this entity (2);
- both "good" and "bad" findings are noted and balanced against each other in the attempt to create
  a picture of the patient´s total bodily resources.

The entire body´s tension and balance status, flexibility and stability are assessed. Great importance is attached to free and spontaneous breathing and to the body´s adaptability, meaning ability to changes. Examination of posture, respiration, movement (function), muscular quality and consistency as well as reaction to the examination are the main elements of assessment. The posture is judged according to a biomechanical model as well as by the general expression, e.g. defensive posture, openess etc. The mobility of the body refers to the ability of body parts to move freely and independently of one another, and to the ability to be tense and relaxed. In the conclusion the individual findings, their interplay and their significance to the whole are weighed and interpreted. In clinical practice the case history, tne patient´s awareness of his/her own body and ability to understand and reflect are taken into account in addition to the physical findings and the reaction to the examination.

The method includes many variables. It uses a structured model of estimates which we have further developed for the project. The variables are treated in a natural scientific way and summarized in an interpretation of a hermeneutic nature.

We wanted to make a scientific scrutiny of this examination method in the form of an Interobserver Reliability test (IOR). We have further developed the examination for the project and named it Resource Oriented Physiotherapeutic Examination (ROPE).

Method

Independently of one another two physiotherapists examined 27 healthy subjects at intervals of a few days. The target was to make the examination as similar as possible to a clinical situation. From this examination method 90 elements were chosen and defined. In some of them both the left and the right side of the body were examined, others consisted of several parts. The total number of variables examined was 149.

The conclusion of examination was simplified. It was made on the basis of the physical findings and the subject´s reactions to the examination. For this purpose a result scale was designed which had not formerly been tried.

As the physiotherapist is very much involved in the examination his/her behaviour towards the subject is of great importance. The examinations were therefore made according to a given structure and the attitude defined as empathic and accepting but neutral as regards the findings.

Statistical processing and assessment criteria

The IOR was calculated both for the individual variables and for the conclusions. In order to limit the analysis only a moderate number of variables for each part of examination have been analysed. The criterion for the choice of variable was in accordance with the PMP theory in so far as flexion and extension patterns were to be illustrated as well as the need for control and the ability to relax. The variables to be analysed were chosen after the examinations had been made but before the statistics were processed.

In this project IOR is expressed as a correlation (Pearson´s product moment correlation r_{xy}) and as a percentage agreement. There is no unequivocal limit for satisfactory results, but the result must always be interpreted against the background of the nature of the examination (3). Several authors claim that in subjective assessments an IOR of $r_{xy} \geq 0.5$ and a percentage agreement of $\geq 70\%$ are satisfactory (4) (5). These limits are recommended for assessment methods largely based on subjective estimates with numerous and complex variables. ROPE is such a method.

Result and discussion

IOR as the correlation r_{xy} and percentage agreement of four variables from each examination are given in the table below.

Tabell 1 % Percentage Agreement and r_{xy} of 16 variables

	Posture				*Respiration*				*Function*				*Musculature*			
	back	shoulder	pelvis	knee	flexib. thorax	restr. line	inspi- ration	move- ment	shoulder	relaxa- tion	flexib. back	arm	quadri ceps	teres	mass- eter	biceps
%	89	74	74	74	77	89	87	70	81	62	85	81	74	69	81	74
p	0.715	0.403	0.766	0.544	0.487	–	–	–	0.529	0.503	0.612	0.711	0.525	0.564	0.073	0.431
	***	*	***	*	*				**	**	**	***	**	**		*

* $p\ 0.05$ ** $p\ 0.01$ *** $p\ 0.001$

14 out of 16 variables in the table show a percentage agreement of $\geq 70\%$ and may consequently regarded as a satisfactory result. In the examination of respiration the estimates are nominal and r_{xy} has not been calculated (6). The table therefore shows only 13 variables with r_{xy}. 9 of these show a correlation of ≥ 0.5 - a satisfactory result. All results except one are significant. We interpret the total result of the individual variables as satisfactory.

We have found that several factors may have influenced the results for the individual variables. For instance a group of healthy subjects shows smaller variations for some of the variables. This may have a negative effect on the correlation.

The time elapsed between the examinations may also affect the body pattern and consequently the correlation.

Each encounter between two individuals is unique. No matter how carefully an assessment procedure has been defined, the meetings with different individuals making the extimates may affect the correlation. We have a strong interest in further studying the significance of the encounter within ROPE.

Regarding the conclusion it turned out that the two physiotherapists have used the newly designed scale differently and the result of IOR was not satisfactory. Anyhow each examiner has used the scale consistently. This indicates that they each had a firm norm for the assessments. This is a positive result for each physiotherapist but negative for the IOR.

The conclusion is an interpretation of findings. Despite the subjectivity it should be possible to develop the conclusion by further structuring and carefully describing the principles for analysis and interpretation.

Our personal experience from this project is that, by comparing one´s ability of assessment with others, one becomes more aware of oneself as an examiner. We consider this an important prerequisite for more accurate assessments. Fox Keller says "Through getting to know the subject, ourselves, we develop our ability to be objektive" (7).

Subjecting oneself and one´s method of examination to scientific scrutiny implies development of the method and of the examiner.

It is difficult but not impossible to study clinical examinations scientifically. The conditions for research and for clinical activities are different, but they are both important and should not be separated.

This project has proved that ROPE has a structure that makes it possible for two examiners to have satisfactory IOR regarding the individual variables when the examinations are made as similar as possible to a clinical situation.

References:

1. Reich W. (1972) Characteranalysis. Tanchstone, N.Y.
2. Bunkan, B (1985) Muskelspenninger og kroppsbilde, Universitets-forlaget, Oslo
3. Hartman, D.P. (1977) Consideration in the choice of interobserver reliability estimates. Journal of Applied Behavior Analysis, 10. 103-116
4. Kazdin, A. (1977) Artifact, bias, and complexity of assessment: The ABC´s of Reliability. Journal of Applied Behavior Analysis, 10. 141-150.
5. Sundsvold, M. (1982) Global fysioterapeutisk muskelundersökelse. Eget förlag, Oslo
6. Öst, L-G. Reliabilitetsmätning vid observationer och skattningar (1979). Nordisk Tidskrift för Beteendeterapi, vol. 8. 133-159
7. Fox Keller, E. (1985) Reflections on gender and science, Yale University Press

PSYCHODYNAMIC BODY THERAPY. THE DEVELOPMENT OF A METHOD IN PSYCHIATRIC/PSYCHOSOMATIC
PHYSIOTHERAPY.

KIRSTEN MONSEN
MELKEVN. 24, 0386, OSLO 3 NORWAY.

PDB integrates a physiotherapeutic and a psychological level of understanding (5). During the
course of treatment interventions are made parallel on a bodily level, through Psychomotor
physiotheraphy (PMT), and on a psychological level through activ psychodynamic psychotherapy.
EMOTIONAL CONFLICT, THE PROBLEMSOLVING APPROACH AND POSTURE.
Within psychodynamic theory, patterns qualities of social individual's relations to himself
(2). The development of habitual behaviour-patterns, postures and traits of character are
understood as a product of specific manners of being together within the family.
Emotional conflicts are understood as a potential drive in the development of new conscios-
ness. This implicates that the individual himself must be able to find real solutions to
contradicitionary and conflict-filled emotional experiences. The ability to solve emotional
conflicts are dependent e.g. on the individuals contact with his emotional experiences, his
ability to recognise and admit to his emotional experiences and to take a conscious choice
of solutions (2).

The human being will also repress and defend himself towards his own information of experiense.
Neurotic traits of character and symptoms are understood as negative problemsolving methods,
where the individual habitually are repressing unpleasant emotions from conscious experience.
Neurotic traits of character do not give a real solution. On the contrary, they protect the
individual against conscious registration of emotions. They also disturb the individuals
vitality and ability to cope in general. The particular approach to problemsolving is
with other words the problem.

W. Reich (6) went thoroughly into how conflictsolving trials and traits of character were
manifested in a paralellel manner on both a physical and psychical level. The body with
its several organsystems will always be a part of such habitual and unreflected ways of
conflictsolving trials. It is therefore reasonably to think that posture, patterns of
respiration, function and evt. other physiological organdistrubances will be a part of an
individual's efforts in problemsolving. Both traits of character, and the bodys total
tensionpatterns, may serve a defensive purpose.

Focus on the therapeutic intervention.
Based on the above postulated connections between posture, emotional conflicts and social
relations, PDB is focused on the following three relations:

1. Relation to ones own body.
2. Relation to emotional experiences.
3. Experiences and actions in relation to important others.

Ad 1. Vitality seen from a bodily point of view means a release of posture, repiration
and function to reach a maximum grade of flexibility. In PMT muscletension and repressed
respiration is released according to biomecanic principles. Each of the body's weight-
bearing segments may act as a fixed base of support for the segments above. The release

will in this manner also have a stabilizing effect. Such a combination of bodily flexibility and stability gives a better basis in tolerating personal emotions. We also know that experiences can get stronger and emotions more obvious when muscletension is released. The emotional content repressed from conscious experience via tense muscles and repressed respiration can get activated. The biomecanical interventions contributes to a release of blocked energy, which also gives the patient a better access to repressed emotional experiences.

Ad 2. To become vitalized on a psycholigical level is achieved through the work on increasing the patient's ability to emotional experience and expressivity (4). With an individuals ability to emotional experience is understood the level of conscious integration of emotional content. Such an integration implies a reasonable high level of attention and tolerance to personal content of emotions. Therapeutic interventions are in the first place conserntrated on the patients attention to personal emotional reactions, and his ability to admit them in relation to himself. The patient must in addition let the emotions affect himself, be moved. In this manner emotional experiences will penetrate easier into consciousness. The content of emotions and particular information from the emotions can now be integrated. The following step is to let the patient try to determine the social relations which the emotions are ment for. When emotional relations are placed in a meaningful context, they can be transferred into ideas, understanding and acceptance. Further-on the patient is encouraghed to express his experiences.

Ad 3. The aim of PDB is to reduse regression and transference. The relationship between the therapist and the patient is not the primarily focus in this treatment. The therapy is directed towards giving the patient a clearer experienced connection between his own body, his emotions and important others outside the therapyroom. Phenomenon such as resistance and transference which is central in all types of therapies, are treated only in the degree it is necessary. More central is increased conscience concerning the patients relationship to his parents and adapted parental picture. It is in relationship to these factor that an individuals basic attitudes to himself and others are made. Through the ability to view his parents more clearly, the patient will also increase his ability to emotional experience. The patient will also get a more open relationship to personal experiences and to other people within his surroundings.

Tecnical aspects:

The bodily methods of intervention (PMT) is descriebed in detail by Berit Bunkan (1). We will briefly look at some psychotherapeutic techniques from active psychdunamic theory: EMPHATIC ABILITY OF UNDERSTANDING, DIRECT INTERVENTION, ACTIVE BUILDING OF HYPOTHESIS, MAKE RESPONSIBLE.

Through the ability of <u>empatic understandin</u> the therapist is trying to discriminate and to articulate precisly and accurate different aspects of the patients experiences. The patient might often not be able to articulate this or is not aware of these aspects. One obvious qualifacation is that the therapist is honest and accepting. <u>Direct intervention</u> means that the patient is given a clear feedback concerning his expressions, regardless if the experience is pleasent or unpleasent. The therapist's directness gives the patient a chance to react. The patient can either confirm or reject the feedback, but he is being forced in an activ manner to relate to what he is expressing himself and to deal with its content. If the patient constantly is avoiding difficult experiences and is rejecting, then therapist activly can introduce certain issues. Insted of getting stuck in this rejecting, the therapist is preparing for an <u>activ guessing</u> and <u>building of hypothesis</u>.

The purpose is to get the process of emotional experience and expression started. The hypothesis is usually formed in such a manner that they simutaneously teaches psychological self—understanding through generalization and knowlegde about psychological connections. With being made responsible is ment to show that the patient himself is always making an active choice regardless if he admits to or represses personal experiences. An emotional "deadmaking" is always something the individual is doing with his own body and ability concerning expression. The purpose is to avoide activation as well as consicious registration of personal emotions.

EFFECTS:

Systematic clinical experience have shown that PDB is a particulary successful method in the treatment of chronic pain-conditions, mild psychosomatic disorders and mild conditions of anxiety and depression. In a successful treatment, the patient have moved from a subconscious way of avoiding emotional conflicts to a conscious way of dealing with them, as well as solving these conflicts. Increased emotional consciousness seem to reduce the tendency to the somatizing of painful emotional experienses. Since the effect of this treatment involves attitude changing both on a physical and psychical level, then the improvement achieved is of a more lasting character.

References:

1. Bunkan, B. (1991): Psychomotor Physiotherapy departs from traditional principles.
2. Horney, K. (1967): Vore indre konflikter. Haase & Søns Forlag, København.
3. Karon, B. & Vandenbos, A. (1981): Psychotherapy of Schizophrenia, Jason Aroson, N.Y.
4. Monsen, J. (1990): Vitalitet, psykiske forstyrrelser og psykoterapi. Tano forlag, Oslo.
6. Reich, W. (1972): Characteranalysis. Tanchstone, N.Y.
5. Monsen, K. (1989): Psykodynamisk Kroppsterapi. Tano, Oslo.

VITALITY IN PSYCHODYNAMIC BODY THERAPY

G Wennerberg, M Weigardh
Department of Physioterapy, Karolinska institutet, Box 60400,
104 01 STOCKHOLM, Sweden

Introduction: Psychodynamic Body Therapy (PBT) is a body psychotherapy which is given by specialist-trained physiotherapists. It is a further development of Norwegian psycho-motoric physiotherapy. What is new is that the physiotherapist is responsible for the psychotherapeutic element as well as the physiotherapeutic. (1) The theoretical background to PBT orginates from the psychoanalysis, particularly W.Reich῀s theories of the close interplay between body and mind. Reich discovered that the human psychological posture had its correspondence in the body. Muscle tensions act as a shield (bodily defence) which inhibits respiration, the production of energy, and vitality. (2)Today the theoretical background has been further developed and influenced by psychodynamic, existential and system theories.(3) In PBT the person is considered as a whole. The treatment is based on anatomical, physiological and psychodynamic principles. It is guided by the patient´s tension patterns, and the whole body is treated each time. Through massage and exercises, respiration flow and locked tension patterns are released. The patient is encouraged to participate actively by feeling his. experiences.

The therapist gives the patient the opportunity to process verbally the experiences and conflict material which are activated in connection with the treatment.

The purpose of PBT is to bring about a bodily and psychological re-adjustment so that vitality increases.

Body vitality implies that respiration can flow freely without interruption from any tense organ, and that it is re-adjustable; that the differnt segments of the body rest in balance whit each other, and that there is an equivalent relationship of tension in the anterior and in the posterior structures. Vitality also implies that the person has a full joint motion range and that joints move freely in relation to each other; and that the person has a homogeneous,flexible, soft and well-toned musculature, and good contact with it. The person should have free bodily functions, i.e. can sigh, yawn, sneeze, belch, have orgasms, etc., without blocking these off with muscular tensions. (1,4).

Psychological vitality implies that a person is able to employ psychological and physical defences when the situation demands, and is able to release these when the danger is over. It means having increased contact with one´s own experiences. Every person has an advanced information system consisting of different forms of experience: Feelings, thoughts,dreams, sense impressions, fantasies and drives. These contain meaningful in-formation and tell the individual about his relationship with himself and his social reality.

All this involves the ability, in one´s daily life to reflect upon, relate to and accept responsibility for one´s problems in a sophisticated way. In PBT we strive to teach patients to be aware of their own feelings and increasingly to accept, and to be able to show, verbally and in body-language, how they feel. (3)

To start the re-adjustment, various massage strokes are used in the treatment. These are divided into two main groups, unprovocative and provocative. The former include effleurage, petrissage and frictions, for stimulating the body and making it more aware. They are also used for calming the patient and apportioning the treatment so that the respiration flow is not released too fast. The provacative strokes consist of pinching tense muscles. The slight pain the pinch causes opens the way for a bodily discharge (e.g. sigh, kick) and an emotional one: It is important that patients express what they feel, both bodily and verbally. The point at which the emotional discharge and the respiratory response coincide brings the greatest physical and psychological re-adjustment. (5)

Aims

Our aims were to study the reactions a patient exhibits during a PBT session, and to try and find signs of vitality (as described above) during the treatment.

Method

We analysed a videorecording of a PBT session. The recording had been made earlier for teaching purposes. The patient was a middle-aged woman who had sought physiotherapeutic help for hypertensive headaches. The session recorded was the thirteenth of thirty. The therapist was a physiotherapist with special training in PBT. We first viewed the whole videotape to gain a general view of its contents and then selected parts we considered relevant for closer analysis. We noted everything the therapist did (massage strokes, etc), the patient's reactions (sighs, kicks, etc), and what the therapist and the patient said. This material was then analysed.

Results and discussion

The therapist treated the whole body in a systematic order (back, left leg and arm, right leg and arm, neck and face), using unprovocative and provocative massage strokes to stimulate the patient to come into contact with her body and her experiences. The patient expressed various reactions during the treatment, most frequently in direct connection with the therapist's provocative message strokes. We observed the following reactions:

Bodily reactions, e.g. sighs, movements, blows and kicks.
Verbal interjections, e.g. ow!, ugh!, oof! and Ahhh!.
Verbal expressions, e.g. Ah, now it's better; I was mostly angry when I kicked out, now I want to cry.
Autonomous reactions e.g. Sobbing, swallowing and vomiting reactions.

We saw how the patient relaxed her muscular respiration blocks by sighing. She expressed her anger clearly with blows and kicks against the couch. Examples from the treatment process were: Patient: "I want to kick (kicks the couch); Oh, now it's better (sighs); I suppose I was a bit angry; I was mainly angry when I kicked". She expressed what she felt with interjections (Ow, ahhh) and how she felt, verbally (Now I want to cry). The vomiting reaction was more frequent than other autonomous reactions. Reich (2) writes that in the vomiting reaction the peristalsis induced in the oesophagus is in the opposite direction to that induced by swallowing in crying or anger. Examples from the treatment process were (vomiting reflex, sticking tongue out) "Now I feel sick. Such a lot of crying. Because that's what I do when I don't want to cry, I get like this in my throat". Considering the whole treatment process in more detail, we could see a clear pattern. In the first part, the therapist gave more provocative massage strokes and the patient showed more bodily reactions than in the second part. From the middle to the end, the therapist intervened more verbally, and the patient increasingly gave verbal expression to feelings and experience. During the whole treatment there was a dialogue in which we could see the therapist prodding and encouraging the patient in her experiences and reactions. Our interpretation is that the therapist, through massage strokes and manner, helped the patient to get into contact with her feelings and experiences via her body, so that she could later process her problems.

We interpret the fact that the patient, during the treatment, gives bodily, emotional and verbal expression to how she feels to mean that she is starting to get contact with her vitality (as described by us) and that a process of re-adjustment has started.

What we belive to be unique in this treatment method compared with other phsyiotherapy methods is that the therapist systematically treats the whole body at each session, and actively encourages the patient to release bodily functions and to express his feelings verbally.

We consider video analysis a good complement for scrutinizing what happens during bodily therapy, as a way of evaluating both the treatment given and the treatment process over time. Using this method of observation, we hope to be able to find and further develop more reliable measurement methods for evaluating the results of treatment. This requires that more patient sessions are analysed and that more people analyse the same session independently of each other.

We believe it is possible to increase vitality and improve health with PBT. We wonder whether it is possible to reverse pathogenic processes with PBT, and hope to be able to investigate this in further research.

References

1. Monsen, K., 1989. Psykodynamisk kroppsterapi (Psychodynamic Body Therapy), Tano forlag, Oslo.

2. Reich, W., 1972. Character Analysis. Simon & Schuster, New York.

3. Monsen., J, 1990. Vitalitet, psykiske forstyrrelser og psykoterapi (Vitality, Psychological disorders and Psychotherapy), Tano forlag, Oslo.

4. Bunkan Heir, B., 1985. Muskelspenninger og kroppsbilde (Muscle Tensions and body image. University Press, Oslo.

5. Bunkan Heir, B., Radoy, L. and Thornqvist, E, 1982. Psykomotorisk behandling (Psychomotoric Treatment). University Press, Oslo.

ACUPUNCTURE TREATMENT IN EPICONDYLALGIA
A comparative study of two acupuncture technique

Eva Haker, RPT and Thomas Lundeberg MD, PhD
Department of Physiology II, Karolinska Institutet, 104 01 Stockholm, Sweden

Tennis elbow or lateral humeral epicondylalgia [1,2] is a painful condition at the lateral aspect of the elbow. There is no general agreement about the etiology but it appears to be multifactorial in origin, and the clinical picture is often fairly uniform [1-3].

Few studies have investigated different acupuncture techniques [4,5]. In 1983 MacDonald suggested that superficial needle insertion might be as effective as classical acupuncture when treating low back pain [4]. In a recent study it was shown that the pain-relieving effect of classical acupuncture was superior to that of superficial acupuncture when treating patients suffering from head and neck pain of varying origins [5].

The purpose of this study was to compare the pain-alleviating effect of two acupuncture techniques in patients suffering from lateral epicondylalgia: *(a) classical "deep" acupuncture*, in which the needles are inserted and manipulated to evoke the sensation of *Teh Chi*, and *(b) superficial needle insertion*, where the needles are merely inserted subcutaneously with no sensation of *Teh Chi*.

PATIENTS and METHODS
Patients included in the study were those who experienced pain over the lateral epicondyle, produced by two or more of the following four tests and a duration of pain of at least 1 month. The diagnostic criteria were as follows: *(1) Palpation of the lateral epicondyle. (2) Resisted wrist extension. (3) Passive stretching of the extensor muscles of the forearm. (4) Resisted finger extension.* Resistance applied on digiti III = *Middle finger test*.

Those excluded were patients demonstrating (a) dysfunction in the shoulder, neck and/or thoracal region; (b) local arthritis, generalized polyarthritis; (c) neurological abnormalities; and (d) radial nerve entrapment [6].

Details were reported of profession, work load, affected and domonant arm, cause, involvement in monotonous and repetitive movements and previous treatment.

All the patients were informed that two different acupuncture techniques were to be tried out and that no fee was to be charged. They were also instructed to " use the arm but avoid painful movements."

Method of assignment
Consecutive cases were randomly assigned to 2 groups.

Group A: 44 patients (28 men and 16 women) with a mean age of 47.5 years (25-68) and a median duration of pain of 7 months (1-60).

Group B: 38 patients (24 men and 14 women) with a mean age of 46.3 years (28-70) and a median duration of pain of 10 months (1-120).

Method of treatment
Group A. Acupuncture needles were inserted at 5 sites corresponding to traditional Chinese acupuncture points related to the elbow [7].

The points used were: LI 10, 11, 12, Lu 5, and SJ 5. All the points are partly innervated by the radial nerve.

The needles were inserted and rotated to elicit the sensation of **Teh Chi**. The sensation of **Teh Chi** was elicited every 5 min during a 20 min period.

Group B received superficial needle insertion. The needles were merely inserted subcutaneously at the same points as used in group A and left there for twenty minutes. The **Teh Chi** was not obtained.

The patients were treated two to three times weekly, 10 treatments in all (one course) [7]. Follow-ups were done at the end of the treatment, after 3 and 12 months.

Method of evaluation

In addition to the four diagnostic criteria *(tests 1-4)*, the patients were evaluated in another 4 tests.

Test 5 and 6. The patients were tested as to whether pain could be produced at the lateral aspect of the epicondyle by isometric pronation and supination of the forearm.

Test 7. The Vigorimeter test. Grip strength can be measured by a vigorimeter. Thorngren and Werner (1979) used the Martin vigorimeter to determine the ratio dominant/non-dominant hand to $1.07 + 0.11$ [8]. According to this result the value of the unaffected arm can serve as a parameter in evaluating the pain-free grip strength. Consequently, we used the Martin vigorimeter to measure grip strength in the unaffected arm, and the pain threshold when gripping in the affected arm.

Test 8. Lifting test. Sitting in the position described above, the patient was also required to lift four different weights 1, 2, 3, and 4 kg, and pain over the epicondyle was recorded as present or absent.

All the tests were performed bilaterally.

After the tenth treatment and at the follow-ups all the eight clinical tests were repeated, and moreover, a subjective assessment completed the clinical examination. A scale of 1-5 was shown to the patients (1, excellent; 2, good; 3, improved; 4, slightly improved; 5, unchanged/worse) and they were asked "How do you assess your pain today compared to the pre-treatment condition?" The patient indicated and described the parameter that most adequately reflected his or her present condition.

Statistical analysis.

Correlation analysis, the Mann-Whitney U test of two independent samples, and chi-square test were used for the statistical analysis.

RESULT

Eighty-two patients completed the study and they had all a similat pre-treatment condition.

Subjective outcome

After the tenth treatment, 22 patients of the 44 in group A and eight of the 38 in group B reported excellent or good results (1-2 on the scale). Seventeen patients in each group reported an improvement (3 on the scale), whereas five in group A and 13 in group B reported slight improvement or unchanged or worse condition (5 on the scale). A comparison between the groups showed a significant difference ($p < 0.01$).

No statistical differences between the groups were found at the 3 month or 1 year follow-up

Objective outcome (Evaluation of the Vigorimeter test)

The pain threshold on gripping (see Methods) was noted before and after the ten treatments and at the follow-ups. The post-treatment values were compared with those obtained at the pre-treatment evaluation and then the median values of the differences were calculated.

After 10 treatments, the pain threshold on gripping the balloon had significantly increased in group A compared with group B ($p < 0.05$). No significant differences were observed at the follow-ups.

Considering the effect of previous treatment on the outcome, neither the steroid injections nor any other of the previous treatments had a correlation to the result.

Finally, no correlation between the subjective outcome or the vigorimeter test on one hand and the pre-duration of pain on the other could be detected. No side-effects were reported during or after the treatment period.

DISCUSSION

In this study we have shown that patients treated with classical "deep" acupuncture reported significantly less pain after 10 treatments than those treated with superficial needle insertion (subjective outcome); the classical acupuncture group had also significantly increased pain-free grip strength.

The patients in both groups reported further reduction of pain during the follow-up period. However, the difference between the groups was not significant.

The pre-treatment condition was similar in both groups, and for that reason the improvement seen in the two groups after 3 and 12 months, probably reflects the spontaneous recovery known to occur. However, explanation of the difference after 10 treatments requires reference to classical acupuncture procedure and/or the placebo effect. Pain alleviation obtained with acupuncture is generally attributed to activation of spinal and central pain inhibitory mechanisms [8-12]. In provoking the sensation of *Teh Chi* during classical acupuncture, a larger number and possibly a different set of receptors are activated compared to superficial needle insertion. By this means classical acupuncture produces more powerful activation of pain inhibitory systems, and the efficacy may depend on the intensity of "Teh Chi" [8].

The placebo effect must be considered, and, for that reason, it is reasonable to assume that the differences seen between the groups are related to a combination of the placebo effect and the therapeutic effects of classical deep acupuncture.

The result of the present study shows that, even if there was no difference between the groups at the follow-ups, classical deep acupuncture is superior to superficial needle insertion in the short-term symptomatic treatment of lateral epicondylalgia. As no correlation was found between the pre-duration of pain (1-120 months) and the result, classical deep acupuncture can be recommended as well for acute as for chronic pain.

REFERENCES.
1. Goldie I. Epicondylitis lateralis humeri. A pathogenetical study. Acta chir scand suppl 339 1964;339:1-119.
2. Coonrad RW. Tennis elbow. Instr Course Lect, Am Acad Orthop Surg 1986;35:94-101.
3. Wadsworth TG. Tennis elbow: conservative, surgical and manipulative treatment. Br Med J 1987;294:621-624.
4. MacDonald AJR, Macrae KD, Master BR, Rubin AP. Superficial acupuncture in the relief of cronic low back pain. Ann R Coll Surg Engl 1983:44-46.
5. Lundeberg T, Hurtig T, Lundeberg S, Thomas M. Long-term results of acupuncture in chronic head and neck pain. The Pain Clinic 1988;2:15-31.
6.Morrison DL. Tennis elbow and radial tunnel syndrome. Differential diagnosis and treatment, J AOA 1981;80:823-826.
7. Essentials of Chinese Acupuncture. Foreign Languages Press, Beijing, China, 1980.
8.Thorngren K-G, Werner CO.Normal grip strength. Acta orthop scand 1979;50:255-259.
9. Chiang C-Y, Chang C-T, Chu H-L, Yang L-F. Peripheral afferent pathway for acupuncture analgesia. Sci sin 1973;XVI:210-217.
10. Chang H-T. Neurophysiological basis of acupuncture analgesia. Sci sin 1978;21:829-846.
11.Melzack R. How acupuncture can block pain, Impact of Science on Society 1973;23:65-75.5.
12.Melzack R, Wall PD. Pain mechanisms: A new theory. Science 1965;150:971-979.5.

A SINGLE BLIND PLACEBO CONTROLLED STUDY OF THE EFFECTS OF ACUPUNCTURE AND TRANSCUTANEOUS ELECTRICAL NERVE STIMULATION ON THE PAIN OF MSELENI JOINT DISEASE.

C.A. Liggins
Departments of Physiotherapy, University of Durban-Westville and King Edward VIII Hospital, Durban, South Africa.

INTRODUCTION

Mseleni joint disease (MJD) is an endemic, crippling and multi-joint arthropathy of unknown aetiology. It causes joint pain and joint destruction mainly in the hips and knees but it may also affect the shoulders, ankles and spine. The disease affects the Black population around the Mseleni and Manguzi areas of northern Kwa Zulu, South Africa.

The disease was first described in the medical literature in 1970[1] . The locals attribute the disease to bewitchment and DDT spraying for malaria control. Current research is examining the possibility of a genetic cause for the disease as well as nutritional causes, including trace element deficiencies[2]. Trace element deficiencies, diet and traditional eating patterns may be factors in a unique, unknown environmental combination which causes the disease.

After studying radiographic evidence, Soloman et al[3] proposed that there are two major disease processes occurring in MJD, namely multiple epiphyseal dysplasia (MED) and a polyarticular osteoarthritis (POA). It has been suggested that MED may be inherited but the aetiology of POA remains obscure.

A survey carried out in 1982 indicated that the overall incidence of MJD was 16,8 per cent of the population. Women constituted the largest number of sufferers with a ratio of 5:1. It has been estimated that there are up to 3 000 persons, in the two areas concerned, who currently have the disease.

CLINICAL FEATURES

Pain is a major feature of MJD and this is the earliest symptom, the hip joints being particularly affected. This is followed by a progressive stiffening of joints with accompanying loss of range of motion.

CONVENTIONAL MANAGEMENT

Medical management consists of analgesics and surgery, a number of sufferers having had total hip replacements. Physiotherapeutic measures include regimens for relieving pain and maintaining mobility.

MERIDIAN THERAPY

This study was initiated after the results of a preliminary, uncontrolled, study had suggested that acupuncture and transcutaneous electrical nerve stimulation (TENS) may be effective in treatment of the pain of MJD.

In the first study the treatment by meridian therapy was directed specifically to the hip. However several patients in both groups reported that they had also obtained relief in other affected joints during the treatment. This led the author to consider the effects of acupuncture and TENS on the overall joint pain of MJD and to compare the results of two treatment groups (acupuncture and TENS) with a control group receiving placebo "therapy". The second study was carried out at the Mseleni Hospital and was designed to test the hypothesis that meridian therapy, using needle acupuncture and TENS applied to acupuncture points, is a more effective form of intervention than placebo for relief of joint pain in MJD.

METHODS

Thirty three patients with a diagnosis of MJD and who gave informed consent, were randomly assigned to one of three groups viz: acupuncture, TENS and placebo. Subjects in all three groups were assessed for pain and tenderness by an independent operator who was not aware of which treatment the subject was to receive. The Simple Descriptive Scale (No Pain - Mild - Moderate - Severe - Very Severe) was used for rating pain intensity and a record was made of all joints where pain was present. The acupuncture procedure consisted of the insertion of stainless steel needles into points GB 30 (7,5 cm), GB 29 (3.75 cm) and GB 34 (2,5 cm). Needles were left in situ for 20 minutes and were given vigorous manual stimulation at five minute intervals. On removal of the needles the pain was re-assessed. Subjects in the TENS group were treated with a dual channel stimulator using silicone rubber electrodes placed bilaterally on points GB 29 and GB 30. Stimulation was given for 30 minutes using the low frequency (2 Hz), high intensity method. Pain intensity was measured pre and post treatment using the same scale as for the acupuncture group. Patients in the placebo group were connected to a de-activated TENS unit (identical to the unit used for the definitive TENS group but adapted so that no current would pass to the electrodes). Before commencing, the subjects in this group were told that they may or may not feel stimulation under the electrodes which were positioned over the same acupuncture points as those of the definitive TENS group. On the termination of treatment all patients were re-assessed by the independent operator who was not told which treatment the subject had received.

RESULTS

In this study 33 subjects (30 female and three male) were assigned to one of three groups (11 in each group) and the pre and post treatment scores are shown in figures 1, 2 and 3. As all subjects had pain in joints other than the hip joint on assessment, the scores are shown as an average for all the affected joints. The data were analysed using the Wilcoxon signed rank test in the Oxstat computer programme.

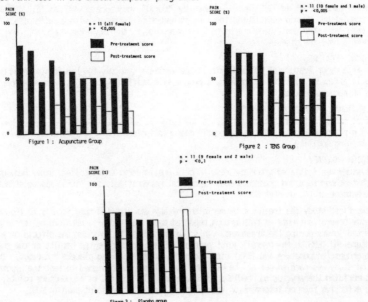

Figure 1 : Acupuncture Group

Figure 2 : TENS Group

Figure 3 : Placebo group

DISCUSSION

Although MJD causes gross deformity and disability the patients major complaint is pain which is mainly located around the hip joints, though other joints are also affected. Patients are given simple analgesics, but these tend to give only short lasting or minimal pain relief. A small number of patients have had total hip replacement surgery (80 replacements on 50 patients). It was with these factors in mind that the author decided on a meridian therapy approach to the pain of MJD. This approach is relatively simple to carry out and is extremely cost effective.

A noteworthy point, which emerged at follow-up treatment sessions after the first study, was that most patients in the acupuncture group indicated that they had experienced sustained relief (ranging from a few days to six weeks) after the initial treatment. A number of patients in both groups also reported relief of pain in joints other than the hip joints.

The second study was carried out at the Mseleni Hospital which is a considerable distance from the area (Manguzi Hospital) where the first study was conducted. This was done to eliminate the procedures of the first study being communicated to potential candidates. The results reported here are from the initial treatment sessions.

In the acupuncture group three subjects were rendered pain-free, seven had a reduction of pain of 50 per cent or more and in one subject there was no change. The overall improvement in this group was 72 per cent. In the TENS group one subject was rendered pain-free, seven had an improvement of 50 per cent or more, two had an improvement of less than 50 per cent and in one subject there was no change. The overall improvement in this group was 51 per cent. In the placebo group one subject was rendered pain-free, one had an improvement of more than 50 per cent, five had an improvement of less than 50 per cent, three were unchanged and one was worse. The overall improvement in this group was only 20 per cent.

An analysis of the data obtained from the pre and post treatment scores of each treatment regimen showed the following levels of significance: acupuncture: $p = <0,005$, TENS: $p = <0,005$, and placebo: $p = <0,1$. Thus the hypothesis was proved valid.

CONCLUSIONS

Although MJD is a relatively rare disease the sufferers have a real problem with the management of their pain. This study has shown that meridian therapy, using needle acupuncture and TENS on classical acupuncture points, may be a useful adjunct to conventional treatment. Although it may not be convenient to give needle acupuncture or TENS to patients in remote areas situated away from hospitals, it is considered that another variant of meridian therapy, namely acupressure, could be given to these patients. Consequently simple acupressure techniques are now being taught to community rehabilitation workers who live among the patients with MJD and the efficacy of acupressure on the pain of MJD is the subject of a current study.

REFERENCES

1. Wittman W and Fellingham SA. (1970). Unusual hip disease in remote part of Zululand. Lancet 1:842-843.

2. Fincham JE, van Rensburg SJ and Marasas WF. (1981). Mseleni joint disease-a manganese deficiency? S Afr. Med. J. 60; 445-447.

3. Solomon L et al (1986). Distinct types of hip disorder in Mseleni joint disease. S. Afr. Med. J. 69: 15-17.

CHRONIC PAIN AS A REFLECTION OF POST-TRAUMATIC STRESS
DISORDER

C J Manheim and D K Lavett, 12 C Carriage Lane, Charleston,
South Carolina, 29407, USA

Chronic pain patients are described as experiencing
depression, confusion, impaired concentration, alcohol and
drug abuse, nightmares, phobias, excessive dwelling on the
cause of their pain, restriction of sexuality, restriction
of activities, a sense of hopelessness and helplessness (1),
and flashbacks (2). Patients with post-traumatic stress
disorder are described as experiencing depression,
confusion, impaired concentration, alcohol and drug abuse,
nightmares, phobias, restriction of activities, sexual
dysfunction, a sense of hopelessness and helplessness,
flashbacks, chronic anxiety, somatization, amnesia for some
life events, and emotional numbness alternating with extreme
emotional sensitivity (3). The diagnosis of chronic pain is
made when the individual has complained of pain for six
months or longer. Post-traumatic stress disorder is
diagnosed after one month of symptoms. The diagnostic
criteria for post-traumatic stress disorder specifies that
the person must have experienced an event that is outside
the range of usual human experience and would be markedly
distressing to almost anyone (4). We contend that being in
an automobile accident, falling from a height, being hit by
an object or another person, being sexually and/or
physically abused or fearing being killed are all adequate
situations to cause both chronic pain and/or post-traumatic
stress disorder. These similarities suggest that some
chronic pain patients are also suffering from post-traumatic
stress disorder.

Fifty-four patients who had not responded to traditional
physical therapy treatments for complaints of chronic pain
were treated with myofascial release (5) and craniosacral
therapy (6). Myofascial release is an interactive stretching
technique that relies on feedback from the patient's body to
determine the direction, the duration and the intensity of
the stretch. This feedback is gained by the therapist
creating a kinesthetic link with the patient through touch.
This link includes matching the rate and rhythm of
respiration, the underlying neurophysiologic tone and the
more overt muscle tone. By matching these inherent tissue
responses, the therapist is able to detect and treat even
subtle restrictions in motion within a myofascial unit.
Craniosacral therapy focuses on decreasing tension on the

nervous system by movement of the cranial bones, the sacrum and the dural tube. Physically facilitated abreactions were experienced by each patient during the course of treatment.

Abreactions, first described by Freud (7), consist of the recall to consciousness of a repressed memory and the appropriate expression of the repressed emotions connected to that memory. When the restriction in the myofascial unit is due to an injury, repositioning that segment in the same position in which the injury occurred may bring back a body memory of the injury. If conscious memory of the injury exists, the patient will recount the injury in detail, being able to recall the circumstances and feelings around the injury. When maximum myofascial tension is achieved in the position of injury, a profound relaxation will occur, removing the residual restriction from that injury. When no conscious memory exists, this body memory may return in its entirety or may return in disjointed fragments of memory. The body memory may be accompanied by unexpressed emotions or may be totally devoid of emotion, indicating a dissociated state of consciousness. The physically induced abreactions are experienced as flashbacks. Flashbacks are a vivid reexperiencing of traumatic events during which a person temporarily cannot distinguish the past from the present. Once an abreaction is completed, the pain associated with that incident also disappears. If the memory returns as a fully defined event complete with all visual details, sounds, smells, and sensations, the person needs only one reexperiencing for pain relief. If, however, only memory fragments are available, then reexperiencing coupled with hypnotic time and age regression is needed to unite the fragments into a completed whole.

Reexperiencing the memory in part or in totality without change results in reinforcing the trauma memory by minimal muscle contraction as the body recreates the movements made during injury. Just as mental rehearsal of movement can improve athletic performance, mental reliving of trauma can reinforce the trauma. Thus, some aspect of the revivification must be changed to remove the pain memory. Permitting or encouraging the patient to fight back while giving strong resistance gives the patient both the mastery over the situation and the maximal muscle contraction needed to release the excess tension. Hypnotic suggestion may be used to make the patient's limbs very heavy when fighting back is needed to create the needed resistance. Permitting and encouraging the verbal expression of anger, pain, hurt and terror is needed when the patient was threatened with greater harm if these noises were made. Physical contact with and physical comforting from the therapist is the final ingredient which will change the outcome of the reexperiencing for the patient.

Both myofascial release and craniosacral therapy can be learned as mechanical techniques, but the therapist who

wishes to use physically facilitated abreactions for the
treatment of chronic pain patients must also have extensive
training in psychology and counseling. Physically
facilitated abreactions aid in the recovery of memory and of
emotions, psychological counseling is needed for the patient
to integrate this knowledge into present reality and to stop
these past events from effecting current behavior.

The first author has found in her practice of physical
therapy that physical and/or sexual abuse in childhood often
results in a chronic pain complaint in adulthood.

1. Osterweis M, (1987) Pain and Disability. Washington, DC,
National Academy Press.

2. Webber TD (1973) Diagnosis and modification of headache
and shoulder—arm—hand syndrome. Journal of the American
Osteopathic Association 72:697–710.

3. Manheim CJ, Lavett DK (1989) Craniosacral Therapy and
Somato—emotional Release: The Self—healing Body. Thorofare,
NJ, Slack Incorporated.

4. American Psychiatric Association (1980). Diagnostic and
statistical manual of mental disorders. (3rd edition).
Washington, DC, American Psychiatric Association.

5. Manheim CJ, Lavett DK (1989) The Myofascial Release
Manual. Thorofare, NJ, Slack Incorporated.

6. Upledger JE, Vredevoogd, JD (1983) Craniosacral Therapy.
Seattle, WA, Eastland Press.

7. Freud S (1961) The Standard Edition of the Complete
Psychological Works. Vol 3. Trans. from German, Strachey J
(ed) London, England, Early Psycho—Analytic Publications.

POINT PERCUSSION THERPAPY

S.I.VINCENT, A.D. BOOTH
NEUROLOGICAL REHABILITATION GROUP PTY LTD
MELBOURNE, AUSTRALIA

Point Percussion Therapy is a manual therapy with its origins in Traditional Chinese Medicine. Its developement has been strongly influenced by Western orthopaedic knowledge, and so it is deliberate blending of Eastern and Western approaches to physical limitation.

Point Percussion Therapy is effective in conditions where there is pain and/or stiffness due to acute or chronic soft tissue damage, where there is a change in muscle tone, reduced circulation, or where there is central nervous system damage leading to movement or sensory disorders, and changes in levels of brain arousal.

This is a potent technique and the contraindications for its use are (1):

1. Haemorrhagic conditions : e.g. haemophila, allergic purpura, haemorrhagic purpura, warfarinisation.
2. Cardiovascular diseases, tuberculosis, malignant tumours.
3. Acute conditions, such as acute stages of pyogenic arthritis, acute infective diseases.
4. Severe dermal conditions.
5. Orthopaedic conditions, e.e. osteoporosis, hips at risk of dislocating.

The particular combination of techniques used had been pioneered in a remote area of China by a local healer and his son Li-hui . Professor Wang Zhao-pu and collagues from the Academy of Traditional Chinese Medicine in Beijing studied this method in 1983 eventually specialising in its use in treating cerebral palsied children.

STIMULATION LINES AND POINTS:

As With accupuncture, Point Percussion Therapy uses a framework of lines and points on the body which are stimulated to effect physical change. There are approximately 100 points used in this method, most of which correspond to standard acupuncture points. Some are derived from pressure points used in martial arts. Trigger points are also used. The 16 stimualtion lines of Point Percussion are closely related to the meridians of accpuncture.

TECHNIQUES:

1. Percussion is performed along stimulation lines over the trunk and lkimbs, using the tips of either one, three or all five fingers. The force of percussion ican be varied between light and medium and strong.

The intensity of percussion depends on: 1. the symptom being treated
2. the size of the part being treated
3. the tolerance of the patient to treatment
4. the anticipated effects of treatment.

Indications for percussion are: 1. Hypertonicity
2. Hypotonicity
3. Pain
4. Sensory disturbance
5. Decreased level of alertness
6. To achieve relaxation

2. Pressing is applied to points on the trunk, head and limbs using the tip of the thumb. The thumb is moved down, side to side and in a small circle over the point, taking care not to let the thumb slide across the skin. A'chi and trigger points are also treated in this way.

Selection of points depends on the symtptoms being treated and the treatment priorities. There are some sets of points for specific problems, e.g. drooling and epilepsy.

Stimualtion of points can: 1. stimulate motor function
2. stimulate function of the viscera and nervous system
3. release muscular tightness
4. relieve pain

3. Pinching uses the thumb and index finger on opposite sides of the patients fingers and toes stimulate martial arts points. "Snapping", a rapid traction applied to each digit is an effective technique for quickly reducing flexor tone.

4. Knocking consists of tapping the head or any body point with the tips of the fingers loosely spread. This is used ofr general stimulation.

5. Clapping with the palm of the hand to the head or back is used to relieve the patients reaction to the treatment or to relieve muscle spasm.

6. Grabbing with finger and thumb along the line of individual muscle bellies and tendons stimulates contraction of those muscles.

7. A Kneading action similar to petrissage is sometimes used to aid muscle relaxation.

8. Three finger massage involves dragging the 3 central digits along the muscle belly in the direction of the fibres.

9. Mobilisation of muscles and peripheral joints (called Supplementary Manipulations by Professor Wang) is achieved by passive stretching techniques and passive movement through joint range.
10. Manipulations are used to treat some foot and back problems.

11. Splinting   Commonly used splints include resting back slabs to maintain knee extension and the plantigrade ankle position, a "frog" splint to maintain hip abduction and external rotation, and a lively hand splint to maintain maximum wrist and finger extension.

12. Exercise is prescribed for both orthopaedic and neurological conditions to strength and re-educate muscles. The authors have found that motor skils learning theroy combines will with the return of muscle function stimulated by Point Percussion Therapy.

PHYSIOLOGICAL EFFECTS:
Results of research conducted in China (2), suggest that physiological effects include:
1. increased conduction speed of the sensory evoked potential;
2. improved circulation through decreased peripheral resistance of blood vessels, decreased diastolic pressure, decreased viscosity of the blood; and
3. increased presence of immunological bodies in the blood.

CLINICAL EFFECTS
1. Range of Movement : In the majority of cases significant increases in passive range have been achieved more quickly than with other techniques available. In one case, a 7 year old child with spastic quadriplegia was due to have a femeral osteotomy with severe pain in his left hip and apparent shotening of 3 inches. After 10 treatments over 3 weeks, his legs were level, and the pain reduced to a point where he was easy to handle.
2. Tone seems to be normalised in cases where it has been either increased or decreased. One 7 month old cerebral palsied child had fixed neck rotation to the left, flexed and retracted arms and adducted and extended legs, with virtually no active movement due to increased tone. After 15 treatments over 4 weeks she was able to kick both legs, had begun to demonstrate isolated eversion in one of her feet, and could turn her head away from the left.
3. Sensation : A 49 year old man who had suffered a head injury 10 years earlier had no propriocetion in his thumb, fingers , wrist and elbow, with 80% accuracy in his shoulder when initally tested. After 18 sessions over 4 months, retesting revealed 50 % accuracy in his thumb, awareness of movement in his index finger but inability to identify direction, wrist 25%, elbow 100%, shoulder 100%. Fifteen months after initial testing, he had 50 % thumb, 75% wrist, elbow and shoulder remained good. Finger agnosia persisted. These changes were accompanied by increased functional use.
4. Pain : Uncontrolled pain affecting the uper limb of a 36 year old farmer who had had a head injury 5 years earlier was sever enough to stop him working. Point Percussion Therapy achieved some pain relief in the first session, which increased over the next fortnight of intensive therapy. Long term follow-up was impossible. Pain was thought to be due to ischaemia resulting from v=severe muscle spasm.
A 54 year old typist and mandolin player was treated once for tennis elbow, which she had had bilaterally for 18 months, during which time she had received conventional physiotherapy. She reported that the problem became negligible in the less severely affected arm, with the other arm initially improving, but regressing when follow-up treatment could not be carried out.
5. Brain arousal : One 7 month old child with hypsarrhythmia was being treated for increased tone and limited range of movement. Points for epilepsy were included in her treatment and she was also receiving medication to control her epilepsy. Medication continued during a break from Point Percussion Therapy, but fitting became more frequent. Treatment resumed and after 1 week her epilepsy was again under control.

SUMMARY

Point Percussion Therapy complements other forms of physiotherpay, especially those which are exercise – based. There is a minimum requirement for equipment, and some of the techniques can be self-administered or carried out by family or helpers.

REFERENCES:
1. Wang 2, (to be published 1991) Accupressure Therpay: Point Persuccion Treatment for Cerebral Birth Injury, Brain Injury and Stroke. Churchill Livingstone.
2. Dixon. S. (1989) Accupiont Percussion Therpay : A Report Submitted to the Spastic Society of Victora.

APPLIED KINESIOLOGY AND REACTIVE MUSCLES

ROALD   AASBOE

Applied Kinesiology (A.K.) was primary developed by
Dr. George Goodheart,U.S.A.,in the 1960's, and has expanded
to become a very thorough system of functional evaluation of
the body and minds balance. A.K. takes care of the physical,
psychological,chemical,thermical,electromagnetical balance etc.,
and is - according to western authors of acupuncture- what
makes acupuncture understandable to people in the western world.
Dr. George Goodheart found a connection between certain muscles
in the body and inner organs,which corresponds with acupuncture
and its laws about yin & yang,energetic balance between inner
organs,etc.
A.K. is based on the fact that body language never lies.Manual
muscle testing as found in the works of Kendall,Kendall and
Wadsworth,remains the primary diagnostic tool in A.K. It
is an indicator of body language and it increases the practicio-
ners ability to observe the body and minds function and change.
This opportunity touse the body as an instrument of laboratory
analysis, is unique in modern therapeutics,because the response
is unerring.
By mastering the techniques of A.K.,the health professionals
will gain extra dimensions in working with health problems.
And with the proper approach, a correct "diagnosis" can be
made, and the body and mind's response is adequate and very
satisfactory to both the therapist and the patient.
Using A.K. is how the healer within is awakened to
heal himself in a sure,practical,reasonable and observable
way. And physiotherapists are the very most suitable group
of health practitioners to work with these techniques.
A REACTIVE MUSCLE is one which only tests weak immidiately after another muscle has been contracted. The muscle
which tests weak, is known as the "reactive muscle", and
the initial muscle as the primary one. The weakening of the
reactive muscle is almost always due to improper signalling
from the neuromuscular spindle cells, or possibly the Golgi
tendon apparatus, of the primary muscle. When there is activation of the primary muscle, the Ia afferent impulses cause
an overabundant inhibition of an antagonist,synergist or
other muscles through inhibitory interneurons.
Triano & Davis studied the "reactive muscle phenomenon"
with electromyography, and the CYBEX II has also been used
for monitoring strength and energetic level.

REACTIVE MUSCLES are found by analyzing the patients problem, and can be present in any structural condition,mostly after traumas such as sports injurys,car accidents (Whip-lash),and people constantly turning their ankles. In Parkinsons Disease and Multiple Sclerosis a reactive pattern is also very often found.
One has to analyze the muscles that are working during a certain activity, and then have the patient contract a muscle, and immidiately afterwards test the muscle(s) which act(s) sequentially. A positive reactive test is when both or more muscles test strong in the clear, but test weak straigth after the primary muscle contracts.

A REACTIVE PATTERN may occur between upper and lower contralateral extremity muscles which have a comparable function in gait. For example muscles in the right shoulder and left hip or vice versa, because of an involvement on the basis of crossreciprocal innervation. Also suspect possible reactive muscle patterns whenever a person exercises regularly, but still is unable to "tone up" certain muscles. This is very often the case in those who are doing their "situps" faithfully, yet are unable to get rid of their "love handles".

THE TREATMENT is nearly always directed to dysfunctioning neuromuscular spindle cells in the primary muscle. This is done by locating those and manipulate the two ends of the spindle cells toward each other to "set down" their activity. Once after the treatment, which is done with very light pressure,- the reactive muscle(s) should test normal. Occasionally, evaluation of the Golgi tendon organs is necessary to achieve a desirable result.

THE BENEFITS from REACTIVE MUSCLE REPATTERNING are release of major energy blockages as well as a better balanced muscle tone and coordination. Other benefits are remarkable recoveries from sports injuries,stroke,scoliosis,improved postural balance,flexibility and mobility, improved vision and athletic performance,release from neck,upper and lower back ache as well as headache and migraine.

This particular approach to REACTIVE MUSCLES makes it possible to reset several sets of muscles with little or no additional trauma, and is extremely beneficial in difficult cases where everything else has been tried.

REFERENCES:

1. GOODHEART,George J.jr.: "Reactive muscle testing",
        Chiro Econ,Vol.21.,No.4.(Jan/Feb. 1979).
2. HAGBARTH,K.E.;"Exitatory and inhibitory skin areas for
        flexor and extensor motoneurons".
        Acta Physiol. Scand.,Vol. 26,Supp 94(1952).
3. HAGBARTH,K.E.;"Spinal withdrawal reflexes in the human
        lower limbs" J. Neurosurg.Psych.
        Vol. 23. (1960).
4. TRIANO,J.& DAVIS,B.P.;"Reactive muscles; Reciprocal and
        cross-reciprocal innervation phenomenon".
        Proceedings of 7th Biomechanic Conference
        on the Spine, University of Colorado at
        Boulder,(1976).
5. WALTHER,David S.;Reactive Muscles,;Applied Kinesiology,
        Synopsis,(1988).

EVALUATING EFFECT OF PSYCHOMOTORIC PHYSIOTHERAPY

A. L. Vangen, leading physiotherapist
Hauger Private Physical Practice, Bærum, Norway

INTRODUCTION
    Little reseach has been done with regard to the effect of
treatment within physiotherapy. Standardized examination methods are a necessity for the provision of a good treatment programme for the patient. In order to adjust the therapy during
its course it is important to be able to measure any changes
in status. The GLobal Physiotherapeutic Muscle method-72
(GPM-72) which is developed and standardized by Marit Østbye
Sundsvold fills this condition.(1,2,3,4.) The GPM-72 is a
valid and reliable examination of muscular deviation of the
entire body.
    Sundsvold et al.(5) showed in a case history how the GPM-
method gave a better evaluation of treatment effect than that
made by the staff. Vangen (6) found in a project A that patients with muscular tension related conditions had the best
effect of Psycho-Motoric Physiotherapy when their total GPM-
72 sumscore was less than 65. The effect of treatment was far
less for those patients with total GPM-72 sumscore equal and
higher than 65.
    In this project B, one wished to find out if patients with
the highest total GPM-72 sumscore would achive a better outcome than in project A, through a more systematic regulated
therapy, adjusted systematically during the treatment period.
MATERIAL AND METHODS
    The material consisted of 27 pasients.
Diagnoses: 6 nevroses, 9 myalgia generalis and tenseness, 1
vertigo, 5 fibroses and 6 myalgia nuchae.
    Patients were examined by the GPM-72 method, which con-
sists of 72 variables evaluating posture, respiration, movements and palpation of musculature and skin. All the 72 examinations are well described and judged by a predefined 15-
steps numerical scale. The results add up to the total GPM-72
sumscore for each person, which correlates with the degree of
problems/psychopathology.(7). An interview of social functioning of the patient is also part of the GPM-72 method. The process and the effect of treatment can be measured by the
difference in the total GPM-72 sumscore at the beginning, during and at the end of treatment. The 27 patients were treated
by Psycho-Motoric Physiotherapy (PMP), which is a somatic
treatment for patients with psychosomatic pains. The 1 hour
treatment of the entire body consists of a special massage-
technique combined with passive and some few active exercises

which influence respiration to become more free. Liberation
of respiration stimulates relaxation and releases feelings.
Prior to treatment all the 27 patients were examined by the
GPM-72 method and divided in two groups.
Group I: Patients with the lowest total GPM-72 sumscore (less
than 65). N=15. They were given liberation of respiration /re-
laxation.
Group II: Patients with the highest total GPM-72 sumscore
(equal or more than 65). N=12. Fig. 2. shows that these patients have the highest degree of problems /psychopathology and
do not tolerate any large reduction of muscular defences in a
short period of time. At start they were treated with PMP
without liberation of respiration. They were given careful,
swift massage and only active exercises. 6 of these patients
were later treated with moderat liberation of respiration.
    Patients were reexamined 1-3 times during the course of
treatment. Treatment was then adjusted in relation to the new
total GPM-72 sumscore and the patients experience of his situation. The patients were treated 1-5 years on an average for
2 years, receiving an average 49 treatments.
RESULTS
    Figure 1 shows: In the first project A, improved treatment
effect was 85% for the patients with lowest total GPM-72 sumscore and only 43% for the patients with highest total GPM-72
sumscore. In the last project B, the results after treatment
were 87 and 43 per cent respectively.
    Figure 2 shows: Prior to treatment the average total GPM-
72 sumscore in the two groups were 54 and 75. On completion
of treatment this fell to 42 and 65 respectively.

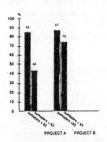

Fig.1. Treatment effect improved, in percentage
in project A and B measured with the
total GPM-72 sumscore. The material is
divided in two: Patients with lower and
higher total GPM-72 sumscore than 65
prior to treatment

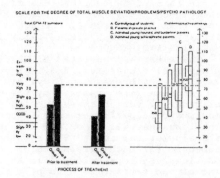

Fig.2. The average total GPM-72 sumscore for 2 groups of patients
prior to and after treatment. N=27

DISCUSSION
    Patients in group II, with the highest total GPM-72 sum-
score /degree of problems /psychopathology were in project B
approached more carefully with no or little liberation of

respiration /relaxation. Compared with project A, selection
of patients in two groups by the GPM method gave a more
differentiated treatment and led to much better treatment for
the patients with the highest total GPM-72 sumscores. Helping
these ill patients is an importalt task. This study shows
that patients with different degree of muscular deviation in
GPM-72 need to be treated differently to reach the same outcome in improvement of total GPM-72 sumscore.

In 21 patients in project B, there was agreement between
the GPM evaluation and the subjective feeling of improvement.
Three of the patients who felt subjectively better at the end
of treatment, without improvement in their GPM scores, had
relapses. The GPM evaluation was more reliable than the patients subjective feeling of improvement. This is in accordance with the results of Sundsvold.

CONCLUSION

This study has documented that selecting patients prior to
treatment and adjusting therapy with the standardized GPM
method led to better outcome for all the patients.

References:
1: Sundsvold,M.Ø., Vaglum,P., Denstad,K.: Global Fysiotera-
            peutisk Muskelundersøkelse. Til bruk i klin-
            isk arbeide og forskning. Eget forlag, pp.212,
            Oslo 1982. Til salgs i Norlis bokhandel, Oslo.
2: Sundsvold,M.Ø., Vaglum,P.: Muscular Pain and Psychopatho-
            logy Evaluation and Treatment planning by use
            of the Global Physiotherapeutic Examination
            (GFM). Chapter in: Hoskins Michel, T.: Inter-
            national Perspectives in Physical Therapy:
            Volume on Pain. Churchill Livingstone, London
            1985.
3: Sundsvold,M.Ø.: Muscle Tension and Psychopathology. Paper
            presented at the 10th European Conference on
            Psychosomatic Reseach, Edinbourogh 1974.
4: Phil,M.: Hvilken plass kan Global Fysioterapeutisk
            Muskelundersøkelse, GFM, ha i videreutdanning-
            en innenfor psykiatrisk/psykosomatisk fag-
            gruppe? Oslo, januar 1988.
5: Sundsvold,M.Ø., Vaglum,P., Friis,S.: Does Psychiatric
            Treatment influence Muscular Deviations as
            much as Psychopathology? Paper presented at
            the 15th European Conference on Psychosomatic
            Research, London 1984.
6: Vangen,A.L.: Valg av behandlingsopplegg i psykomotorisk
            fysioterapi etter grad av muskulære avvik og
            sosial fungering. Undersøkelse av behandlings-
            resultater. Særoppgave i psykomotorisk fysio-
            terapi 1987.
7: Sundsvold,M.Ø.: Muskelspenning og psykopatologi. Fysiotera-
            peuten 1972, 39, 33-51.

CORTICO-STEROID INJECTION THERAPY

Stephanie Saunders MCSP

Society of Orthopaedic Medicine
London, England

The role of cortico-steroid injection
therapy in orthopaedic conditions treated by
the physiotherpist is controversial. Abuse
and overuse of these drugs has led to confusion
and reluctance to employ them in suitable
cases.

This paper attempts to put into perspective the claims and counterclaims surrounding
the choice of this type of therapy. It add-
resses the merits of the different preparations,
the indications, contraindications and complications, the technique of application and review
of the most recent literature.

SIMULTANEOUS ACUPUNCTURE AND UV-RADIATION IN LUMBOSACRAL OSTEOCHONDROSIS

O N Narbekov, Ye D Troshina, Yu Tsaryov

Centre of Balneology & Traditional Medicine, Frunze, Kirghiz SSR, USSR

Introduction : A mutually potentiating effect of simultaneously administered acupuncture and erythematously dosed UV-radiation(UVR) procedures in patients with lumbosacral osteochondrosis was studied.

Treatment : The urinary bladder meridian-oriented points were selected in lumbosacral pain zones. In cases of lumbar ischialgia the treatment was effected on the femur and crus areas along the route of the schiatic nerve of the affected leg. The daily treatment involved only a single pain zone with a total of 2 to 4 sessions per each zone.

Results : The clinical and functional studies showed an apparent therapeutic effect as evidenced from the improvement of bioelectric muscular activity, vascular tone, the reduction of thermoasymmetry and restoration of cutaneous reflexes in distally spaced parts of lower limbs.

Conclusion : It is concluded that the high therapeutic effect of simultaneous acupuncture and UV-radiation in lumbosacral osteochondrosis is due to synergism of the cure factors and their optimum dosage. The method is registered as innovation in the USSR.

REFLEXTHERAPY---THE VALIDITY and POTENTIAL in PHYSIOTHERAPY
PRACTICE.
C B Jones
Midland School of Reflextherapy
5 Church Street, Warwick. United Kingdom.

Reflextherapy is a development of an ancient art of healing
which has a recorded history of over five thousand years and
is rapidly increasing in recognition both in its own right
and as complementary to the more modern therapies.
As Physiotherapists our skills are employed in areas of
great diversity. We are involved in an extensive range of
physical trauma and disease, in the aid and support of those
with mental disturbance, emotional damage, learning
difficulties, terminal illness, and in veterinary care, as
well as everyday life procedures - childbirth and natural
departure and in the promotion of health.
This space allows only a brief introduction to a therapy
which in clinical practice shows a profound effect on the
healing and health within most of these avenues.
The history and principles of the science of reflexology are
readily available in a growing number of texts. For the
purpose of this presentation it is necessary to recount the
re-instigation and development during this century. In the
early 1900's Dr.W.Fitzgerald, an American E.N.T. specialist,
noted that trigger points distal to a site of trauma and in
the same longitudinal line reflected a similar sensitive
sensation; manipulation of the associated area relieved the
pain in the original trauma site.
He devised a grid system in vertical sections noting all
connections and effects. 'Zone Therapy' saw the greatest
response within the most distal tissues. His work was
furthered by colleagues Dr's Riley and Bowers and a
therapist working with Riley, Eunice Ingham. The work of
these pioneers is well recorded and used today. The
twentieth century approach to this ancient art of healing is
known as Foot and Hand Reflexology.
The charts show the body divided into ten longitudinal zones
extending from the top of the head to the fingers and toes.
The feet and hands are also found to be micro-organs which
mirror exactly a miniature representation of the state of
the body tissues.
Any trauma, congestion, tension or other circumstance which
prevents full healthy function reflected within the hands
and feet in a most accurate manner.

Manipulation of the image affects the associated trauma site and assists the natural process of healing. The first effect is a release of tension leading to decongestion and elimination. Improved circulatory flow brings the necessary healing nutrients (subject to availability).

Science now proves that All is Energy. The Universe is filled with it. All life forms are subject and influenced by these energies - including man. The mind is also recognised as a powerful energy force, one which, as with all energy, may have a positive or negative influence.

Quantum Physics accepts and explains the influence of the Mind of the Observor, a realization which holds the greatest responsibility for the therapist, and may also hold the answer to the very essence of movement which brings with it the living process of healing.

The body is now accepted as a structure bonded and influenced by energy forces obtained from the surrounding environment. The quality of the nutrients of earth, water, air, the solar rays and cosmic energy and that of the mind all directly influence the physical being - and this with its own genetic tendency, inherent healing and subtle universal awareness.

This collective vital force passes throughout the body tissues in an organised manner, influencing all in its path. It is further influenced by the ionic particles of the circulatory and nervous flow. This vital force (simply termed in China as Chi) is itself subject to the variable resistance offered by the tissues through which it flows.

The flow of Chi is aided by any approach which assists relaxation and encourages movement of fluids. Reflexology works to stimulate or sedate the level of Chi so to restore harmony and homeostasis to the body as a whole.

Eastern philosophy has also maintained the integral and interwoven bonding of the body and mind. Imbalances such as the "irritable liver", to "vent ones spleen" amongst other phrases suggest that the west has not entirely divorced body from mind. A great benefit of reflexology is the restoration of the associated emotional and mind balance.

My first encounter with reflexology was in desperation some twenty years ago. The unexpected benefit both to my own symptoms and general health gave the incentive to learn, research and to use such a remarkable approach to healing. Patients, both two and four-legged, responded well. It was exciting and rewarding and gave energy to my determination to see the therapy accepted within the scope of Physiotherapy Practice. To this end, I now find myself in the realms of a minefield of research and appreciate more the difficulties of 'proving' the efficacy of a hands-on-therapy, that it is more than 'a foot massage and a cosy chat!' The work with unconscious patients, babies and animals has provided evidence in single case studies; more detailed studies are progressing and results should provide suitable evidence in the near future.

The first part of this presentation is deliberately based on the more 'orthodox' approach to reflexology. It is used extensively, effectively and safely by numerous professional and lay practitioners throughout the world. However, during early years in clinical practice, several patients' general constitutions seemed too sensitive or their trauma too extensive for such a procedure. I applied the laws of healing and body functions, and instead of concentrating on the zones, I decided on a more gentle and more physical approach encouraging circulation and elimination of surface toxins before activating deeper chronic or more sensitive areas. The more sensitive or sick the patient, the more gentle the approach. This often produced a totally unexpected response - a recall of some childhood or pre-birth trauma, a forgotten accident or emotional disturbance - the patient releasing the shock from the conscious or subconscious mind, and so too the linked trauma in the body tissues. This softer but more extensive approach became known as Reflextherapy.

In searching for explanation, research has shown the interwoven relationship of mind and body which stores the memory of all events; the more gentle touch seems to trigger the release of the original trauma.

The varying effects of Reflextherapy therefore may be useful for patients with most disorders which cause pain, strain, tension, congestion, reduced vitality, poor assimilation, misalignment or imbalance whether of body or of mind.

The choice of words in the title for this paper was deliberate in its in-depth definition: 'Validity' as 'having some foundation, force or power' (as well as 'legality or authority'); 'Potential' as 'embryonic, inherent, undeveloped, unrealized' (as well as the more usual 'capacity or possibility'); 'Physical' from the Greek 'phuein'- to make grow; and 'Therapy'-to be in attendance. These give a subtle appreciation of the individual latent ability of each patient. If there is no expectation at any session - the patient will respond according to his or her own timing and needs. The therapists desire to help with a predetermined 'plan' for the patient may indeed limit the process of the deeper healing of the inner mind. The therapist is responsible for providing a safe, knowledgable, caring and healthy environment, recalling that we are also bonded and influenced by energy forces, our own vitality, energy and balance of mind will also influence all in our path.

It is some twenty years since I encountered Reflextherapy. I have found it a privilege and an approach rewarding and beneficial beyond expectation. It well deserves its place within the scope of Physiotherapy Practice.

PHYSICAL THERAPIST AS HEALER: EMERGENCE OF A TRANSPERSONAL HEALING PHENOMENON

Ronald Bugaj
Graduate School for the Study of Human Consciousness, John F. Kennedy University
6045 Skyline Boulevard, Oakland, California, 94611, U.S.A.

Cross Disciplinary Research Evidence: Recent scientific interdisciplinary research results (1) in a variety of life and health science disciplines, parapsychology and consciousness studies are providing supportive evidence for the fundamental theoretical principles of modern quantum physics. The basic principles of quantum physics reveal a model of reality which suggests that we are all subtly interconnected with one another and with all things in the universe. These findings provide evidence of the transpersonal healing phenomenon in which an individual's "human touch," energized by mind, emotions and intention, can facilitate the healing process and promote health in another individual.

An investigative report of current and future science and technology issues, prepared by the Committee of Science and Technology for the United States House of Representatives, stated that recent experiments (2):

suggest that there exists an "interconnectiveness" of the human mind with other minds and with matter. This interconnectiveness would appear to be functional in nature and amplified by intent and emotion.

With regard to the implications for health care, the report suggested a potential advancement by the blending of traditional medical cures with mind-initiated cures.

The emergence of this revolutionary view of a fundamental connective link between mind, matter and one another requires an extension of previous perspectives regarding the importance of the therapeutic relationship and patient-practitioner interactions. The Cartesian/mechanistic view of ourselves and the world, and the kind of human values represented by traditional scientific belief systems undergo basic transformation and enhance prospects for the potential convergence of science and spirituality. Sperry, one of the world's most acclaimed neuroscientists and Nobel laureate in medicine and physiology for his split-brain research, affirms that natural science, religion and philosophy are merging, and states (3):

Instead of excluding mind and spirit, as had been the rule for all of us in brain-behavior science for many decades, my new logic requires that mental and spiritual forces be reinstated at the top of the brain's causal control hierarchy as real interactive "emergent" properties of brain processes and given primacy in determining what a person is and does.

The application of this understanding and knowledge will potentially promote the efficacy of a wide variety of therapeutic practices and interventions.

The Perennial Wisdom: The preceding research findings and conclusions parallel the world-view referred to as the "perennial philosophy,"(4) which lies at the heart of the world's great spiritual traditions. The perennial wisdom implies that our true natures are something greater . . . an aspect of a universal consciousness . . . being . . . mind or God; the view that all phenomena are interconnected and a part of a unified whole and that an individual is also part of this unity. The awakening to this expanded nature of being is the direct awareness or realization that the universe and God are not external to us, but exist within us. According to the spiritual traditions, this realization, which is acquired through meditation or other self-regulation strategies, is the primary objective of human existence.(5,6)

Dimensions of Transpersonal Being: Transpersonal refers to the transcendental as manifested in and through an individual for the purpose of evoking that individual's highest potential and performance levels. The "transpersonal self," or Self, is a self-sense that transcends the egoic and existential identifications, but is not yet absolute spirit.(7) The transpersonal self is the divine spark, or the Godself, within each individual, the place where we are all interconnected and one with God and the universe. This transpersonal or higher self can be discovered by turning one's attention inward, often through the practice of meditation, prayer or other self-regulating practices, but it can also be uncovered spontaneously. According to the perennial philosophy, knowledge of this higher self within is an essential evolutionary stage on the path toward transcendental wisdom and universal consciousness.(8) Vaughan provides us with a clear description of the transpersonal self (9):

> . . . as holistic and ecological, recognizing the interrelatedness of all phenomena. As an integrated harmonious whole, it defends no boundaries and sees no separate parts. As limitless transcendental being, it partakes of infinite wisdom and compassion, understanding, allowing and forgiving all things, without exception and without reservation. As a manifestation of absolute spirit, it is capable of unconditional love.

In reviewing the qualities above, it becomes apparent that the heart in individuals is the center of spiritual or transpersonal consciousness, and the head is the center of intellectual (superegoic) consciousness. Through meditation, prayer, contemplation and other self-regulation strategies, one moves from the intellectual into the spiritual. Our task is to bring all our consciousness and energies into the heart, for the heart is the threshold to the transpersonal self.

Transpersonal Dimensions of Healing: Following the practice of self-regulation techniques, transpersonal healers often report the ability to balance their personal life energies by attuning to a universal force, source or field. According to these healers, the ability to attune with the universal energy source is crucial to the effectiveness of the transpersonal healing, for it is through the attunement process that the healer becomes conditioned to be a conduit or channel through whom the healing energies flow. One of the most frequent metaphoric themes, among a variety of prominent transpersonal healers recently reviewed,(10) concerns the attainment of harmony for the healee (patient). The healer, while in an altered state of consciousness, maintains a world-view in which there is an harmonious interconnectedness of the universe, and the healer and healee are simply parts of it. Within this world-view, there are vast forces and energies that maintain stability, order and harmony in the universe. Through an alteration of one's consciousness, the healer is able to focus and intentionally channel these energies to enhance the condition of the healee.(1) Although the variety of transpersonal approaches to healing are methodologically different, the objective is generally similar . . . to restore harmony and order to the healee, who is perceived to be in a state of disharmony.(10)

During the process of establishing this harmonious healing connection, the healer detaches or "lets go" of the normal sensory or space-time reality mode of everyday living by attuning or synchronizing his or her inner (wave-like) rhythms with the oneness or harmony of the universe. Following this centering or attunement process, the healer, focusing on a deep level of love and caring for the healee, then attempts to merge with and flow into the healee. Physical contact with the hands may or may not be established during this merging process. The healer then gradually shifts into an altered state of consciousness in which he views himself and the healee as one entity within the harmony of the universe. While assuming this condition of intense love and compassion, the healer does not attempt to directly affect the healee, but merely tunes into, connects and becomes one with the healee. The healer, functioning as a channel for the universal healing power, directs the force to flow unconditionally through his own fields to those of the healee. Through this subtle connection between the harmonious forces of the universe, the attuned healer and the healee . . . harmonization is achieved and healing occurs.(10)

Although a variety of methods exist for channeling the healing energy, love has been recognized as the healing force.(10) The primary role of the healer is to assist the healee in becoming conscious of and in recognizing his or her own innate potential for healing. By expanding his or her own state of consciousness, the healee can learn to connect with the inner healer, or transpersonal self within, and then become aligned with the universal healing source. From this perspective, the healer is simply a channel that facilitates the healee's own self-healing potential by expanding the healee's awareness of the higher self and the universal source of healing.

Physical therapy practitioners concerned with promoting health and human function can no longer neglect these subtle bio-energetic field and/or information transfer effects on an individual's performance. Practitioners are challenged to recognize, explore and integrate these emerging dimensions of healing into their own lives and professional practices.

References:

1. Bugaj, R (1991) The Emergence of the Healing Connection in Clinical Practice: Ancient Insights, Modern Discoveries and Future Directions for the Health Care Professions. (In Press)
2. Committee of Science and Technology: Survey of Science and Technology Issues, Present and Past. Staff Report, U.S. House of Representatives, Ninety-seventh Congress, First Session, Washington, D.C.: Superintendent of Documents, U.S. Government Printing Office (June), 1981, pp. 411-416, 144, 59.
3. Sperry RW (1987) The New Mentalist Paradigm and Ultimate Concern. Perspectives in Biology and Medicine 29(3):413-422, 1986.
4. Huxley A (1945) The Perennial Wisdom. New York: Harper and Row.
5. Miller JP (1985) Curriculum: Perspectives and Practice. New York: Longman, 118.
6. Wilber K (1979) Physics, Mysticism and the New Holographic Paradigm: A Critical Appraisal. Re-Vision J 2(2):43-55.
7. Vaughan F (1985) The Inward Arc: Healing and Wholeness in Psychotherapy and Spirituality. Boston: Shambhala, 39-40.
8. Walsh R, Vaughan F (1985) Toward an Integrative Psychology of Well-Being. In Walsh R and Shapiro (Eds.): Beyond Health and Normality. New York: Van Nostrand, 404-405.
9. Vaughan F (1985) Healing and Wholeness in Psychotherapy and Spirituality. Boston: Shambhala, 42-43.
10. Bugaj R (1983) Cross Cultural Review of Prominent Psychic/Spiritual Healers Demonstrating Transpersonal Abilities. Unpublished manuscript. John F. Kennedy University, Orinda, California, 38, 42-44.

A CLOSER LOOK AT EMPATHY - THE MOMENT OF CROSSING OVER

C.M. Davis Ed.D. P.T.
University of Miami School of Medicine, Department of Orthopaedics and
Rehabilitation, Division of Physical Therapy, Coral Gables FL 33146, USA

Empathy, a concept that is not universally understood, nonetheless has
been characterized as a positive and powerful intersubjective force facilitative to healing.[1] When empathy or compassionate rapport is allowed to
develop, a deep bond is created that is reported to form the real basis of
effective healing therapy. Precisely how empathy facilitates healing is not
known. This paper delves more thoroughly into the experiencing of empathy
as first described phenomenologically by Stein[2] and expanded by Davis[3] in
the physical therapist-patient interaction. Two aspects of Stein's description that she asserts make empathy unique will be carefully explored:
1) the fact that empathy happens to us and we discover ourselves as having
been granted the experience nonprimordially, or after the fact, and 2) the
powerful second stage of the three stages of empathy, the moment of
"crossing over." These characteristics will be compared first to Martin
Buber's concept of dialogue in the "I Thou" interaction, and second with
the theory of the body as comprised of energy flow, a central belief of all
of the major Eastern philosophies, and now being emphasized by western
quantum physics. I will then venture an explanation of what happens to us
in the moment of crossing over when we find ourselves experiencing empathy,
and suggest how that experience is perceived as a healing one.

Empathy is not simply a product of intentional thought. The nature of
empathy as described by Stein is that of an absolutely unique intersubjective process, a part of which seems to come from beyond. Also, it happens
to us in not one step, but in three quickly overlapping stages. These two
characteristics make empathy significantly more complex than sympathy, or
fellow feeling, than identification, or self transposal, the cognitive
"thinking of ourselves" into the place of the other (most often confused
with empathy).

In my dissertation research, 10 physical therapists described their experiencing of empathy with their patients quite similarly to Stein. In the
first stage of empathy they described themselves as using active listening
to better understand the patient's experience. Then quite suddenly, they
reported feeling a "blow to the gut" or an intense emotional shared moment
of meaning with the patient, the moment where they forgot for a millisecond
that they and the patient were separate. This seemed to happen to them, and
they reported that they felt as if a part of the experiencing self had
truly "crossed over" or merged into the space of the other. In the third
stage they felt as if they regained the feeling of separateness and that
they and the patient shared common feelings about the incident, or were in
sympathy with one another. In sum, the three overlapping stages seem to
resemble first, self transposal, followed by a powerful and emotional
identification, followed by sympathy.

Stein claims that, in the second stage, I grasp the other's experience by allowing myself to be transferred into it, but that I don't realize what is happening until after the fact. It happens to me, or it is <u>nonprimordially</u> given, unlike a memory. This crossing over, or "fusion of intuition" (2 p. 25) makes possible a true feeling of oneness with the other, a deeper and richer sharing of experience than is possible through the unifaceted fellow feeling of sympathy. Because empathy "catches" us, we cannot make it happen, but we can block it from happening. For one to experience empathy, one must be truly present in the interchange, and be open and willing to come outside of oneself to experience the crossing over. And because this happens to us, it might be described as a "gift" that comes to us from beyond, or a transcendent moment, much as occurs with forgiveness.

Martin Buber is well known for his description of the therapeutic effect of the "I-Thou" relationship, wherein I relate to the other person as a unique person rather than as an object, as in an "I-It" interaction. What happens to two people in an I-Thou relationship is not located in either of the two people, but lies "between" the two in the power of the dialogue.[4] In genuine dialogue I try to make the other truly present, experience the other as a unique whole rather than an abstraction or a stereotype. For true dialogue to take place, one must be fully present and be willing to be completely open. In the monologue of the "I-It" relationship, people talk past each other, "they are centered in themselves, not in the relationship." (4 p. 111) When one lives life preferring "I-Thou" relating, one becomes open to what it means to be authentically human, for the truly human, according to Buber, is found in the authentic meeting of person with person, and person with the world. And to Buber, a Jewish theologian, it is God who makes possible such meeting, and who is present in every human meeting. When we are directed to life in an "I-Thou" perspective, we have our ears and hearts open to hear the "word" of God expressed to us, thus we are open to sense a universal meaning in all that speaks to us. Thus Buber says it is foolish to seek God, for God is already present in the authentically human interaction, the interaction that would allow for the crossing over of empathy to take place.

Although the various schools of Eastern mysticism vary, they share in common the view of the basic unity of the Cosmos, and whether Hindu, Buddhist or Taoist, the highest aim is to become aware of the unity and mutual interrelationship of all things.[5] A vital force or energy composes all of the universe, and pervades the human organism. Termed <u>prana</u> in Sanskrit, <u>Ch'i</u> by the Chinese, this force is described as moving throughout the body in channels or meridians, and when blocked, disease results. Advocates of this philosophy believe it is possible to transfer and balance energy through a healer's touch. Common alternative forms of healing that utilize this concept include therapeutic touch, reflexology, Reiki, Traeger, Rolfing, Jin Shin Do, cranio-sacral therapy, polarity balancing, acupuncture and acupressure, Shiatsu massage, and many others.[6]

Quantum physicists explain to us that all matter is made up of atoms and molecules that structurally are composed of 99% air. In reality, our bodies are more accurately portrayed in the stippled style of the Impressionistic artist, a series of submicroscopic dots separated by submicroscopic space. As energy is added to or withdrawn from this system the dots can be seen to undulate in waves. The shadow of our energy waves (the aura) has been captured by Kirlian photography, and high energy foci up the midline are described as <u>chakras</u> in the Yoga tradition. The root of the word "heal" is the Anglo-Saxon word <u>haelen</u>, to become whole. Health and healing have to do with wholeness, with harmony of body, mind and spirit. For healing to take place, the healer would best be wholly present to the other, physically and emotionally, bringing about balance and harmony. Perhaps the healing power of dialogue, and the healing power of the moment of "crossing over" has to do with a shift in energy within the two people. It is unlikely that the energy of one actually "crosses over" to the other, but perhaps what happens is that, at the emotional shared moment of meaning, there is a resonance of energy such that the waves of energy of the two people flow in such synchrony that the experience feels like a fusion of the experiencing self, or of the intuition, one with the other. And if Buber is correct, perhaps this resonance lifts the experience higher, closer to a recognition of the unity of all of the Universe, and the presence of God, or the power of the Universe, for one brief moment is brought closer to us in transcendent grace. With it would undoubtedly come a balancing, a perception of wholeness, the basis for healing. Life force in its highest form is made manifest in a shared moment of grace. The intentional healer empowers the other not with the quick "fix" of the "I-It" relationship, but with the confident and competent willingness to experience meaningful physical touch and emotional touch through empathy, and herself is healed in the process. For as in touch, one cannot touch without being touched, in empathy, one cannot cross over without being affected by the shared moment of meaning.

1. May R (1989) The empathic relationship: a foundations for healing. In Carlson R, Shield B (1989) Healers on Healing. Los Angeles, Jeremy Tarcher, p 109

2. Stein E (1970) On the Problem of Empathy. The Hague, Martinus Nijhoff

3. Davis CM (1982) A Phenomenological Description of Empathy as it Occurs in Physical Therapist for Their Patients. Boston University, Unpublished Dissertation

4. LeFever P (1966) Martin Buber - Man in dialogue. In Understandings of Man. Philadelphia, Westminster Press

5. Capra F (1985) The Tao of Physics. Boston, Shambahala New Science Library

6. Tappan FM (1988) Healing Massage Techniques. (2nd ed) Norwalk, Connecticut, Appleton and Lange

PELVIC PAIN

PELVIC PAIN: AN UNDERREFERRED CONDITION?

V.R. Harding,   C.E. Pither,   M.K. Nicholas,   A.C.deC. Williams.
INPUT,   St. Thomas's Hospital Pain Management Unit
London SE1 7EH   U.K.

Pain in the pelvic region is not a condition frequently seen in Physiotherapy Departments. A review of physiotherapy journals 1975-1990 produced only 2 articles on the subject, in pregnancy. In the medical literature however, pelvic pain is well documented. A literature search of the last 10 years produced 318 articles on pelvic pain.

Chronic Pelvic Pain (CPP) comprises 2-10% of out-patient gynaecologic referrals and ranks amongst the most common complaints (1). 41% of laparoscopies in an American survey(2) and over 50% in a British survey(3) were performed in an attempt to diagnose the cause of pelvic pain. 20-92% of diagnostic laparoscopies for pelvic pain however reveal no abnormality(4,5) Some of the "pathologies" found at laparoscopy are found in asymptomatic subjects undergoing tubal ligation viz large pelvic veins/varicosities, endometriosis ($\frac{1}{3}$ subjects with endometriosis are asymptomatic), adhesions and retrodisplacement of the uterus. Thus, a clear-cut cause for the pain is not found in most subjects. The frustration of this situation is demonstrated in a review(6) of 200 CPP cases where clinical assessment failed to produce positive findings in 17% and only 13% improved as a result of gynaecological treatment. Unfortunately the author takes this to mean that CPP has psychological rather than organic origins in the vast majority of cases

Treatment is also a problem area. The success rate 6 months after laparoscopic ventrosuspension for retroverted uterus varies from 18.6%-46.5% (7). In the U.S. 12% of hysterectomies are performed for CPP(8), yet its value is unproven. In view of those cases who develop CPP post-hysterectomy, - in one series(9) 30% of subjects presenting with CPP had already undergone hysterectomy - there are risks with this operation.

In recent years there has been a surge in the number of cognitive/behavioural multidisciplinary pain management (C/BMPM) centres. Rather than searching further for an elusive diagnosis or magic cure, patients are taught to come to terms with their pain and to get back to a normal healthy and active lifestyle. The long term results from C/BMPM centres is extremely encouraging, with dramatic and maintained improvement in fitness, function and depression despite the continuance of pain. Even this may in time reduce somewhat. C/BMPM programmes for CPP are also proving successful.

In the U.K. a grant aided research project assessing in-patient C/BMPM called INPUT has been running for $2\frac{1}{2}$ years. This study was undertaken to assess the frequency of CPP in a C/BMPM programme, and to investigate the role of exercise and manual therapy in the management of these conditions.

METHOD: A retrospective analysis of the history and examination findings by the unit physiotherapist on the first 159 patients attending INPUT was performed. All patients underwent a Maitland-type examination on the evening of the 1st or 2nd days of the 4-week programme.

The following data was collected:
1. Details of patients' sex and age on entry to the programme.
2. The presence of pelvic, coccygeal, rectal, perineal and low abdominal/ bladder pain (pelvic+ pain) on the physiotherapist's pain drawing. Pelvic+ pains were further categorised into:
   a) Only pain   b) Worst pain   c) Secondary pain
3. Details of past physiotherapy treatment. Patients' responses were categorised into:
   a) None
   b) Active – ANY single therapy involving some activity from the patient i.e. exercise, hydrotherapy etc.
   N.B. Joint Mobilization/Manipulation and out-patient traction were included in this category.
   c) Passive – Heat, massage and other electrotherapy not involving any movement by the patient.
4. The number of operations for pain.
5. The number of previous low abdominal, pelvic, perineal and coccygeal operations.
6. The presence of the following physical signs:
   a) Dural stretch reproduced the patient's presenting worst pain.
   b) Dural stretch reproduced one of the patient's secondary presenting pelvic+ pains.
   c) Dural stretch –ve for pain but very tight compared with lumbar flexion.
   d) Dural stretch –ve for pain but localised lumbar movements reproduced patient's pelvic+ pain.
   e) Less than one quarter of the expected range of total lumbar flexion /extension present with either a fixed lumbar flexion or fixed lumbar extension deformity.
   f) A totally solid spine unable to move 5° in any direction.

RESULTS: 64 (40%) of 159 subjects had some pelvic, coccygeal, perineal or low abdominal/bladder pain. For 27 (17%) this was their worst pain and for 6 (4%) their only pain. These patients did not differ from the 95 patients without pelvic+ pain in age – mean age of pelvic+ pain patients = 53.5; mean age of non-pelvic pain patients = 51.7. There were sex differences however, with 51 female pelvic+ pain patients (80% of the group), and 60 female non-pelvic pain patients (63% of the group).

Spinal Biomechanical Findings

A retrospective study of the physiotherapy assessments of the 64 pelvic+ pain patients produced the following findings:
- 17 (27%) patients had pelvic+ pain reproduced on dural stretch, and 6 (9%) on localised lumbar spine movement.
- 15 (23%) patients had gross spinal dysfunction or dural tightness, with fixed deformity or only a quarter of the expected range, despite no alteration of pelvic+ pain on dural or lumbar tests. 3 (4%) had developed completely rigid spines. N.B. There were no cases of diagnosed Ankylosing Spondylitis, though there were 5 spinal fusions in 4 patients.

No patient who was classed as a rigid spine had had a spinal fusion. 59% of these patients therefore had signs that could indicate the musculoskeletal (M/S) system as either of primary cause, secondary cause or at least a maintaining factor in a complex chronic pain state.

Previous Operations

The mean no. of operations <u>for pain</u> for the pelvic+ pain patients was 1.2 (range 0-4) and for the non-pelvic pain patients 1.3 (range 0-6). There was a significant difference (p>=0.025) in the number of previous abdominal pelvic, peroneal or coccygeal surgery whether for pain or other conditions (excluding laparoscopies). Of the 64 pelvic+ pain patients, 39 (61%) had had 105 operations (mean 1.64) whereas 47 of the 95 non-pelvic pain patients (50%) had had 82 operations (mean 0.57). 51 female pelvic+ pain patients had had 24 hysterectomies (47%) whereas the 60 female non-pelvic pain patients had had only 13 (22%).

Previous Physiotherapy

19 pelvic+ pain patients (30%) said they had never been referred to physiotherapy for their complaint and 29 (45%) said they had had no active physiotherapy. Only 12 said they had had active treatment and only 4 (6%) said they had had active physiotherapy to the tissue that referred to their pain area. This is in contrast to 39 (70%) who had had operations for pain (excluding laparoscopies). Of the 27 whose pelvic+ pain was their worst pain, 16 had had no physiotherapy yet 9 had their pain reproduced on dural or spinal movement and 10 had a gross spinal/dural dysfunction.

<u>DISCUSSION</u>: Patients with pelvic+ pains are clearly not usually referred to physiotherapy either initially or when chronic. These patients, especially females, are usually referred to surgeons, so tend to receive operations. From the literature, surgeons who operate for CPP are unaware that the spine is capable of referring to the abdomen, pelvis, perineum or coccyx. The only papers mentioning the link between spine and CPP are 4 produced by a chiropractor (10). Shorter times in hospital after abdominal surgery mean patients are experiencing less contact with physiotherapists who might prevent tightening of scars and adhesions. Surgeons are also unaware that there is any treatment for pain and movement limitation due to adhesions other than surgical division.

Some pain specialists have become interested in trigger points of the abdomen or perineum in CPP patients but tend to see this as a condition in itself(11). Their treatment is directed at the trigger points and not one paper suggests a spinal biomechanical assessmnet or treatment. Some very welcome interest in the mechanics of the pelvic floor muscles and the relationship between pain and function is starting, with research into the use of the pelvinometer and performance of appropriate muscle re-ed. exercises.

Papers that address multidisciplinary treatment of women with CPP uniformly suggest that the team include gynaecologists and psychologists, as well as specialists in the areas of urology, gastroenterology and anaesthesiology. Not one of these specialists includes a M/S examination in their usual clinical practice. Few even come into contact with physiotherapists who evaluate M/S function. The author of a study(12) of subjects with coccygeal pain and/or depression proposed that rectal digital examination evoked coccygeal pain is an objective diagnostic sign for masked depression. Some women and of course men, may be referred to general chronic pain management clinics where they will have access to physiotherapists. Now however the emphasis may be on the behavioural approach and fitness generally rather than more specific biomechanical evaluation and treatment.

Physiotherapists clearly need to assert their role in the evaluation and treatment of the pelvic pain patient. The physiotherapist is the only health professional trained in M/S and biomechanical diagnosis. A physiotherapy assessment for the pelvic pain patient could easily be fitted in while waiting for a laparoscopy. This would also give the patient the opportunity to be advised on a programme for healthy functioning of the pelvic floor and bowels as well as appropriate exercises/ergonomics for the spine. Once referral patterns are improved, the role of the spine and meninges in pelvic pain will become more apparent as will the value of exercise and manual therapy to the intestines. Use of the Behavioural approach in treatment is also essential as these patients are at great risk of becoming chronic pain sufferers(13).

<u>CONCLUSIONS</u>: Pelvic pain patients are a distinct group in a Pain Clinic population who have been rarely referred to physiotherapy. They are usually referred first to surgical specialists who have no knowledge of biomechanical diagnoses. Once on this treadmill they don't get off it until they achieve the label "CPP" and are referred for pain management.

Physiotherapists need to be aware of the problem, liase with Family Practitioners, Gynaecologists and the Obstetric team to encourage early physiotherapy referral for assessment, then treat and advise where appropriate.

Bibliography
1. Reiter C (1990) A profile of women with chronic pelvic pain. Clin.Obstet.Gynecol. 33(1):130-136.
2. Peterson HB, Hulka JF, Phillips JM (1990) American Association of Gynecologic Laparoscopists' 1988 membership survey on operative laparoscopy. J.Reprod.Med. 35(6):587-9.
3. Royal College of Obstetricians and Gynaecologists. Gynaecological laparoscopy. Report of the working party of the confidential enquiry into gynaecological laparoscopy. Chamberlain G, Brown JC, eds. London 1978.
4. Levitan S, et al (1985) The value of laparoscopy in women with chronic pelvic pain and a 'normal pelvis'. Int.J.Obstet.Gynaecol. 64:672-4.
5. Kresch AJ, Seifer DB, Sachs LB, Barrese L (1984) Laparoscopy in evaluation of 100 women with chronic pelvic pain. Obstet.Gynecol. 64:672-4.
6. Yoong AF (1990) Laparoscopic ventrosuspensions. A review of 72 cases. Am.J.Obstet.Gynecol. 163(4 pt1):1151-3.
7. Dicker RC, et al (1982) Complications of abdominal and vaginal hysterectomy among women of reproductive age in the United States: the collaborative review of sterilization. Am.J.Obstet.Gynecol. 144:842.
8. Guirgis RR (1988) Referral of women with chronic pelvic pain. J.Roy.Coll.G.P. 38(317):567.
9. Slocumb JC (1990) Operative management of chronic abdominal pelvic pain. Clin.Obstet.Gynecol. 33(1):196-204.
10. Browning JE (1988) Chiropractic distractive decompression in the treatment of pelvic pain and organic dysfunction in patients with evidenceof lower sacral nerve root compression. J.Manip.Physiol.Ther.11(5):426-32.
11. Slocumb JC (1984) Neurological factors in chronic pelvic pain: Trigger points and the abdominal pelvic pain syndrome. Am.J.Obstet.Gynecol. 149(5):536-543.
12. Maroy B (1988) Spontaneous and evoked coccygeal pain in depression. Dis.Col.&Rect. 31(3):210-5.
13. Collett B (1990) Personal communication.

DIAGNOSTIC SIGNS, SYMPTOMS AND EXPERIENCES OF TREATMENT OF MECHANICAL
PELVIC DYSFUNCTION SYNDROME.

Lennart Silverstolpe
Department of Clinical Neurophysiology, Karolinska Hospital
S-104 01 Stockholm, Sweden

INTRODUCTION

The term Mechanical Pelvic Dysfunction Syndrome, MPDS, was introduced
by our Swedish research group as a general term for non inflammatory disorders in the pelvis independent of whether the primary cause is thought
to be in the sacroiliac joints, ligaments or muscles (1,2). First a description of diagnostic signs and treatment of MPDS:

Diagnostic signs: The diagnostis of the MPDS is based primarily on a
triad of signs: a) The Silver-reflex (S-reflex), i.e. palpation of the
erector spinae in the lower thoracic region (Th8-11) elicits a pathological
reflex with a contraction in the lower part of erector spinae (1,2), varying from a weak within a few segments to a strong more painful contraction,
involving neck and leg muscles. b) A tender point on the upper part of the
buttocks. c) A tense and tender sacrotuberous ligament, STL (pararectal
palpation). The two first signs are usually unilateral and positive on the
same side as the affected STL. The latter phenomenon has earlier been described by Midttun and Bojsen-M öller (3) as well as following often present signs: positive Patrik, affected sacroiliaca joint, torsion of the
pelvis and secondary scoliosis.

Treatment: Therapeutic massage treatment of the STL is performed at its
upper part (coccyx level), from the skin surface, for 2-3 minutes, till the
ligament get slacked and painless. Both the S-reflex and tender point disappear simulataneously with a decrease or relief of symptoms of MPDS (see
below). Most of the tense muscles will be relaxed. The compensatoric scoliosis, locked joints and remaining tense muscles are treated by MET (Muscle-
Energy-Technic).

The purpose of this study, on a material of 373 cases with MPDS, was to
investigate the presence of typical diagnostic signs, symptoms and effect
of specific treatment.

MATERIAL

A totally of 373 cases were studied; 232 females and 141 males. The
mean age (and range) were 49 (16-82) and 46 (13-85) years respectively.

RESULTS

Before treatment a positive S-reflex was present of all studied patients;
for 69% on the left side of the body, 4% on the right and 9% on both sides.
18% changed from left to right side during treatment of STL. A tender point
of the buttocks was present before treatment in 98% of the patients and
then at the same side as the S-reflex. A tense and tender STL was present
in all patients on the same side of the body as the S-reflex. All these
three signs (S-reflex, gluteal tender point and tense and tender STL) disappeared by massage of the STL for all patients.

All different categories of symptoms and effect of treatment for each
category are shown in Table 1-7. Of the 373 studied patients 284 showed

only spinal symptoms (Tab. 1 and 2), 89 exhibited also cranial (Tab. 3 and 5) and/or visceral symptoms (Tab. 4 and 5). The cranial symptoms included voice disturbances (Tab. 6), craniomandibular and tongue disorders (Tab. 6 and 7).

Table 1. Only spinal symptoms were found in 284, i.e. in 76% of all cases with MPDS. Astonishing is that in this group neck symptoms are found in as much as 76% and shoulder symptoms in 60%, but lumbar symptoms only in 10%.

SYMPTOMS

A. CERVICAL	No.	%		B. THORACO	161	56.7		D. SACRAL		218	76.76
NECK	217	76.4		SHALLOW BREATHING	19	6.7		GLUTAE		187	65.8
SHOULDER	169	59.5						SITTING DIFFICULTIES		63	22.2
ARM	81	28.5		C. LUMBAR	28	9.8		LEG		161	56.7
HANDS	18	6.3						KNEE		33	11.6
								FEET		37	13.0

RESULT	No.	%
CURED	195	69
IMPROVED	80	28
STATUS QUO	7	2
WORSE	2	1
	284	100

Table 2. Result of treatment in MPDS cases with only spinal symptoms (n=284). Mean observation time was 11 months. Mean number of visits during this period was 2,5. Two cases ("worse") got sacroilitis and seven patients ("status quo") were in beginning of treatment.

SYMPTOMS	MALE	FEMALE	TOTAL
NAUSEA	13	18	31
VERTIGO	18	28	45
HEADACHE	19	28	47
SHALLOW BREATHING·	11	16	27
CRANIOMANDIBULAR DYSFUNCTION	14	33	47
DEVIATION OF TONGUE	10	37	47
BLURRED VISION	16	24	40
LOSS OF HEARING	11	17	28
PHONASTHENIA	12	36	48

Table 3. Cranial symptoms was found in 89 cases (24% of all with MPDS). Most common symptoms were phonastenia, headache, craniomandibular dysfunction and deviation of the tongue. In the group of phonasthenia there are a lot of professional singers.

From the table it is evident that most patients had more than one cranial symptom. Of the 89 patients 54 had also visceral symptoms.

SYMPTOMS	MALE	FEMALE	TOTAL
DYSPHAGIA	8	17	25
GLOBUS SENSATION	17	28	45
ABDOMINAL TENESMS	2	15	17
SENS. OF PERIENAL PROLAPSE		6	6
DYSURIA	3	13	16

Table 4. Visceral symptoms were found in 54 cases (14% of all with MPDS). Most common symptoms were globus sensation and difficulties in swallowing. No organic disease to explain these symptoms were found. Abdominal tenesms had brought several patients to emergency wards. A feeling of perineal prolapse was a common symptom for women, described also in the Danish report (3).

RESULT	No.	%
CURED	74	83
IMPROVED	13	15
STATUS QUO	2	2
	89	100

Table 5. Result of treatment in MPDS cases with cranial and/or visceral symptoms. After a mean observation time of 1 year and a mean number of visits of 2,7, about 80% were cured in the sense that they had resumed their work and were free from symptoms. 15% were still under treatment. The two last patients had other complications (sacroilitis and coxarthrosis).

It may be noticed that in 3 cases with increased diastolic blood pressure (110-120) this pressure was found to be normalized (80-90) after only treatment of STL.

CLINICAL SYMPTOMS	NO.	REDUCED AT LEFT SIDE	REDUCED AT RIGHT SIDE
DIFF. BETWEEN VIBRATION VOCAL CORDS	16	7	9

		TO THE LEFT	TO THE RIGHT
DEVIATION AT JAW OPENING	16	7	9
TONGUE DEVIATION	16	7	9

NECK PAIN	8
CHEST PAIN	3
LOW BACK PAIN	8

Table 6. Vocal disturbances for 16 singers with MPDS (of the above mentioned 89 cases) The group consisted 3 males and 13 females with a common mean age af 31 years. This group is of special interest. The lack of symmetry in vibration between the two vocal cords can be demonstrated by simultaneously palpation of the lateral sides of the throat, while the patient is talking or singing. These patients also exhibit deviation at jaw-opening, as well as deviation of the tongue to the side of reduced vibration. All of them were improved by treatment of their MPDS and they could sing again which was important especially for those who were professionals.

	BEFORE TREATMENT	AFTER TREATMENT
DEV. JAW	14	1
DEV. TONGUE	9	0
CLICKING	5	2
CREPITATION	6	3

Table 7. Craniomandibular disorders in 17 cases. The group consisted 5 males and 12 females with a common mean age of 40 years. This group resisted local therapy earlier given by dentists. All these cases proved to have MPDS. However, interesting the different symptoms disappeared in most cases on proper treatment of the pelvic dysfunction. Mean of increase of jawopening ability after treatment was 9,5 mm. This study was made in cooperation with M.D. Gustav Hellsing, specialist in oral physiology.

Thus, on the studied 373 cases, the triad of basic signs which the diagnosis of MPDS is based on: 1) the S-reflex in erector spinae, 2) a tender point on the upper part of the buttock and 3) an increased tension and tenderness of the STL, appears to diminish or abolish simultaneously with the symptoms by treatment of the sacrotuberous ligament.

REFERENCES

1. Silverstolpe, L. (1989). A pathological erector spinae reflex - a new sign of mechanical pelvic dysfunction. A proposal of treatment. J Manual Medicine 4:28.
2. Skoglund, C.R. (1989). New physical aspects on the pathological erector spinae reflex in cases of mechanical pelvic dysfunction. J Manual Medicine 4:29-30.
3. Midttun, A. and Bojsen-Möller, F. (1986). The sacrotuberous ligament pain syndrome. In: Modern manual therapy of the vertebral column (ed Grieve G P). Churchill Livingstone, Edinburgh, London and New York, pp 915-918.

PROGRAM FOR SELF-MOBILIZATION AND MUSCLE TRAINING FOR THE MECHANICAL
PELVIC DYSFUNCTION SYNDROME

Asta Eriksson
Department of Clinical Neurophysiology, Karolinska Hospital
S-104 01 Stockholm, Sweden

Among patients with low back pain it is possible to define a subgroup exhibiting the following characteristic signs and symptoms: (I) A tender and tens sacrotuberous ligament, STL, (II) an increased tension and tenderness of the erector spinae muscle at the thoracic level, (III) a pathological erector spinae reflex and, as a rule, positive Patrick´s and Derbolowsky´s tests.

This type of back pain has been referred to as "Mechanical Pelvic Dysfunction Syndrome" (1) successfully treated with massage of the STL. The treatment usually abolishes the pathological erector spinae reflex and, as a rule, Patrick´s and Derbolowsky´s tests are normalized.

Even if good immediate results usually are obtained with this form of treatment many patients experience a relapse of their lumbar pain after some days. In an attempt to obtain a more long-lasting result a therapeutic exercise program was developed and tested. The program is based on conventional exercises for self mobilization and stabilization.

Material and method. The patients were all diagnosed on the basis of case history and clinical examination including the tests by Patrick and Derbolowsky, the erector spinae reflex test and the recording of gluteal trigger point.

The exercis program consists of two parts, self-mobilization and muscle training. These are explained to the patient at three initial consultations. After additional two treatment sessions, during which the performance is checked, the patient is expected to be capable of exercising the different techniques at home. The treatment program includes a protocol in which the patient, before and after each treatment, records the results of self-applied Patrick´s and Derbolowsky´s tests as well as the level of experienced pain by rating on a visual analog scale (VAS).

Great emphasis is placed on making the patient more aware of the musculo-skeletal functions and the importance of taking his own responsibility for a lasting, good result. The mobilizing exercises shown in Figs 1-6 in three consecutive steps involve the pelvis, the thoracolumbar spine and cervical spine. The muscle exercises are aimed at stabilizing the pelvis. The two parts of the program should consistently be combined and carried out twice a day for five weeks.

Results. Out of 249 patients referred to physiotherapeutic treatment during one year 120 were found to fulfil the criteria of mechanical pelvic dysfunction. Following the treatment program all the applied tests for pelvic dysfunction were negative. The VAS-rating (scale of 10) varied between 0 and 1 after the treatment period (five weeks) as compared to 5 to 7 initially.

50 patients were followed-up after one year, 15 of them by physical examination and 35 by telephone interviews. 40 declared themselves painfree. Most of them, however, had experienced one or several relapses. All of these patients had treated themselves successfully with the treatment program they had been taught. 10 patients who were pain free after finishing the initial five weeks treatment period declared that they now had daily

lumbar pain again. None of these patients had continued the treatment program as originally planned.

Comments. It should be pointed out that the therapeutic exercises cannot be readily applied in all cases. Hypermobile patients may often experience an increased pain some hours after performing the mobilizing exercises. In such cases the massage of the sacro-tuberal ligament descibed by Silverstolpe (1) is of particular value as an initial (or an alternative) treatment. The ligament massage treatment is preferable for pregnant patients but should in these cases be followed by a muscle training program.

The pathophysiological mechanisms underlying the so-calle mechanical pelvic dysfunction are unknown. An attempt has been made, however, to elucidate the neurophysiological aspects of the concomitant pathological erector spinae reflex (2). With the good results from the mobilizing exercises described here it would seem resonable to assume that the pathophysiological explanation of this type of lumbar pain syndrome may be some kind of neuromuscular inbalance maintaining a disturbed pattern of muscular tone. The therapeutic exercises described could be assumed to readjust the balancing points for the multilevel, and very intricate, control system for the position and movements of the pelvis and the vertebrae.

Mobilization program.

1.

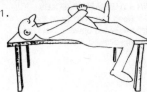

1.MOBILIZING ILIUM. Start in supine position with half the pelvis outside the couch. Pull the knee of the healthy side up against the abdomen and let the leg showing positive Patrick´s sign hang down for 7 s. Then lift the leg to a hip flexion of 60° if possible. Hold the leg in this position for 7 s. Relax. Repeat 3 times.

2.

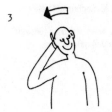

2. MOBILIZING THORACOLUMBAR SPINE. Lie on left side, hold right knee on the couch with left hand and look down at the couch. Inhale. Rotate to the right while exhaling and looking at right hand. Hold this position for 7 s. Repeat 3 times. Then lie on your right side and repeat the exercise in the opposite direction.

3

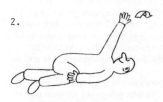

3. MOBILIZING COSTA I. Sit with your head slightly tilted to the right. Push head to the right and keep right hand firmly against head. Press against the head with the hand. N movements allowed. Look to the left. Hold still for 7 s. Repeate three times. Perform the same exercise in the opposite direction.

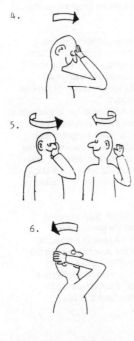

4.

4. ACTIVATING THE SCALENE MUSCLES.
Look down. Press head down against
firmly held hand on the forehead. No
movements allowed. Relax. Repeat 3 times.

5.

5. MOBILIZING THE CERVICAL SPINE.
Rotate head against right hand firmly
pressed aginst the right side of the
face. Look to the right. No movements
allowed. Relax. Turn head in the opposite
direction as far as possible. Repeat 3
times. Perform the same exercise in the
opposite direction.

6.

6. ACTIVATING THE NAPE MUSCLES.
Look upward. Keep hands firmly on the
occiput. Push backward-upward. Hold for 7
s. No movements allowed. Relax.

Summary. Out of 249 patients referred to physiotherapy 120 patients proved to fulfil the
criteria established for MPDS. At five sesssions these 120 patients were taught a home
exercise program for self-mobilization and muscle strength training based on conventional
techniques but applied according to a special schedule. Great importance was attached to
the control of the patient´s ability to learn the program. The patients were instructed to
assess the effects of the treatment by performing Patrick´s and Derbolovsky´s tests and by
rating their pain on the VAS.

Out of 50 patients followed up after one year 40 were free from symptoms, 5 had
intermittent recurrences whereas 5 had not improved. The later group had not been able to
carry through the program for various reasons.

References.
1. Silverstolpe L. A pathological erector spinae reflex. A new sign of mechanical pelvis
   dysfunction. J Manual Medicine 1989, 4: 28.
2. Skoglund C R. Neurophysiological aspects on the pathological erector spinae reflex in
   cases of mechanical pelvic dysfunction. J Manual Medicine 1989, 4: 29-30.

INTERACTIONS BETWEEN MUSCLES AND LIGAMENTS ON CENTRAL REFLEX EXCITABILITY IN MAN - EMG TESTS BEFORE AND AFTER TREATMENT

Eva Andersson, Carl Rudolf Skoglund, Lennart Silverstolpe and Asta Eriksson.
Dep. of Physiol. III, Karolinska Institute, Lidingövägen 1, 114 86 Stockholm and Dep. of Clin. Neurophysiol., Karolinska Hospital, 104 01 Stockholm, Sweden.

INTRODUCTION

In patients with skeletomuscular symtoms and signs there seems to be a complex interaction between ligaments and muscles. However objective analysis with neurophysiological methods on neuromuscular dysfunctions associated with disturbances in the biomechanics of the pelvis is scarce.

Mechanical pelvic dysfunction syndrome, MPDS, has been introduced as a general therm for disturbances of pelvic functions independent of their assumed pathogenetic origin (1, 2). The syndrome compromises also secondary symtoms on spinal and cranial levels. The diagnosis of MPDS is based primarily on a triad of signs; 1) the Silver-reflex (S-reflex), i.e. brisk perpendicular pressure over the erector spinae, ES, in the lower thoracic region (Th5-11) elicits a pathological reflex with a contraction in the lower part of erector spinae (1), varying from a weak within a few segments to a strong more painful contraction, involving neck and leg muscles, 2) a gluteal trigger point and 3) a tense and tender sacrotuberous ligament, STL. The latter sign has earlier been described by Midttun and Bojsen-Möller (3).

In a S-reflex test has earlier been recorded an electromyographic, EMG, respons for the lumbar ES (2). The sign disappeared by massage of STL. If this EMG reflex answer can be spread to several muscles is so far unknown, as well as an abolishment with treatment.

METHODS

Seven cases (6 males and 1 female) with initially positive S-reflex were studied. For the males the mean (and range) of age, weight and height were 35 (21-79) years, 76 (68-85) kg and 1.80 (1.65-1.90) m, respectively, and for the female: 25, 53 and 1.64.

The reflex responses were recorded with electromyogaphic (EMG) technique bilaterally with indwelling electrodes from the iliacus portion (IL) of the iliopsoas muscle and with surface electrodes from the lumbar erector spinae, L4 level, (ES), (7 cases); and from gluteus maximus (GM), hamstrings (HAM), hip adductor (ADD), trapezius (TRA) and triceps brachii (TRI) muscles (2 cases), before and after massage of STL. All EMG-signals were amplified 1000-5000 times, band-pass filtered at 10-1000 Hz and recorded on an ink recorder (Mingograf 803). For each muscle was performed a static maximal voluntary contraction, MVC, for comparison of the EMG amplitude.

RESULTS

Bilaterally in ES and iliacus EMG reflex answers for all patients could be recorded. The reflexes were also electromyographic recorded in all other examined muscles (except in the hamstrings for one patient and in the hip adductor muscles for another). After massage of STL, for 3 to 5 minutes, the reflex responses were diminished or abolished in all muscles. The S-reflex was present on both sides of the body for all patients. The EMG reflex answer in the ES was usually greater on the same side as the S-reflex test was performed for all patients. The EMG-amplitude in a S-reflex answer was about 25-75 % of the amplitude during a static MVC for each recorded muscle.

<u>Figure 1.</u> EMG recordings during S-reflex test performed on the left ES before and after treatment with massage of the STL. For the abbreviations of the muscles see above. L=left and R=right side. Note that EMG amplitude can not be compared between different muscles. However the changes in amplitude for each muscle before and after treatment is obvious. Exact latencies indeterminable (ref. 2). ECG-artefacts are seen for ES, TRA and TRI muscles.

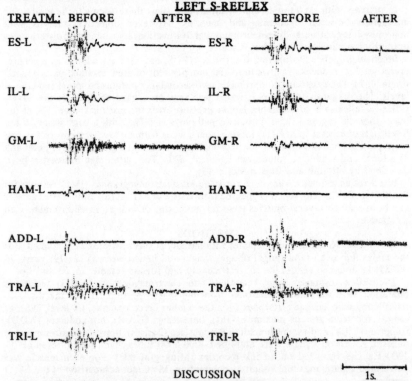

LEFT S-REFLEX

DISCUSSION

The results of the study has shown that the S-reflex may activate several widely spread muscles of the body bilaterally, thus, indicating may be due to enhanced excitability of spinal reflexes that can be influenced from the sacrotuberous ligament.

The mechanism behind the increased central reflex excitability is hard to explain but could possible be caused by an abnormal afferent inflow at different segmental levels (2, 4). Possible sources of such an inflow might be the different affected muscles or ligaments, such as a tense STL. That there could be a complex neurophysiological

738

interaction between the muscles and ligaments is supported by studies on cat showing the role of the ligamentum cruciata for tonus in the muscles sourronding the knee joint (5). Another mechanism which can contribute to an increased reflex excitation of the muscles can be due to supraspinal influence. The supraspinal influence results in a momentary status with a decrease of the normal central inhibition on the motor neurons in the anterior horn in the spinal cord. This theory is based on findings from a study by Leonard et al. (6), who found more widely spread reflex excitation of muscles in the lower extremities (at patellar- and achillestendon reflexes) in persons with cerebral palsy as compared to normals.

The present results has shown that the increased reflex excitability can be spread to several segmental levels and muscles independent of the primarily source. Except an increased reflex excitability as a reason to increased muscle tone in erector spinae (4) and in other muscles sourronding the pelvis there is also a clear mechanical affection on the muscles through the change in the biomechanics of the pelvis. The possibility that disturbances in the mechanics of the pelvis can be secondary to muscle tension has been suggested by Lewit (7). With adequate treatment of STL massage together with mobilisation exercises and/or a self-mobilization programme (8) for the muscles at the pelvis, spine, neck and the legs these momentary neuromuscular and also biomechanic dysfunctions can be abolished together with the symtoms.

In comparison with the clinical routine testing of muscle reflexes in legs and arms, surprisingly little attention has been paid to the possibility of eliciting reflexes in back muscles. The presence of a distinct pathological S-reflex is a sign indicating an increased muscle excitability primarily in the erector spinae muscle, but also can be widely spread to other muscles; for example during a S-reflex test the patient lifts the head (neck muscles) and/or lift the leg (hip and leg muscles). Thus, the S-reflex is of great value in the clinics for diagnosis of musculo-skeletal disorders.

REFERENCES

1. Silverstolpe, L. (1989). A pathological erector spinae reflex - a new sign of mechanical pelvic dysfunction. A proposal of treatment. J Manual Medicine 4:28.
2. Skoglund, C.R. (1989). New physical aspects on the pathological erector spinae reflex in cases of mechanical pelvic dysfunction. J Manual Medicine 4:29-30.
3. Midttun, A. and Bojsen-Möller, F. (1986). The sacrotuberous ligament syndrome. In: Modern manual therapy of the vertebral column pp 815-818 (ed Grieve G P). Churchill Livingstone, Edinburgh, London and New York.
4. Skoglund, C.R., Andersson, E. and Eriksson, A. (1989). Syndromet mekanisk bäckendysfunction - neurofysiologiska aspekter. Sjukgymnasten 12:24-31, Sweden. English summary.
5. Sjölander, P (1989). A sensory role for the cruciate ligaments. Thesis. Umeå University, Sweden. Medical Dissertations, New series no 245.
6. Leonard, C.T., Hirschfeldt, H. and Forssberg, H. (1988) Gait acquisition and reflex abnormalities in normal children and children with celebral palsy. Elsevier Science Publishers B.V. (Biomedical Division). Posture and gait: Development, adaption and modulation. B. Amblard et al., editors, pp 33-45.
7. Lewit, K (1987). Beckenverwringung und Iliosacralblockierung. Manuelle Medizin 25;64-70.
8. Eriksson, A. and Skoglund, C.R. (1989). Program för självmobilisering och muskelträning vid mekanisk bäckendysfunktion. Ettårsuppföljning av 50 patienter. Sjukgymnasten 12:32-38. Sweden. English summary.

PAIN RELIEF

THE EFFECT OF INTERFERENTIAL THERAPY IN THE RELIEF OF EXPERIMENTALLY INDUCED PAIN : A PILOT STUDY.

Scott, S.M. & Purves, C.E.
Queen Margaret College, Edinburgh.

INTRODUCTION

There has been limited and inconclusive investigation of the ability of Interferential Therapy (IFT) to reduce pain perception. In contrast, Transcutaneous Electrical Nerve Stimulation (TENS) has been well researched both clinically and in the laboratory[1]. The aim of this study was to investigate the affect of IFT on experimentally induced pain perception using a protocol similar to one that has previously been used to investigate TENS. Experimentally induced pain is useful for studying the affect of a modality on pain as the pain is not complicated by clinical disease or injury.[1]

There is little consensus to be found in the literature as to the optimum IFT frequency for pain relief. Thus, to ascertain clinical practice a short questionnaire was sent to physiotherapists working in the NHS in south east Scotland. 34 replies from the 38 distributed revealed that a great range of frequencies are used to treat the similar symptoms arising from the same condition. 130Hz constant was indicated as the most commonly selected frequency (13 replies,38 %). This frequency was investigated in this trial.

The following null hypothesis was set; there is no difference in the pain perception of an ischaemic stimulus between a treatment group (IFT, 130Hz, constant), a placebo group and a control group.

METHOD

First year physiotherapy students volunteered to take part in the trial (n=15, f=10). The subjects were unfamiliar with IFT and were not experiencing any pain at the time of the trial. The subjects were randomly allocated into three groups; IFT group, Placebo group, Control group. All subjects had the same Tourniquet Test (TT) applied both before and after intervention. The TT was based on a modified version of the touniquet test developed by Smith et al (1966)[2]. The test produces ischaemic pain which has been likened to clinical pain[3]. The procedure of the TT was as follows: a previously calibrated sphygmomanometer

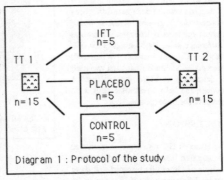

Diagram 1 : Protocol of the study

cuff was attached above the elbow and inflated to 250mmHg to occlude bloodflow to the forearm. 20 seconds after cuff inflation a standardised exercise test was commenced using a hand ergometer. The exercise involved hand contractions held for 25 seconds at 25% of maximal voluntary grip strength followed by two seconds rest. The rate of contractions were paced by a calibrated metronome and continued until the subject terminated the test due to pain. The time to test termination was recorded with a stop watch and the pain perception of the ischaemic pain in the forearm at test termination was recorded using a Visual Analogue Scale (VAS). After the initial TT there was a break of 90 minutes to allow the dispersal of accumulated metabolites. Before the next TT one of three test procedures were implemented: IFT group (n=5) received moderate intensity IFT from an Endomed 433 via 4 small plate electrodes attatched to the forearm at a frequency of 130Hz C for 7 minutes prior to the test and for the duration of the TT. The placebo group (n=5) followed the same procedure as the IFT group but the intensity was not turned on. The Control group (n=5) sat in the standardised position for 7 minutes before the TT started.

RESULTS

One Way Analysis of Variance was used to determine wether there was a difference in the test duration times of the IFT, Placebo and Control groups. A student's T Test was applied to the before and after TT duration times to determine differences between the 3 groups. Kruskal-Wallis analysis was used to determine if there was a difference in the VAS ratings of the IFT, Placebo, Control groups. Wilcoxon's Matched Pairs Signed Ranks test was used to determine if there was difference between the before and after pain scale ratings of the three groups.

DISCUSSION

The effect of IFT on ischaemic pain was investigated using a TT. Statistical analysis of the results revealed that there was no difference in the VAS rating or the TT duration time after application IFT at 130Hz compared with either the placebo or control interventions and therfore the null

TOURNIQUET TEST

GROUP	VAS RATING	DURATION OF TEST
IFT:PLACEBO	ns	ns
IFT:CONTROL	ns	ns
PLACEBO:CONTROL	ns	ns
BEFORE:AFTER IFT	ns	ns
BEFORE:AFTER PLACEBO	ns	ns
BEFORE:AFTER CONTROL	ns	ns

p>0.05

Table !: Statistical Analysis of the VAS ratings and TT duration times.

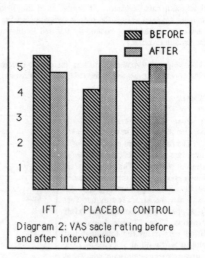

Diagram 2: VAS sacle rating before and after intervention

744

hypothesis can be accepted. However, the results of this pilot study cannot be extrapolated to the use of IFT in general. This study involved a small sample size and interesting, although not significant, trends can be seen in the VAS ratings. A larger sample size is required to investigate these trends further. Also only one of the many possible frequencies was studied and an area of future work must be to clarify the the present confusion of which frequency should be used for pain relief.

FUTURE USE OF THE TT

The results from this study suggest that the TT may be a suitable method of evaluating the pain relieving properties of IFT. This conclusion was reached because all groups started with similar pre-test measures in response to a standard stimulus which indicates that the test provides a reliable measure. However, the fact that no intervention altered the pain perception may possibly indicate that this test is not sensitive to changes in pain perception. This test protocol involved a rapid transition from a condition of no pain to one of intense pain i.e. the test duration was approximately 2-3 minutes. A TT that has a slower onset of pain may be more sensitive to detecting any effects of IFT.

CONCLUSION

Interferential is a widely used[4] and expensive modality, but its effectiveness as modality to alter pain perception has still to determined.

REFERENCES

1 Roche P.A., and Wright A., (1990) An Investigation into the Value of Transcutaneous Electrical Stimulation (TENS) for Arthritic Pain. Physiotherpay Theory and Practice 6 25-33.

2 Smith, G.M. Egberg, L.D. Markowitz, R.A. Mostller, F. Beecher, H.K. (1966) An Experimental method Sensitive to Morphin in Man; the Submaximal Effort Tourniquet Test. J Pharmacol Exp Ther 154 326-331.

3 Roche P.A., Gijsbers K., Belch J.J.F., Forbes C.D., (1984) Modification of Induced Ischemic Pain by Transcutaneous Electrical Stimulation. Pain 20 45-52.

4 Ide L., and Partridge C.J. (1989) Survey of Electrotherapy Equipment in Physiotherapy Departments and Private Practice. Centre for Physiotherapy Research, King's College London.

A COMPARATIVE TRIAL IN ELECTROANALGESIA: CODETRON VS TENS FOR SHORT TERM PAIN RELIEF

T. MAROVINO
P.W. STRATFORD

SUSSEX PHYSIOTHERAPY, MISSISSAUGA, ONTARIO, CANADA
McMASTER UNIVERSITY, HAMILTON, ONTARIO, CANADA

PATIENTS SUFFERING FROM ACUTE LOW BACK PAIN OF MUSCULO-SKELETAL ORIGIN WERE GIVEN TWO MODES OF ELECTROSTIMULATION ON ALTERNATE SESSIONS RANDOMIZED IN BLOCKS OF SIX TREATMENTS. EACH SUBJECT RECEIVED EITHER THE CODETRON OR TENS PACKAGE FIRST, FOLLOWED BY THE OTHER TREATMENT ON A SUBSEQUENT VISIT. PATIENTS WERE BLINDED TO TREATMENT TYPE. BOTH MODALITIES WERE EVALUATED FOR THEIR ABILITY TO REDUCE PAIN INTENSITY, PAIN DURATION AND IMPROVE GENERAL FUNCTIONAL STATUS IN PATIENTS SUFFERING FROM AN ACUTE EPISODE OF LOW BACK PAIN. AN ANALYSIS OF COVARIANCE DEMONSTRATED THAT THE PRE-TREATMENT VAS SCORE WAS A STRONG PREDICTOR OF THE AFTER TREATMENT PAIN SCORE $P < 0.001$. THE SESSION NUMBER DID NOT INFLUENCE THE AMOUNT OF PAIN RELIEF. ALSO, NO STATISTICALLY SIGNIFICANT DIFFERENCES WERE EVIDENT BETWEEN THE CODETRON AND TENS TREATMENT FOR EITHER OUTCOME MEASURE. THE RESULTS WOULD INDICATE THAT CODETRON IS NO LESS EFFECTIVE THAN CONVENTIONAL TENS IN THE SHORT TERM MANAGEMENT OF ACUTE LOW BACK PAIN.

LASER MEDIATED INCREASES IN NERVE CONDUCTION LATENCIES: LONG TERM EFFECTS

Baxter, G.D.[1], Bell, A.J.[2], Allen, J.M.[1] & Ravey, R.[3]
[1]Biomedical Sciences Research Centre, [2]Dept. Occupational Therapy & Physiotherapy, [3]Dept. Psychology, UNIVERSITY OF ULSTER, Jordanstown, BT37 0QB, N. Ireland.

Introduction

Low Level Laser Therapy (LLLT[1]) has recently become a popular treatment modality in physiotherapeutic practice, its most common applications being in the photobiostimulation of wound healing and the relief of pain[2]. Despite their apparent popularity, the use of these devices remains contentious, not least because of contradictory findings from basic and clinical research and the poor quality of a large number of the published papers[3].

Given the analgesic use of LLLT, a number of studies have investigated the neurophysiological effects of laser with contradictory findings. *In vitro* preparations have shown increased acetylcholine release[4] and altered neural firing patterns[5] after laser irradiation. In contrast, other groups have failed to observe any such laser-mediated effects[6]. Similarly, in studies on healthy human volunteers, a report of apparent photosensitivity in the median nerve[7] was found to be impossible to replicate using an identical protocol[8]. Nerve conduction studies are a relatively common test of peripheral nerve function in clinical neurophysiology[9], and have been used recently by a number of groups to assess the effects of low level laser irradiation upon the human radial nerve *in vivo*. Once again, the results of these studies are contentious with some finding no effect[10], while others report increase in conduction latencies after relatively short periods of irradiation[11].

We have reported previously that irradiation over the course of the human median nerve in resting subjects using low intensity continuous wave infrared laser (830 nm, 1.2 J/cm[2]) produced an increase in antidromic conduction latencies[12]. This effect was not observed in the contralateral limb[13]. The current study was designed to assess the duration of this laser-mediated increase in nerve conduction latency and to assess the concomitant effects upon (peak to peak) amplitude of the compound action potential. Preliminary results from this work have already been reported elsewhere[14].

Methodology

For the current study, which was approved by the University's ethical committee, healthy human volunteers (n=27) were recruited and screened for peripheral neuropathy. The experimental procedure was explained, a simple consent form signed, and subjects allowed to rest for 20 minutes. After this, the skin over the forearm was prepared with alcohol to remove surface lipids and an abrasive (Omniprep) used to clean the stimulation and recording sites. A bipolar muscle stimulator was then used to identify the course of the median nerve in the forearm and at the elbow for antidromic stimulation. The site was marked and hydrogel electrodes affixed. A velcro supported earth was then fastened approximately 8 cm above the wrist. Finally, digital ring electrodes prepared with conducting gel were positioned on the second digit, approximately 3 cm apart.

Electrodes were attached to the patient connection unit of a Mystro[+] MS20 neurophysiological stimulation and recording apparatus (Medelec, Woking). Stimulation consisted of 100 µs pulses, using voltages of 55-85V (nominal). Stimulus voltage was increased until response amplitude was maximum. At this point, 16 stimuli were delivered at a frequency of 1 Hz and the responses averaged and stored. This procedure was repeated at 2 minute intervals until a stable recording was obtained.

Subjects were randomly allocated to experimental (laser), placebo, or control conditions. For the experimental condition, subjects were irradiated at ten points along the course of the nerve between the electrodes for 30 s each point, using a continuous wave 40 mW laser diode operating at 820 nm (1.2 J/cm^2). For the placebo condition, the procedure was repeated without switching on the laser diode. These two groups of subjects were unaware of whether actual or sham radiation was delivered during this part of the experiment. In the control condition, subjects rested for five minutes. At the end of this period, all subjects had nerve conduction tests repeated in the manner described above, and again at 5 minute intervals for a total period of 60 minutes. On conclusion of the experiment, all electrodes were removed, the subjects' arms cleaned and examined for any sign of injury.

Stored recordings were analysed to determine the latency (in ms) to the positive peak of the evoked compound action potential, and peak to peak amplitude (in µV).

Results

Subsequent analysis of results showed a small but reproducible increase in conduction latency at the digital recording site after laser irradiation(see table). No such increases were observed for control or placebo conditions. This difference was found to be significant at the 0.05 level using analysis of variance. In contrast, as can be seen from the table, amplitude scores showed a small but insignificant decrease after laser irradiation.

Table: Summary of Results

NB: "Pre" = first recording, "Post" = after 1 hour. Values given are means +/- sem.

Condition		Latencies (ms)	Amplitudes (µV)
Control	Pre:	7.17 +/- 0.14	21.32 +/- 3.69
	Post:	7.15 +/- 0.15	21.13 +/- 4.06
Placebo	Pre:	6.96 +/- 0.13	24.82 +/- 3.24
	Post:	6.98 +/- 0.14	25.14 +/- 3.91
Laser	Pre:	7.00 +/- 0.13	29.02 +/- 4.51
	Post:	7.46 +/- 0.14	26.73 +/- 3.05

Discussion

This study showed a significant increase in median nerve conduction latencies after laser irradiation of the skin over the course of the nerve. No significant concomitant changes in amplitude were seen. This finding of laser-mediated increases in conduction latency is in keeping with those of Snyder-Mackler and Bork[11], who observed similar latency shifts in the radial nerve. In contrast, Greathouse and colleagues[10] failed to find any such effects. The reason for these contradictory findings are unclear, but may be due in part to the dissimilar irradiation parameters employed.

While the results of this study demonstrate the neurophysiological effects of LLLT used at the irradiation parameters specified, the precise mechanism of action underlying this phenomenon are unclear. Certainly the observed results cannot be explained in terms of a possible photothermal effect, as increases in temperature would tend to reduce nerve conduction latencies[9]. Further work is already underway in this laboratory using microneurography and evoked potential techniques in an attempt to further characterise the neurophysiological effects of laser at peripheral and central levels.

Acknowledgements

This work was supported by the Department of Education for Northern Ireland. Assistance was also received from a charitable trust connected with the University. The help and advice of Dr. J.D. Cole, Consultant Clinical Neurophysiologist, Poole General Hospital is gratefully acknowledged.

References

1. Ohshiro, T. & Calderhead, R.G. (1988). Low Level Laser Therapy: A Practical Introduction. Wiley, Chichester.
2. Baxter, G.D., Bell, A.J., Allen, J.M. et al (1991). Physiotherapy 77, 171-8.
3. Basford, J.R. (1989). Lasers Surgery Medicine 9, 1-5.
4. Vizi, E., Mester, E., Tisza, S. et al (1977). J. Neural Transmission 40, 305-8.
5. Fork, R. (1971). Science 171, 907-8.
6. Lundeberg, T. & Zhou, J. (1988). American J. Chinese Medicine 16, 87-91.
7. Walker, J. & Akhanjee, L. (1985). Brain Research 344, 223-5.
8. Wu, W., Ponnudurai, R., Katz J. et al (1987). Brain Research 401, 407-8.
9. Ma, D.M. & Liveson, J.A. (1983). Nerve Conduction Handbook. F.A. Davis, Philadelphia.
10. Greathouse, D., Currier, D. & Gilmore, R. (1985). Physical Therapy 65, 1184-7.
11. Snyder-Mackler, L. & Bork, C. (1988). Physical Therapy 68, 223-5.
12. Baxter, G.D., Bell, A.J., Allen, J.M. et al. (1991a). Irish J. Medical Science, in press.
13. Baxter, G.D., Bell, A.J., Allen, J.M. et al. (1991b). Irish J. Medical Science, in press.
14. Baxter, G.D., Allen, J.M. & Bell, A.J. (1991). J. Physiology, in press.

The Effect of Low Power Laser on Lateral Epicondylitis Measured by
Infrared Thermography

van Scheers R, Hauger E, Selim A

Hans & Olaf Fysioterapi A/S, Torggata 16, 0181 Oslo 1, Norway

Early low power laser research, especially clinical research, did not
necessarly tell the complete story concerning its efficiency. Published
reports lacked control groups, used group sizes that where too small,
and showed no signs of treatment parameter standardization (1). In
addition, all treatment variables used were basically all "subjective" in
nature allowing for large differences in reported laser treatment results.

In order to do our initial project differently, we looked for tools that
could measure treatment variables more "objectively". We found infrared
thermography, an already established measurement approach which has been
found to be quite effective in measuring the state of inflammatory
conditions such as tendonitis (2,3).

Our pilot study involved nine subjects all showing clinical signs of
lateral epicondylitis. They had increased pain at the epicondyle with
wrist extension and with stretching of the forearm extensors. They had
a palpable tender point at the lateral epicondyle as well.

An Inframetrics 600 infrared thermography system was used to measure the
usual 1-3°C increase in heat detected at the epicondyle (3). All of the
nine subjects had "hot spots" within the range described on the involved
side. The palpable tender point correlated with the location of the
"hot spot" in all nine cases. However, the "hot spot" appeared larger in
size.

Due to their size, the "hot spots" were divided into four squares, each
square receiving an equal amount of laser radiation using an Omega
820nm, 50mW CW laser diode. Each square received a dose of 38.4 J/cm2.
Spot size was .125cm2. Power density was 400mW/cm2. Radiation time was
96sec per square. In addition, the forearm extensor group received two
minutes of radiation using a 46-diode cluster probe. The cluster probe
contained 1x25mW 820nm laser diode in the middle. The laser diode was
surrounded by three rings of superluminous diodes (SLD) containing the
following wavelenghts: 10x870nm, 10x880nm, 10x950nm, and 19x940nm. The
average power of the cluster probe was 75mW/cm2. The cutaneous dose was
9 J/cm2. Spot size was 20cm2. All radiation was given at 5000Hz. Diodes
were in contact with the skin during treatment.

We used two different thermographic measurements as our treatment
variables in this study, the "maximal" and the "average" temperature of
the "hot spots". Measurements were taken before and after a series of
nine laser treatments given three times per week.

Results: Thermographic measurements showed significant changes in both the "maximal" and the "average" temperatures towards normal:

Table I

	Before	After	Change
No. of subjects	9	9	9
Mean (SD)	32.1 (0.8)	31.5 (0.7)	0.6 (0.6)
Median with 95%	32.1	31.3	0.7
Confidence int.	(31.1-32.8)	(30.9-31.6)	(0-0.9)
Min-max	30.8-33.5	30.8-33.2	-0.1-1.9
P-value			$P_2 = 0.02$

Tabel 1: Shows the results of maximal temperature changes measurements

Table II

	Before	After	Change
No. of subjects	9	9	9
Mean (SD)	31.8 (0.8)	31.3 (0.9)	0.5 (0.3)
Median with 95%	31.9	31.3	0.6
Confidence int.	(31.1-32.4)	(30.5-31.6)	(0.1-0.8)
Min-max	30.2-33.2	30.1-33.2	0-0.8
P-value			$P_2 = 0.01$

Table 2: Shows the results of the average temperature measurements

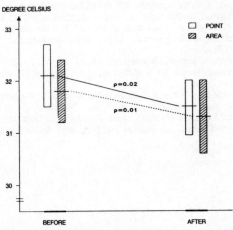

Figure 1: Shows how the maximal and the average temperatures decreased from the pre to the post measurements

Discussion: It appears that the thermograph is able to detect a change in temperature where an inflammatory reaction is taking place. It is invitable to say that as the temperature decreases, which obviously can be detected, must mean that the underlying inflammatory process is resolving. This may or may not be true. However, Dyson et al. has proven that laser and SLD light has an effect on macrophages and mast cells accelerating their action in areas of repair (4,5). Tendonitis involves an area of repair, being repaired by our own immune system. It therefore may be that changes in temperature reflects the state of repair sub-cutaneously.

Seven out of nine subjects showed significant changes between pre and post measurements. Only four out of these seven subjects felt improved. This may imply that the improvement is not always recognizable by the subject. Or, they may not see the improvement as significant and therefore neglect to report it. The two subjects that did not improve appeared more involved clinically showing signs of dysfunctions in their cervical spines with pain referred into the ipsilateral upper extremities. However, they had the usual signs of tendonitis already described and "hot spots" at the epicondyle were observed.

Conclusion: It appears that the low power laser is able to improve the condition of lateral epicondylitis. We look at our pilot results as encouraging. This pilot study is the basis for a larger double blind study presently in progress at our clinic.

References:
1. Basford JK (1986) "Low-energy laser treatment of pain and wounds: Hype, hope, or hokum?" Mayo Clinic Proctor 61:671-675
2. Mangine RE, Siqueland KA, Noyes FR (1987) The Use of Thermography for the Diagnosis and Management of Patellar Tendonitis. The Journal of Orthopaedic and Sports Physical Therapy 9(4):132-140
3. Binder A, Parr G, Page T, Hazleman B (1983) A Clinical and Thermographic Study of Lateral Epicondylitis. British Journal of Rheumatology 22(2):77-81
4. Young S, Bolton P, Dyson M, Harvey W, Diamantopoulos C (1989) Macrophage Responsiveness to Light Therapy. Lasers in Surgery and Medicine 9:497-505
5. El Sayed SO, Dyson M (1990) A Comparison of the Effect of Multi-wavelenght Light Produced by a Cluster of Semiconductor Diodes and of Each Individual Diode on Mast Cell Number and Degranulation in Intact and Injured Skin. Lasers in Surgery and Medicine 10:00-00

A DOUBLE BLIND PLACEBO CONTROLLED TRIAL TO ASSESS THE EFFICACY OF LOW POWER LASER IN
CHRONIC RHEUMATOID ARTHRITIS OF THE FINGER JOINTS

Jane HALL and A K CLARKE

Royal National Hospital for Rheumatic Diseases, Bath

INTRODUCTION
Rheumatoid Arthritis (RA) is the most common chronic inflammatory arthropathy affecting 1.5
million in the United Kingdom. Due to the disabling effect of the disease, the lack of
fully effective medication and the frequent side effects of drugs, new and non-invasive
methods of treatment are constantly sought. Low power laser has recently been introduced
into physiotherapy departments and it may be useful in controlling the inflammation and
pain associated with RA.
BACKGROUND
Reports in the literature suggest that laser may be effective in a wide variety of
conditions, including wound healing [1], soft tissue injury [2], pain relief [3], and rheumatic
disorders [4-9]. The findings from studies conducted on patients with RA are, on the whole,
indicative of improvement in terms of pain relief and some studies report physical benefits.
However it is difficult to draw firm conclusions due to the use of different equipment,
doses and treatment schedultes [10].
AIM OF STUDY
The aim of this study was to evaluate the efficacy of low power laser in terms of
functional and health status, and disease activity in patients who have chronic RA.
METHODOLOGY
This study utilised a randomised, double blind and placebo controlled design.
Equipment:
The low power laser Biotherapy 3, manufactured by Omega Universal Technologies, was used.
The device consists of a power supply unit fitted with 2 detachable probes. One probe
is fitted with one 820 nm, linearly polarised, 50mW narrow profile galium aluminium
arsenide, continuous wave laser diode with a beam divergence of 6^{0}, and pulsed at 5000Hz
with an 80% duty cycle. The diode area is 0.1256cm and the applied radiant exposure per
treatment is 11.9 Joules/cm on each lateral side and 5.9 Joules/cm on the dorsal and
ventral surfaces of each treated joint. A second cluster probe contains an array of 31
diodes (1*820nm, 10*870nm, 10*880nm and 10*950nm). Each diode contained with the cluster
probe produces a maximum average power density of 120mW/cm and a minimum power density
at a single plane at the dermal surface of 10mW/cm.
The laser and dummy laser probes were coded (A and B). For the duration of the trial only
the statistician and the manufacturer knew which machine was which.
The treatment schedule was devised to allow comparisons with other studies. Approximately
80% of patients with RA suffer symptoms in the metacarpophalangeal (MCP) and proximal
interphalangeal (PIP) joints, and these joints were therefore selected on the basis that
recruitment would be propitious. In addition the available wavelengths allow
penetration depths of 3-4cms [11] only and treating small joints would appear to offer the
best chance of demonstrating a positive therapeutic effect.
Patients:
Thirty adult patients with stage II orIII classical or definite RA and who presented with
active synovitis of some or all of the MCP and PIP joints as characterised by pain,
tenderness, swelling and stiffness were recruited to the trial. Patients who were not

on stable medication for a minimum of 30 days prior to the start of the trial or whose joints were incapable of a response for mechanical reasons were excluded. Patients were recruited from the out-patient clinics at the Royal National Hospital for Rheumatic Diseases, Bath following their informal verbal consent.

Treatment Procedure:

Prior to entry to the trial patients underwent a detailed examination by a research physiotherapist to assess the patient's suitability. Following a successful assessment patients were randomly allocated to treatment either with active or placebo laser in a 4-5 week, 12 treatment design.

The 1st to 5th MCP and PIP joints of the most affected hand were treated 3 times a week for 4 consecutive weeks. A standardised treatment in which the radial, ulnar, dorsal and ventral aspects of the MCP and PIP joints were lased with the single and cluster probes for a total of 18 minutes was given by a specially trained physiotherapist.

Measurements:

The following measurements were completed on 4 occasions: before, immediately at the end of the trial, 1 month and 3 months after the treatment at follow-up to evaluate changes. An independant assessor "blind" to the treatment condition obtained the measurements. Patients completed the measures on each occasion at the same time of the day to account for circadian rhythms. Both hands were assessed; the non-treated hand being assessed to investigate the possibly systemic effect.

Measures of physical function included grip strength and three finger chuck pinch, a standardised 9 hole peg test and range of movement of the MCP and PIP joints. Measures of disease activity included laboratory measures (haemoglobin, C-reactive protein, platelet count and alkaline phosphatase, infra red thermography[12], morning stiffness, the Ritchie Index[13] and swelling of the MCP and PIP joints[14]. Subjective measures of health status were recorded by self-report and inlcuded visual analogue scales for the measurement of pain and the Health Assessment Questionnaire[15].

ANALYSIS

The data has been compiled on a micro computer and will be analysed using SPSSX. Comparisons between the groups will be made using two way analysis of variance for a repeated measures design. This will allow an examination of the overall effects of treatment and time. A significance level of 0.05 will be used for all statistical testing.

COMMENT

The results and implications from this study will be presented at the WCPT. Further information may be obtained from the first author.

We wish to thank Omega Universal Technologies for their support and partial funding of this project.

REFERENCES

1. Dyson M and Young S (1986). Effect of laser therapy on wound contraction and cellularity in mice. Lasers in Medical Science, 1, 2:125-130.

2. England S M, Coppock J S, Struthers G R and Bacon P A (1985). An observer blind trial of I.R.ceb mid-laser therapy in biciptal tendonitis and supraspinatus tendonitis. Procedings of the International Congress on Laser and Medicine, Bologna.

3. Walker J (1983). Relief from chronic pain by low power laser irradiation. Neuroscience Letters, 43: 339-344.

4. Goldman J A, Chiapella J, Casey H et al (1980). Laser therapy of Rheumatoid Arthritis. Lasers in Surgery and Medicine, 1:93-101.

5. Palmgren N, Jensen G F, Kaae K, Windelin M and Colov H C (1989). Low-power laser therapy in rheumatoid arthritis. Lasers in Medical Science, 4:193-196.

6. Bliddal H, Hellesen C, Ditlevsen P, Asselberghs J and Lyager L (1987). Soft-laser therapy of rheumatoid arthritis. Scand J Rheumatology, 16:225-228.

7. Asada K, Yutani Y and Shimazu A (1989). Diode laser therapy for rheumatoid arthritis: A clinical evaluation of 102 joints treated with low reactive-level laser therapy (LLLT). Laser Therapy, 1,3:147-151.

8. Obara J, Yanase M, Motomura A et al (1987). The pain relief of low energy laser irradiation on rheumatoid arthritis. Pain Clinic, 8,1: 18-22.

9. Walker J, Akhanjee L, Cooney M, Goldstein J, Tamayoshi S and Sgal-Gidan F (1987). Laser therapy for pain of rheumatoid arthritis. Clinical Journal of Pain, 3:54-59.

10. Kitchen S S and Partridge C (1991). A review of low level laser therapy. Physiotherapy, 77, 3: 161-168.

11. Kolari P J (1985). Penetration of unfocused laser light into the skin. Arch Dermatol Res, 277: 342-44.

12. Bacon P A, Collins A J, Ring F J and Cosh J A (1976). Thermography in the assessment of inflammatory arthritis. Clinics in Rheumatic Diseases, 2,1: 51-65.

13. Ritchie D M et al (1968). Clinical studies with an articular index for the assessment of joint tenderness in patients with rheumatoid arthritis. Quarterly Journal of Medicine, New Series, 37, 147: 393-406.

14. Webb J, Downie W W, Dick W C and Lee P (1973). Evaluation of digital joint circumference measurements in rheumatoid arthritis. Scand. J of Rheumatology, 2:127-131.

15. Fries J F, Spitz P W and Young D Y (1982). The dimensions of health outcomes: the health assessment questionnaire, disability and pain scales. J Rheumatol. 9:789-793.

AN INVESTIGATION OF THE EFFECT OF LOW LEVEL LASER THERAPY UPON ERB'S POINT SOMATOSENSORY EVOKED POTENTIALS

Mokhtar, B., Baxter, G.D., Bell, A.J. & Allen, J.M.
Dept. Occupational Therapy & Physiotherapy, Biomedical Sciences Research Centre, UNIVERSITY OF ULSTER, Jordanstown, BT37 OQB , N. Ireland.

Introduction

Low Level Laser Therapy (LLLT) has recently been promoted as an analgesic modality, yet it's efficacy remains contentious and its underlying mechanisms of action unclear[1]. As part of an extensive research programme on the neurophysiological effects of LLLT, the present study was carried out to investigate the effect of this relatively new modality upon Erb's point Somatosensory Evoked Potentials (SSEPs).

Background

Over the last several years, a number of studies have attempted to determine the neurophysiological effect of LLLT. At the peripheral level, experiments have shown that Argon laser (488 nm) alters the firing pattern of ganglion cells in Aplysia[2], and that Ruby laser (694nm) increases acetylcholine release in guinea pig Auerbach's plexus[3]. Others have recorded an increase in Na-K-ATPase activity in rat saphenous nerve after Gallium-Aluminium-Arsenide (Ga-Al-As, 830 nm) laser application[4], and normalisation of action potential in crushed rat sciatic nerve following Helium-Neon (He-Ne, 632 nm) laser exposure[5]. Contrary to these findings, Lundeberg and Zhou found that neither of the above lasers had any effect on the generation of sensory potentials in Crustacean receptor cells[6].

Studies on human volunteers have produced similarly mixed results, with some workers finding no effect[7], while others report an increase in sensory nerve conduction latency in the superficial radial nerve[8], and the median nerve[9] after laser irradiation. More interestingly, Walker and Akhanjee reported that stimulation of the median nerve with an He-Ne laser initiated a propagated action potential which could be recorded at Erb's point[10]. Unfortunately, these results could not be confirmed by other investigators who attempted to replicate the above study[11].

Given the reports of increased antidromic latencies after laser irradiation, it was the purpose of this study to investigate the peripheral neurophysiological effects of LLLT upon Erb's point SSEPs

Methods

Subjects

Fifteen healthy volunteers, aged 20-28 years (mean=23years) were recruited to carry out the current investigation, and randomly assigned to one of three experimental conditions: laser, placebo or control. Subjects were briefed on experimental procedure, screened for relevant neuropathology, and asked to sign a simple consent form. The project was approved by the University's ethical committee.

Procedure

Subjects rested supine for 10 minutes before the procedure was commenced. After this period, subjects' arms were exposed and the skin over the wrist, the biceps and the ipsilateral Erb's point was prepared with alcohol, and an abrasive (Omniprep) to remove surface lipids. A bipolar muscle stimulator was then used to identify the precise location of Erb's point and the median nerve at the wrist. Silver/Silver chloride electrodes were affixed firmly to the marked Erb's point and referenced to the contralateral clavicle as described by Walker and Akhanjee[10]. A ground electrode was also attached securely over the biceps. Finally, two hydrogel electrodes were affixed over the median nerve at the wrist for orthodromic stimulation. All the electrodes were connected to a Mystro+ MS 20 stimulation and recording apparatus (Medelec,Woking).

The median nerve was stimulated with 2 ms pulses at 5Hz. The intensity (V) was adjusted to produce comfortable thumb twitch. Each recording consisted of 256 averaged responses. The filter was set at band-pass frequencies between 20-2000 Hz. Recordings were taken at 5 minute intervals for a further 20 minute period. Laser (or placebo) when used was applied between the first and second recordings. For the laser condition, a multiwavelength, multidiode "Cluster" array (Omega Universal Technologies, London), operating at wavelengths between 660-920 nm, was used to irradiate the median nerve at three equidistant points in the forearm for 30s per point. This cluster array delivers a total of 600 mW of incident power across a 12 sq.cm area, giving an average energy density of 1.5 J/sq.cm. For the placebo condition, a "dummy" treatment head was used to deliver sham irradiation.

Results

The stored data was analysed using analysis of variance. Mean latencies obtained pre and post-test for all three experimental conditions, as well as standard errors of the mean (SEM) are summarized in the table.

Table: Summary of Results (NB: Latencies in ms)

condition		-5	0	5	10	15 (min)
L	Mean	9.70	9.76	9.79	9.81	9.83
	SEM	0.15	0.16	0.16	0.16	0.15
P	Mean	9.92	9.94	9.97	9.97	9.98
	SEM	0.12	0.13	0.11	0.11	0.12
C	Mean	9.72	9.70	9.70	9.70	9.74
	SEM	0.13	0.13	0.12	0.12	0.14

Discussion

The purpose of this study was to investigate the effect of low level laser irradiation of the median nerve upon the latency of Erb's point SSEPs elicited by innocuous electrical stimulation. From the data presented above it can be seen that latencies are increased following laser application. Note that 15 minutes post laser, the mean latency has increased from 9.701+/-0.153 to 9.837+/-0.157 ms. This difference is significant at the 0.05 level. No such increase was observed in placebo or control conditions.

The results suggest that laser irradiation of the skin overlying peripheral nerves at therapeutic doses has a direct neurophysiological effect. This finding provides further evidence of laser-mediated neurophysiological effects in vivo.

References

1. Baxter, G. D. , Bell, A. J., Allen, J. M. et al. (1991). Physiotherapy 77, 171-178.
2. Fork, R. (1971). Science 172, 907-908.
3. Vizi, E., Mester, E. & Tisza, S. (1977). J. Neural Transmission 40, 305-308.
4. Koduh, C., Inomata, K., Akajima, K. et al. (1988). Laser Therapy, Pilot Issue, July 1988.
5. Rochkind, S., Nissan, M., Razon, N. et al (1986). Acta Neurochir. 83, 125-130.
6. Lundeberg, T. & Zhou, J. (1988). American J. Chinese Medicine XVI, 3-4, 87-91.
7. Greathouse, D., Currier, D. & Gilmore, R. (1985). Physical Therapy 65, 1184-1187.
8. Snyder-Mackler, L., & Bork, C. (1988). Physical Therapy 68, 223-225.
9. Baxter, G.D., Bell, A.J., Allen, J.M. et al (1990). The 4th International Biotherapy Laser Association Seminar, Guy's Hospital, London.
10. Walker, J. & Akhanjee, L. (1985). Brain Research 344, 281-285.
11. Wu, W., Ponnudurai, R, Katz, J. et al. (1987). Brain Research 401, 407-408.

THE EFFECT OF UHF-CURRENTS IN PATIENTS WITH LUMBER OSTEOCHONDROSIS

A Ye Asheraliyeva

Centre of Balneology & Traditional
Medicine, Frunze, Kirghiz SSR, USSR

Introduction :The effect of UHF-currents on re-
flex(Re) and radicular(Ra) syndromes in patients
with lumber osteochondrosis was studied.
Treatment   :60 Re- and 70 Ra-syndrome patients
received UHF-currents in the continuous mode of
operation using 12 cm-diameter condenser-type
plates in lumbar and leg zones, a 1.5 cm clearance being left between the plates and the surface of the affected zones. The treatment consisted of ten 15-min daily sessions and was started with an initial dosage of 5.5 wt which was
increased to 13 to 30 wt after two sessions. The
controls (20 subjects) received a placebo, i.e.
an imitation of electric procedures. Occasionally, an additional treatment of sulfurated hydrogen baths, massage and physical exercise were
prescribed to Ra-syndrome patients to relieve
persistent exacerbation due to radicular irritation and compression.
Results:The positive effect was achieved in 69%
of Re-patients and 47% of Ra-patients, the placebo group showing only a 25% improvement.
Conclusion : The UHF-currents are an effective
treatment modality in lumbar osteochondrosis,
particularly in patients with reflex syndromes.

CONTROLLED STUDY TO MEASURE THE EFFECTIVENESS OF PULSED SHORT WAVE FOR PAIN RELIEF IN OSTEOARTHRITIC HIPS

JA KLABER MOFFETT MSc, MCSP, H FROST MCSP & PH RICHARDSON PhD
Physiotherapy Research Unit, Nuffield Orthopaedic Centre, Oxford

INTRODUCTION

THE USE OF PULSED SHORT WAVE IN PHYSIOTHERAPY

Pulsed short wave therapy (PSW), since it has been introduced from the USA about 20 years ago, has more recently gained considerable popularity in this country (Goats 1989). Pulsed short wave (PSW) consists of bursts of alternating high frequency (HF) current, interspersed with a cut-off phase, during which time any heat formed in the tissues can be dissipated. It is used for the treatment of soft tissue injuries and also for more chronic conditions, including osteoarthritis. Clinicians have found it to be beneficial in reducing swelling and inflammation, assisting the healing process and relieving pain. The high frequency electromagnetic field is claimed to act at a cellular level, having the ability apparently to restore the membrane potential of a damaged cell. It may also influence the healing process, by helping to re-establish the sodium and potassium ionic balance (Hayne 1984).

THE EFFECT OF THE PULSED SHORT WAVE ON THE TISSUES AT A CELLULAR LEVEL

Many different hypotheses have been put forward to explain the apparent effect of a PEMF on tissue healing at a cellular level. When tissue damage occurs some cells will die and it is possible that PEMF could assist the process of phagocytosis (Evans 1980).

During tissue damage, many surviving cells suffer a reduction in their cell membrane potential. Collis and Segal (1988) carried out a series of well-designed in vitro experiments, which provide evidence of a specific effect of PEMF on the cell membrane, using the same field type (15Hz) as was used for the healing of un-united fractures.

A number of animal studies have provided some evidence in favour of the effectiveness of PSW (27MHz) in accelerating healing or regeneration of living tissue (Eg. Wilson & Jagadeesh, 1976).

CLINICAL TRIALS

A number of placebo controlled studies in a clinical population claim positive effects of PSW on pain, disability and swelling (eg Barclay et al 1983), but none of these studies appear to have used a blind or independent assessor.

Two studies included an independent assessor blind to the treatment provided. However, differences in the parameters used in the application of the PEMF make it difficult to compare the results of these studies, directly with the above trial results. Binder et al (1984) obtained significantly good results in patients with chronic and recalcitrant rotator cuff tendinitis using a lower frequency (75Hz) PEMF which was applied for 5-9 hours daily. Barker et al (1985), who like Wilson (1974) and Pasila (1978) treated sprained ankles, found no significant difference between the treatment and control groups but this could be due to the application of a lower intensity dosage. This last study appears to be the only study to date that used a truly double blind design, where the therapist is also blind to the treatment. In other trials where this is not the case the results of the study are laid open to interpretation.

There are no studies to date on the use of PSW for the relief of pain in osteoarthrosis of the hip, although this form of treatment is claimed by clinicians to be very beneficial. A double blind placebo controlled trial is now underway to study the effects of PSW used for this purpose. But since there are no established guidelines as to which method of application or dosage is most effective, a pilot study (Phase I) was necessary and is described in this paper.

METHOD

DESIGN

The study was a randomised controlled trial with patients allocated to one of three different methods of application/dosage. Measures of pain and disability were taken pre-treatment, post-treatment and at 3 month follow-up.

PATIENTS

45 Patients (22 males, 23 females, mean age 64.5 years) with osteoarthrosis of the hip, currently on a waiting list for total hip arthroplasty, or referred to out-patient clinics of the Nuffield Orthopaedic Centre or were invited to take part in the study if they met the inclusion/exclusion criteria. Radiological changes in the hip reported as degenerative or arthritic, pain predominantly confined to one joint and the ability to walk 50 metres, were the main inclusion criteria. Principal exclusion criteria were previous arthroplasty on the joint to be treated, or any physiotherapy or surgery to this joint in past 6 months.

PROCEDURE

Drug therapy was stabilised as far as possible during a two week baseline period, prior to entry into the study. At this stage, advice on weight and dieting and the use of a walking aid were given if appropriate.

Treatment: A pulsed short wave machine Ultramed (supplied by medical students' charitable funds,) with a drum-type applicator, called a "Circuplode" containing a coil, provides the PEMF. It was placed in contact with the patient, directly over the centre of the joint being treated. PSW was administered three times a week for 15 minutes, over a period of three weeks, unless the patient was completely painfree sooner. No other form of physiotherapy treatment was given. The attention placebo factor, including the amount of time spent with the patient, was carefully controlled and standardised, so that these factors can be taken into account.

Three variations in application/dose were given depending on which the patient was allocated to: "Dose" A = 200 pulses/sec x 3, "Dose" B = 110 pulses/sec x 5, or "Dose" C = 82 pulses/sec x 7.

A second physiotherapist set up the dials according to the application that the patient had been randomly allocated to, so that in this way the therapist who provided the treatment did not know which dosage was being used.

Outcome measures

1) Pain diaries were completed by the patient daily, recording pain intensity and pain distress, using a numerical rating scale (0-100).

2) Functional disability, (related to 6 problem areas) was recorded on an 11-point scale verbal rating scale.

3) Active range of hip motion using specially developed equipment, based on a very large goniometer for greater reliability.

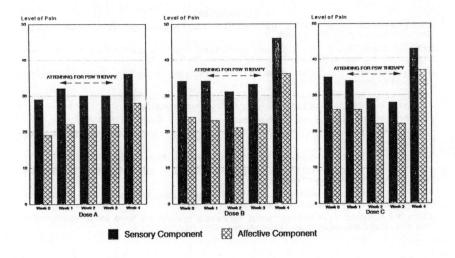

Pain Reports from Diaries

761

RESULTS

<u>Statistical Analysis:</u> Analysis of Variance for Repeated Measures over time was used to analyse the data (generated from the outcome measures from each patient on 3 occasions). This procedure allows the effect of interaction of the different treatments with the time factor to be studied.

<u>Pain:</u> Pain reported 4 times daily was averaged out over the day, and then over the weeks, keeping the affective and sensory components separate. Repeated measures analysis of variance over time showed no significant difference between the groups for either of these. Mean scores of the two components of the pain reports for each of the 3 dosages are shown on the figure.

<u>Functional disability:</u> Each activity was analysed separately but no significant difference between groups over time was found.

<u>Range of Movement:</u> Abduction, medial and lateral rotation also showed no significant difference between the groups over time.

DISCUSSION

Since there were no significant differences between the treatment groups over time for pain, functional disability or range of movement, the dosage and application of treatment was decided on, by analysing the best mean improvement in pain reports. On this basis it was decided to use "Dose" C for Phase II.

Although there was no statistically significant improvement over time according to these results, it was necessary to proceed to phase II to compare the active treatment with the placebo and a no treatment control group. It was possible, since these patients were suffering from a chronic condition and most of them were on the waiting list for total hip surgery, that without any treatment, they would have got worse. Any treatment effect can only be ascertained by comparison with a control group.

Phase II of the study is therefore now in progress, using "Dose" C in its active mode, comparing it with the dummy application and a control group who do not attend the hospital.

ACKNOWLEDGEMENTS

Thanks are due to the Oxford medical students who donated £3,000 for the pulsed short wave machine, the Oxford Regional Health Authority, who funded the first year of the study and current support from the Arthritis and Rheumatism Council.

REFERENCES

Barclay V, Collier RJ & Jones A (1983). Treatment of various hand injuries by pulsed electromagnetic energy (Diapulse). Physiotherapy 69, 6, 186-188

Barker AT, Barlow PS, Smith ME et al (1985). Double blind clinical trial of low power pulsed short-wave therapy in the treatment of soft tissue injury. Physiotherapy, 71, 12, 500-504

Binder A, Hazleman B, Parr G, Fitton-Jackson S (1984). Pulsed electromagnetic field therapy for persistent rotator cuff tendinitis. Lancet , 695-98

Collis CS & Segal MB (1988). Effects of pulsed electromagnetic fields on Na+ fluxes across a stripped rabbit colon epithelium. Journal of Applied Physiology American Physiological Society, 65, 1, 124-130

Evans P (1980). The healing process at cellular level; a review. Physiotherapy, 60, 256-259

Goats GC (1989). Pulsed electromagnetic (short wave) energy therapy. *British* Journal of Sports Medicine, 23, 4, 213-216

Hayne CR (1984). Pulsed high frequency - its place in physiotherapy. Physiotherapy, 70, 12, 459-466

Pasila M, Visuri T, Sundholm A (1978). Pulsating shortwave diathermy: value in treatment of recent ankle and foot sprains. Arch Phys Med Rehabil 59, 383-86

Wilson DH (1974). Comparison of shortwave diathermy and pulsed electromagnetic energy in the treatment of soft tissue injuries. Physiotherapy, 60, 10, 309-310

Wilson DH, Jagerdeesh P (1976). Experimental regeneration in peripheral nerves and the spinal cord in laboratory animals exposed to a pulsed electromagnetic field. Paraplegia, 14, 12-20

A COMPARISON OF THE ANALGESIC EFFECT OF T.E.N.S AND ENTONOX

Jones A.Y.M & Hutchinson R.C.
Dept. of Rehabilitation Sciences, Hong Kong Polytechnic, Hung Hom, Kowloon, Hong Kong.

INTRODUCTION:

The aims of post-operative respiratory physiotherapy are to regain and maintain the expansion of the alveoli and prevent chest complications. Post-operative wound pain however, seems to be the most common obstacle to an effective physiotherapy procedure. Adequate pain relief allows the patient to take deeper breaths and restore a higher lung volume. It was suggested that Entonox inhalation during post-operative chest physiotherapy would allow a more vigorous and effective treatment programme[1], however, the efficacy of Entonox in chest physiotherapy has not been previously reported.

Entonox (50% nitrous oxide and 50% oxygen) has a quick analgesic on and off-set time[2]. Although it has minimal effects on the normal cardiovascular and respiratory systems, mild side effects such as light-headedness and headache are not uncommon. Clinically, Entonox is a very popular analgesic modality in pain management[4,5,6], but in physiotherapy, Entonox is usually chosen as a last resort when other analgesic modalities are unsatisfactory. Transcutaneous electrical nervous stimulation (TENS) has been a popular adjunct to pain relief in patients for over 15 years. Reports of the efficacy of TENS in post surgical patients however are contradictory[7,8,9].

To determine the analgesic effect of Entonox in physiotherapy and compare this effect with TENS in the management of post operative wound pain, a prospective randomised placebo controlled study was undertaken.

METHOD:

Thirty-one patients admitted for upper abdominal surgery were seen by the physiotherapist on the evening prior to surgery and informed consent obtained. The research procedure was explained and a visual analogue scale (VAS) and peak flow meter were introduced. Those who were unable to understand or use the VAS or peak flow meter were excluded from the study.

Three chest physiotherapy treatments were given to the same patient on the first day post operation by the same physiotherapist. Each session lasted twenty minutes and consisted of a standarised treatment programme of relaxed breathing exercises, percussion and vibration to both lungs. During each physiotherapy session, analgesia was provided in random order by: a. Entonox via a face mask (Entonox group), b. paraincisional TENS (TENS group) and c. TENS with the electrodes attached to one of the patient's legs, below the tibial condyles (TTL group)

The TENS machine was a Medtronic Selectra, programmed to produce a square wave with a pulse width fixed at 175 microseconds and frequency at 99Hz. Intensity was varied according to individual patient's tolerance. Before, immediately post and 30 minutes post treatment, the patient was positioned in the half-lying position, and asked to mark the VAS, and the PEFR was measured.

This study used the patient as his own control to eliminate between patient variation. A 'sham' application was not possible but a distant TENS stimulation to the leg was used as a "modified placebo".

The data was analysed with SPSS PC+ statistic package, using non-parametric Wilcoxon matched-pairs signed-ranks test to determine a significant difference ($p < 0.05$) in the pain score, and a paired t-test to determine a significant difference in peak expiratory flow rate, before and after each treatment session. The group difference was also determined.

RESULTS:

A. Pain Score analysis:
1.   Time effect (Figure 1 & Table 1) -
      There was a significant decrease in pain score immediately after treatment in all

three groups. At 30 minutes after treatment, the decrease in pain score was only significant in the Entonox and TENS groups.

2. **Effects of the different analgesic modalities (Table 2) -**
The analgesic efficacy of the three treatment modalities was compared by calculating the difference in pain scores pre-treatment and immediately after treatment. The pain reduction by the TTL modality was significantly less than the other two methods. There was however no significant difference between the Entonox and the TENS groups. The results are similar when the pain reduction levels derived from pre-treatment and 30 minutes post treatment were compared.

B. PEFR analysis

1. **Time effect (Figure 2 & Table 3) -**
The PEFR measured immediately after treatment increased significantly in both the Entonox and TENS groups, but **not** in the TTL group. At 30 minutes post treatment, the PEFR in the TTL group **decreased** significantly when compared to both pre- and immediately post-treatment.

2. **Effects of the different analgesic modalities (Table 4) -**
Immediately post treatment, TENS significantly improved the PEFR more than the TTL therapy. At 30 minutes after treatment the PEFR improvement level was significantly less in the TTL patients compared to the other two groups. There was no difference between the TENS and Entonox groups.

Three patients complained of dizziness after Entonox inhalation. There were no other side effects of any of the treatments.

DISCUSSION:

This study demonstrates that the subjective pain scores decreased significantly immediately after physiotherapy treatment in all three analgesic modalities. An analgesic effect is expected in the TENS and Entonox group but to a lesser extent in the TTL group. The improvement in pain scores in the TTL group may be a psychological response to treatment or the electrical current may have induced endorphins which provided endogenous pain relief. The objective assessment of PEFR immediately after treatment demonstrated an increase **only** in the TENS and Entonox groups, but **NOT** the TTL group. Therefore we postulate that the subjective improvement in pain score in the TTL group was most probably mediated psychologically. During physiotherapy treatment, the physiotherapist's explanation, empathy, encouragement and tactile reinforcement, reduce the awareness of the patient to his pain[10] and reinforce a placebo effect[11]. This is probably why the improvement in pain score in the TTL group was not significant at 30 minutes after treatment when the patient was left alone.

In both the TENS and Entonox groups, the pain scores at 30 minutes post treatment were higher than the score immediately after treatment, although they were significantly lower than the pre-treatment score. This demonstrates that the analgesic effect of TENS and Entonox is of relatively short duration. We showed that there was a significant increase in PEFR immediatley after physiotherapy treatment in the TENS and Entonox groups, but not the TTL group. We hypothesise that this improvement was due to both the pain relief and the relaxing effect of the deep breathing exercises. The increase in PEFR was higher in the TENS group, suggesting that clinically TENS may provide a more effective pain relief. The PEFR significantly **decreased** in the TTL group at 30 minutes post treatment, suggesting that physiotherapy without analgesia may have an adverse effect.

A comparison of measured falls in VAS and changes in PEFR between different groups showed a significant difference between the TTL group and the other two groups, but not between the TENS and Entonox groups. This suggests that TENS and Entonox were both equally effective in providing pain relief and in helping to improve PEFR in our patients.

Our study showed that TENS was free from any side effects, but Entonox inhalation was associated with dizziness in 10% of our patients. The TENS machine was also easier to handle and subjectively preferred by our patients. We therefore suggest that TENS is superior to Entonox as a supplementary form of analgesia during chest physiotherapy.

REFERENCE:

1. Parbrook G D, Rees G A, Robertson G S, (1964). Relief of Post - operative Pain: Comparison of a 25% Nitrous-oxide and Oxygen Mixture with Morphine. Brit. Med J; 2:480-482
2. Paul A Sloan, (1986). Nitrous Oxide / Oxygen Analgesia in Palliative Care. Palliat Care, 2:1:43-48

3. Steward R D, Paris P M, Stoy W A, Cannon G, (1983). Patient controlled inhalational analgesia in prehospital care: a study of side effects and feasibility. Crit Care Med; 11:851-5
4. Goodard J M,(1986). Postoperative nitrous oxide analgesia. Anaesthesia; 41:915-8
5. Ruben H,(1972). Nitrous oxide analgesia in dentistry: its use during 15 years in Denmark: Br Dent J; 132:196-6
6. Arthurs G J, Rosen M,(1981). Acceptability of continuous nasal nitrous oxide during labour: a field trial in six maternity hospitals. Anaesthesia; 36:384-8
7. Ho A, Hui P W, Cheung J, Cheung C, (1987). Effectiveness of Transcutaneous Electrical Nerve Stimulation in Relieving Pain Following Thoracotomy. Physiotherapy; 73:33-35
8. Jones A, Lee Y W, Holzeburger D, Jones R D M, (1990). A Comparison of Different Electrode Placements on the Effectiveness of Pain Relief in TENS in Post-cholecystectomy patients. Physiotherapy; 76:9:567-570
9. Navarathnam R G, Wang I Y S, Thomas D, Klineberg P L,(1984). Evaluation of Transcutaneous Electrical Nerve Stimulator for Postoperative Analgesia following Cardiac Surgery. anaesth Intensive Care; 12:345-50
10. Weinman J, (1987). An Outline of Psychology as Applied to Medicine. 2nd ed, John Wright, Bristol.
11. French S,(1989). Pain: Some psychological and sociological aspects. Physiotherapy; 75:5:255-60

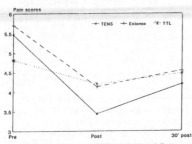

Figure 1 - Pain score at different treatment times

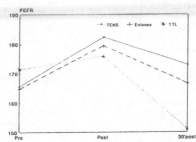

Figure 2 - PEFR at different treatment times

Table 1 -   Pain Scores for each treatment modality before, immediately after and 30 minutes after treatment

	TENS	ENTONOX	TTL
Pre	5.47 (0.37)	5.71 (0.32)	4.82 (0.35)
Post	3.44 (0.39)	4.14 (0.35)	4.21 (0.33)
30' post	4.21 (0.43)	4.55 (0.37)	4.48 (0.35)

Treatment time comparison	P values		
	TENS	ENTONOX	TTL
Pre-post	p < 0.0001	p < 0.0001	p < 0.02
Pre-30' post	p < 0.0005	p < 0.0001	p > 0.2 (NS)
Post-30' post	p < 0.005	p < 0.02	p > 0.05(NS)

Results are mean (SEM). Significance level at p < 0.05

Table 3 -   PEFR for each treatment modality before, immediately after and 30 minutes after treatment

	TENS	ENTONOX	TTL
Pre	165.6 (14.3)	164.8 (12.8)	171.3 (13.6)
Post	132.4 (14.3)	179.4 (16.2)	175.8 (14.1)
30' post	172.9 (13.6)	166.6 (13.6)	151.1 (11.7)

Treatment time comparison	p values		
	TENS	ENTONOX	TTL
Pre-post	p < 0.001	p < 0.04	p > 0.4 (NS)
Pre-30'post	p > 0.2 (NS)	p > 0.7 (NS)	p < 0.007
Post-30'post	p > 0.2 (NS)	p < 0.04	p < 0.001

Results are mean (SEM). Significance level at p < 0.05

Table 2 -   Comparison of the improvement in pain score between the three treatment modalities before immediately after and 30 minutes after treatmen

Groups	Difference of means	p value
Pre - immediately post treatment		
Entonox-TENS	- 0.46 (0.31)	p > 0.27 (NS)
TTL-Entonox	- 0.96 (0.34)	p < 0.006
TTL-TENS	- 1.43 (0.34)	p < 0.0006
Pre - 30' post treatment		
Entonox-TENS	- 0.09 (0.4)	p > 0.9 (NS)
TTL-Entonox	- 0.83 (0.34)	p < 0.02
TTL-TENS	- 0.93 (0.42)	p < 0.04
Post - 30' post treatment		
Entonox-TENS	0.36 (0.28)	p > 0.3 (NS)
TTL-Entonox	0.14 (0.26)	p > 0.8 (NS)
TTL-TENS	0.50 (0.37)	p > 0.3 (NS)

Results are mean (SEM). Significance level at p < 0.05

Table 4 -   Comparison of the improvement in PEFR between the three treatment modalities before, immediately after and 30 minutes after treatment

Groups	Difference of means	p value
Pre - immediately post treatment		
Entonox-TENS	2.26 (7.9)	P > 0.8 (NS)
TTL-Entonox	10.00 (7.68)	P > 0.2 (NS)
TTL-TENS	12.26 (5.49)	P < 0.03
Pre - 30' post treatment		
Entonox-TENS	5.48 (6.49)	P > 0.4 (NS)
TTL-Entonox	21.93 (7.32)	P < 0.005
TTL-TENS	27.42 (8.69)	P < 0.004
Post - 30' post treatment		
Entonox-TENS	3.23 (6.37)	P > 0.6 (NS)
TTL-Entonox	11.93 (6.94)	P > 0.1 (NS)
TTL-TENS	15.16 (8.75)	P > 0.1 (NS)

Results are mean (SEM). Significance level at p < 0.05

THE ROLE OF PULSED SHORT WAVE DIATHERMY IN THE MANAGEMENT OF UNDISPLACED
FRACTURE OF NECK OF HUMERUS

A. A. MUGGLESTONE, P.J. LIVERSLEY, J. WITTON
CROW HILL REHABILITATION CENTRE, CROW HILL DRIVE, MANSFIELD, NOTTINGHAMSHIRE. U.K.

Abstract
Fracture of the neck of the humerus is a common injury, the incidence of which increases with
age. 85% of fractures of the neck of the humerus are minimally displaced. Treatment with
physiotherapy is reported to produce a satisfactory outcome. Early treatment is thought to
produce a better outcome (1,2,3) although this approach may be limited by pain. Many
electrotherapeutic measures are employed by physiotherapists to reduce pain and swelling,
pulsed high frequency electromagnetic energy (PHFE) being the most commonly employed (4). To
establish the efficacy of this treatment to permit earlier mobilization of minimally
displaced humeral head fractures a prospective double blind controlled trial has been
conducted.

Introduction
Electrical treatments of various types have been used to treat painful skeletal disorders
since the discovery of electricity. Shortwave radiation, 27.12M Hz, delivers both electrical
and magnetic energy 180 degrees out of phase. Although such energy may cause heating the
therapeutic effect is thought to result from the electromagnetic changes, not from the
heating effect (5). Golden et al (1981) suggest that the mechanism of action may be the
restoration of cell membrane potentials damaged by inflammation, such changes leading to
physio-chemical changes resulting from osmosis secondarily to the passage of ions (7).
Pulsed systems of delivery (PHFE) have been developed to exploit the electromagnetic
phenomena whilst allowing heat to dissipate between burst of energy. Such systems are
widely used in physiotherapy departments (4,8).

Numerous trials in the use of PHFE have been undertaken to demonstrate its role in the
reduction of inflammation, pain and swelling as well as its ability to enhance healing.
PHFE has been used in podiatric surgery with good results (9,10,11). However the trials
included multiple diagnosis with subjective methods of assessment. Wilson (1972)
demonstrated a minor improvement in recovery of sprained ankles employing PHFE. Golden et
al (1981) showed an improved rate of healing with PHFE treatment of donor sites for split
skin grafts. Both studies were well conducted double blind trials, although assessments
were made on subjective criteria alone. Other studies (13,14) of back pain and minor hand
injuries, although less well conducted, gave similar positive results.

Barker et al (1985) applied PHFE to acute sprains of the lateral ligament of the ankles in a
well set up double blind trial, but was unable to demonstrate any benefit. Treatment was
given in one 45 minute session per day for the first three days only, whereas most authors
express the opinion that an effect will not be seen in under five days of treatment (4).

Method
We have conducted a double blind trial of PHFE in minimally displaced fractures of the
neck of the humerus.

During an eighteen month period all patients who sustained minimally displaced fractures of the neck of humerus and who were able to co-operate were referred immediately to physiotherapy. The patients were randomised into two groups, one group received PHFE from a 'Curapuls' machine, the other group sham treatment with a de-activated machine.

Treatment was administered for 30 minutes per session for the first 10 working days following referral.

The machine settings were pulse repetition frequency 35 intensity 3. Pulse power is listed at 300w. Pulse duration is 0.4 ms per pulse.

Employing the capacitance method medium size electrodes were applied to the shoulder in a contraplanar technique. Movement of the injured shoulder was commenced immediately also and to enable standardisation a performance based algorithmic approach to physiotherapy treatment was developed.

Assessment was carried out using the Nottingham shoulder chart and European shoulder assessment chart by an independent assessor. Assessments were carried out at one, two and six months. Assessments at a later stage being deemed unnecessary (3).

After six months the codes were broken and the results were analyzed by means of unpaired t-tests, Mann Whitney U test and Spearman rank correlation coefficient.

Results

Sixty seven patients were referred - 16 did not meet entry requirements. Randomisation placed 22 patients in the treatment group and 26 in the control group. The two groups were comparable in age/sex and side injured. There were no differences between the time of starting treatment and discharge of the two groups. 51 patients entered the study, 3 failed to complete follow up, one of whom was from the treatment group.

All the 48 patients who completed treatment and review attained a good result. There were no poor results. Good being defined as useful power in the limb - abduction beyond 60^{0} and ability to place hand behind neck (3).

No significant difference was found between the two groups at any stage of the trial by any means of the assessments. No difference was found in the patients subjective opinion of the treatment, none of the patients receiving PHFE noted a heating effect.

A strong correlation between the time to beginning treatment after the fracture and time to discharge (correlation coefficient 0.4236 P <0.02) was seen. No correlation was seen between functional outcome at 6/12 and time of starting treatment. Older patients complained more of pain (cc 0.489 P <0.001) and loss of function an inverse correlation being found between age/outcome. Younger patients continued to improve after discharge from physiotherapy; older patients did not.

We have been unable to demonstrate any benefit with the use of PHFE in this series. The value of such machines remains unproven in the management of acute injuries to the shoulder.

References

1 Brostrom, F. (1943) Early mobilization of fractures of the upper end of the humerus. Arch Surg 46:614

2 Maitland (1980) Peripheral Mobilizations. pub: Butterworths London

3 Young, T.B., Wallace, W.A. (1985) Conservative treatment of fractures and fracture dislocations of the upper end of the Humerus J.B.J.S. 67B:373

4 Haynes, C. (1984) Pulsed high frequency energy - Its place in physiotherapy.
Physiotherapy 70(12):459

5 Nagelschmidt, K.F. (1940) Specific effects of high frequency currents and magnotherapy.
B.J. Phys Med November 201

6 Golden, J.H.   Broadbent, N.R.G.   Nancarrow, J.D. et al (1981). The effects of dispulse
on healing wounds: A double blind randomized clinical trial in man. Br J Plastic Surg 34:267

7 Binder, S.A. (1981) Application of low and high voltage electrotherapeutic currents in
electrotherapy. in: Electrotherapy. ed: Wolf, S.L. pub: Churchill Livingstone P 1 - 24

8 Oliver, D.E. (1984) Pulsed electromagnetic energy - What is it? Physiotherapy 70(12):458

9 Steinberg, M.D. (1964) Diapulse in general Podiatry practice. A preliminary report.
J of Am Pod Assoc 54(12) :849

10 Kaplan, E.G. Weinstock, R.E. (1964) Clinical evaluation of dispulse as adjunctive therapy
following foot surgery. J of Am Pod Assoc 58(5) :218

11 Bentall, Eckstein. (1975) A trial involving the use of pulsed electromagnetic therapy on
children undergoing Orchodipexy. Kinderchir 17(4) :380

12 Wilson, D.H. (1972) Treatment of soft tissue injury by pulsed electrical energy.
BMJ ii:269

13 Wagstaff, P. Wagstaff, S. Downey, M. (1986) A Pilot study to compare the efficacy of
continuous and pulsed magnetic energy (short wave diathermy) on the relief of low back
pain. Physiotherapy 72(11) :563

14 Barclay, V. Collier, R.J. Jones, A. (1983) Treatment of various hand injuries by pulsed
electromagnetic energy (Diapulse). Physiotherapy 69(6) :186

15 Barker, A.T. Barlow, P.S. Porter, J. et al. (1985) A double blind clinical trial of
low powered short wave therapy in the treatment of soft tissue injury.
Physiotherapy 71(12) :500

SOFT LASER IN PATIENTS SUFFERING FROM ANTERIOR KNEE PAIN.

P.Petriccione di Vadi, ^D.Minden and *M.Dyson.
Pain Relief and *Tissue Repair Units, Guy's Hospital, London
^Dept of Physiotherapy, Queen Elisabeth Hospital, London.

INTRODUCTION.

In the last few years low level laser (LLL) irradiation has been used as a procedure to promote pain relief in patients suffering from different diseases. Clinical trials have shown contradicted results in terms of pain relief (1,2,3).
It has been proposed that LLL irradiation produces analgesia in a manner similar to that obtained by transcutaneous electrical nerve stimulation by provoking the "gate phenomenon". It has also been suggested that LLL irradiation has a serotoninergic action with consequent potentiation of the inhibit discending pathway. This suggestion lies on the observation of a large increase of 5-hydroxyindoloacetic acid (5-HIAA), a degradation product of 5-hydroxytryptamine (5-HT), in the 24-hours urine of subjects receiving LLL irradiation (3). It should be noted, however, that the excretion of 5-HIAA is increased after consumption of serotonin containing-foods such as bananas, tomatoes etc. and after intake of various drugs such as caffeine and nicotine.
Experimental studies have reported that exposure to low power laser alters neuronal activity (4). On the contrary another study reported a failure to confirm propagated nerve action potentials in response to a laser light stimulus (5).
Aims of the study were:
-to estimate the validity of LLL irradiation over the affected knee in patients suffering from anterior knee pain
-to evaluate whether there is any additional relief by bilateral LLL irradiation of the radial, median, saphenous and deep peroneal nerves, following an established method.

METHOD.

Patients suffering from anterior knee pain for at least three months were admitted to the study. They were of either sex and aged between 18 and 50. Exclusion criteria were pregnancy and general illness. A written consent form was obtained. The patients were divided in four groups by randomization.

Single 820 nm 50 mW 0.4 W/cm probe (active or dummy) was installed on the apparatus and placed on slight contact vertically over the skin surface. The length of the irradiation was of 60 sec at each points (24 J/cm). The probe was applied to:

A. Each area of skin overlying the following anatomical points:
  -Medial and lateral aspect of the base of the patella.
  -Pole of the patella at the origin of the patella tendons.
  -Medial and lateral femoral condyles immediately adjacent to   the edge of the patella.

B. Each area of skin overlying the saphenous nerve at the anterior aspect of the medial malleolus, the superficial and deep peroneal nerve at the midpoint of the lateral aspect of the shaft and the radial and median nerve at the dorsal side of the second phalanx of the thumb bilaterally.

In the first group (A) the patients received LLL irradiation on the affected knee and to the skin overlying the thumbs and both shaft.

In the second group (B) the patients received LLL irradiation on the affected knee and placebo irradiation to the peripheral nerves.

In the third group (C) the patients received placebo irradiation to the affected knee and LLL irradiation to the thumbs and both shafts.

In the four group (D) the patients received placebo irradiation on the affected knee and on the peripheral nerves.

The total time of the treatment was three times a week for 3 weeks, followed by one month of follow up.

A week before the beginning of the course the patients was asked to follow a diet deprived of food containing 5-hydroxytriptamin. They also completed a Mc Gill questionaire, a Pain Index and a Visual Analogue Scale at the beginning of the trial, after the 5th treatment, at the end of it and at the end of the follow up period.

The concentration of 5-HIAA in 24-hour samples was measured twice before the beginning of the trial. Samples were then collected after the 5th laser application, at the end of the treatment and at the end of the follow up period.

Clinical assessment was performed by a physician unware of patients' treatment before the course of the treatment, at the end of it and one month later at the end of the follow up period.

Drugs requirement was also monitored during the study.

REFERENCES.

1.Walker JB, AKhanjee LK, Cooney MM, Tamayoshi S, Segal-Gidan F. Laser therapy for pain of trigeminal neuralgia. Clin J Pain 3, 183-7, 1988
2.Hansen HJ, Thoroe U. Low pawer laser biostimulation of chronic oro-facial pain. A double-blind placebo controlled cross-over study in 40 patients. Pain 43, 169-79, 1990.
3.Walker J.. Neusci. Lett. 43, 339-44, 1983.
4.Walker J, Akhanjee K. Laser-induced somatosensory evoked potentials: evidence of photosensitivity in peripheral nerves. Brain Research 344, 281-5, 1985.
5.Wu W, Ponnudurai R, Kalts J, Pott CB, Chilcoat R, Uncini A, Rapoport S, Wade P, Mauro A. Failure to confirm report of light-evoked response of peripheral nerve to low power helium-neon laser light stimulus. Brain Research 401, 407-8, 1987.

POSTER PRESENTATIONS

NON-INVASIVE ACUPUNCTURE ANESTHESIA POINT STIMULATION TO
REDUCE POST-SURGICAL HIP-PAIN DURING EXERCISE

E.H. Groll, PT, AP
Department of Physical Therapy, Manor Pines Convalescent
Center, 1701 NE 26th Street, Wilton Manors, Florida 33305

Acupuncture Anesthesia (AA) is based on the theory that
acupuncture has the effect of easing pain and regulating
physiological functions of the human body. AA safely and
effectively reduces, or entirely eliminates the pain
experienced by the patient (PT) during surgical procedures.
Also PT's, who because of advanced age, debility, critical
illness or allergic reactions to conventional medications,
are unable to safely tolerate conventional modes of
anesthesia, may be a candidate for AA as an effective
substitute. Needle-less electric stimulation analgesia
(NESA) makes use of electrode plates to conduct electric
pulsations into the acupuncture points (AP) to give
stimulation to certain parts of the body for the purpose
analgesia. With this method of analgesia, as opposed to
the use of needles that penetrate the skin surface, there
exists a certain degree of incomplete anesthesia and
insufficient muscle relaxation. For the Physical Therapist
who routinely treats Post-Surgical Patients that rely on
pain medication to reduce pain during exercise, NESA may be
an effective tool for pain reduction during therapeutic
exercise where complete anesthesia required for surgical
procedures is not paramount.

The Post Surgical Hip Fracture and Hip Replacement PT was
selected in our Pain Study at MPCC[1]. The selection of NESA
AP were taken from traditional books of acupuncture[2]. AP
selected were ST-36 (Zusanli), ST-40 (Fenglong), B-59
(Fuyang), GB-36 (Waiqiu), GB-39 (Xuanzhong), SP-6
(Sanyinjiao), GB-40 (Qiuxu), ST-43 (Xiangu), all
ipsilateral stimulation [Figure 1]. Auricular AP (AAP),
Shenman, Lung, Sympathetic, Kidney, all Bilateral
Stimulation [Figure 2]. NESA point location is not as
critical as is that for needle insertion, owing to the fact
that a larger area of coverage is treated by the surface
electrode. AAP location, however, must be as exacting as
possible for successful stimulation. Difficulty arises
because the size and shape of the auricles of each
individual vary, making AAP location on some PT's
difficult. Also the multitude and closeness of AAP's add
to the location problem. An acupuncturist's auricular
point locator may be of value. AP locators are also found
on some Electric Stimulators (ES). In our study, a IC-1107

Electro-Acupuncture Unit and a WQ-10 Acupunctoscope were used for NESA of the affected leg. A Neuroprobe and the WQ-10 were used for AAP ES. The Neuroprobe was more effective in AAP ES because of its more sensitive point locator. The surface electrodes used in NESA were medtronic snapease and magnet electrodes of the type used in Magnet Therapy. Not to embellish the claims made for Magnet Therapy, the electrodes worked very well and gave a more pinpoint, needlelike, stimulative effect. During NESA treatment the frequency of the stimulation should be adjusted to patient comfort. For AAP stimulation, we followed the Neuroprobe guidelines for pain control. On the initial treatment, the PT is placed in the supine position. All selected NESA points are identified and skin cleaned with TENS skin cleaner. AMMT and ROM Test[3] are given. Pain sensitivity is noted in all ranges of allowable motion of the post surgical hip using a pain scale [Figure 3] for progress noting.

Most of the PT's [14] had pain through their entire joint ROM. The formation of pain itself is influenced by a large extent from psychological factors. The PT's acceptance of this procedure is extremely important. The spoken word from the Physical Therapist that can have a positive effect on the mood of the PT cannot be overemphasized. Stimulation of the AAP is done first, bilaterally. To save time the NESA electrodes can be attached ipsilaterally while the AAP are stimulated by the Physical Therapist. Most ES have 3 terminal split leads; therefore 6 AP's can be prepared for stimulation. After auricular stimulation the post-operative leg can be stimulated. The intensity is increased as the patient becomes used to the intensity given. Stimulation is given for 15 minutes before exercises are started. The hip ROM or exercise is given within the patient's pain threshold, increasing the intensity of stimulation on increases of hip pain.

It was found that definite increases in pain diminished ROM occurred using this method with almost every PT treated [Figure 3]. All types of exercises can be given with the only restriction being the leads themselves which are attached to the extremity exercised. In our study of 18 painful Post-Surgical Hip PT's, medication was required to reduce pain on Hip-Movement. NESA and AAP started 15 minutes before and carried out during exercises of the Post-Surgical Hip did effectively reduce Hip pain in most cases. Medications used to control this pain during exercise were either reduced or eliminated which was very beneficial to the PT's health and well being.

Footnotes

1. From the Department of Physical Therapy, Manor Pines Convalescent Center, 1701 NE 26th Street, Wilton Manors, Florida 33305.

2. Acupuncture, A Comprehensive Text. Shanghi College of Traditional Medicine, Eastland Press, USA.

   Acupuncture Anesthesia, A Translation from Chinese. U.S. Directory Service, USA.

   Essentials of Chinese Acupuncture. Foreign Languages Press, Beijing, China.

3. Muscle Testing Manual, Daniels L., Williams M., Worthingham C. W.B. Saunders Company, London.

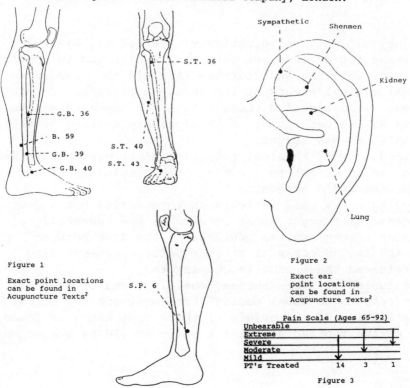

Figure 1

Exact point locations can be found in Acupuncture Texts[2]

Figure 2

Exact ear point locations can be found in Acupuncture Texts[2]

Pain Scale (Ages 65-92)			
Unbearable			
Extreme			↓
Severe			
Moderate	↓	↓	
Mild			
PT's Treated	14	3	1

Figure 3

777

A MYOFASCIAL TRIGGER POINT THAT CAUSES GASTROINTESTINAL SYMPTOMS

C J Manheim, D K Lavett

Carol J Manheim, MS, PT, Physical Therapy
Charleston, South Carolina, USA

Object   : Twelve patients referred to physical
therapy for chronic low back pain were found to complain of
nausea, vomiting and diarrhea that did not respond to the
usual medical treatment for these complaints. Careful
questioning revealed these complaints appeared at the same
time as the back pain. A physical explanation of these
complaints was sought.

Method   : Physical palpation of trigger points was
used in an effort to reproduce the complaints of nausea,
vomiting and diarrhea.

Results   : All patients in this series had a deep
myofascial trigger point located on the underbelly of the
lumbar erector spinae proximal to the disc between
L4 and L5. Successful trigger point treatment also
eliminated these somatic complaints.

Conclusion : When nausea, vomiting, and/or diarrhea does
not respond to usual medical treatment and no medical
explanation of the origin of these complaints is found,
an active myofascial trigger point should be suspected.

The effect of physiotherapy in patients with eleva=
ted brucella antibody titres, vertebral pains and
headaches.

Maria Wichura Krause

Department of Physiotherapy
Province of the Orange Free State, Republic of
South Africa

Introduction: Brucellosis sufferers complain of pains in the
vertebral column, peripheral joints and headaches. References
to physiotherapy treatment for these symptoms are non-specific
and negative.

Aim: To assess whether passive mobilisation to vertebral joints
given to patients with diagnosed brucellosis relieves or ex=
acerbates symptoms.

Treatment: Thirty diagnosed cases were randomly placed into
three equal groups. After assessment one group received spe=
sific physiotherapy without medication, one non-specific phy=
siotherapy without medication and one only medical interven=
tion.

Results: Both the Wilcoxin test and Fisher's Exact test were
used to process the data. A graph was plotted to demonstrate
the change in symptoms.

Conclusion: Specific physiotherapy relieves vertebral pains
and headaches, non-specific physiotherapy has no effect.
Medication is an effective long-term treatment for vertebral
pains, but not for headaches.

COMPARISON OF RELATIVE EFFECTIVENESS OF THERAPIES
FOR CHRONIC PAIN: AN 8 YEAR EXPERIENCE OF A
MULTIDISCIPLINARY PAIN CENTER

Cora Huitt, Amir Rafii, Ann Dunbar and Donald D.
Price.

Department of Anesthesiology, Medical College of
Virginia, Richmond, Virginia 23298-0001   USA

The effective management of chronic pain often requires a
combination of different treatments by different health care
providers. Single treatments, regardless of their rationale
or possible validity, are often ineffective. Different combinations of treatments have been evaluated by the MCV Pain Management Center over the past 8 years. Three groups of consecutively referred patients with chronic musculoskeletal pain
disorders each received one of the following: 1.) TENS alone
(N=18), 2.) TENS alone for 2 months followed by a combination
of TENS and weekly or bi-weekly electroacupuncture treatments
(N=23), and 3.) TENS, Amitriptyline, and physical therapy,
patient education, therapeutic exercise) (N=24).

The composition of the 3 groups were very similar with
regard to diagnoses, duration of pain, age, sex, number of
symptoms, and initial sensory and affective VAS ratings of
pain intensity. TENS alone was ineffective both in Group 1
and in the first 2 months of treatment of Group 2. The combination of electroacupuncture therapy and TENS produced small
(16%) but significant reductions in usual and maximum pain ratings related to the previous week (paired t tests). Reductions in VAS sensory and affective ratings of Group 3 (35-49%)
were all highly statistically reliable and clearly greater
than those in Groups 1 & 2 (p 0.01). Results show combinations of treatments are definitely more effective and that VAS
monitoring of pain is useful in revealing these differences.

THE SEMANTICS OF PAIN

Margaret H MOON
Private Practice, P O Box 21 244, Christchurch, New Zealand.

THE SEMANTICS OF *PAIN*

The word *pain* came into the English language somewhere between 1150 & 1350. It came from the Old French, & had acquired a richness of meaning by that time. The earlier derivation was from the Latin word, *poena*, meaning *penalty* & *punishment*.

Five meanings of *pain* as a noun, three as a verb, & the meanings of the related words, *pine*, *patient* & *patience*, are given. (Source: Oxford Dictionary) Literary extracts will illustrate the presence through history of these meanings.

1. PAIN means *suffering or loss inflicted for an offence, punishment or penalty or a fine.*
    1387   Christ has paid a pain for his all. *(Trevisa)*

2. PAIN means *a primary condition of sensation or consciousness, the opposite of pleasure; the sensation felt when hurt in body or mind; suffering, distress.*
    1598   Every pleasure has a pain they say. *(Chapman, Blind Beggar Alexandria, Plays 1873 I. 29)*

3. PAIN is used in a specifically physical sense meaning *bodily suffering; distressing sensation; soreness.*
    1377   For pain of the palm powered them [the fingers] to fail to clutch or to claw. *(Langl P. PL. B. xvii, 187)*

    The suffering or throes of childbirth are a more specific meaning of **pains** within the physical sense.
    1388   But when she has borne a son, she thinks not of the pain but of love, for a man is borne into the world. *(Wyclif, John xvi, 21)*

4. PAIN is used in a specific psychical sense, meaning *mental suffering, grief, trouble, sorrow.*
    1656   Of all the pains the greatest pain, it is to love but love in vain. *(Cowley, Misc Gold)*

    In this psychical sense, **pain** can mean *distress felt by possible evil, anxiety; apprehension.*

> 1688 I am in great pain to know how my horses have
> performed on the journey. *(R Montagu in
> Buccleuch MSS)*

5. **PAINS**, can mean *trouble taken for the accomplishment
    of something; labour, toil, exertion, or effort taken
    in order to secure a satisfactory result.*
    1542 The pains of teaching is worthy of great wages.
    (Udall Erasmus Apoph 51 margin)

    Also, the notion of recompensing is not new.
    1598 Give this sweet Nan this ring: there's for thy
    pains. *(Shakespeare, The Merry Widow iii,iv,103)*

6. **TO PAIN** means *to inflict a penalty, to torture by way
    of punishment, to fine.*
    1620 If there is anything pained at the last court to
    be done & yet is not done, you must enquire who
    has made default therein. *(J Wilkinson Courts
    Baron 148)*

7. **TO PAIN** means *to inflict pain upon, to cause to
    suffer, to hurt, to distress. This may be mental pain,
    as to inflict suffering upon, to afflict, to give pain
    to; to grieve, to hurt the feelings of.*
    1591 So shall you cease to plague & I to pain.
    (Daniel, Sidney's Astra & Stella etc Soun.xi)

8. **TO PAIN** means *to endeavour, to strive; to exert
    oneself with effort with care & attention.*
    1596 She pained with womanish art to hide her wound.
    (Spencer Fairie Queen, iv, vi, 40)

9. **TO PINE** is an earlier form from the Latin *poena* & in
    obsolete Middle English meant *punishment, torment,
    torture, the penal sufferings of hell & purgatory.*
    Present meanings of *pine* as a verb are, *to exhaust or
    consume by suffering of body & mind; to cause to
    languish; to wear out, emaciate; to fret; to mourn.*

10. **PATIENT & PATIENCE** are Middle English words, coming
    from Old French, from the Latin stem, *pati, to suffer.
    Patience is the quality of suffering or enduring pain
    with calmness & composure. A patient is one who
    suffers patiently, or who is under medical treatment.*

THE SIGNIFICANCE OF THE MEANINGS OF *PAIN.*

A child who grazes its knee, cries & runs to mother for a
cuddle - the emotional comfort seems to reduce the pain.

The medical, biomechanistic model has responsibility for the
identification & amelioration of tissue damage, but is the
need for the cuddles recognised? Is the environment caring

enough?

Pain/3, the physical sense, is only a portion of the experience, and although it must receive sound medical attention, the recognition of **pain/2,** the primary sensation that is the opposite to pleasure, is necessary.

When acute pain does not go away, **pain/4** creeps into the situation aligned with anxiety, apprehension, worries about not sleeping, work, money, operative procedures, family reactions & so forth. As the losses in life that are consequential to the onset & continuation of the pain become apparent **pain/4,** with its meanings of trouble & sorrow, become apparent. The person may be **pining/9** over losses of mobility, jobs, recreational activities, & changes in relationships.

Pain/1 may compound the situation, as for the young man who had a brachial plexus lesion, & also was on court charges for having caused the accident. This aspect of pain related to the punishment for that offence.

Pain/5 in the rehabilitative phase, is when sufferers exert themselves to learn coping skills that will ensure mastery of every day living. People with severe chronic pain take great **pains/5** to regain control of their own lives, & to re-establish themselves in society.

People are **pained/7** when they have to undergo medical procedures like epidurals & surgery and are **pained/7** when they are not believed, or their integrity is threatened. They are **pained/6** when they suffer penalties, as when their earnings related compensation is stopped in a manner perceived as inappropriate by the accident victim. They are **pained/8** by the trouble they have to take to go through review & court processes. They **pain/8** themselves to hide their disability in order to be accepted as normal people in the community. Children, often, are **pining/9** for the parent who previously had energy & was fun & active.

Over the past century, **pain/3** has dominated; **pain** has become medicalised, almost to the exclusion of all other meanings. But when semantics is considered, the *complexity* of **pain** becomes apparent. If appropriate rehabilitation is to occur for people who are suffering from complex, chronic pain syndromes, then the medical model alone cannot suffice because it admits to only a fraction of the meaning of the word *pain*. Communication, emotion, behaviour, beliefs, & philosophy assume importance if the **patient/10** is to learn to suffer less & to become more able to handle chronic pain with increasing calmness & composure.

*This paper is followed by **Pain as a Process & Chronic Pain Rehabilitation.***

THE FREQUENCY OF JOINT HYPERMOBILITY SYNDROME IN CHRONIC PAIN PATIENTS

V.R.Harding

INPUT
St.Thomas' Hospital Pain Management Unit
LONDON SE1 7EH
U.K.

A pilot survey was undertaken to assess the proportion of subjects attending a behavioural programme for chronic pain sufferers who also had evidence of past or present Joint Hypermobility Syndrome (JHS).
 METHOD: The Beighton and Contompasis (modified) 9-point scoring systems were used. The subjects were 36 Caucasians of a mean age of 53.2 (range 24-77). Hypermobility was deemed to be present with a Beighton score of 4 or more (range 0-9), OR a Contompasis score of 26 or more (range 18-56). OR a past history of being able to place the hands flat on the floor when bending forwards. All subjects in the study were assessed by the same physiotherapist.
 RESULTS: From the sample of 36 patients 18(50%) met the criteria for JHS. 7 patients (19.4%) met the Beighton criteria, 11(30.5%) met the Contompasis criteria and 18(50%) met the past history criteria. In contrast, studies on normal samples typically report proportions ranging from 4% to 7%.
 CONCLUSIONS: From these preliminary observations, there appears to be a larger proportion of JHS subjects amongst the sample of chronic pain patients used in this study than might be expected from normal population studies. A larger study is in progress to investigate this relationship, and possible implications of these findings will be discussed.

WOUND HEALING

THE EFFECT OF PULSED ELECTROMAGNETIC FIELDS ON SOFT TISSUE REPAIR

N Nirsimloo, S R Young, R E Smith*, M Dyson

Tissue Repair Research Unit, United Medical and Dental Schools, Guy's Hospital, London, England. (* Professorial Surgical Unit, St Bartholomew's Hospital, London, England.)

The repair of skin wounds consists of three overlapping phases: inflammation, proliferation and remodelling. The stage the wound has reached can be identified by performing differential cell counts (DCC) of polymorphonuclear leucocytes and macrophages (cells characteristic of the inflammatory phase) and of fibroblasts and endothelial cells (which characterise the proliferative phase). During remodelling, total cellularity decreases.

The effect of therapeutic pulsed magnetic fields (PMF) on healing of skin wounds was studied in 1 cm^2 full-thickness lesions in the flank skin of anaesthetised female CD1 mice using three groups, one PMF-exposed at frequency 16.7 Hz, a second to PMF at 25 Hz (both at an amplitude of 3.4 mT), and a third which was a sham-exposed control. Differential cellularity of the injured tissue was monitored at 2, 3, 5 and 7 days post-operatively. A significantly higher number of fibroblasts was observed in PMF-treated wounds at 3 days ($p < 0.05$) suggesting that PMF treated wounds entered the proliferative phase more quickly. The observation that by 7 days the 16.7 Hz treated wounds contained significantly fewer macrophages than in 25 Hz and control wounds ($p < 0.05$) provides more evidence of less time spent in the inflammatory phase by this group of wounds.

In conclusion, both 16.7 Hz and 25 Hz PMF seem to accelerate wound healing.

Accelerated Healing of Chronic Dermal Ulcers with Pulsed Electrical Stimulation

L.C. Kloth and J.A. Feedar
Program in Physical Therapy
Marquette University, Milwaukee, WI   USA

Since 1969, a number of publications related to the clinical use of electrical stimulation for treatment of chronic dermal ulcers have reported accelerated rates of healing of 13 to 46 % per week during an average of 6.6 weeks compared to small numbers of control wounds which have healed between 5 and 15 % per week.[1-4] In all of these studies the polarity of the wound electrode was changed periodically during the study period. All of these studies delivered 200 to 1000 µA of either direct current[1-3] or time averaged pulsed current[4] to the wound tissues.

Although there is lack of agreement on the effects of polarity, many animal studies have reported that µA stimulation from direct[5-7] and time-averaged µA pulsed current devices[8] produce faster closure of acute induced wounds[5-8] and greater tensile strength of the wound scar tissue[5,6] compared to control wounds. Recently, studies on induced wounds in pigs have reported that electrical stimulation can improve the survival of skin flaps,[9] significantly increase the rate of wound epithelialization[7] and contraction[10,11] and the proliferation of fibroblasts.[10] Some of these findings are in turn supported by in vitro studies which have reported that isolated epidermal cells, cell clusters and cell sheets demonstrate galvanotaxis in migrating toward the cathode.[12,13]

The purpose of this clinical study was to compare healing of chronic dermal ulcers treated with pulsed electrical stimulation with healing of similar wounds treated with sham electrical stimulation. Based on the available information regarding the use of therapeutic electricity for enhancing wound repair, we hypothesized that chronic dermal ulcers treated with pulsed electrical current would demonstrate greater rates of healing and percentage of healing than ulcers treated with sham electrical stimulation.

METHOD

Subjects

Fifty-nine patients with 67 Stage II, III, or IV chronic wounds were enrolled at nine investigational sites. Patients were required to participate in the study for four weeks, since it was felt that some measurable effect on healing would occur in that amount of time. Patients were excluded if they had cardiac pacemakers, had peripheral vascular disease disposing them to thrombosis, were pregnant, had active osteomyelitis, or were on long-term radiation, steroid or chemotherapy. Following the initial evaluation to determine if the wound and the patient met the selection criteria, the patient was asked to sign an informed consent form. Patients were than randomly assigned to either an electrical stimulation treatment group or to a sham electrical stimulation group.

Wounds

Wounds could be Stage II, III, or IV pressure sores, vascular insufficiency ulcers, or wounds caused by trauma or surgery. Wounds excluded from the study were those with immeasurable length and width, those which were completely occluded by eschar, were hemorrhaging or were of cancerous etiology.

Instrumentation

The electrical stimulator device used in this study was at the time the commercially available Vara/Pulse*R which delivers monophasic pulsed current, having a duration of 132 µS and of 3.9 µC. For this study, a pulse amplitude of 29.2 mA (output dial set at 35 mA) and pulse frequencies of 128 and 64pps were used. At these frequencies the pulse period was 7.74 mS and 15.5 mS respectively. Thus, the accumulated pulse charge was 499.2 µC/S at the higher pulse frequency and 249.6 µC/S at the lower frequency.

Procedure

This study was conducted as a randomized, double-binded clinical trial. Each consecutive numbered patient at each center was randomly assigned a sham or active electrical stimulation device by serial number. Neither investigators not patients were aware of which type of device was used for a particular wound during the four week study period. Patients in the treatment and sham groups received identical treatment during the study period except that active stimulators were used on the treatment group and sham (inactive) stimulators were used on the sham group.

Once a week the wound appearance was documented and length and width of the wound were recorded on a wound diagram. A color photograph was taken, to provide a permanent record and for monitoring purposes every two weeks. The protocol consisting of two 30 minute active or sham stimulation sessions was given seven days a week with no fewer that four hours and no more that eight hours between sessions. The protocol was based on the method used in previous clinical studies by other investigators[1-4] and consisted of the following:

   a. irrigation of the wound bed with saline solution before each treatment and maintenance of a saline moistened wound environment between treatments.
   b. application of clean, saline moistened gauze sponges directly over stage II or into stage III and IV wounds.
   c. application of a 16 x 16 cm non-treatment sponge electrode moistened with tap water and secured to the skin a minimum of 12 inches from the wound site.
   d. application of a 7.5 x 7.5 cm sponge electrode on top of the saline moistened gauze covering the wound.
   e. Vara/Pulse stimulation controls were set at a pulse frequency of 128pps, an amplitude of 35mA and the polarity switch was set to deliver negative charge to the electrode placed on the wound.
   f. daily treatments were continued until the wound debrided spontaneously or a serosanguinous drainage appeared. After three additional days the polarity of the wound electrode was changed every three days until the wound healed to a stage II classification. At that time the pulse frequency was deceased to 64pps and the polarity of the wound electrode was alternated daily until the wound closed.
   g. if a wound entered the study as a clean stage II wound, treatment was started as described in step f. above.

Patients who were randomized to receive a sham stimulator were treated for a four-week sham trial and then were given the opportunity to switch to an active stimulator. Patients who chose to crossover to an active stimulator were followed and treated in the same manner as if they were newly enrolled in the study. Wounds which were randomized to an active stimulator were treated for at least four weeks or until wound closure occurred. All sham and treatment wounds were assessed at weekly intervals for four weeks after the study protocol was terminated.

Data Analysis

Wound length and width were measured at weekly intervals during the treatment period. Since there are wound measurement values for both the treatment and sham control groups each week for four weeks, we used the wound size data (defined as the length-width product) at the four-week point as the definitive endpoint for comparison purposes. A reduction in the length-width product was taken as an indication of wound healing.

These changes in wound size were assessed by expressing each wound's length-width product at each week as a percentage of its initial length-width product, which allows comparisons of all wounds regardless of their absolute size. The means of the individual percentages for each group of wounds were compared, using the two sample t-test (one-tailed) to evaluate the null hypothesis of no treatment differences. For the sham wounds that were crossed over to active stimulation, a paired t-test (one-tailed) was used to compare four weeks of active treatment to four weeks of sham treatment.

Results

Of the 67 wounds initially enrolled, 17 wounds on 12 patients were not included in the analysis, leaving 50 wounds (26 treatment, 24 sham control) on 47 patients which were available for data analysis. Patient ages ranged from 29 to 91 years. The mean ages of the treatment and control groups were 66.6 and 60.7 years respectively. There were 52% males and 48% females, and they were equally distributed between the groups. Two of the wounds were stage II, 39 were stage III, and 9 were stage IV.

After four weeks, the 26 wounds in the stimulation treatment group were 44% of their original size while the 24 wounds in the sham group were 67% of their initial size (p<0.02). This is an average healing rate of 14% per week for the treatment group versus 8.25% per week for the sham control group. None of the treatment ulcers increased in size, while 5 of the sham ulcers did so.

Fourteen of the wounds in the sham control group were crossed over to nonrandomized active electrical stimulation after completing the four weeks of sham treatment, and their data are presented in Table 3. After four weeks of sham treatment these 14 wounds were 88.7% of their initial size, and had healed at a rate of 2.9% per week. After four weeks of electrical stimulation, these same wounds were 49% of their size at the time of crossover, and had healed at a rate of 12.8 % per week. The reduction in wound healing is fourfold greater when receiving active stimulation, and this difference is significant (p=0.005). These wounds continued to be treated for a mean total treatment time of 10.8 weeks; all but two continued to improve, and 43% (6/14) of them healed completely.

After the four week double blind portion of the study, 17 of the actively treated wounds continued to be treated. After a mean of 8 weeks total treatment time, the wounds had healed to 23.6 % of their original size, on the average. In addition, 38.5% (10/26) had healed completely or nearly completely (>95% healed) and 61.5% (16/26) had healed more than 80%.

Discussion

In this study we found that at four weeks wounds in the treatment group healed a mean of 44% of initial size at a mean healing rate of 14% a week. In contrast during the same time period wounds in the sham control group healed a mean of 69% of their original size at a mean healing rate of 8.35% a week. These findings are supported by the rates of healing per week reported in other clinical studies.[1,4] Furthermore, the results of this study provide support for changing polarity during the course of treatment, a procedure initially used by Wolcott et al[1] and subsequently by others.[2,4] In addition, the significant increase in rate of healing of treated compared to sham control wounds in this study produced by 7 hours of electrical stimulation a week, confirms a suggestion by Kloth and Feedar from their previous report,[4] that electrical stimulation treatment time required to satisfactorily enhance tissue healing does not need to exceed 60 minutes five to seven days a week. This trend away from the 20 to 42 hours of electrical stimulation treatment time reported in other studies[1-3] further suggests that between 3.7 hours of treatment a week reported by Kloth and Feedar and 7 hours a week reported in this study may decrease the length of patients institutional stay and wound treatment costs. Further evidence supporting the use of pulsed electrical stimulation as an efficacious treatment of chronic wounds is obtained from the 14 wounds in the sham group of this study that were crossed over after four weeks to a nonrandomized active electrical stimulation treatment group. After four weeks of treatment these wounds healed at a mean rate of 12.8 a week to 49% of their pretreatment size. Kloth and Feedar reported a similar response by a small group of crossover wounds in a previous study.[4]

The wounds in the sham group healed a mean of 67% of their initial size after four weeks is not surprising to us because each of these wounds received an intensive amount of additional care including maintenance of a moist microenvironment as part of the sham treatment. Thus, despite the improvement of the sham wounds after four weeks, it is clearly evident that the treated group of wounds benefited not only from maintenance of a moist wound environment but also from electrical stimulation which very likely accounts for the fact that the treated wounds healed 56% compared to only 33 % for the sham wounds during the four-week double-blind study.

There is growing evidence that exogenous electrical currents can augment the healing process of dermal ulcers perhaps by mimicking the body's own bioelectric signals. However, additional studies are needed to identify the mechanisms involved in the promotion of wound healing with electrical stimulation and to determine the stimulus variables that most efficaciously accelerate tissue repair.

Conclusion

The healing rate of 14% a week of chronic wounds in the treatment group falls within the range of 13% to 5% reported in the literature. Therefore, since both the treated group and the sham group received otherwise identical care, the differences between the healing rates of the two groups can be attributed to the electrical stimulation. We conclude that the use of electrical stimulation in the dosage and manner used in this study is a safe and effective way to treat Stage II, III and IV chronic dermal ulcers.

References

1. Wolcott LE, Wheeler PC, Hardwicke HM, (1969) Accelerated healing of skin ulcers by electrotherapy: Preliminary clinical results. Southern Medical Journal 62:795-801.
2. Gault WR, Gatens PR Jr. (1976) Use of low intensity direct current in management of ischemic skin ulcers. Physical Therapy 50:265-269.
3. Carley P, Wainapel S (1985) Electrotherapy for acceleration of wound healing: Low Intensity direct current. Archives Physical Medicine Rehabilitation 66:443-446.
4. Kloth LC, Feedar JA (1988) Acceleration of wound healing with high voltage, monophasic, pulsed current. Physical Therapy 68:503-508.
5. Assimacopoulos D (1988) Wound healing promotion by the sue of negative electric current. American Surgeon 34(6):423:431.
6. Bigelow JB, Al-Hussein SA, Von Recum AF et al: Effect of electrical stimulation on canine skin and percutaneous device - skin interface healing. In Brighton CT, Black J, Pollack SR (eds), Electrical Properties of Bone and Cartilage: Experimental Effects and Clinical Applications. New York, Grune and Stratton, 1979; pp 289-310.
7. Alverez OM, Mertz PM, Smerbeck RV (1983) Healing of superficial skin wounds is stimulated by external electrical current. Journal Investigative Dermatology 81:144-148.
8. Brown MB, McDonnel MK, Menton DN, (1989) Polarity effects on wound healing using electric stimulation in rabbits. Archives Physical Medicare Rehabilitation 70:624-627.
9. Im MJ, Lee WPA, Hoppes JE (1990) Effect of electrical stimulation on survival of skin flaps in pigs. Physical Therapy 70:37-40.
10. Cruz NI, Bayron FE, Suarez AJ (1989) Accelerated healing of full-thickness burns by te use of high voltage pulsed galvanic stimulation in the pig. Annals Platic Surgery 23(1):49-55.
11. Stromberg BV (1988) Effects of electrical currents on wound contraction. Annals Plastic Surgery 21(2):121-123.
12. Cooper MS, Schliwa M (1985) Electrical and ionic control of tissue cell locomotion in a DC electrical field. Journal Neuroscience Research 13:223-244.
13. Erickson CA, Nuccitelli R (1984) Embryonic fibroblast motility and orientation can be influenced by physiological electric fields. Journal Cell Biology 98:296-307.

THE EFFECT OF LOW LEVEL LASER ON MACROPHAGE - LIKE CELLS IN VITRO

T D Sheilds, B M Hannigan, W S Gilmore, J M Allen, A J Bell.
Biomedical Sciences Research Centre, Dpt Occupational Therapy
& Physiotherapy, University Of Ulster, BT37 0QB.

INTRODUCTION

Since the 1960s, low level laser therapy (LLLT) has become a popular treatment modality, typically being used for the promotion of wound healing. Consequently, the most prolific area of research is the effect of LLLT on cell function. Numerous reports exist in which laser irradiation of various cell types in culture has produced significant alterations in a number of cell functions e.g. collagen synthesis (1) ATP synthesis (2) cell proliferation (3) and altered immune response (4). However the lack of basic information on possible mechanisms of action has lead to much controversy surrounding the clinical value of LLLT as a therapeutic device.

Macrophages constitute a significant proportion of wound fluid and are implicated in a multiplicity of wound healing processes, including wound debridement, fibrosis and the release of soluble factors involved in host defence and inflammation. The fundamental protective function of macrophages is related to the cells' unique ability to generate large amounts of oxidants e.g. superoxide (O2-), when adequately stimulated. There is considerable evidence that the increment in cytochrome C is an adequate biochemical correlate for activation (5). Activation of the macrophage enhances important aspects of cell function, such that the cell assumes a new significance in immunoregulation, phagocytosis, bactericidal defence and inflammation. This offers one possibility through which acceleration of wound healing observed following LLLT might be mediated.

The purpose of this investigation is to determine whether LLLT activates U-937 in vitro, using the production of O2- as an indicator of activation. U937 cells are a pre-monocytic and relatively indifferentiated cell line. Nonetheless, this cell line is a well established and popular model of macrophages in vitro.

MATERIALS AND METHODS

U-937 cells were maintained in culture in RPM1 1640, supplemented with 10% foetal calf serum, and 1%

penicillan/streptomycin, at 37 degrees C, 5% CO_2 .Cells were
routinely sub-cultured approximately every 3 days. The
microassay for O2- production is based on the reduction of
ferricytochrome C by O2-, measured as a function of absorbance
over a 90 minute period. The laser used was an Omega
Biotherapy 3ML (Omega Universal Technologies). Power = 15mW,
wavelength = 660nm, pulsing frequency = 5000Hz, area
irradiated = 0.125cm.sq. Irradiation times, = 10, 30 or 60
secs, energy densities = 1.2, 3.6, or 7.2J/cm.sq,
respectively.

Cells were grown to an exponential concentration of 4-6 x 10
cells/ml in a large volume of medium (80 - 100 mls). The
sample was centrifuged (1200RPM x 5mins) and cells resuspended
in phosphate buffered saline (PBS), supplemented with 2mMCacl
, 4mM glucose at a concentration of 4×10^{-6} cells/ml. Cells
were removed to a 96 well flat-bottomed microtitre plate (100
ul, 4×10^{-6} cells/100 ul). Test wells were irradiated with
10, 30 or 60s irradiation. Following irradiation cytochrome C
was added (60 uM, 40ml) Control wells contained an additional
20ml of superoxide dismutase (10,000ng/ml). Total volume in
the wells was 200ml using PBS to supplement volume.

A positive control using phorbol myristate acetate (PMA)
(10,000 ng/ml), a known inducer of respiratory burst, was
included in this investigation to ensure that cell samples
were in a position to respond by O2- production. A microtitre
plate reader (Dynatech) was used to read absorbance in the
wells at 550nm, at 15 minute intervals, for 90 minutes.
Absorbance values observed represent the colour change which
occurs in Cytochrome C as it becomes reduced by O2-. These
are converted to nanomoles of O2- based on the extinction
coefficient of cytochrome C (E 550 = 2.1 x 10 M cm-) (5).

This study was repeated on cells exposed to dimethyl
sulphoxide (DMSO) to induce cell differentiation. DMSO (3%,
v/v) was added and the cells incubated (37 degrees c) 24 hours
prior to the experiment.

Results

In this study, U937 cells did not respond to PMA or laser
irradiation by O2- production. Further, cells pre-treated
with DMSO to induce differentiation did not respond to either
stimulant.

DISCUSSION

The results suggest that laser irradiation and PMA stimulation
do not induce O2- production in U937 cells in vitro.
Other studies investigating the ability of U937 cells to
generate O2- after stimulation with PMA and opsonized zymosan

also found that the cells produced no superoxide anion. (6, 7). However, in these studies U937 cells cultured in medium containing soluble factors released by activated lymphocytes or pre-treated with a bacterial lipopolysaccaride produced significant O2- when stimulated with PMA and zymosan. It is suggested that the ability of macrophages to produce O2- is variable and determined by state of differentiation and the influence of moodulatory factors (5).

U937 cells are a relatively immature, undifferentiated cell line. The precise stage of differentiation at which monocytes acquire the ability to generate O2- is uncertain. In this study it may be suggested that U937 cells were not adequately mature to show any O2- production following laser irradiation or PMA stimulation. Superoxide production was not enhanced in cells pre-treated with DMSO to induce differentiation. However studies conducted at this university indicate an increase in O2- production in U937 cells treated with DMSO over a 2 week period, thus allowing cells to fully differentiate. Little or no change in O2- production occurred over 24 hours. (P. Mullan, unpublished observation). Also it was shown that fully differentiated mouse peritoneal macrophages produce considerable amounts of O2- with PMA stimulation following treatment with heat treated bacteria to prime the cells. (S. Eason, unpublished observation).

Macrophages generated in the wound healing process are, in terms of cell differentiation and functional abilities, more mature than the macrophage - like cell line used in this study. Hence, they may be in a position to respond to PMA and laser irradiation by O2- production. The latter study is ongoing at this University, investigating the effect of laser irradiation on peripheral blood monocytes. Preliminary results suggest that LLLT does indeed induce macrophage activation in vitro. This might implicate the laser as an effective therapeutic device in the wound healing process.

References

1. CASTRO D J, ABERGEL D, MEEKER C. et al (1983).
   Annals of Plastic Surg. 11, (3) 214-222.
2. PASSARELLA S. (1988). Abstract.
   Omega Laser Conference, Guys Hospital, London, 1988.
3. BOULTON M, MARSHALL J. (1986).
   Lasers in Life Sciences. 1 (2) 125-134.
4. INOUE K, NISHIOKA J, HUKUDA S. (1989).
   Clin Exp Rheum, 7, 521-523.
5. DICK E. (1986). Meth. of Enzymol. 132, 409-21.
6. FRUEND M, DICK M. (1984).
   'Thymic Hormones + Lymphokines' p. 335 Dlenum, N-1.
7. CLEMENT L T, LEHMEYER J E. (1983).
   J. Immunol. 130, (6) 2763-2766.

EFFECT OF THERAPEUTIC PULSED MAGNETIC FIELDS ON KERATINOCYTE PROLIFERATION *IN VITRO*

N Nirsimloo, R E Smith*, M Dyson

Tissue Repair Research Unit, Department of Anatomy, United Medical and Dental Schools, Guy's Hospital, London, England. *Professorial Surgical Unit, St Bartholomew's Hospital, London, England.

Exposure to therapeutic pulsed magnetic fields (T-PMF) is used by some physiotherapists to treat both hard and soft tissue injures. The latter including skin lesions, in the repair of which keratinocyte proliferation is generally involved. This research involves the application of T-PMF to spontaneously transformed keratinocytes *in vitro*. The period of exposure was 30 minutes and performed at room temperature. The T-PMF applied were 10, 16.7, 25 and 50 Hz with a constant intensity of 5.1 mT or intensities of 0.6, 2.3, 4.2, 4.9 or 5.1 mT with a constant frequency of 16.7 Hz.

Proliferation was assessed daily for five days using photometry. Keratinocytes exposed to T-PMF showed an increase in proliferation with a peak at day 3. All frequencies gave a significant ($p < 0.05$) increase over the control at day 3, the most efficacious being 16.7 Hz, the least 10 Hz. At 16.7 Hz, this increase was significantly greater than the control level at all intensities ($p < 0.05$). The largest increase was obtained at 5.1 mT, the smallest at 2.3 mT. By day 5, cell number had decreased to control levels. This may be due to the depletion of essential nutrients by the cells. This is pertinent to injured tissue which, in the early stages of repair, has less nutrition available and may even be necrotic.

McIntosh J.M. Grant A. Sleep J.
Physiotherapy Dept. Royal Berkshire Hospital, Reading, RG1 5AN.

A RANDOMISED PLACEBO-CONTROLLED TRIAL TO COMPARE ULTRASOUND AND
PULSED ELECTROMAGNETIC ENERGY GIVEN IMMEDIATELY POST-PARTUM FOR
THE TREATMENT OF THE SEVERELY TRAUMATISED PERINEUM.

Previous research [2] has shown that 70% of women suffer trauma
to the perineum at delivery, and that pain following this
trauma may persist for months [3]. In the light of previous
research into the effects of ultrasound [4,5,6,7,8] and pulsed
electromagnetic energy [9,10] on healing, the following hypotheses
were tested. It was hoped to prove that ultrasound and pulsed
electromagnetic energy:- a) reduced pain at 10 days, b) reduced
the time to resumption of intercourse, and c) increased the
incidence of painfree intercourse at 3 months.
Patients were recruited on the post natal wards at the Royal
Berkshire Hospital, over a 10 month period, always by the same
midwife researcher, within 12 hours of delivery. All women who
had forceps or ventouse assisted deliveries, or sustained
severe trauma, and those who had extensive oedema and/or
bruising, and/or haemorrhoids were considered eligible. 419
women were approached and only 5 declined to take part, these
received treatment as normal.

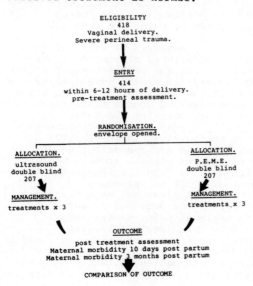

ELIGIBILITY
418
Vaginal delivery.
Severe perineal trauma.

ENTRY
414
within 6-12 hours of delivery.
pre-treatment assessment.

RANDOMISATION.
envelope opened.

ALLOCATION.
ultrasound
double blind
207

ALLOCATION.
P.E.M.E.
double blind
207

MANAGEMENT.
treatments x 3

MANAGEMENT.
treatments x 3

OUTCOME
post treatment assessment
Maternal morbidity 10 days post partum
Maternal morbidity 3 months post partum

COMPARISON OF OUTCOME

Prior to the first
treatment the midwife
researcher assessed the
patients' condition and
collected the following
data:- maternal age,
parity, mode delivery,
anaesthesia, type of
trauma, method of
repair, gestation and
birth weight. She also
recorded the extent of
bruising and/or oedema,
size and number of
haemorrhoids, and the
patients mobility. The
patient filled in a
questionnaire which
included a linear
analogue. The patients
were then randomly
allocated to an ultra-
sound or pulsed electro-.
magnetic energy group
by means of a sealed

opaque brown envelope. The midwife researcher handed the
envelope to an obstetric physiotherapist and left the ward. All
patients received three treatments within the next 48 hours.
Following the third treatment the midwife researcher returned
to the ward and re-assessed the patient's condition as before,
also recording analgesic requirements. At 10 days the women
were visited in their own homes by their community midwife who
assessed the condition of the perineum, recent analgesic
requirements, and general maternal morbidity. The woman filled
in a further questionnaire. At three months the women were sent
a postal questionnaire to assess post natal maternal morbidity,
resumption of intercourse, urinary and faecal incontinence. A
response was received from 91% of those approached. The
community midwives and the midwife researcher were not aware
which type of treatment the women had received.
The treatment regimes prescribed were in line with current
practice throughout the United Kingdom, and also with the
manufacturer's specifications. Current practice was established
prior to implementation of the trial by means of a postal
questionnaire sent out to 120 obstetric physiotherapists. The
chosen treatment modalities were as follows: Ultrasound 3MHz,
intensity $0.5w/cm^2$, pulsed 1:4, treatment time was 2 minutes
per head size of trauma. The treatment was given in contact
using the E.M.S. couplant as recommended by the manufacturer.
Pulsed electromagnetic energy was set at an operating frequency
of 27 MHz, a pulse repeat rate of 100 pulses per second, and a
pulse width of 65μs, pulse ratio normal, duration of treatment
10 mins. The machines used were the E.M.S. Therasonic 1030 Unit
and the E.M.S. Megapulse Unit. Three treatments only were given
as, in the majority of Maternity Hospitals in the United
Kingdom, following a vaginal delivery, women are generally
discharged after 48 hours.
The double blind placebo effect was achieved by means of an
additional switch on both machines with 12 digits, 8 of which
were operative and 4 inoperative, but the physiotherapists were
not aware of the code which was kept in sealed envelopes by the
manufacturer for the duration of the trial period. These codes
were changed by the manufacturer every 2 months to further
minimise the risk of the therapists breaking the code. Both
machines were tested each week by a physiotherapist employed
elsewhere in the hospital and not involved in the trial.
Results. All groups were well matched for randomisation and
comparability. The results of the two placebo groups were so
similar that they were amalgamated to form a third group. At
the post treatment assessment over 90% of the women in all
three groups felt that the treatment given had made them feel
better. This is in line with all other previous research [1,2].
There were no differences in perineal pain, oedema and
haemorrhoids in the three groups immediately following
treatment, however in the ultrasound group bruising was found
to be more extensive. At 10 days post partum the ultrasound
group had the lowest prevalence of bruising, although this was
not statistically significant. All other findings at 10 days

were similar between the three groups except that the pulsed electromagnetic energy group reported more pain than the ultrasound or placebo group. At three months there was no statistical difference between the three groups.

Discussion. These findings showing no clear benefit within the two treatment groups were unexpected. (With hindsight a fourth 'no treatment' group might have shown an interesting placebo effect of physiotherapy per se.) A possible explanation is that the wrong operating frequencies were chosen, however the number and duration of treatments, frequencies and intensities used were in line with current practice.

Conclusion. This trial urgently needs to be replicated using alternative treatment parameters.

References.
1. Grant A., Sleep J., McIntosh J.,(1989) Ultrasound and pulsed electromagnetic energy for perineal trauma. A randomised placebo-controlled trial. Br. J Obs & Gynae96:434-439.
2. Sleep J.,Grant A.et al (1984) The West Berkshire perineal management trial Br Med J 289:587-590.
3. Sleep J.,Grant A.(1987) The West Berkshire perineal management trial: 3 year follow-up. Br Med J 295:749-751.
4. Binder A., Hodge G. et al (1985) Is therapeutic ultrasound effective in treating soft tissue lesions? Br Med J 290:512-514.
5. Callam M.J.,Harper D.R. et al (1987) A controlled trial of weekly ultrasound therapy in chronic leg ulceration. Lancet ii: 204-206.
6. Dyson M.(1987) Mechanisms involved in therapeutic ultra-sound. Physiotherapy 73: 116-120.
7. El Hag et al (1985) The anti-inflammatory effects of dexamethasone and therapeutic ultrasound in oral surgery. Br J Oral Maxillofacial Surgery 23:17-23.
8. Partridge C.J.(1987) Evaluation of the efficacy of ultrasound. Physiotherapy 73:166-168.
9. Bewley E.L.(1986) The Megapulse trial at Bristol. J Assoc Chart Physiother Obstet Gynaecol. 58:16.
10. Hayne C.(1984) Pulsed high frequency energy-it's place in physiotherapy. Physiotherapy 70:459-466.
11. Creates V.(1987) A study of ultrasound treatment to the painful perineum after childbirth. Physiotherapy 73:162-165.
12. McLaren J.(1984) Randomised controlled trial of ultrasound therapy for the damaged perineum. Clin Phys Physiol Meas 5:40.

Myers, RS High Voltage Pulsed Current Enhancement Of Chronic Dermal Wound And Ulcer Healing: A Meta-Analysis, American Physical Therapy Association, 1111 N. Fairfax Street, Alexandria, VA 22314, USA

Evidence is mounting that high voltage pulsed current (HVPC) is effective in promoting the healing of chronic wounds and ulcers. In this paper the result of a study of a number of randomized controlled clinical trials will be presented. The technique used to analyze the results of the five clinical trials is meta-analysis. Meta-analysis is the use of formal statistical techniques to sum up a number of separate, (but similar) experiments. It is a quantitative synthesis of all available data in contrast to the usual qualitative review conducted by an expert in the field (Light and Pillmer 1984; Mann 1990). The Mantel-Haenszel Chi-Square Statistic, one of the most commonly used statistics in the evaluation of epidemiologic data, was used in this analysis (Woolson 1987).

METHOD
Sample:
Five studies were chosen for this analysis based on the following criteria.
1) randomized controlled clinical trial
2) HVPC was applied for a total of 45 - 60 minutes a day
3) sufficient data was contained in the article or manuscript to determine the results of treatment based on predetermined categories whether or not the author(s) chose to report the data in this manner
4) article was either published, accepted, or submitted for publication
5) wounds and ulcers included in the study were Stage II, III, or IV
6) the treatment and the control group received good wound care during the course of the study

Five studies met all of the criteria and are therefore included in the analysis. Kloth and Feedar (1988), Mulder (accepted for publication), Feedar and Kloth (submitted for publication), Unger and Eddy (submitted for publication), Griffin (accepted for publication).

Three studies used a double-blind randomized controlled design (Feedar and Kloth, Mulder, and Unger and Eddy), one a modified double-blind randomized controlled design (Griffin), and one a randomized controlled design (Kloth and Feedar). Three studies were conducted for a short specified period of electrical stimulation, four weeks (Feedar and Kloth, Mulder, and Griffin) and the remaining two studies for longer treatment periods with the goal of complete healing in a reasonable period of time (Unger and Eddy and Kloth and Feedar).

Procedure:
The results of the clinical trial were either reported in the manuscript or were assigned from the reported results to one of three categories based on the percentage of the initial wound size.

Classification	Criteria
Excellent	0 - 25 percent of the initial wound size
Good	26 - 75 percent of the initial wound size
Poor	76 - 100 percent of the initial wound size

For the purpose of calculating the Mantel-Haenszel Chi-Square Statistic the categories were further collapsed into two categories. Three of the studies were conducted for four weeks and two for longer periods of time. Therefore the assigned categories were as follows to account for a healing response that would likely occur within the four weeks of the trial.

1) non-healing or no response (poor)
2) healing or response (excellent and good)

A 2 x 2 table was constructed and the observed outcome (O), expected number (E), and variance (V) were calculated for each study included in the analysis. The Mantel-Haenszel Chi-Square Statistic and an odds ratio (OR_{M-H}) were then calculated to determine whether to accept or reject the Null-hypothesis that there was no difference between the experimental (HVPC) group and the control group and the alternative hypothesis that there was a significant difference between the groups.

	Treatment Group	Control Group
No Response (Non Healing)	a	b
Response (Healing)	c	d

$$\text{O or } A_{i}^{\cdot} = a$$

$$E(A_i) = \frac{(a + b)(a + c)}{N}$$

$$V(A_i) = \frac{(a + c)(b + d)(a + b)(c + d)}{N^2(N-1)}$$

$$\text{M-H Chi-Square} = \frac{(|\sum_{i=1}^{s} A - \sum_i E(A_i)| - 1/2)^2}{\sum_{i=1}^{s} V(A_i)}$$
1 df

$$OR_{M-H} = \frac{(\sum_{i=1}^{s} A_i D_i)/N_i}{(\sum_{i=1}^{s} B_i C_i)/N_i}$$

From the 2 x 2 tables the following values were calculated and used in calculating the Mantel-Haenszel Chi-Square statistic and the odds ratio using the formulas above.

Study	Obs Outcome	ExpNumber	Variance	Odds Ratio	
				AD/BC/N	
Feedar & Kloth	2	6.76	2.4	.52	5.28
Griffin	0	.94	.44	0	.94
Kloth & Feedar	0	3.38	.92	0	3.38
Unger & Eddy	1	3.18	.97	.18	2.35
Mulder	2	6.76	2.4	.52	5.28
	5	21.02	7.13	1.22	17.23

Calculation of the Mantel-Haenszel Chi-Square Statistic yielded a Chi-Square value of 38.28 which was significant at p = .001 level. The odds ratio (.07) was less than one. The Null-hypothesis was rejected and the alternative hypothesis was accepted.

Discussion:

A meta-analysis has been employed to assess five clinical trials which addressed the same question of whether patients' wounds and ulcers treated with HVPC would respond better than a control group given only good nursing care. Taken together 150 wounds and ulcers were treated in the five studies, 78 wounds were treated with HVPC and 72 wounds served as controls. In the studies carried on for longer periods of time the majority of the treated (HVPC) wounds healed and in the three studies of four weeks duration the wounds in the HVPC group healed to a significantly greater degree than the control groups' wounds. In all five studies the HVPC groups responded significantly better than the control groups. The results indicate that HVPC is an effective treatment for patients.

References

Feedar JA, Kloth LC Chronic dermal ulcer healing enhanced with mmonophasic pulsed electrical stimulation. Submitted for publication Physical Therapy.

Griffin JW, Tooms RE, Mendius RS, Clifft JK, Vander Zwaag R, El-Zeky F, (1991) Efficacy of high voltage pulsed current for healing of pressure ulcers in patients with spinal cord injury. Physical Therapy, 71

Kloth LC, Feedar JA, (1988) Acceleration of wound healing with high voltage, monophasic, pulsed current. Physical Therapy, 68:503-508

Light R, Pillmer D, (1984) SUMMING UP: THE SCIENCE OF REVIEWING RESEARCH. Harvard University Press, Cambridge

Mann C, (1990) Meta-Analysis in the Breech, SCIENCE, 249:476-480

Mulder GD, Treatment Of Open Skin Wounds With Electrical Stimulation. Archives Of Physical Medicine And Rehabilitation, accepted for publication

Unger PG, Eddy JG, A controlled study of the effect of high voltage pulsed current (hvpc) on wound healing. Submitted for publication Physical Therapy

Woolson R, (1987) STATISTICAL METHODS FOR ANALYSIS OF BIOMEDICAL DATA. John Wiley & Sons

THE PLACEBO EFFECT OF SOFT LASERS

A.Y. Bélanger
Department of Physiotherapy, Faculty of Medicine, Laval University,
Ste-Foy (Québec), Canada, G1K 7P4

The placebo effect is defined as the effect of a treatment which cannot be attributed to characteristic treatment factors but rather to incidental treatment factors (1). The experimental evidence provided in the literature suggests that the placebo effect results from two main components of the treatment, i.e. the complexity of the treatment and the therapist-patient relationship (1). The placebo effect may therefore be potentially important in Physiotherapy because many of the treatments provided are complex in nature and often require a close and prolonged therapist-patient relationship. Studies have shown that the use of electrotherapeutic modalities, such as TENS (2-3) and ultrasound (4-5) can evoke a powerful placebo effect. Over the past few years, the interest of physiotherapists for soft lasertherapy has grown considerably (6-15). The often beautiful and futuristic designs of laser machines, coupled with the mysterious effect of pure light on cells and tissues, are likely to induce a placebo effect. The purpose of this paper is to compare the therapeutical efficacy of true and placebo lasers in Physiotherapy. To attain this goal, an exhaustive and critical review of the English and French literature was undertaken. The analysis focuses only on the results of in-vivo human randomized controlled studies, single or double blind, published in peer-review journals.

Results and discussion

Table 1 summarizes the true and placebo effects of soft lasers. As might be expected from a new and controversial modality, the research literature on low power laser is limited, fragmented and conflicting. Nevertheless, the results of the present study suggest that incidental treatment factors associated with the use of soft lasers has a powerful placebo effect on patients. The placebo effect of any therapeutical treatment is important. However, the answer to the question of whether the placebo effect is directly attributable to the application of placebo laser perse or to the passage of time alone is equally important. To answer this question, comparisons between a placebo laser group and a control group not submitted to any treatment are necessary. Evidence that placebo laser can mimic physiological responses of characteristic treatment factor (true laser) will require that the placebo group gets significantly better than the control group. The only study of this kind reported no significant difference between the two groups (14; Table 1). Further research is needed in the field of lasertherapy.

Table 1: True and placebo efficacy of soft lasertherapy

AUTHOR	LASER	CASE	PHENOMENON	CHANGE LASER	PLACEBO
Walker, 1983	HeNe	Mixed	Chronic pain	↓	
			5-HIAA urine	↑	
Waylonis et al, 1988	HeNe	Myofascial	Chronic pain	–	–
Kreczi et al, 1986	HeNe	Mixed	Chronic pain	↓	
Klein et al, 1990	IR	Back	Chronic pain	–	–
			Disability score	–	–
			Spinal ROM	–	–
			Back strength	–	–
Basford et al, 1987	HeNe	Thumb	Joint tenderness	↓	
			Pain	–	–
			ROM	–	–
			Grip strength	↑	
			Activity level	–	–
			Medication	–	–
Lundeberg et al 1987	HeNe IR	Tennis elbow	Pain (at rest)	–	–
			Pain (wist ext.)	–	–
			Pain (susp. weight)	–	–
			Grip strength	–	–
			Sensory radial nerve		
			. latency	–	–
			. ampl. potential	–	–
			Skin temperature	–	–
Siebert et al, 1987	HeNe IR	Tendinopathies	Pain (at rest)	–	–
			Pain (movement)	–	–
			Pain (pressure)	–	–
Snyder-Mackler et al, 1986	HeNe	Trigger point	Skin resistance	↑	
Snyder-Mackler et al, 1989	HeNe	Trigger point	Skin resistance	↑	
			Pain	↓	
DeBie et al, 1989 . Inclusion of a control group . No difference between control-placebo	IR	Ankle sprain	Pain : (5 days)	↓	
			: (17 days)	–	–
			Sports participation		
			: (5 days)	↑	
			: (17 days)	–	–

- : No difference (statistical or not) between the laser and placebo groups

REFERENCES

1. Geilen F (1989) Discussion of placebo effect in physiotherapy based on a noncritical review of the literature. Physioth. Can. 41: 210-216

2. Abelson K, Langley GB, Shappeard H, Vlieg M, Wigley RD (1983) Transcutaneous electrical nerve stimulation in rhumatoid arthritis. New Z. Med. J. 96: 156-158

3. Thorsteinsson G, Stonnington HH, Stillwell GK, Elveback LR (1978) The placebo effect of transcutaneous electrical stimulation. Pain, 5: 31-41

4. Hashish I, Harvey W, Harris M (1986) Anti-inflammatory effects of ultrasound therapy: Evidence for a major placebo effect. Br. J. Rhumatol. 25: 77-81

5. Binder, Hodge G, Greenwood AM, Hazleman BL, Page-Thomas DP (1985) Is therapeutic ultrasound effective in treating soft-tissue lesions. Br. Med. J. 290: 512-514

6. Walker J (1983) Relief from chronic pain by low power laser irradiation. Neurosc. Letters 43: 339-344

7. Waylonis CW, Wilke S, O'Toole D, Waylonis DA, Waylonis DB (1988) Chronic myofascial pain: Management by low-output helium-neon lasertherapy. Arch. Phys. Med. Rehab. 69: 1017-1020

8. Klein RG, Bjorn CE (1990) Low-energy laser treatment and exercise for chronic low back pain: Double-blind controlled trial. Arch. Phys. Med. Rehab. 17: 34-37

9. Basford JR, Sheffield CG, Mair SD, Ilstrup DM (1987) Low-energy helium-neon laser treatment of thumb osteoarthritis. Arch. Phys. Med. Rehab. 68: 794-797

10. Siebert W, Seichert N, Seibert B, Wirth CJ (1987) What is the efficacy of "soft" and "mild" lasers in therapy of tendinopathies? Arch. Orthop. Trauma. Surg. 106: 358-363

11. Lunberg T, Haker E, Thomas M (1987) Effect of laser versus placebo in tennis elbows. Scand J. Rehab. Med. 19: 135-138

12. Snyder-Mackler L, Bork C, Bourbon B, Trumbore D (1986) Effect of helium-neon laser on musculoskeletal trigger points. Phys. Ther. 66: 1087-1090

13. Kreczi T, Klinger D (1986) A comparison of laser acupuncture versus placebo in radicular and pseudoradicular pain syndromes as recorded by subjective responses of patients. Acupuncture and Electro-Therapeutics Res. Inter. J. 11: 207-216

14. DeBie RA, Steenbruggen RA, Bouter LM (1989) Effects of laser therapy on ankle sprains. Ned. T. Fysiotherapie 99: (spec. ed.): 4-7

15. Snyder-Mackler L, Barry AJ, Perdins AI, Soucek MD (1989) Effects of helium-neon laser irradiation on skin resistance and pain in patients with trigger points in the neck or back. Phys. Ther. 69: 336-341

AN EXPERIMENTAL AND CLINICAL STUDY OF THE He-Ne LASER RADIATION ON HEALING OF NONSPECIFIC ULCERS: AN ANALYSIS OF 160 CASES

J. Y. Li

Department of Rehabilitation, Affiliated Hospital, Shandong Medical University, Jinan, Shandong, The People's Republic of China

Nonspecific ulcers are a common surgical disease including ulcers due to injury, burn, scald, cold injury, malnutrition, and infection, neurotrophic ulcers due to nerve injury and ischemic-necrotic ulcers. The clinical manifestations are mainly tissue defect and edema of granulation tissue with dark gray or pale color. The surface is covered with purulent secretion and its surrounding tissue has various degrees of inflammation and pigmentation. Doctors of physiotherapy and rehabilitation usually treat them with He-Ne laser radiation or ultraviolet radiation with definite therapeutic effect. For the purpose of selecting the best physiotherapeutic modality, an experimental study was carried out and 160 cases were analysed.

I. Animal Experiment

1. Methods

In this study fifteen pairs of rabbits of similar condition were selected and divided into 3 groups, each group having 5 pairs of rabbits. An area of the skin about 3x3 cm of the buttock of each rabbit was scissored off to the depth of muscular layer. The wounds were then painted with pus and E. Coli. Twenty four hours later local ulcers were formed. The first group was treated with He-Ne laser radiation. The distance between the ulcer and light source was 50 cm. Each ulcer was radiated at five spots with laser and each spot was radiated for 5 minutes. Treatment was given once daily until healing of the ulcer. The average number of treatments was 15.4 times.

The second group of 5 pairs of rabbits were treated with ultraviolet radiation. The therapeutic procedure was that a local ultraviolet radiation with a second degree erythema dose was given daily until the ulcer healed. The average ultraviolet radiation treatment was 17.9 times.

The third group of 5 pairs of rabbits received no treatment and the average duration of ulcer healing was 53.3 days

2. The experimental results are shown in Table 1.

Table 1. The comparison of the therapeutic effect of these 3 groups

Comparison	t value	P value
Group 1 compared with group 3	11.28	< 0.001
Group 2 compared with group 3	10.13	< 0.001
Group 1 compared with group 2	0.732	> 0.2

The results indicated that ulcers treated with He-Ne laser radiation healed the most rapidly, those treated with ultraviolet radiation healed less rapidly and ulcers without treatment healed slowly. Statistically, there was no significant difference between He-Ne laser radiation and ultraviolet radiation.

3. Pathological Changes

The pathological changes are the same in experimental groups and controls. The pathological changes indicate that the ulcers produced in these 3 groups are almost the same but the healing process is comparatively more complete in the group treated with He-Ne laser radiation, next in the group treated with ultraviolet radiation and poor in controls.

II. An Analysis of Therapeutic Effect

1. Materials

Among these 160 patients 106 were referred to our department from the surgical department, 37 from the department of stomatology and 17 from the department of gynecology and obstetrics. The sex distribution was 68 males and 92 females. Nine patients were under 1 year old, 10 in 1-10 years, 15 in 11-20 years, 42 in 21-30 years, 19 in 31-40 years, 24 in 41-50 years, 30 in 51-60 years, 9 in 61-70 years, and 2 over 70 years old. The causes were trauma in 36 cases, surgical operation in 28 cases, vasculitis in 15 cases, burn in 19 cases, infection in 52 cases, cold injury in 8 cases and unknown in 2 cases. The duration of illness was within 1 month in 85 cases, 1-6 months in 37 cases, 6 months-1 year in 4 cases, 1-5 years in 20 cases, 5-10 years in 7 cases, 10-20 years in 4 cases, 20-30 years in 1 case and 30-40 years in 2 cases. The distribution of ulcer is shown in Table 2.

Table 2. The site of ulcer

Site	No. of cases	%
Oral cavity	37	23.13
Lower leg	28	17.5
Foot and ankle	25	15.62
Head and face	13	8.12
Other sites	57	35.63

2. Therapeutic Method

One hundred and four cases were treated with He-Ne laser radiation. The apperatus used was the same as for animal models. During treatment the patient was sitting or lying on his back. The distance between ulcer and the source of light was 50 cm. Several points of the ulcer were radiated locally and each point was radiated for 5 minutes. The treatment was given once daily. The shortest duration of treatment was one day and the longest duration was 42 days, averaging 8 days. Fifty six patients were treated with ultraviolet radiation. The apperatus was the same as for animal models. The ulcer was radiated locally. The dosage given was first degree erythema dose to start with and the treatment was given once daily. The shortest duration was 4 treatments and the longest one was 28 treatments, averaging 9.4 treatments.

3. Therapeutic Effect

The criteria of therapeutic effect are: (1) Recovery Symptoms subside and the ulcer has healed. May have some pigmentation of the skin over the healed ulcer; (2) Marked improvement Symptoms almost subside and the ulcer has decreased to ⅓ of its original size; (3) Improvement Symptoms are alleviated and the size of ulcer decreases somewhat; and (4) Failure There is no change of original symptoms and signs. Statistically the response rates of He-Ne laser radiation and ultraviolet radiation are significantly different by using significance test (P< 0.05) and the He-Ne laser radiation is superior to ultraviolet radiation.

III. Discussion

1. Both low power He-Ne laser radiation and ultraviolet radiation have anti-inflammatory properties. Their anti-inflammatory mechanism is to stimulate the immune function of the host defense mechanisms such as the increase of bactericidal function of humoral immunity, the increase of serum IgG and IgM, the increase of the function of adrenal cortex, the increase of the capacity of lymphocyte transformation, the promotion of blood and lymph circulation and the resolution and absorption of pathological metabolic products. In our series, 160 patients had various degrees of inflammatory infiltration and these two methods of treatment showed marked anti-inflammatory infiltration, which was proved by the results of animal experiment.

2. Both low power He-Ne laser radiation and ultraviolet radiation can promote tissue regeneration. Studies indicate that these 2 therapies can increase the regeneration of collagen fibers and capillaries which is beneficial to the healing of an ulcer and enhance the anabolism of epithelial cells such as the increase of the content of DNA, RNA and protein. These responses are beneficial to the proliferation of the epithelial cells and promote the healing of an ulcer.

The results of animal experiment and the therapeutic effect of 160 cases indicate that both therapies can promote the healing of an ulcer and He-Ne laser radiation is superior to ultraviolet radiation in the treatment nonspecific ulcers.

IV. Summary

1. The animal experiment indicates that both therapies are superior to controls. Statistically, these 2 therapies had no marked difference (P> 0.2). The histologic findings reveal that the tissue repair is most complete in He-Ne laser radiation, next in fltraviolet radiation and poor in controls.

2. Clinical analysis of the therapeutic effect of 160 cases reveals that the cure rate of the 104 cases treated with He-Ne laser radiation is 73.08% and that of 56 cases treated with ultraviolet radiation is 42.86%. Statistically, the difference is marked (P< 0.05). Thus, for the treatment of nonspecific ulcers He-Ne laser radiation is superior to ultraviolet radiation.

A DOUBLE BLIND TRIAL OF LOW LEVEL LASER THERAPY FOR SOFT TISSUE INJURY

Alison Clark
Trent Health Authority, Fulwood Road, Sheffield S10 3TH

INTRODUCTION

Research into the effects of low and mid power laser is still in its infancy. Many clinical studies have, however, shown some promise in its possible effectiveness as a therapeutic tool in physiotherapy and in the laboratory setting it has been reported to induce various biological effects at a cellular level [1]. Never the less these results are difficult to interpret as different workers have used different parameters in their studies, and rarely is the same dose and treatment regime repeated.

Soft tissue injuries are a significant contributor to temporary disability and a loss of man hours. This study seeks to establish whether the healing and recovery of such injuries are expedited by the use of Low Level Laser Therapy (LLLT) in conjunction with conventional physiotherapy exercises. Further to this it seeks to establish whether or not the pulsed frequency of the laser energy emitted influences the final outcome. If it could be demonstrated that healing and recovery could be maximised by using LLLT, then the introduction of this treatment for routine therapy may have an important impact upon these very common soft tissue injuries.

MATERIALS AND METHODS

Inversion sprains of the lateral ligament the ankle have been used as the study group. Patients meeting the selection criteria, having sustained an injury within the previous 3 days were referred from the consultant from accident and emergency department. Each patient gave signed consent and was randomly assigned into one of three treatment arms.

Descriptive statistics of trial group (table 1)

Laser setting	No x	Age (mean)	Sex % male	Ankle %left	Time/ treat.	Degree sprain(%2)	%previous injury
Low	22	31.3	77.0	63.2	36.4	36.2	36.4
High	16	30.0	68.8	56.2	31.2	56.2	62.5
Placebo	17	29.4	76.5	64.7	34.2	58.8	52.9

Equipment

Laser Unit:An Omega 3ML AlGaAs Biotherapy laser, 50mW, wavelength 820nm with a 12 frequency capability has been utilised. The unit has been altered to enable only 2 frequencies to be emitted, and these were randomly organised such that either 5000Hz (treatment arm I), 2.28Hz (arm II) or placebo (arm III) laser was administered. The output was blind to both the patient and the therapist.

Treatment

The probe of the LLLT laser was placed over the 5 most tender points of the lateral ligament of the affected ankle for 2 minutes per area, this being the dose recommended by the manufacturer. Each subject received an identical ankle exercise regime, incorporating muscle strengthening exercises, proprioception re-education and finally stretching. All patients were issued with elbow crutches to be used for the first 3 days post initial assessment, and with a double thickness tubigrip to be used throughout the trial period. Each subject attended five treatment sessions.

b **Assessment of Outcome**

The outcomes of the patient treatment were measured on the 1st, 3rd, 5th and 6th visit. The first 5 visits occurred within 8 days of initial assessment. The final assessment was carried out on day 15. Each assessment was carried under the same conditions in the same order, regardless of treatment.

Initial Assessment :

In the initial assessment the following parameters were recorded:

a) Subjective assessment.

The manner in which the injury occurred. The immediate care of the injury, and whether any immediate medical self help was administered; Past medical history of lower limb injury.

b) Objective assessment :

The injury was judged to be a 1st or 2nd degree sprain [2]. Medial Tenderness noted; The Injured structures were located by the physiotherapist and the most tender areas marked, identified and recorded. These areas were used throughout the treatment period.

Objective parameters:

a) Active PF/DF was measured using a Penny and Giles electronic goniometer.

b) The degree of swelling occurring in the foot/ankle was quantified using the water displacement technique [3] and a supplementary girth measurement.

c) Pain experienced by the patient in the injured ankle during the walkway measurements. (vide infra) was quantified using a VAD assessment scale [4].

d) Gait was assessed electronically by recording the position and timing of the feet whilst the patient walked along a purpose built walkway. [5]

be) Time elapsed to full return to work/ADL was noted.

Follow on assessments

All Objective assessments were repeated on subsequent assessment days.

Analysis of preliminary results

bAssessments of 60 patients who completed the course of physiotherapy were analysed. Descriptive statistics of the subjects participating in the trial are presented in table 1. The ratios and log of all the results were calculated, and were analysed using anova, t-test and a non-parametric analysis - the Kruskall-Wallis test. In addition summary measures [6] were calculated by obtaining the area under the graph of each subject analysis. In this way the results were given a weighted average.

Preliminary Results

Anova analysis of the area measurements are presented in table 2:

ANOVA table of area measures. (table 2)

	Swelling	ROM	Pain	Contact Time	Step Length	Velocity
p- value	0.360	0.319	0.847	0.664	0.840	0.139

Non parametric analysis of these results had similar levels of significance. Similarly, statistical analysis of each assessment stage exposed no significant differences between groups.

DISCUSSION

The study population in this clinical trial reported to date here was small, hence there is the possibility that a relevant effect of the laser therapy was not revealed. These preliminary results, however, indicated that the Null Hypothesis has been confirmed and that the rate of recovery of ligament healing is not influenced by Low Level Laser Therapy. That is, using the present assessment parameters, with the described routine, no significant difference could be reported between placebo, high and low frequency laser. These findings are to some extent backed by De bie et al [7] and Kumer et al [8].

Evaluation of the efficacy of treatment for sprained ankles is difficult. There are various factors influencing the healing process. These include the initial mechanics of the injury; the severity of injury; structures involved; the initial treatment of the ankle prior to physiotherapy; and compliance to the physiotherapy regime. In addition, initial levels of fitness, job type and speed of return to work may markedly influence treatment outcome.

The depth of penetration also requires to be considered. It has been estimated that at a depth of 1cm, only 0.1% of the initial intensity, can be detected, and thus most of the LLLT is restricted to the uppermost layers of the skin [9]. The lateral ligaments of the ankle, although relatively superficial structures, will be virtually untouched by the laser in the presence of substantial swelling. A systemic effect of the LLLT has been reported [10]. Blood supply, on the other hand, may be compromised by swelling, further reducing this effect. These clinical factors require to be clarified.

CONCLUSION

Given the vast combination of treatment frequencies and duration possible with laser, these results can be considered conclusive only with regard to the specific course of treatment given, and of the parameters measured. Much more clinical investigations are required to verify the clinical effects if any, of 'soft' lasers.

References

1 Enwemeka C.S., (1988) Laser Biostimulation of Healing Wounds: Specific Effects and Mechanisms of Action. The journal of Orthopaedic and Sports Physical Therapy.9(10);33-337

2. Dupont M., Beliveau P., Theriault G., (1987) The efficacy of Anti-inflammatory Medication in the treatment of the acutely sprained ankle. American journal of sports medicine. 15(1):41-45.2.

3.Millson S., Haughen G.B., (1987) The efficacy of Anti-inflammatory Medication in the treatment of the acutely sprained ankle and foot. J Oslo City Hospital, 31:11-15.

4 Revill S., Robinson J.O, Rosen M., Hogg M.I.J. (1976) The reliability of a linear analogue for evaluating pain. Anaesthesia, 31(1):1191-1198.

5. Arenson J.S, Ishai G, Bar A. (1983) A system for monitoring the position and time of feet contact during walking. J. Med. Eng. and Technology. 7(6):280-284

6. Mathews J.N.S., Altman D.G., Campbell M.J., Royston P.(1990) Analysis of serial measurements in medical research. BMJ 300:230-235

7. De Bie R.A., Steenbruggen R.A., Bouter L.M., (1989) Effects of Laser therapy on Ankle Sprains. Ned. T. Fysiotherapie. 99:4-7 .

8. Kumar P.S., Jayakumer C.S., Kentworthy J., Moor K.S., Hira M., Ohshiro T., (1988) A comparative study of low level laser therapy and conventional physiotherapy for treatment of inversion injuries of the ankle. Lasers in Medicine Science Abstract 289.

9.Kolari P.J., (1985) Penetration of Unfocused Laser Light into the Skin. Arch.Dermatol.Res 277:342-344

10 Rochkind S., Rousso M., Nissan M.,Villarreal M., Barr-Neal., Rees D.G.,(1989) Systtemic effects of Low Power Laser Irradiation of the peripheral and CNS, cutaneous Wounds and Burns Lasers in Surgery and Medicine 9:174-182

Acknowledgements: This study was supported by Trent Health Authority. The author would like to thank staff and patients of Rotherham District General Hospital.

TRIAL OF LOW LEVEL LASER THERAPY IN THE OUT-PATIENT TREATMENT OF DIABETIC ULCERS.

Vice, P.A., Walters, J.S. and Robinson, B.J.
Departments of Chiropody and Medicine, Royal Preston Hospital,
Preston, Lancashire, England.

Diabetes mellitus may result in ulceration of the feet. The patients are vulnerable because of a variety of factors; increased susceptibility to infection, impaired circulation, loss of sensation, and deformity. They heal more slowly than non-diabetic subjects.

Low level laser increases the speed at which wounds heal. Research has shown an increase in collagen sythesis[1-4] and an increase in tensile strength[4]. The vascularity of grafts has improved[5], and there is greater epidermal growth[1].

Omega Universal Technologies Ltd. recommend that lesions are treated three times per week. This schedule is not possible in our Out-Patient clinic. The company supplied a 3ML medical laser for an eight week trial of one application of the laser per week.

The patients treated were those attending the combined chiropodial/ medical clinic, which runs each week. All patients continued in their routine care of good diabetic control and antibiotic cover, combined with debridement and dressings. The dressings used were either alginate or polymer gel, designed to provide a moist environment into which granulation tissue will grow.

The same regimen for the laser was applied to all patients. The pencil probe (660 n.m.) was applied for 20 seconds at 2 cm intervals around the edge of the lesion. The cluster probe (31 diode) was applied for 2 min. to the ulcer and surrounding skin. All applications were at setting F5. The ulcers were photographed to document healing.

It was quite apparent within two to three weeks that the ulcers were healing more quickly. The amount of exudate increased. The granulation tissue looked more vascular. At the time of the trial, those patients whose ulcers were the most recent, responded the most dramatically.

Our experience has modified our management of diabetic ulcers. Low level laser is a routine part of our treatment. The patients themselves have provided the funds. We now own a 3ML and a 2001 Biotherapy laser.

1. Braverman, B., McCarthy, R.J., Ivankovich, A.D., Forde, D.E., Overfield, M. and Bapna, M.S. (1989).
   Effect of Helium-Neon and Infrared Laser Irradiation on Wound Healing in Rabbits.
   Lasers in Medicine and Surgery, 9:50-58.

2. Lyons, R.F., Aberger, R.P., White, R.A., Dwyer, R.M., Caster, J.C., and Uitto, J. (1987).
   Biostimulation of Wound Healing In Vivo by a Heluim-Neon Laser.
   Annals Plastic Surgery, 18:47-50.

3. Rochkind, S., Rousso, M., Nissan, M., Villarreal, M., Barr-Nea, L. and Rees, D.G. (1989).
   Systemic Effects of Low Power Laser Irradiation on the Peripheral and Central Nervous System, Cutaneous Wounds and Burns.
   Lasers in Medicine and Surgery, 9:174-182

4. Yew, D.T., Li, W.W.Y., Pang, K.M., Mok, Y.C. and Au, C. (1989).
   Stimulation of Collagen Formation in the Intestinal Anastomosis by Low Dose He-Ne Laser.
   Scanning Microscopy, 3:379-386.

5. Ohshiro, T., Calderhead, R.C., Fujino, T., and Maruyama, Y. (1989).
   The Role of Low Reactive Level Laser Therapy in Revitalising Failing Grafts and Flaps.
   American Society for Laser Medicine and Surgery Abstracts.
   No. 126 p. 31.

LASER PHOTOSTIMULATION MODULATES COLLAGEN SYNTHESIS IN REGENERATING TENDONS.

Chukuka S. Enwemeka, Ph.D., P.T.

Division of Physical Therapy, Department of Orthopaedics & Rehabilitation, University of Miami School of Medicine & Veterans Affairs Medical Center, 5915 Ponce de Leon Blvd, 5th Floor, Miami, FL, U.S.A.

Introduction

Accumulating evidence indicates that laser photostimulation accelerates the healing process of skin wounds,[1-3] and fractures.[4,5] Although the mechanisms by which these beneficial effects are produced remain ill-understood, available data indicate that photostimulation facilitates fibroplasia and collagen synthesis,[3,6,7] augments the levels of types I and III procollagen mRNA pools,[8] and promotes ATP synthesis.[9] Because tendons heal mostly by collagen synthesis and are 86% collagen by dry weight,[10] we exposed regenerating rabbit calcaneal tendons to low doses of He-Ne and Ga-As lasers, to determine the biomechanical, ultrastructural and morphometric effects of laser therapy on surgically repaired tendons.

Methods

Ninety rabbits were used for this study. Under adequate anaesthesia, the right calcaneal tendon of each rabbit was surgically isolated, transected, sutured, skin sutured, then immobilized in a hard solid cast that maintained the knee at 90° and the ankle in full plantarflexion. Thereafter, the rabbits were randomly assigned to groups (Table I).

Beginning from the first post-operative day, treated tendons were exposed to varying doses of either He:Ne or Ga:As laser beam of 632.8 nm and 904 nm wavelength respectively. The 11 mW He:Ne laser device was pulsed 50% of the time at a rate of 50 pulses per second, and the beam delivered transcutaneously via a 1.82 mm^2 applicator at a divergence angle of 30°. To irradiate the immediate 1.0 cm^2 area overlying the site of tenotomy, the applicator was clamped to maintain a vertical distance of 9.76 mm between the tip and the skin. This method was used to treat the tenotomized tendons of five groups of rabbits everyday. The tendons in each group received the same energy density of laser treatment, thus five doses, namely, 1,2,3,4, and 5 mJ cm^{-2} were utilized. Since each dose level was determined from the formula:

$$\text{Energy Density} = \frac{\text{Average Power X time}}{\text{Area}}$$

only the duration of treatment was varied from one group to the next. Using the same approach, each of another 2 groups of rabbits were exposed to the Ga:As laser beam. Treatment with the 7 mW Ga:As laser device was timed to yield energy densities of 1 or 2 mJ cm^{-2}. One more set of rabbits served as surgically tenotomized non-treated controls (Table I).

On the 14th post operative day each tendon was excised. Tendons designated for biomechanical test were excised and immediately frozen in 0.09% NaCl and kept at -70°C but thawed to room temperature before they were tested on an Instron materials testing system (Instron Inc., Houston, TX). Those designated for electron microscopy were fixed *in situ* with 2% paraformaldehyde/2.5% glutaraldehyde (pH 7.4) before they were excised and processed for electron microscopy, then visualized and photographed with a JOEL 100CX electron microscope as previously described.[11] To objectively compare the ultrastructural morphometry of the collagen fibrils in each tendon, the electron micrographs obtained were digitized; then, the cross-sectional area of the collagen fibrils were measured as detailed in previous reports.[11,12]

Analysis of variance was then used to compare the tensile strength, tensile stress, energy absorption capacity and cross-sectional area of the tendons. Where significant differences were found, Student-Neuman-Keul procedure was used to identify groups that differ. To analyze the morphometric data, first the normality of distribution of the collagen fibrils was determined by Kolmogorov-Smirnov D statistic. This test revealed that the distribution of each group of fibrils differed significantly from a normal distribution, therefore, non-parametric ANOVA was used to compare the area and diameter of the collagen fibrils. Thereafter, Mann-

Whitney U tests were performed to distinguish groups that differ in diameter and cross-sectional area.

Table I: **Experimental Design**

Group	Number of Rabbits	Surgery	Treatment
1	14	Yes	None
2	13	Yes	1 mJ cm^{-2}, He:Ne Laser
3	11	Yes	2 mJ cm^{-2}, He:Ne Laser
4	10	Yes	3 mJ cm^{-2}, He:Ne Laser
5	11	Yes	4 mJ cm^{-2}, He:Ne Laser
6	11	Yes	5 mJ cm^{-2}, He:Ne Laser
7	10	Yes	1 mJ cm^{-2}, Ga:As Laser
8	10	Yes	2 mJ cm^{-2}, Ga:As Laser

Note: In each group, the surgically tenotomized tendons of 3 rabbits were used for electron microscopic studies; the remaining tendons were tested biomechanically.

Results

Notwithstanding the type of laser used, biomechanical tests showed that exposure to laser beam enhanced tensile stress but not the ultimate tensile strength and energy absorption capacity of the tendons (Table II). Electron microscopy and subsequent morphometric analysis revealed denser collagen fibrils that were significantly smaller in area and diameter than controls. Whereas, control matrix was mostly in disarray; the collagen matrix of laser-treated tendons were often aligned in the longitudinal axis of the tendon (Fig. 1).

Table II: **The biomechanical effects of low doses of He:Ne and Ga:As lasers.**

Group	Treatment	Area (mm^2)	Strength (N)	Stress (Ncm^{-2})	Energy (mJ)
1	None (control)	35.6±4.69	65.4± 7.32	185.0±20.45	261.0±3.26
2	1 mJ cm^{-2} He:Ne Laser	16.8±8.31*	73.8± 5.82	498.1±52.59*	254.4±2.76
3	2 mJ cm^{-2} He:Ne Laser	21.3±8.91*	71.2± 4.66	375.3±45.54*	337.6±4.82
4	3 mJ cm^{-2} He:Ne Laser	14.0±2.77*	59.3± 9.09	412.3±50.71*	217.6±4.23
5	4 mJ cm^{-2} He:Ne Laser	14.8±1.60*	68.8±11.84	471.6±83.44*	206.2±3.26
6	5 mJ cm^{-2} He:Ne Laser	17.0±3.03*	91.9± 8.26	542.6±49.15*	347.6±4.02
7	1 mJ cm^{-2} Ga:As Laser	15.0±1.00*	53.4± 6.97	354.4±42.90*	255.0±7.01
8	2 mJ cm^{-2} Ga:As Laser	15.0±1.00*	59.2± 6.01	394.0±31.11*	346.2±5.60

*Significantly different from control ($P < 0.05$).

Discussion

These findings indicate that He:Ne and Ga:As laser photostimulation modulates collagen synthesis in healing tendons. As part of the remodelling process of tendons, collagen fibrils polymerize and align in the longitudinal axis of the tendon.[11-12] The more orderly arrangement of collagen fibrils in photostimulated tendons suggests that exposure to laser beam augments tendon remodelling. During collagen synthesis, fibrils of relatively small cross-sectional area are produced initially.[11] As fibrils polymerize, larger more mature fibrils are produced progressively. The presence of denser but smaller fibrils in laser-treated tendons suggests that laser therapy enhanced synthesis of large quantities of fibrils, perhaps at the expense of fibril maturation. Previous studies have shown elevated type I and type III procollagen mRNA levels in He:Ne laser treated skin wounds,[8] and increased ATP synthesis in cultured mitochondria.[9] Similarly, it has been shown that laser photostimulation augments fibroplasia and the strength of healing skin wounds in several animal models.[3] These findings are consistent with our present results, since increased fibrillogenesis will necessitate elevated

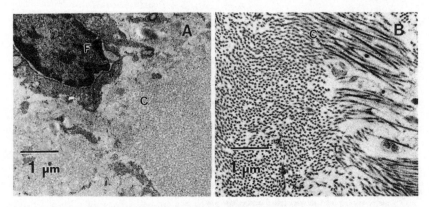

Fig. 1: Representative electron micrographs showing cross-sections of collagen fibrils in laser-treated tendons (A), and non-treated controls (B). Note the more orderly arrangement of fibrils in the laser-treated tendon and the larger sizes of control fibrils. Both electron micrographs have the same magnification (14,400X).

procollagen mRNA levels and increased ATP synthesis. Whether a greater number of relatively small-sized fibrils will strengthen the tendon better than fewer relatively large-sized fibrils deserve further experimentation. Since the present findings pertain to a narrow range of doses, the possible effects of other doses of both lasers deserve further studies because of the need to identify an optimal dose.

References

1. Mester E, *et al.* (1971) Effect of laser rays on wound healing. Am J Surg 122:532-535
2. Bosatra M, *et al.* (1984) In vitro fibroblast and dermis fibroblast activation of laser irradiation at low energy. Dermatologica 168:157-162
3. Mester E, *et al.* (1985) The biomedical effects of laser application. Lasers Surg Med 5:31-39
4. Tang XM, Chai BP (1986) Effect of CO_2 laser irradiation on experimental fracture healing: A transmission electron microscopy study. Lasers Surg Med 6:346-352
5. Trelles MA, Mayayo E (1987) Bone fracture consolidates faster with low power laser. Lasers Surg Med 7:36-45
6. Lam TS, *et al.* (1986) Laser stimulation of collagen synthesis in human skin fibroblast cultures. Laser Life Sci 1:61-77
7. Abergel RP, *et al.* (1987) Biostimulation of wound healing by lasers: Experimental approaches in animal models and in fibroblast cultures. J Dermatol Surg Oncol 13:127-133
8. Saparia D, *et al.* (1986) Demonstration of elevated type I and type III procollagen mRNA levels in cutaneous wounds treated with Helium-Neon laser. Biochem Biophys Res Comm 138:1123-1128
9. Passarella S, *et al.* (1984) Increase of proton electrochemical potential and ATP synthesis in rat liver mitochondria irradiated in vitro by helium-neon laser. FEBS Lett 175:95-99
10. Williams IF (1985) Cellular and biochemical composition of healing tendons In: Jenkins DHR (ed.) Ligament injuries and their treatment. Rockville MD, Aspen Publications pp 43-57
11. Enwemeka CS (1989) Inflammation, cellularity and fibrillogenesis in the regenerating tendon: Implications for tendon rehabilitation. Phys Ther 69:816-825
12. Enwemeka CS, *et al.* (1990) Morphometrics of collagen fibril populations in He:Ne laser photostimulated tendons. Journal of Clinical Laser Medicine and Surgery 8:47-52.
13. Parry DAD, Barnes GRG, Craig AS (1978) A comparison of the size distribution of collagen fibrils in connective tissue as a function of age and a possible relation between fibril size distribution and mechanical properties. Proc R Soc Lond [Biol] 203:305-321

Supported by the Foundation for Physical Therapy

EFFECTS OF TNS ON PAIN, SKIN CIRCULATION AND WOUND HEALING IN CASES OF
PERIPHERAL VASCULAR DISEASES

Asta Eriksson, Carl Rudolf Skoglund
Department of Clinical Neurophysiology, Karolinska Hospital,
104 01 Stockholm Sweden

In addition to its well-established pain relieving effect, electrical
stimulation of the spinal cord has been found to increase peripheral blood
circulation(1). This effect has been used in the treatment of vascular
disease and severe limb ischemia(2). Some investigatiors have studied the
obvious alternative, i.e. transcutaneous nerve stimulation (TNS). Kaada
(3) showed that low frequency TNS could improve the healing of chronic leg
ulcers. However, these results with low frequency TNS have not been regularly reproducible.

In an attempt to improve the effect of TNS on the healing of ulcers in
varicose or ischemic legs we have studied the effect of high frequency,
instead of low frequency, TNS with the electrodes applied in the immediate
vicinity of the leg ulcer. Preliminary results of these studies have been
reported previously (in Swedish, 4).

Patients and methods. The study includes 25 patients, 37-83 (average 67)
years old, with leg ulcers of different etiology. The circulatory insufficiency was of arterial type in 7 cases, 4 had venous stasis, 8 were diabetics and 6 showed circulatory insufficiency of a more general arterio-
sclerotic nature. The patients had all received conventional local treatment for their leg ulcers which had not been healed during the last 2-3
months or more (up to 3 years).

TNS (100 Hz, pulse duration 0.2 ms) was applied through electrodes
placed on the leg, the negative electrode above the peroneal nerve at the
head of the fibula and the positive electrode 2-3 cm distal to the ulcer.
The stimulus strength was adjusted upward until the patient experienced
mild parasthesias but no pain. The TNS was applied for 25 minutes twice
daily. The patients were asked to rate their pain before and after each
treatment in an analog scale of 10. The healing process was documented
with colour photographs and measurements of the size of the open ulcer.

Results. When present, pain was relieved shortly after the application
of the stimulation. The most dramatic effects were obtained in patients
with a arterial ischemia and less so in diabetics who already at the beginning reported little or no pain (diabetic neuropathy). The pain relief
in connection with the electrical stimulation lasted for about 4 hours.

During the TNS treatment an increase in skin temperature (by thermography) and in superficial blood circulation (by laser-Doppler flow measurements) was observed.

In some instances, by coincidence or arranged for control, the daily
treatment schedule was interrupted for a couple of weeks. When after this
time the daily observations and measurements of the size of the ulcers was
continued, it was observed that during the "rest period" the surface of
the ulcers had increased. When the daily TNS treatment was recommenced the
healing was again improved. A typical case is presented in figure 1.

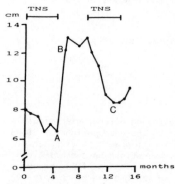

T.N. 83 years old. Ulcer on right lower leg since 3 years. Size of ulcer (longest diameter in cm) when TNS treatment was interrupted for 4 months after an initial treatment period of about 4 months. When treatment was recommenced the size of the ulcer again decreased.

TNS treatment for a duration varying from a few months to one and a half year resulted in complete healing of the leg ulcers in 12 cases, definite improvement in 6 and no effect in 3. The treatment could not be carried out as planned in 4 cases, 3 due to sudden deaths (ischemic heart disease or stroke) and 1 due to hospitalization.

Discussion. In this study no attempts were made to determine the optimum frequency and duration of the TNS treatment periods. A more frequent treatment than twice a day may well have been more effective. In clinical practice the best result will be obtained if the treatment schedule is in-dividually adjusted.

It has been recognized clinically for a long time that pain may increase peripheral vasoconstriction. The effect of TNS stimulation could therefore possibly, at least in part, be a secondary one due to the reduction in pain. However, the observation that diabetic ulcers with no or very little pain responded equally well indicates that some other mechanism may be more important.

Neurophysiological experiments in animals have shown that a reflex inhi-bition of the outflow of vasoconstrictor impulses may be produced by stim-ulation of afferent nerves. These observations would seem to be in line with the observations in man that TNS apparently reduces the sympathetic tone of cutaneous vessels as indicated by thermographic recordings (5).

Theoretically, the ulcer healing could also be influenced by electrical currents produced by the locally applied electrodes. This possibility has not been further analyzed in this rather small number of patients.

The good results obtained by high frequency TNS as regards pain reduc-tion as well as ulcer healing would seem to justify further studies in which the optimum treatment schedule as well as the mechanism of action may be further elucidated.

References:
1. Cook A W, Oxygar A, Baggenstos P et al. (1976) Vascular disease of extremities: Electrical stimulation of spinal cord and posterior roots. NY State J Med 76:366-8.
2. Augustinsson L E, Carlson C A, Holm J, Jivegård L. (1985) Epidural electrical stimulation in severe limb ischemia. Pain relief, increased blood flow and a possible limb-saving effect. Ann Surg 202:104-10.

3. Kaada B. (1982) Behandling av perifere sirkulasjonsforstyrrelser og kroniske sår med trankutan nervestimulering. Tidskr Nor Laegeforen 102:1563-70.
4. Eriksson L, Skoglund C R. (1988) Smärtlindring och förbättrad sårläkning genom TNS vid perifera cirkulationsrubbningar. Läkartidningen 85(14):1237-41.
5. Owens S, Atkinson E R, Lees D E. (1979) Thermograhic evidence of reduced sympathetic tone with transcutaneous nerve stimulation. Anesthesiology 50:62-5.

TRAUMA

CAUSALGIA: A NEN APPROCH TO ITS TREATMENT

S.M.Hashemi

Department of physiotherapy,faculty of rehabilitation Medical faculty University of Tehran,Iran.

Introduction: This most disturbing clinical condition which is
called CAUSALGIA it is not a common disease or disorder one comes
cress it.Many specialist,general practitioners and physiotherapists may never see this condition during the while yers of thier
practice,but if one see the real case of causalgia will   never
forget the case,the most agonising pain andburning sensation with
spasific facial expression of these patients.Causalgia is occas-
sionally seen in injuries caused in accidents but most often seen
and first reported in patients being injured in the war by bullet
or different type of injuries caused by explusions of pieces of
high temprature penettrating metals.To relief the symptoms   all
approches reported have not always been fully effective.

Treatment: During the 8 years of war in Iran when we used to have
hundreds of addmission of injured at one time I had eight cases
of Reflex sympatetic dystrophy (causalgia).Treatments used was
T.N.S. andultrasend & one group with Sinosidal current,the result
with sinosidal current was not only satisfactory but most marked
after the first session.

Result :
        Due to the sensory effect of the sinosidal current and
the countra-irritation effect the symptomwas reliefed in   all
patients among which ,all methods suggested were applied,patient
who never slept for over six month

conclusion:There are still needs to work with this current.

818

BURNS: INCIDENCE AND PHYSICAL THERAPY IN LAGOS

MRS. M.R. RAJI & DR. I.O. OWOEYE

LAGOS UNIVERSITY TEACHING HOSPITAL, LAGOS,
NIGERIA.

The objectives of this study were to study the pattern of the incidence of burns in Lagos as typical of a developing country and to identify the most beneficial physical therapy procedures for the management and prevention of contracture deformities of burns.

In this study, 10 cases were randomly selected and studied. Various physical therapy procedures were utilized in the physical management of the cases.

The most threatening causes of burns were found to be kerosine explosion and hot water scalding. The commonest place of occurrence of burns was found to be in the homes.

Following physical therapy, all the patients fully recovered without any contracture deformity. Breathing and coughing exercises, good positioning, graduated mobilizing exercise, saline bath and lanoline massage of scar tissues when applied at appropriate periods during the course of management as reported in this study enhanced very speedy recovery without the complication of contracture deformities.

It was concluded that the rate of incidence of burns can be reduced very drastically by improvement on the domestic life styles in the developing countries. Also when physical therapy is administered early and as reported in this study, burns can be managed without any residual deformities.

MEASUREMENT

A FUNCTIONAL RATING SCALE FOR THE LOWER EXTREMITY

U. Öberg, County Hospital of Eksjö-Nässjö, P.O. Box 1007, S-575 28 Eksjö, Sweden

A new 20-variable functional rating scale for the lower extremity is presented. The scale has been tested on patients with coxarthrosis and gonarthrosis. The variables have been tested with regard to their descriptive capacity, and with regard to validity and reliability.

In the scientific literature some 20-30 rating scales for the lower extremity have been reported, e.g. Harris' hip score, the HSS-scale, the Merle d'Aubigné scale and in Sweden the Larsson scale for patients with arthrosis deformans and rheumatoid arthritis. However, almost all of these scales have been designed for the needs of the physician and not for the physiotherapist. Almost none of the scales have been tested for reliability and validity. The aim of my study has been to construct a rating scale which fulfils the needs of the physiotherapist. The scale must evaluate traditional hard variables such as joint movement, muscle strength, but also functional and social variables related to the daily life of the patient. The scale shall also be tested for reliability and validity with different methods. This paper is a short presentation of the scale and some of the results from clinical tests.

Material and Methods: The rating scale is a 20-variable functional rating scale for the lower extremity (see appendix). The scale is semiquantitative, where the disability of the patient is rated from 0 to 4 in every variable. The rates are plotted into a diagram to make a functional profile. The scale has been tested on 42 patients, 21 with coxarthrosis, 21 with gonarthrosis. The mean age was 70 (55-87) years. There was no major differences between diagnosis groups and sexes. Grouping of the variables have been made by factor analysis with varimax rotation. Two independent physiotherapists made the evaluations. Inter-observer reliability has been tested with different non-parametric correlation methods (Spearman rank correlation, Kendall's tau and Goodman-Kruskal's gamma).

Results: The scale is presented as an appendix. The ratings in the different variables for coxarthrosis and gonarthrosis respectively are presented in fig 1 and 2. Correlation coefficients illustrating the inter-observer reliability were very high, 0.92-1.00 for the different variables. Factor analysis with varimax rotation grouped the variables in five relatively distinct factors: hip variables, knee variables, functional variables, social variables and pain. There was a minimal overlap between the factors.

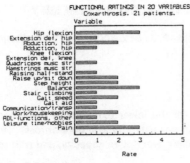

FUNCTIONAL RATINGS IN 20 VARIABLES
Coxarthrosis. 21 patients.

Fig 1   Median scores

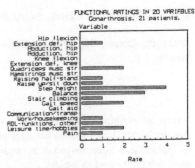

FUNCTIONAL RATINGS IN 20 VARIABLES
Gonarthrosis. 21 patients.

Fig 2 Median scores

Discussion: In the diagram are plotted: the needs of the patient and his actual ability. The deficit between need and actual ability is the same as the needs for improvement by operation and-or training. It easy to see from the diagram, what variables to train. The scale is made primarily to evaluate patients with coxarthrosis and gonarthrosis, but it can also be used for patients with other diagnoses. It can also be used by the physician. The reliability tests show a very high correspondence between two independent observers. Factor analysis is made for simplification and to examine the explanatory value of the variables. In this study it was possible to group the variables in five practical groups.

This paper is only a short preliminary presentation. I intend to make further publications concerning details of every variable in the scale, reliability testing and validity testing. The scale has also been tested on a healthy control group.

References: Can be given on request.

APPENDIX

CIVIL STATUS: M SEX: Female	
AGE: 72 HEIGHT: 1.64 WEIGHT: 80	M. S.
☒PREOP [ ]POSTOP	
☒TGRP [ ]CGRP MPAIR·	DATE: 91 03 25 SIGN: MS

FUNCTIONAL RATING SCALE FOR THE LOWER EXTREMITY		
DIAGNOSIS: COXARTHROS	☒R	[ ]L

VARIABLE	0	1	2	3	4
HIP FLEXION					
EXTENSION DEFICIT, HIP					
ABDUCTION, HIP					
ADDUCTION, HIP					
KNEE FLEXION					
EXTENSION DEFICIT, KNEE					
QUADRICEPS MUSCLE STRENGTH					
HAMSTRINGS MUSCLE STRENGTH					
RAISING UP FROM HALF-STANDING					
RAISING UP/SITTING DOWN					
STEP HEIGHT					
BALANCE STANDING ON ONE LEG)					
STAIR CLIMBING					
GAIT SPEED (M/S)					
GAIT AID					
COMMUNICATION/TRANSPORT					
WORK/HOUSE KEEPING					
ADL-FUNKTIONS, OTHER					
LEISURE TIME/HOBBIES					
PAIN					

825

GONIOMETRIC MEASUREMENTS OF HIP AND PROXIMAL INTERPHALANGEAL JOINTS FLEXION RANGES OF MOTION IN NORMAL SUBJECTS

Hano Okeke & Wen Ling
Physical Therapy Department, New York University,
New York, NY 10010. USA

INTRODUCTION

Joint limitation is often an indication of biomechanical disorder. Joint motion measurement is, therefore, used by physiotherapists and other clinicians as part of techniques of arriving at decisions on diagnosis, determination of baseline limitations before treatment is commenced, progress of treatment, level of disabilities in addition to provision of research data.

Many devices for and methods of measuring joint motions exist. This study utilized not only goniometric measurements but also specifically used universal goniometer mainly for its widely accepted validity and reliability.

Even with use of valid and reliable goniometric instruments, reliability studies in the past had resulted in varying levels of reliability coefficient[1]. Comparison of range of motion measurement reliability of polyaxial joint with that of a uniaxial joint was not available in the literature. The purpose of this study was to compare the reliability of active flexion measurements of the right hip joint with that of interphalangeal joint of the right middle finger on normal subjects. The authors hypothesized that due to a higher degree of freedom of movement, it was more difficult to reliably measure a polyaxial joint than a uniaxial joint.

Literature

Results of few studies had implied that uniaxial joint motion measurements were more reliable than those of polyaxial joints. Low[2] compared estimation with goniometric measurements and intratester with intertester reliability in elbow and wrist joints. He concluded in part, without explaining the methodology used or stating the problem, that reliability of measurement with a goniometer varied in different joints.

Gajdosik, et al[3] reviewing literature on validity and reliability concluded, again without reporting investigation on that line, that complex joint motion reliability was different from that of "simple hinge joints".

Methods

Twenty-one healthy subjects with the mean age of 28.1 and standard deviation of 3.4 years participated in the study. With proper control and stabilization, right hip joint flexion motion and proximal interphalangeal joint of the right middle finger flexion motion of the subjects were measured by one experienced physiotherapist in two different sessions. During each session, three measurements of each joint were taken. Common to procedures used in the measurement of the two joints include that determination of range of motions was active, motions were carried out against gravity, positioning and stabilization were rigidly standardized and that 0° - 180° system of notation was used. Pearson Product - Moment Correlation Coefficient was used to examine the data.

Results

In order to compare the test and the retest measurements of the right hip joint and the proximal interphalangeal joint of the right middle finger, Pearson Product -Moment Correlation for intratester reliability was employed. This yielded 0.93 for hip flexion and 0.99 for proximal interphalangeal joint flexion. Coefficient of variance for hip flexion was 11.8% and for PIP joint flexion 8.8%.

The researchers then used one-way analysis of variance (ANOVA) to determine whether there was a difference between the differences of measurements in each session of the two joints. There was a significant difference (P 0.005). Based on the findings, the researchers rejected the null hypothesis which stated that there was no difference between the goniometric range of motion measurement reliability in the hip joint flexion and that of PIP joint flexion motion.

Discussion

The study was designed to determine the comparative reliability of goniometric measurements of a complex joint with that of a simple joint.

High correlation coefficients were obtained in the two joint flexion motions. Although the design of the study was not intended primarily to test measurement precision, the high correlation values in the two joints had two implications: 1. The coefficient values formed part of the data on which comparisons were based 2. Measurement error was minimal indicating proper control of test environment and methodology.

The results of Boone, et al[4] goniometric reliability study on three joints of the upper extremity and three of lower extremity appeared to have contrasted with the result of this study. However, considering that they were more preoccupied with comparison between the upper and lower extremity joints rather than with the types and behaviours of individual joints making up the group, their methodology and control focused more on group comparison perhaps, at the expense of measurement of individual joints. Results of other previous studies notably by EKStrand, et al[5], Rothstein, et al[6] and Miller[1] supported the outcome of the present study.

The study has shown that, in addition to obvious structural and functional differences in joints, there could be other inherent confounding variables peculiar to each joint which make consistency of some joint measurements less consistent.

Conclusion

The result of this study indicated that as a simple uniaxial joint, the proximal interphalangeal joint could be more reliably measured than the more complex polyaxial hip joint in normal subjects using universal goniometer. These findings should interest clinicians who need to be aware of the idiocyncracies of joints when conducting range of motion measurements on their patients.

References

1. Miller PJ: Assessment of Joint. In Rothstein JM (Ed): Measurement in Physical Therapy. Churchill Livingstone, New York, 1985

2. Low JL: The Reliability of Joint Measurement. Physiotherapy 62: 227 - 229, 1976

3. Gajdosik RL, Bohannon RW: Clinical Measurement of Range of Motion: Review of Goniometry Emphasizing Reliability and Validity. Phys Ther 67: 1867-1872, 1987

4. Boone DC, Azen SP, Lin C-M, et al: Reliability of Goniometric measurements: Phys Ther 58: 1355-1360, 1978

5. EKStrand J, Wiktorsson M, Oberg B, et al: Lower Extremity Goniometric Measurements: A Study to Determine Their Reliability. Arch Phys Med Rehabil 63: 171-175, 1982

6. Rothstein JM, Miller PJ, Roettger RF: Elbow and knee Measurements. Phys Ther 63: 1611-1615, 1983

AN INNER RANGE HOLDING CONTRACTION: AN OBJECTIVE MEASURE OF STABILIZING
FUNCTION OF AN ANTIGRAVITY MUSCLE

C A Richardson, K Sims
Department of Physiotherapy, University of Queensland Q 4072 Australia

Gluteux Maximus (GM) forms part of the antigravity musculature
responsible for stability of the trunk and pelvic regions. Although some
functions of GM can be assessed through hip extensor torque production
against manual or mechanical resistance, its role in stabilisation is
considered to be reflected more in its ability to perform prolonged static
contractions. Stengel et al [1] suggest that the ability to generate a
tonic holding contraction as opposed to a phasic contraction is the
critical function for antigravity competency.

The testing of this function of muscle becomes even more important
when one considers evidence of the changes which can occur in skeletal
muscle as a result of disuse or lack of appropriate sensory input. The
tonically firing motor units change, over time, to display more phasic
erratic firing patterns. Evidence of this comes from animal studies
[2,3,4,5,6] and human research [7,8,9]. This research explains why weak muscles
are seen clinically to have a phasic quality and most significantly lack
the ability to control a tonic static contraction.

When developing a test for loss of function in an antigravity muscle
such as GM, the most important aspect of the assessment would be the
estimation of the length of time a static hold could be maintained and
controlled without jerky (phasic) movements occurring.

Sullivan et al [10] suggest that it is particularly important to
assess this stabilising, antigravity function when the muscle is in its
shortened (inner range) position. Positions used for classic muscle tests
for the large antigravity muscles such as GM confirm the significance of
such clinical observations [11].

For this study a test was designed to assess loss of stabilising
(tonic) function of GM. It measured the ability of GM to statically hold
the thigh in extension from the prone position (an eccentric contraction)
and estimate the length of time this muscle could hold and control the
thigh in this shortened position without jerky (phasic) movements
occurring.

In order to begin to evaluate the significance of such an
assessment, subjects with no pathology or pain but with consistent
observations of GM 'weakness' were selected for comparison with matched
normal subjects. Detailed observation of road cyclists, who train for long
hours on their bikes indicated that their GM muscles were usually
underactivated and weakened. Due to apparent functional deficits in their

GM, cyclists were chosen as the experimental group for this initial study.

METHOD

A group of 13 cyclists (who trained in excess of six hours per week and who had been riding for at least six months) and 16 normal subjects of similar age, weight and height and with no excessive muscle tightness were compared for their ability to maintain a static inner range GM contraction.

Subjects were positioned in prone (trunk support only) with arms at their side and the non test leg supported with slings attached to springs (Figure 1). Such a non-stable support was important to allow pelvic stabilisation through active trunk muscle contraction rather than allow the leg to be supported on a stool. Pilot trials established that a stable support of the non test leg allowed more substitute movements to occur and hence the test became less discriminatory.

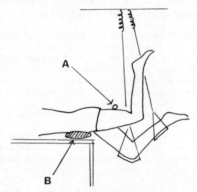

Figure 1 The test position
A - the horizontal bar placed on top of the thigh
B - the pressure biofeedback devices used to detect trunk movement

The test leg (knee at 90°) was taken passively into the horizontal position and the subject asked to hold the leg steady. The timing of the static hold continued until subjects lost contact with a horizontal bar which had been placed above the thigh (Figure 1). Timing also ceased if substitute trunk movements occurred. These were monitored through the use of two pressure biofeedback devices placed under the pelvis on each side.

RESULTS

The mean holding time was 37.06 seconds for normal subjects and 5.08 seconds for the road cyclists. The difference was significant at the .0001 level. For all cyclists it was a movement of the thigh away from the bar (often due to phasic muscle contraction) which terminated the test. In the normal subjects with longer holding times, 25% lost trunk stabilisation before thigh position.

DISCUSSION

The results of this study confirmed that the ability to control an inner range static contraction does provide a means of depicting a marked functional loss in GM. Clinical assessments using this type of testing procedure have proved useful for other antigravity musculature such as the deep neck flexors and lower scapular stabilisers. In all testing procedures the importance of eliminating trick or substitute movements is essential.

Although the functional changes of the neuromuscular system are extremely complex and not possible to determine at the cellular level, it is still important to develop clinical tests which best illustrate functional loss of particular aspects of muscle function which are essential for the assessment of rehabilitation procedures. Clinical evidence to date suggests that these testing procedures do give an indication of the success of rehabilitation techniques used to activate and develop the stabilising role of antigravity musculature.

REFERENCES

1. Stengel TJ, Attermeier SM, Bly L, Heriza CB (1984) Evaluation of sensorimotor dysfunction. In Clinics in physical therapy: Paediatric neurologic physical therapy. SK Campbell (Ed), Churchill Livingstone, London
2. Henneman E, Olson CB (1965) Relations between structure and function in the design of skeletal muscles. Journal of Physiology 29:581-598
3. Fischback GD, Robbins W (1969) Change in contractile properties of disused soleus muscles. Journal of Physiology 20:305-320
4. Ianuzzo CD (1976) The cellular composition of human skeletal muscle. In Neuromuscular mechanisms for therapeutic and conditioning exercise. Knuttgren HG (Ed), University Park Press, Baltimore
5. Templeton GH, Sweeney HL, Himson BF, Badalino M, Dudenhoeffer GA (1988) Changes in fibre composition of soleus muscle during rat hind limb suspension. Journal of Applied Physiology 65(3):1191-1195
6. Leiber RL, Johansson CB, Vahlsing HL, Hargens AR, Feringa ER (1986) Long term effects of spinal cord transection on fast and slow rat skeletal muscle. Experimental Neurology 91:423-434
7. Grimby L, Hannerz J (1976) Disturbances in voluntary recruitment order of low and high frequency motor units on blockade of proprioceptive afferent activity. Acta Physiologica Scandinavia 96:207-216
8. Oganov V, Skuratova S, Potapov N, Shirvindkaye M (1980) Physiological mechanisms of adaptation of skeletal muscles of mammals to the weightless state. In Advances in physiological science. F Cuba, G Maredal, O Takacs (Eds). Pergamon Press, Hungary
9. Richardson CA (1987) Atrophy of vastus medialis in patello-femoral pain syndrome. Proceedings of the 10th International Congress of the World Confederation for Physical Therapy, Sydney p400-403
10. Sullivan PE, Markos PD, Minor MA (1982) An integrated approach to therapeutic exercise. Reston Publishing Co, Reston, Virginia
11. Daniels L, Worthingham C (1980) Muscle testing: techniques of manual examination 4th edn WB Saunders, Philadelphia

MEASURING MOVEMENT CONTROL WITH TRACKING SCORES

James R. Carey, Ph.D., P.T.
Program in Physical Therapy, Mayo School of Health-Related Sciences
1104 Siebens Building, Rochester, MN 55905, USA

Introduction

Measurement of active range of motion at a joint is important in evaluating patient function. However, this parameter gives no indication of the patient's ability to produce well-controlled bodily movements toward a target. Such aiming control is a vital motor skill in daily function; yet, it has been underemphasized in the evaluation of patients with neurological and orthopedic conditions. This report describes a system that quantifies control of index finger movements.

Instrumentation

A computer screen displays a stationary sine wave that serves as a target for the subject to track with the computer screen cursor. The controlling device for the cursor is an electrogoniometer attached to the index finger metacarpophalangeal (MP) joint. The voltage signal from the electrogoniometer is directed to the computer through an analog-to-digital converter, which samples the signal at 100 samples/second.

At the start of the test, the cursor moves from left to right across the screen and during this time the subject attempts to track the sine wave target by careful movement of the MP joint; finger extension moves the cursor upward and finger flexion moves the cursor downward. For the figures that follow, full active flexion is defined at 0° and the range of full active extension is indicated. The target track begins at the midpoint of the subject's predetermined flexion-extension range. The extension (upper) and flexion (lower) peaks of the target track are set at 85% and 15% of this range, respectively.

Measurements

The computer is programmed to calculate three scores from the tracking performance that are important in analyzing control of the finger movement. First, the computer calculates the root-mean-square (RMS) error[1] between the response line and the sine wave target. To allow comparison between individuals, this overall error score is converted to an accuracy index (AI) that is normalized to the vertical scale of each individual's target track.[2] The maximum possible AI score is 100%.

For further description of the tracking response, the computer also calculates the constant error (CE) and variable error (VE), which are two separate components that comprise the overall error within a tracking response.[3] Briefly, CE is the average error in a response and indicates whether the subject is generally undershooting or overshooting the target. Conversely, VE measures the variability of the subject's response around the mean response. Since CE and VE are related to the overall RMS error (E) according to the following equation: $CE^2 + VE^2 = E^2$, the relative proportions of CE and VE contributing to the total tracking error can be calculated. Knowledge of these proportions may be valuable in understanding the impaired tracking responses of patients with different disorders.

Figure 1 shows the tracking response of a healthy subject whose full MP range of motion was 109°. The above scores were calculated separately for the extension phases (upper half) and the flexion phases (lower half) of the sine wave. For the extension phases the AI score is 73.48% The fraction of the tracking error that is formed by CE is 0.14, while the fraction formed by VE is 0.86. The tracking response for the flexion phases has an AI of 77.72%. The fraction that CE contributes to the tracking error is 0.13, while the fraction formed by VE is 0.87.

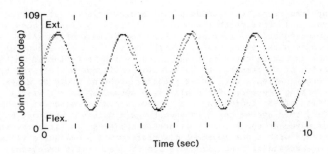

Fig. 1.   Tracking response of a healthy subject.

By contrast, Figure 2 shows the impaired tracking response of an individual with spastic hemiparesis. Even though the tracking target is well within the subject's range, the response shows difficulty in reaching the extension peaks in the time required, which is consistent with the hypertonicity observed in her finger flexor muscles. The AI score for the extension phases is only 16.63%. Compared to the healthy subject's response, tracking error in the hemiplegic subject is dominated more heavily by CE with a fraction of 0.40, while the VE fraction is 0.60. The AI for the flexion phases is closer to normal at 59.0%. The CE fraction of the tracking error during the flexion phases is closer to normal at 0.09, while the VE fraction is 0.91.

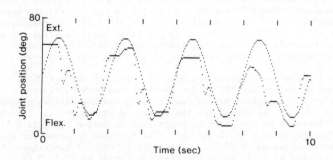

Fig. 2. Tracking response of a spastic hemiparetic subject

Discussion

The impaired tracking response of the hemiparetic subject during the extension phases is considerably subnormal and this finding is consistent with the common functional problem in these individuals of impaired release of objects following grasp. Furthermore, the great amount of undershoot error during the extension phases, which is reflected in the higher fraction of CE compared to normal, is consistent with flexor hypertonicity. Other patients with motor planning problems would be expected to show a tracking response with a similarly subnormal AI but with a higher fraction of VE, indicating a much more variable response.

Thus far, this system has been used to gain valuable information about finger movement control in hemiparetic subjects.[2,4] Tracking studies on patients with other movement disorders could prove quite valuable in further understanding such disorders and in quantifying treatment effects.

References

1. Poulton EC (1974) Tracking skill and manual control. New York: Academic Press

2. Carey JR (1990) Manual stretch: Effect on finger movement control and force control in stroke subjects with spastic extrinsic finger flexor muscles. Archives of Physical Medicine and Rehabilitation 71:888-894

3. Schmidt RA (1982) Motor control and learning: A behavioral emphasis. Champaign, IL: Human Kinetics Publishers

4. Halaney ME, Carey JR (1989) Tracking ability of hemiparetic and healthy subjects. Physical Therapy 69:342-348

THE EFFECT OF LEG LENGTH DISCREPANCY AND LEG DOMINANCE ON THE MUSCULAR
FUNCTION OF THE LEGS

AKK Chow-Gardner, PC Leung
Physiotherapy Section, Department of Rehabilitation Sciences
Hong Kong Polytechnic, Hung Hom, Kowloon, Hong Kong.

The majority of individuals have minor leg length discrepancies (LLD) at maturity. LLD alter the base of support and disturb the biomechanical balance, produce abnormal stress on related joints and soft structures, predisposing the individual to a variety of symptoms: backache[1], unilateral degenerative changes of the hip joint[2,3,4] disordered gait and running injuries[5] Studies investigating the effect of LLD reported the greatest amount of electro-myographic activities on the long legs with LLD 0.5cm[6], a lateral shift of weight bearing centre to the short leg side in individuals with LLD < 0.6cm, and a shift to the long leg side with LLD > 0.6cm[7] and the shorter leg (LLD > 0.5cm) was consistently the weaker in total leg strength (TLS)[8].

Specific investigation in the effects of cerebral dominance of the legs on the strength of the legs cannot be found. Conflicting views were presented as by-products of the main studies during investigations of muscular capacity of the lower extremity. Smith et al[9] evaluating the lower extremity torque output of professional and Olympic ice hockey players, reported no significant difference between the right and left leg. Wyatt et al [10] while comparing knee torque values of normal males and females reported a significant difference between the dominant and non-dominant legs in male subjects. Goslin & Charteris[11] presenting the normative isokinetic data of young adults concluded that there was no difference between the right and left legs but the dominant legs were stronger. The definition of leg dominance was also inconsistent. Goslin defined the dominant leg as the stronger leg, while Wyatt's definition is the kicking leg.

The purpose of this study was to determine whether any differences in muscle function exist in the legs of young adults with respect to LLD and leg dominance.

Subjects

51 physiotherapy students (25 females, 26 males) participated in this study. Interviews and postural examinations determined their suitability. Criteria for selection required that subjects have normal health without history of back pain, hip, knee or ankle pain in the past two years. Individuals with primary scoliosis were excluded.

Procedure

1.   LLD: LLD were determined by a modified indirect method[12]. Subjects stood on a specially designed platform, the movable portion was raised or lowered until the spirit level pressed against the iliac crests indicated a levelled pelvis. LLD were measured with a mechanical depth gauge.

2.   Leg dominance: Dominant legs were defined as the ones which perform fine coordinated movements. Subjects kicked a shuttle cock ten times. The kicking legs were recorded as dominant and the supporting legs as non-dominant.

3.   Muscle function: Cybex II, with a dual channel recorder and Data Reduction Computer was used for measuring muscle function. After a five minutes standardized warm up period, subjects were tested in pairs for hip abduction/adduction, hip flexion/extension, knee flexion/extension, ankle plantarflexion/dorsiflexion at 180° per second according to the recommended test protocols. The dominant leg was tested first. There were five minutes rest periods while the apparatus was positioned for the contralateral leg and ten minutes rest periods while the other subject was tested. The same procedure was repeated for each joint motion.

Data Analysis

TLS was computed by summation of average power of all joint motions recorded. TLS body weight ratio was used for inter-individual comparison. Right and left leg data was analyzed first, then the data were grouped into long/short; dominant/non-dominant; long and dominant (LD)/short and non-dominant(SN); short and dominant (SD)/long and non-dominant (LN); and male/female groups. Two-tailed paired t-test tested the difference in means of the grouped data with respect to the TLS and individual joint motion. Significance was accepted at the $p < 0.05$ level.

Results

The mean LLD obtained was 0.58 ± 0.30cm (range 0.20-1.50). There were 21 (41%) subjects with right long legs; 46 (90%) with right dominant legs; 24 (47%) with ipsilateral LD legs, 27 (53%) ipsilateral LN legs, 11 (44%) male subjects with ipsilateral LD legs; 13 (50%) female subjects with ipsilateral LD legs; and 15 (48%) with LL > 0.5cm.

Table 1 presents the means of TLS % body weight for all subjects, male and female subjects. Although the means of TLS % body weight suggested differences in the mean strength of the legs, paired t-test analysis indicated no significant difference except in the male subjects with ipsilateral LLD legs (n=25, TLS % body weight, p=0.028).

Table 1. Means of TLS % Body Weight

Legs	TLS % Body Weight (All) (Mean $\pm$ SD) n=51	TLS % Body Weight (Male) (Mean $\pm$ SD) n=25	TLS % Body Weight (Female) (Mean $\pm$ SD) n=26
Right Left	1224.78 $\pm$ 310.87 1207.38 $\pm$ 312.11		
Long Short	1214.68 $\pm$ 308.45 1217.48 $\pm$ 314.75	1434.46 $\pm$ 256.97 1420.59 $\pm$ 272.77	1003.36 $\pm$ 179.29 1022.18 $\pm$ 213.97
Dom Non Dom	1259.42 $\pm$ 313.34 1202.74 $\pm$ 309.30	1446.52 $\pm$ 253.04 1408.53 $\pm$ 275.24	1020.67 $\pm$ 206.01 1004.87 $\pm$ 188.53
Long & Dom Short & NonDom	1182.00 $\pm$ 286.12 1156.63 $\pm$ 284.47	1400.65 $\pm$ 224.61* 1341.73 $\pm$ 259.34*	996.99 $\pm$ 184.27 1000.01 $\pm$ 202.66
Long & NonDom Short & Dom	1243.73 $\pm$ 329.68 1271.57 $\pm$ 335.67	1461.02 $\pm$ 285.27 1482.55 $\pm$ 276.09	1009.72 $\pm$ 181.44 1044.35 $\pm$ 230.75

* paired t-test $p = 0.028$

DISCUSSION

The difference in means of TLS suggests that short legs were marginally stronger than the long legs (3% body weight), however, statistical analysis proves otherwise. This study did not support Bolz's finding that the short legs were the weaker legs. Bolz did not report any statistical analysis and his conclusion was based on eight subjects. In general, the male subjects appeared to have more strength in their lower extremity than the female subjects. This study suggests that TLS is not a good indicator of muscle function in the lower extremity. Initial analysis of the individual joint motion suggests differences may exist in strength, endurance and power of specific muscle groups. Detailed analysis is beyond the scope of this paper.

In general, most people believe that the dominant upper extremity is stronger and the same must be true of the lower extremity. If one defines the dominant extremity, according to neurology studies, as the one more equipped to perform fine coordinated movements which may not require strength or power, one may not be born with a stronger dominant extremity. The strength may have been acquired later in life with practice and endless use of the dominant extremity. The primary function of the lower extremity is to support the body for locomotion, thus the alternate cycles of stance and swing during gait ensures equal opportunities for both lower extremities to develop strength. Any difference in strength may be due to specific training or constant unilateral use of one lower extremity. In the male subjects, a significant difference is found in TLS % body weight between the LD and SN legs. It is possible that the finding reflects the extracurricular activities the male subjects participate in, such as soccer, which would require more use of the dominant leg during the kicking of a ball. The female group shows a slightly different pattern. The mean strength of the LD legs are slightly weaker than the SN legs but the difference is insignificant.

Further analysis with independent t-test confirmed no difference between the leg which is dominant and the leg which is non-dominant. The same is true of the short legs. Amongst the dominant and non-dominant legs, length also has no effect on the strength.

CONCLUSION

This study concludes that LLD or dominance have no effect on the muscle functions of the leg and that dominance and length has no effect on each other in the lower extremity, and that dominance does not have a significant effect on TLS of non athletic, healthy individuals. TLS is not a good indicator of muscle balance, as specific weakness in muscle groups could be camouflaged when one summates the average power of the whole leg. Clinicians should evaluate each muscle group to fully understand the complex function of the legs. Differences in muscle function may be more related to activities than length or dominance.

REFERENCES

1. Giles LGF, Taylor JR (1981) Low back pain associated with leg length inequality. Spine 6:5:508-521
2. Gofton JP, Trueman GE (1967) Unilateral idiopathic osteoarthritis of the hip. Canadian Medical Association Journal 97:1129-1132
3. Gofton JP, Trueman GE (1971) Studies in osteoarthritis of the hip. Part II. Osteoarthritis of the hip and leg length disparity. Canadian Medical Association Journal 104:791-799
4. Gofton JP, Trueman GE (1971) Studies in osteoarthritis of the hip. Part IV. Biomechanics and clinical considerations. Canadian Medical Association Journal 104:1007-1011
5. Subotnick SI (1981) Limb length discrepancies of the lower extremity (The short leg syndrome). JOSPT 3:11-16
6. Strong R, Thomas BE, Earl WD (1967) Patterns of muscle activity in leg, hip and torso during quiet standing. Journal of American Osteopathic Association 66:1035-1038
7. Lawrence W (1984) Lateralization of weight in the presence of structural short leg: A preliminary report. Journal of Manipulative Physiotherapy 7:2:105-108
8. Bolz S, Davies GJ (1984) Leg length differences and correlation with total leg strength. JOSPT 6:2:123-129
9. Smith DJ, Quinney HA, Wenger HA, Steadward RD, Sexsmith JR (1981) Isokinetic Torque outputs of professional and elite amateur ice hockey players. JOSPT 3:2:42-47
10. Wyatt MP, Edwards A (1981) Comparison of quadriceps and hamstrings torque values during isokinetic exercise. JOSPT 3:2:48-56
11. Goslin BR, Charteris J (1979) Isokinetic dynamometry normative data for clinical use in lower extremity (knee) cases. Scandinavia Journal of Rehabilitative Medicine 11:105-109
12. Gardner A, Tam E, Evans JH, Leung PC (1990) The validity of three different methods for measuring leg length discrepancy. Proceedings of 3rd International Physiotherapy Congress Hong Kong 262-267 (paper presentation)

POSTER PRESENTATIONS

A COMPARISON OF PRE AND POST CALCULATION SMOOTHING METHODS.

Derek Littler and Andrew Harrison.
Salford College of Technology.

ABSTRACT

A comparison was made between two methods of applying a Butterworth low pass filter to data derived from both 16mm film and video sources. The raw data of Pezzack and Winter [1] was firstly smoothed and then differentiated twice using finite differences to produce acceleration data (ie. pre-smoothing). This produced identical results to Pezzack's original experiment. The same data was then differentiated twice and the noisy acceleration data was smoothed using the same frequency cut-off as before (ie. 6Hz). Comparisons were made between unsmoothed acceleration data and pre-smoothed data, unsmoothed and post-smoothed data and pre-smoothed and post-smoothed data by calculating the RMS difference between each data set. The results indicated that there is good comparison between the pre-smoothed and post smoothed data sets RMS difference = 6.00). The RMS difference values for pre-smoothed vs. unsmoothed and post-smoothed vs. unsmoothed obviously generated higher but similar values of 16.14 and 15.23 respectively.

Further comparisons were made between both methods using data derived from video sources which might be regarded as "less ideal" than Pezzack's original data. Visual inspection reveals that the post-smoothing method produces a more marked smoothing effect which is arguably closer to reality. The post calculation smoothing method should therefore be given serious consideration since it produces similar if not better results than the conventional pre-smoothing method. It also has the advantages of allowing the user to specify different cut-off frequencies for different body segments in the same movement sequence and it requires less computing time.

INTRODUCTION.

The issues of data smoothing and estimation of derivatives have been, and are still subjects of much discussion in biomechanical analysis. The process of calculating derivatives of raw displacement data from film or video sources tends to amplify the effects of small errors in the raw data (ie. "noise") and can distort the true nature of the velocity/time and acceleration/time curves. Over the years a number of techniques have been used to obtain more accurate estimates of the derivatives. These techniques include ;

- ❏ The use of least squares polynomial approximations which can provide a degree of smoothing in themselves, and can be differentiated directly. Miller & Nelson [2].
- ❏ The use of cubic or quintic spline functions. These consist of a number of low order polynomials which are linked together at points in time called "knots". Woltring [3].
- ❏ The use of Fourier Transforms which express a function as a weighted sum of sine and cosine terms of increasing frequency. Wood [4].
- ❏ The use of moving averages (ie. Hanning or 3 point moving average) and digital filters. Winter [5].

Literature can be found which supports the application of all of the above techniques. (see Wood G.A. 1982 for a full review.) One of the most popular techniques has been the application of the 4th order zero phase shift filter on raw displacement data followed by finite differences as recommended by Pezzack [1] and

Winter [5]. This filter has the advantage of allowing the user to selectively remove frequencies in excess of a specified value. Given that most gross human movement does not contain frequencies greater than 5 or 6 Hz, it is not surprising that this filter is well suited to biomechanics applications. Pezzack [1] showed that prior smoothing of angular displacement data using a Butterworth filter followed by finite differences provided more realistic results for angular acceleration than either Chebyshev Polynomials or finite differences on raw data. Whilst the results produced by this method are generally good, in practical terms the method is not particularly efficient. If a number of limb segments are involved in an analysis, ALL of the raw data will be smoothed before any calculation of derivatives is carried out. In computing terms this is relatively time consuming and extravagant on the use of memory, but more importantly, prior smoothing commits the user to a single cut-off frequency for all body segments. The Butterworth filter also presents a certain amount of undesirable end point distortion which demands that the user should collect raw data for several additional frames at the start and end of a movement sequence of interest. Finally, whilst the application of a digital filter will sharply attenuate high frequencies in the displacement data, it will not remove them completely.

A more efficient method would be to apply the smoothing algorithm AFTER the calculation of derivatives. (ie, Post smoothing). The same cut-off frequency can be used for post smoothing as would normally be used in smoothing raw data since differentiation with respect to time has no significant effect on the frequency of the derivatives. This can be proved by considering the effects of successive differentiation on the periodic function SIN O . The first derivative of SIN O = COS O, and the second derivative is -SIN O , both of which have the same frequency as the original function.

COMPARISON ON PRE AND POST SMOOTHING

Comparisons were made between the following data taken from Pezzack [1] :
- ☐ Unsmoothed acceleration data and pre-smoothed data.
- ☐ Unsmoothed and post-smoothed data.
- ☐ Pre-smoothed and post-smoothed data.

This was done by calculating the RMS difference between each data set. The results indicated that there is good comparison between the pre-smoothed and post smoothed data sets RMS difference = 6.00). The RMS difference values for pre-smoothed vs. unsmoothed and post-smoothed vs. unsmoothed obviously generated higher but similar values of 16.14 and 15.23 respectively. Clearly then, there is little difference between pre and post smoothing techniques in this case, but this will not always be the case, particularly if the raw displacement data contains more noise than Pezzack's original data.

Figures 1 and 2 show a comparison of pre and post smoothing techniques applied in the analysis of a backflip using The Biomechanics Workstation video analysis system. Littler & Harrison [6]. In this case the post-smoothed acceleration graph is clearly smoother than the pre-smoothed graph. The pre-smoothed graph still contains some high frequency elements which may be assumed to be unattenuated noise in the raw data. The post-smoothed graph does not contain these higher frequency elements and it may be argued that the post smoothing procedure

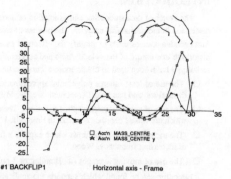

Figure 1. Effects of Pre-smoothing on acceleration data of a backflip.

842

performs better.

CONCLUSIONS.

Clearly further work is required to verify the findings of this research, however the indications are that the process of post-smoothing produces similar if not better results than the more commonly used pre-smoothing procedure. Given the advantages of greater efficiency, and the ability to select different cut-off frequencies for different body segments in the same movement sequence, the post-smoothing method is well worth consideration.

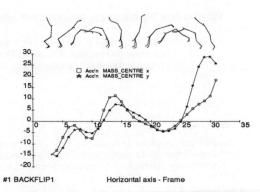

#1 BACKFLIP1   Horizontal axis - Frame

Figure 2. Effects of Post Smoothing on acceleration data of a backflip.

REFERENCES.

1. Pezzack, J.C. (1977) An Assessment of Derivative Determining Techniques used for Motion Analysis. Journal of Biomechanics Vol. 10 pp 377-382.

2. Miller, D.I. Nelson, R.C. (1977) Biomechanics of Sport. Lea & Febiger.

3. Woltring, H.J. (1985) On Optimal Smoothing and Derivative Estimation from Noisy Displacement Data in Biomechanics. Human Movement Science Vol 4. pp229-245.

4. Wood, G.A. (1982) Data Smoothing and Differentiation Procedures in Biomechanics. Exercise and Sports Science Reviews (USA) Vol. 10 pp308-362.

5. Winter, D.A. (1982) Biomechanics of Human Movement. John Wiley & sons

6. Littler, D.A. & Harrison, A.J. (1990) A Description of the Biomechanics Workstation. B.A.S.S. Annual Conference Cardiff (1990).

SEATING FOR THE DISABLED, WITH SPECIFIC REFERENCE TO THE ACTIVITY OF RISING

Kerr, K.M.*, Barr, D.A.**, Baird, H.E.*, Mollan, R.A.B.**, White, J.A.*
*Department of Occupational Therapy & Physiotherapy, University of Ulster
**Department of Orthopaedic Surgery, Queen's University of Belfast

Introduction

The activity of rising from the seated position is a fundamental characteristic of everyday living in normal individuals. However, for many disabled individuals, this activity presents considerable difficulty, to the extent that many potentially ambulant patients remain prisoners in their chairs (1,2). Research into the activity of rising has been limited in extent, both with regard to normal and disabled individuals.

Many of the biomechanical studies, while producing definitive numerical data on moments of force generated at the joints and muscles of the lower extremity during rising (3,4,5,6) have demonstrated substantial complexity in study design, involving highly technical equipment and considerable manipulation of subjects, which may preclude the application of such procedures to large samples of disabled subjects. Electromyographic studies (7,8), while providing useful information on phasic muscle activity during the activity of rising, appear to have little to offer in evaluating the relative ease or difficulty in performing the activity. Similarly, while results from kinematic studies have suggested minimal hip and knee range of motion compatible with independent in rising from standard chairs (9,10,2) there is little evidence of identification of specific problems experienced by patients with definitive joint limitations in hip and knee. Furthermore, there is even less evidence of investigations into the stand-to-sit phase of the total activity.

This study aimed to develop a method of obtaining objective and quantitative data from the analysis of the sit-stand-sit movement, which might also provide an indication of the relative ease or difficulty experienced, and which can be applied to large and discrete samples of the specifically disabled population.

Method

Three measurement systems were used to obtain information on the sit-stand-sit activity, namely vector stereography, accelerometry, and electrogoniometry. The vector stereograph (VS) (11), is a non-optic device capable of providing information on the amount and pattern of displacement of a wand, in all three planes. The accelerometry method involves three accelerometers, orientated in the sagittal, vertical and coronal planes, to provide information on the pattern of change in acceleration in the three dimensions; initial trials indicated that both of these sytems demonstrated consistency in the patterns of displacement and acceleration and that there was a relationship between the changes within the pattern and the phases of the movement. The electrogoniometer, positioned at the knee, provides a useful means of indicating the time at which contact with the seat is lost, and also the time at which lower limb contribution to the rising phase is complete.

From the initial trials, it was concluded that although each system could provide useful information, each on its own was of limited value. Consequently, a seven channel amplifier was constructed to enable simultaneous recording of acceleration and displacement in three planes, and angular displacement at the knee.

Procedure

Ten normal, healthy female subjects, aged between 20.1 and 35.1 years (mean 25.02 ± 4.4) heights between 154.0 and 167.5 cm (mean 161.23 ± 3.7) with no known neurological or musculoskeletal disorders, participated in the study.

Each subject sat on a wooden box, topped with styrofoam blocks, which were used to adjust the seat height, to standardise knee angle to between 95 - 100 (10) and the angle between the shank and the vertical to 18 (6). Heels were positioned 10cm apart (6), and the arms were folded across the chest (6,5)

A poly-propylene back slab, with an attachment for placement of the VS wand, and a housing unit to enable the accelerometers to be placed in mutually perpendicular planes, was strapped to each subject. The point of the VS wand, and the accelerometer unit was positioned at the level of C7. The electrogoniometer was positioned on the lateral aspect of the knee, with the alignment units placed along the axes of the femur and shank.

Subjects practiced standing up and sitting down between six and ten times to familiarise themselves with the equipment, after which knee and shank angles were rechecked. Each experimental trial consisted of two sit-stand-sit cycles, and a total of three trials were performed by each subject. Verbal instructions to 'stand' and 'sit' were given at six second intervals, at which time the subject performed the movement at their own pace. The intervening standing and sitting positions were maintained for approximately four seconds, the total trial time being 25 seconds.

Results and Discussion

Results of the study were obtained in both graphical and numerical form, for all seven parameters measured. Graphical representation of a single trial indicated a definitive pattern of activity in all seven parameters, which showed consistency both within and among subjects. The sequential relationship among the parameters also demonstrated consistency within and among subjects.

Numerical data in terms of linear displacement in three dimensions, angular displacement at the knee, and the time scale of the activity was obtained for analysis. For the purposes of this paper, time scales for forward lean in rising, total time to stand, forward lean in descending and total sitting time were analysed. In addition, the ratios of overshoot (forward displacement beyond the final resting position) to forward trunk lean in standing, and overshoot to backward trunk recovery in sitting were calculated. The results of these analyses can be seen in Tables I and II.

Table I

| | Rising | | | | Descending | | |
| Lean time (s) | | Total time (s) | | Lean time (s) | | Total time (s) | |
mean	S.D.	mean	S.D.	mean	S.D.	mean	S.D.
0.59	0.13	1.96	0.27	0.99	0.10	1.75	0.13
0.53	0.03	1.61	0.32	1.07	0.19	1.72	0.17
0.58	0.05	1.86	0.14	1.14	0.10	1.87	0.14
0.47	0.41	2.04	0.34	1.26	0.87	1.84	0.85
0.57	0.02	1.70	0.42	0.80	0.11	1.41	0.12
0.46	0.03	1.93	0.79	0.78	0.04	1.46	0.12
0.48	0.01	1.73	0.15	0.76	0.03	1.39	0.07
0.58	0.06	1.47	0.08	0.77	0.04	1.52	0.06
0.48	0.07	1.52	0.14	0.78	0.10	1.32	0.13
0.51	0.03	1.57	0.60	0.75	0.02	1.28	0.03
Total 0.52	0.05	1.74	0.19	0.91	0.18	1.56	0.21

Results in Table I demonstrate a mean forward trunk lean time (rising) of 0.53 ± 0.05 s, total standing time of 1.74 ± 0.19 s, forward lean time (descending) 0.91 ± 0.18 s, and total descending time 1.56 ± 0.21 s. The total time to stand is in agreement with previous studies (3,10); the other times cannot be compared as no information on these has been found in the literature. The large standard deviation noted with some subjects is probably related to experimental design, as some subjects were noted to prepare in advance of the 'stand' and 'sit' commands.

Table II demonstrates the ratios of the overshoot phases to total sagittal displacement in both the rising and descending phases of the sit-stand-sit cycle. One subject demonstrated a negative value in the descending phase, which may be due to experimental error. When this subject's scores are eliminated, the mean ratios become 0.28 ± 0.04 (rising) and 0.21 ± 0.07 (descending), indicating relative consistency.

Table II		
	Rising	Descending
	0.35	0.28
	0.25	0.25
	0.32	0.29
	0.10	-0.07
	0.23	0.11
	0.25	0.24
	0.34	0.25
	0.27	0.16
	0.24	0.13
	0.23	0.14
mean	0.26	0.18
S.D.	0.07	0.10

Conclusions

The results from this study indicate that the development of a measuring system, which integrates displacement and acceleration in three dimensions, and angular displacement of the knee, can yield much useful information regarding the analysis of the sit-stand-sit activity.

The limitations of this paper preclude more extensive and detailed analysis, which will be reported elsewhere.

Recommendations include further refinements of the experimental design, and the application of the system to larger groups of both normal male and female subjects (young and elderly) to define normative data, and eventually to specific groups of the disabled population.

References

1. Kerr, K M; White J A; Mollan, R A B; Baird, H E (1991), Rising from a chair: A review of the literature., Physiotherapy 77:1: 15-19.
2. Fleckenstein S J; Kirby R L; MacLeod D A (1988), Effect of limited knee flexion range on peak hip movements of force while transferring from sitting to standing, Journal of Biomechanics 21, 11: 915-918.
3. Yoshida, K; Iwakura, H; Inoue, F (1983), Motion analysis in the movements of standing up from and sitting down on a chair, Scandanavian Journal of Rehabilitation Medicine 15;133-140.
4. Ellis, M I; Seedhom B. B. , Wright, V (1984), Forces in the knee joint whilst rising from a seated position, Journal of Biomedical engineering 6 (April) 113-120.
5. Kralj, A; Jaeger, R. J; Minih, M (1990), Analysis of standing up and sitting down in humans; definitions and normative data presentation, Journal of Biomechanics, 23; 11: 1123-1138.
6. Riley, P. O; Scheukman, M. L; Mann, R. W; Hodge, W. A (1991), Mechanics of a constrained chair rise, Journal of Biomechanics. 24:1 77-85.
7. Kelley, D; Dainis, A; Wood, G. K (1976), Mechanics and muscular dynamics of rising from a seated position, Biomechanics V (B) (ed Komo P) 127-134.
8. Munton, J S; Ellis, M. I; Wright, V (1984), Use of electromyography to study leg muscle activity in patients with arthritis and in normal subjects during rising from a chair, Annals of the Rheumatic diseases, 43; 63-65.
9. Laubenthal, K. N. ; Smidt, G. L; Kettlekamp, D. B (1972), A quantitative analysis of knee motion during activities of daily living, Physical Therapy 52:1 34-43
10. Nuzik,S; Lamb, R; Van Sant, A; Hirt, S (1986), Sit to stand movement pattern., Physical Therapy 66:11: 1708- 1713.
11. Morris, J. R. W; Harris, J R (1976), Three dimensional shapes., The Lancet 1189-1190.

COMPUTER ASSISTED EVOKED POTENTIAL ANALYZING SYSTEM FOR
FUNCTIONAL EVALUATION IN PHYSCAL THERAPY

M Aoki*, T Fujiwara, N Nishimura, S Takahashi, M Matsumoto, J Suzuki,
M Hanaoka** Dept. of Rehab., Shinshu Univ. Hospital*
Kissei Comtec Co. Ltd.** Matsumoto, 390 JAPAN

Introduction
    Recently, electrophysiological examination has become available for
Physical Therapy evaluation : For instance, there is now a measuring method of
nerve conduction velocity(NCV), Hoffmann wave(H-wave), and somato-sensory
evoked potential(SEP). Fujiwara[1] said that the feasibility of using H-wave
observation includes a suitable indication of muscle tone and spinal moto-
neuron excitability. However, its disadvantage was a difficulty in clinical
application due to its complexity in operation and high cost. Therefore, the
purpose of this report is to demonstrate that we have promising evaluation
tools in PT developed by an evoked potential(EP) analyzing system which are
simple operate with less cost.

Subjects & Method
(Subject)
    A total of 10 healthy adults (age: 19-37, a mean of 25) were subjected in
this investigation.
(Method)
    The instrumentation used was : photic stimulator, EMG amplifier, strain
guage, strain amp., nerve stimulator, isolator, P300 stimulator, EEG amp.,
counter, data recorder and a newly developed computer assisted evoked
potential analyzing system, EP-WORKS, for analyzing various evoked potentials.
    The researach items were as follows;
1. Photo-stimulated motor reaction time (M-RT).
    The paradigm which made the subject push a button with a motion as fast
as possible when photo-stimulate signal recognized. This was recorded by
potential from finger flexor muscles and strain guage output triggering with
photo-stimulation. EMG-RT and M-RT were averaged 10 times of 20 trials.
2. H-wave.
    Following the method by Hugon[2] and Fujiwara[3], the electric stimulations
to the tibial nerve were applied on the middle popliteal area. EP taken from
the electrodes were placed on the surface of the soleus muscle. Stable H-wave
were obtaind by an average of 32 times.
3. Event related potential (ERP, P300)
    Auditory oddball paradigm which made the subject count and discriminate
were generated by stimulator as non-target(1kHz:frequent) and target(2kHz:rare)
stimuli. Probability of target sound were maintained approximately 10 %. P300
(positive EP with latency range between 250-500msec) were obtaind by EP taken
from different electrode(Cz) which averaged 32 times.

Results

The results were as follows ;
1. The range of EMG-RT was shown from 93.0 to 147.0 msec.
   The mean EMG-RT of total subjects was shown 111.2 msec.
   The range of M-RT was shown from 137.0 to 214.5 msec.
   The mean M-RT of total subjects was shown 165.9 msec. (see Fig.1)
2. At the contralateral stimulation as conditioning and STNR increased H-wave
   amplitude compare the control prone. (see Fig.2)
   The mean latency of H-wave of total subjects was shown 29.5± msec.
3. The mean peak latency of P300 of total subjects was shown 330.6 msec.
   (see Fig.3)

Discussion

1. The M-RT represents the latency from photo-stimulation to the initiation of
   actual movement. It is necessary for M-RT to be as short as possible in order
   to do smooth voluntary movements. A shortest EMG-RT was recorded in this
   measurement(78.0 msec). Relatively study[4] investigating EMG-RT in human
   subject which limitation of physiological RT was below 105 msec. The data was
   omitted in this study. M-RT can be use as an examination that reflects
   sensory-motor integration and coordination of movement. Therefore, M-RT study
   was usefull to lead an individual follow up.
2. Even if the condition is constantly stimulated, the H-wave amplitude will
   fluctuate. When the obtained waveforms are stable, it is still necessary to
   take the average of the evoked potential. The EP-WORKS was aqcuired easily.
   It was used to record and analyze the latency and maximum and minimum
   amplitude of H-wave. Fujiwara[1] reported that threshold variation of H-waves
   compared with normal and hemiplegic subjects added various loads to their
   neck and extremities. He referred to postual reflex, muscle tone, and spinal
   moto-neuron excitability. Therefore, it is helpful in the clinical
   application of physical therapy.
3. In various environmental tasks, P300 related to decision making processes
   and reacted to each task accordingly. As clinical application of P300 becames
   possible, we can take advantage of the examination of higher brain
   dysfunctions with dementia and decide a therapeutic goal in physical therapy
   more easily.

Conclusion

A computer assisted evoked potential analyzing system, EP-WORKS, was used for
analyzing various evoked potentials. The result of this study indicated that
the system will be usefull for functional evaluation in physical therapy.

References

1) Fujiwara T : Evoked potentials 2.Clinical application in physical tehrapy.
   Journal of Physical Therapy 5:141-147, in JPN 1988.
2) Hugon M : Methodology of the Hoffmann reflex in man. Karger,Basel,3:277-293,
   1973.
3) Fujiwara T et al : Hoffmann Reflex Activity Modified by Facilitation Tecni
   -ques on Human Subjects. Sogo Rehabilitation 10:1009-1014, in JPN 1982.
4) Inoue I et al: Learning effects on reaction time among healthy subjects.
   Journal of Exercise Physiology 6:1-4, in JPN 1991

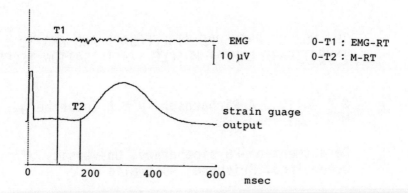

Fig. 1 Photo-stimulated RT (The representative of subjects)
EMG-RT shows 93.0 msec.
M-RT shows 166.0 msec.

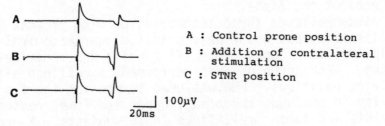

A : Control prone position
B : Addition of contralateral stimulation
C : STNR position

Fig. 2 H-wave (The representative of subjects)

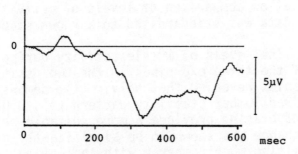

Fig. 3 P300 (The representative of subjects)
Peak latency shows 332.0 msec

THE USE OF PRESSURE BIOFEEDBACK AND EMG TO INVESTIGATE LUMBAR MUSCLE STABILISATION TECHNIQUES

G A Jull, C A Richardson, R M K Toppenberg, M J Comerford

Department of Physiotherapy, University of Queensland, Brisbane, Australia

Instructors commonly teach clients to contract their abdominals to protect their lumbar region prior to loaded movements of the limbs.

This study reviewed three techniques used to promote lumbar stabilisation; posterior pelvic tilt, lower abdominal 'hollowing' with lumbar spine flattening and abdominal bracing. Each technique was performed in reclined sitting and lying positions. EMG was used to monitor the muscle activity in obliquus abdominus, upper and lower rectus abdominis and lumbar multifidus in 15 subjects. A pressure biofeedback was inserted between the lumbar spine and the supporting surface to monitor the pressure change with each exercise. To allow comparison of levels of activity in each exercise, EMG data was standardised to a known stabilisation pattern.

Results : The levels of muscle activity during the performance of the three exercises in the two positions was analysed. Results revealed that pelvic tilt demonstrated least the desired lumbar stability pattern ($p < 0.02$). Both 'hollowing' and bracing provided a more suitable pattern. The pressure change was shown to be significantly greater with pelvic tilting when compared with 'hollowing' and bracing ($p < 0.0001$). The pressure biofeedback proved a useful clinical instrument to differentiate the more neutral lumbar position during 'hollowing' and bracing from the marked lumbar flexion of posterior pelvic tilting.

CHEDOKE-McMASTER STROKE ASSESSMENT: A COMPREHENSIVE CLINICAL AND RESEARCH MEASURE

C Gowland, W Torresin, P Stratford, N Plews, S VanHullenaar, J Moreland, J Sanford. McMaster University and Chedoke-McMaster Hospitals, Chedoke Campus, Bldg. 74, P.O. Box 2000, Stn "A", Hamilton, Ontario, Canada

This poster will describe the Chedoke-McMaster Stroke Assessment and the research study* which is being carried out to determine its reliability and validity as both a discriminative and evaluative measure.

The Chedoke Assessment provides a comprehensive patient evaluation system that is for use in both clinical and research settings. It was first developed by physiotherapists on the Stroke Programme at the Chedoke Rehabilitation Centre and has undergone revision and validation for over a decade and a half. It is suitable as a discriminative, predictive and evaluative measure of impairment and disability post stroke. Its first purpose is to determine the presence and severity of common physical impairments in order to classify patients when planning and selecting interventions. Second, it predicts expected rehabilitation outcomes including who is at risk for shoulder pain and permanent upper limb impairment, and third, it measures clinically important change (outcome assessment) in motor impairment and physical disability. It is designed to be used in conjunction with the Uniform Data System for Medical Rehabilitation (UDS) which includes the Functional Independence Measure (FIM).(1) The Chedoke Assessment has four sections, the first of which, along with the UDS provides prognostic information. Data include description of the lesion, complications, level of consciousness, perception, upper extremity function and somatosensation. In the second section which deals with impairment, six dimensions of motor recovery are scored on a 7-point scale. The dimensions are: shoulder pain, postural control, arm, hand, leg and foot. Although the assessment of motor recovery is based on the stages originally described by Brunnstrom,(2) the definitions have been substantially modified and added to, and new test items have been selected.(3) The third section deals with disability and provides the principle information on functional outcome. Fourteen items of gross motor function and walking are each scored on the same 7-point scale as the FIM. A standardized two-minute walk test(4) is included to assess change in gait efficiency for ambulating patients. The last section of this assessment contains equations for determining the prognosis following rehabilitation.(5) A manual explaining the theoretical basis and giving detailed instructions on administration, scoring and interpretation accompanies this measure. The assessment takes on average one hour to complete. A treatment manual(6) also accompanies this assessment. Using the data on the nature and severity of impairment and disability, it guides the therapist in selecting appropriate goals and activity protocols.

* Funded by National Health Research and Development Programme, Canada

THE VALIDATION STUDY

This study is being carried our in two parts. Initial results from the first set of objectives are partially available and are reported here.

Objectives: The objectives of the first part of the study are to determine: (i) the inter- and intra-rater reliability of the impairment section, (ii) the inter-rater and test-retest reliability of the disability section, (iii) the responsiveness of the disability section, and (iv) the concurrent validity of both the impairment and disability sections.

Method: Subjects include stroke patients undergoing inpatient rehabilitation who are (i) between 21 and 80 years of age, (ii) with a diagnosis of completed stroke of less than six months, and (iii) who are both able and willing to participate. Patients are assessed by both a treating and research therapist during the first week of admission. Random assignment is used to determine who will handle the patient during the assessment. Handling is alternated for subsequent assessments of the same patient. The disability section assessment is reassessed by both therapists within three days. Within the first week, a Fugl-Meyer(7) assessment is completed by the research therapist and a FIM assessment by the treating therapist. The impairment section of the admission assessment is videotaped, and after a minimum wait of two weeks the treating therapist scores the videotape. At discharge, impairments are reassessed by the treating therapist and disabilities by both therapists. The FIM is scored by the treating therapist.

Data Analysis: Data from 16 of the 28 cases needed to complete this part of the study is now available with the exception of discharge scores which are needed to determine responsiveness. To determine reliability, intraclass correlation coefficients (ICC) were calculated using an analysis of variance model.(8) Concurrent validity coefficients were derived from the Pearson product moment correlations.

Results: Results are summarized in the following two tables.

INTER-RATER, INTRA-RATER AND TEST-RETEST RELIABILITY COEFFICIENTS N=16					
Impairment	Inter rater	Intra rater	Disability	Inter rater	Test-retest
shoulder pain	0.97	0.99	gross motor		
postural control	0.94	0.96	function	0.98	0.98
arm	0.88	1.00			
hand	0.92	1.00	walking	0.97	0.97
leg	0.88	0.97			
foot	0.95	1.00	2 min. walking	0.99	0.86
TOTAL	0.97	0.98	TOTAL	0.99	0.99
Overall interrater reliability (impairment + disability) R = 0.99					

CONCURRENT VALIDITY WITH THE FUGL-MEYER AND FIM ASSESSMENTS			
Impairment: (Fugl-Meyer)	Pearson correlation	Disability: (FIM)	Pearson correlation
postural control	0.83	gross motor function	0.88
upper limb	0.95	locomotion	0.94
lower limb	0.82		
TOTAL	n/a	TOTAL	0.85

The complete dataset for this part of the study including responsiveness measures will be reported on the poster.

Discussion: The results to date are extremely heartening, indicating that the Chedoke Assessment is both a reliable and valid measurement instrument for assessing impairments and disabilities in stroke patients. When the second part of this study is complete we will also have information on (i) the test-retest reliability and the responsiveness of the impairment section, (ii) the criterion (both concurrent and predictive) validity and relative responsiveness of the disability section when compared to two other disability measures, and (iii) family and patient perceptions of the importance of the functional changes made on the degree of burden and quality of life. This measure will then add to the physiotherapy domain a comprehensive measure of the physical status of victims of stroke that is suitable for both the clinical and research setting.

References:

1. Data Management Service of the Uniform Data System for Medical Rehabilitation. Uniform Data System for Medical Rehabilitation, Buffalo, Research Foundation - State University of New York, 1990.
2. Brunnstrom S. Movement therapy in hemiplegia: A neurophysiological approach. New York: Harper & Row, Publishers, 1970:1-182.
3. Gowland C. Staging motor impairment after stroke. Stroke 1990; Supplement:II19-II21.
4   Butland RJA, Pang J, Gross ER, Woodcock AA, Geddes DM. Two-, six-, and 12-minute walking tests in respiratory disease. Br Med J 1982; 284:1607-1608.
5. Gowland C. Predicting sensorimotor recovery following stroke rehabilitation. Physiother Can 1984; 36(6):313-320.
6. Gowland C, Torresin W, VanHullenaar S, Best L. Therapeutic exercise for stroke patients. In: Basmajian JV, Wolf SL, eds. Therapeutic exercise. Baltimore:Williams & Wilkins, 1990:207-229.
7. Fugl-Meyer AR, Jaasko L, Leyman I, Olsson S, Steglind S. The post-stroke hemiplegic patient. I: a method for evaluation of physical performance. Scand J Rehab Med 1975; 7:13-31.
8. Streiner DL, Norman GR. Health measurement scales: a practical guide to the their development and use. New York: Oxford University Press, 1989.

ANALYSIS OF STANDING UP: INFLUENCE OF GOAL DIRECTED MOVEMENT ON
PERFORMANCE

E J Clough, S M Kelly, B Richardson, N Virji-Babul
Cambridge School of Physiotherapy, Addenbrooke's Hospital,
Cambridge UK

Introduction

The motor relearning program (1) emphasizes that organization of movement
is dependant on the environmental context in which the action is to take
place and the goal of the action. This approach encourages therapists to
train standing up using a goal orientated approach based on knowledge of
the components of normal movement.

One of the essential prerequisites for functional independence is the act
of rising from a seated position. Although there have been a number of
studies investigating the activity of rising from a chair, (2) there does
not appear to be any literature available on how the act of rising may
differ depending on the purpose of standing up. Traditionally therapists
have trained standing up as a separate, isolated activity without much
consideration of the ultimate goal. The underlying assumption is that the
patient stands up in the same manner whether the goal is to simply stand
up or to stand up and walk. As a result, although the goal may be to walk,
this movement or task is broken down into two components: standing up,
followed by walking (3), each of which is practiced separately. (4)

In order to explore the issue, a descriptive study was undertaken to
examine the influence of changing goals on the performance of standing up.
We were specifically interested in investigating whether there is any
difference in the task of standing up when the goal is simply to stand
up, as opposed to stand up to walk to perform a functional task.

Method

Subjects: 10 female physiotherapy students were recruited on a voluntary
basis from the Cambridge School of Physiotherapy. The subject's age
ranged from 19-26 years (x=20.9 SD+/-1.9). None of the participants
reported any prior musculoskeletal disease or injury.
Apparatus: A standard tripod, recorder and television monitor were used
to record the subject's movements. A Panasonic F10 video camera was
placed 290cms from a standard height (46cms) chair without arms. A
(71x61cms) table was placed 136cms away from the chair. A cup and saucer
were placed 5cms apart on the table, 8cms from the edge.
Procedure: Each subject was barefoot and wore a swimsuit while being
filmed. Body markers were placed on the following points: fifth
metatarsal head, lateral surface markings on the ankle, knee and hip
joints and lateral border of acromion. Each subject was asked to sit back
against the backrest with feet flat on the floor and hands on their lap.
No other attempts were made to correct/adjust their posture. Each
subject was asked to perform 2 tasks, one at a time in a random sequence.

In Task A the subject was asked simply to "stand up". In Task B the subject was asked to "stand and walk to the table and put the cup on the saucer". Each subject was given one practice trial and the second trial was recorded on film.

Analysis: Movement Pattern – Measurements were taken from the television screen using acetates (5). The first observable frame in which the subject's back moved away from the back of the chair was chosen as the beginning of the movement. Data points were taken from every third frame (separated by .06sec). The final point was determined when rising was completed and the subject demonstrated maximal hip extension. Timing – The time taken from the first frame to the last was recorded and the total movement time was then calculated.

Results
On the average, subjects stood up 12% faster (T=3.682, p .003) when standing up to perform a functional task. Figure 1 illustrates the difference in the movement patterns during standing up in each condition. In Task B there is an obvious overlap between the action of standing up and walking, i.e. subjects did not complete the task of standing up before initiating walking. The resulting differences in movement organization is further illustrated in Figure 2. In Task A the knee starts to extend before the hip completes flexion; in Task B, the hip and knee appear to begin extension at the same time. In addition, the hip is flexed to a greater extent (5°) when performing Task B.

(i)   (ii)

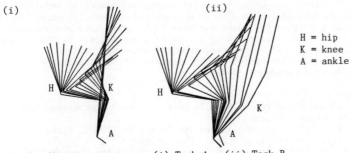

H = hip
K = knee
A = ankle

Fig 1.   Movement patterns   (i) Task A   (ii) Task B

Discussion
The results of this pilot study appear to indicate that movement organization and timing are highly dependant on the goal of the action. When the goal was to stand up, the action involved an overlap of the trunk forward flexion and upward extension phases with knee extension beginning while the hip was still flexing. This flexion action of the hip is thought to facilitate knee extension to lift the buttocks off the chair (6). When the goal was to walk there appeared to be less overlap between the two phases with hip and knee extension beginning at the same time. Following lift off there was a greater degree of hip extension than knee extension with the knee moving primarily in a forward direction.

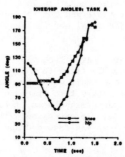
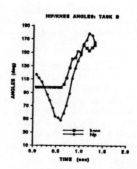

Fig 2. Movement organisation

In addition, the difference in velocity between the two tasks suggests
that the demand for the development of tension is different (for the
involved muscles) in each activity (7).

The above results question the validity of traditional therapy which
trains components of standing up without consideration of the goal.
Davies (3) has suggested that in preparation for walking, patients should
learn to first stand up, assuming an upright position prior to walking.
Our findings suggest that normal subjects do not assume a fully extended
position when the goal of standing up is to walk. Thus, by breaking this
task into smaller components, the relationship and timing between various
joints may be compromised leading to an abnormal movement pattern. It
appears that goal directed tasks may need to be taken into account when
devising therapeutic strategies to aid skill acquisition. By conducting
simple analyses of both, normal and impaired movement, valuable
information can be obtained which can ultimately help to validate
physiotherapeutic management models.

References
1. Carr, JH and Shepherd, RS (1982)A motor relearning programme for
stroke. Heinemann: London
2. Kerr, KM, Whilee, JA, Mollan, RA and Baird, HE (1990) Rising from a
chair: A review of the literature. Physiotherapy 77, 1: 15-19
3. Davies, PM (1985) Steps to Follow: A guide to the treatment of
adult hemiplegia. Springer Verlag: Berlin 146-171
4. Hollis., M (1989) Re-education: Practical Exercise Therapy.
Blackwell Scientific Publications: Oxford 130-140
5. van Vliet, P (1988) Kinematic analysis of videotape to measure
walking following stroke: A case study. Australian Journal of
Physiotherapy 34, 1: 48-51
6. Carr, JH (1987) Analysis and training of standing up. Proceedings
of the World Confederation for Physical Therapy. Sydney 383-388
7. Galley, PM and Forster, AL (1987) Human movement.
Churchill Livingstone: Edinburgh, 21-39

A CLINICAL MEASUREMENT SYSTEM FOR THE MOVEMENTS OF RISING TO STAND AND SITTING DOWN

B. R. DURWARD, P. J. ROWE.

QUEEN MARGARET COLLEGE
EDINBURGH
SCOTLAND

A new clinical measurement system has been developed to assess the functional movements of rising to stand, standing balance and sitting down in a rehabilitation setting. The system comprised a four section force measuring steel platform onto which patients stood and a modified chair with force measuring arm sections. The system measures the vertical forces generated under the hands and feet during the various movements. 2 low profile switches attached to the chair indicate specific phases of the movements. The measuring equipment is linked via a set of amplifiers to an Archimedes micro-computer. Purpose written software has been developed to control the patient test, data storage and data presentation. Hard copy of the results can be produced for immediate entry into patient records.

Some examples of test data from hemiplegic patients are presented to demonstrate the force/time graph display options and their clinical relevance. Lateral and antero-posterior sway graphs are of particular relevance in assessing the hemiplegic patient where asymmetry at different stages of the movement can be identified. The data collected from the platform and chair sections can be further processed to calculate relevant parameters such as variation of impulses and velocity during the different phases of movement.

THREE-POINT MEASUREMENT OF VARUS DEFORMITY

SATOSHI MIYASHITA, NOBORU SEKIYA, KEN YANAGISAWA,
School of Physical Therapy, GOTO College, Tokyo-Eisei Gakuen,
4-1-1 Omori-KIta Ota-ku Tokyo 143, JAPAN

《INTRODUCTION》

Equinovarus of the legs is common among stroke patients with hemiparesis, due to the influence of synergy patterns and associated reactions. The legs come into direct contact with the ground, and receive ones full body weight. It is generally understood that in comparison with the pes equinus, pes varus has a greater effect in hindering movement of the center of gravity, or the ability to bear weight. Futher, changes in muscle tone, brought about by synergy patterns or associated reactions, themselves change according to the location of the upper limbs, trunk, pelvic girdle, and lower limbs etc., yielding a major difference in the amount of equinovarus between an immobile and a mobile state. The level of equinovarus can be examined using a ROM test, but this is at best an assessment in an immobile state, and as there are many unclear points, such as the setting of the axis, measurement errors can easily be made by the examiner. Further, use of PT equipment or corrective surgery is proposed when treatment using leg braces proves unsatisfactory. For this decision, there are many points for which examination and observation must be made in order to determine the proper method of treatment. However, until tne present, there has been no way to test these decisions. If quantitative analysis in a mobile state were possible for equinovarus, one could determine standards for use of physical therapy equipment, or standards for when surgery is the proper response.

At this time the following is a proposal for a more accurate method for measurement of pes varus which can also assess a mobile state, we are reporting our basic data which we have gathered.

《OBJECT》

Normal Adults: Twenty-four males, sixteen females eighty legs, average age 21.3(SD=2.9).

Strok Patients with Hemiparesis: Forty-two, Forty-two legs (right side paralysis 15, left side paralysis 27) average age 72.1(SD=8.6).

In addition to these, in order to obtain an error differential we tested an additional twenty-eight physical therapy students, sixteen males, twelve females, average age 23.6(SD=4.4).

《METHOD》

For the purpose of ease in examination of the inside of the leg, we selected the three base points of the Tibia Malleolus medialis, the Calcaneus Tuber calcanei, and the Tuberositas ossi navicularis, and labeled them respectively as A, B, and C. Then using a measure, we obtained the distance between these three points. Using B as the base point, in order to measure the difference in size of the leg, we took the distance between B-C to equal 100 as a coordinate, and obtained A (X, H). Theoretically, when pes varus occurs, there will be a reduction in ABC. H/X, in other words the tangent, centers around ABC (fig-1).

For normal adults we measured the four values of the mid-flex leg joint value, the 40° planter-flexion value, the inversion value, and the 40° planter-flexsion value excluding causes for inversion (with the leg held flat to the ground, and the lower heel extended).

For the group of stroke patients with hemiparesis, we divided them into the orthotic group and the surgery group, based on examination of treatment, had them stand on their healthy leg, and took the average of three measurements assuming a swing phase.

《RESULT》
1) Concerning Reproduction:
    For four of the stoke patients, we made three examinations on differing days, and
    obtained a coefficient of reliability for the obtained values of 0.91.
2) Result of Examination of Normal Adults:
    The H/X value for the each of the ankle joints was an average of 0.43(SD=0.04) for the
    mid-flex leg joint value. For the 40° planter-flexion value this was an average of 0.38
    (SD=0.06), for the inversion value this was an average of 0.35(SD=0.04), and for the 40°
    inversion value excluding causes for pes varus this was an average of 0.41(SD=0.06). No
    discrepancy was noticeable between men and women for the mid-flex leg joint values, the
    mid-flex values, or the planter-flexion values. Further verification was carried out by
    X-ray, verifying that there was no change in bone location. However, for the inversion
    values, there was a significant reduction due to pes varus (P<0.05).
3) Result of Examination for Stroke Patients:
    The H/X value for each of the leg joints of the orthotic group was an average of 0.30
    (SD=0.07). For the surgery group this was an average of 0.25(SD=0.09). In comparison
    with the inversion values for the normal adults, the H/X of the orthotic group was
    noticeably lower (P<0.01), with a further reduction in the surgery group (P<0.001).
4) Examination of discrepancy in measurment between the former ROM test and the present method,
    using the physical therapy students:
    The same pes varus measurement was made as for the normal adults. For the ROM test this
    showed an average value of 26.5°(SD=5.5), while under this method an average value of 0.37
    (SD=0.05) was obtained. Through this we were able to ascertain that the present
    examination yields a lower margin of error (P<0.05).

《ASSESSMENT》
    The measurement points for the three point measurement of the medial hindfoot were set for
the purpose of easy examination. Further, by reproducing this distance as a coordinate, and
taking the distance between B and C as a uniform value of 100, we were able to eliminate the
influence caused by differing leg sizes.
    For the normal adults, we compared the 40° planter-flexion excluding causes for inversion
(with the leg held flat to the ground, and the lower heel extended), and the 40° planter-
flexion value. For the first, almost the same value was obtained as for the mid-flex leg
joint value. As during this planter-flexion motion, the ankle moves the Trochlea tali to the
rear, the bend in the Chopar joint and the Lisfranc joint supplements this motion, and the
M.tibialis anterior lifts the Os naviculare to the top. For this reason, it can be assumed
that there is little change in location in the Talus, Calcaneus, or Os naviculare.
    For the 40° planter-flexion value, the H/X values tended to be lower than the mid-flex
values. One reason for this is that for the ankle joint, the ankle joint axis is higher than
when held level. Futher, when the work relating to leg inversion is great for the joints, the
M.gastrocnemius, the M.soleus, the M.tibialis posterior, the M.flexor digitorum longus are
separated from the M.tibialis anterior. The joints relating to the planter-flexion movement
are the M.gastrocnemius, the M.soleus, the M.peroneus longus, the M.peroneus brevis, the
M.tibialis posterior, the M.flexor hallucis longus, and the M.flexor digitorum longus.
Therefore during planter-flexion movement, the causes for pes valgus appear, and show up as
numerical values.
    Some deviation in the data for the H/X values for normal adults was attained for each leg
joint value. However, the respective coefficient of reliability for this method yields a
lower margin of error, than that for the former ROM test, a more accurate examination can be
made, with greater possibility for reproduction; both important factors in examination.
    The parameter X in this method changes back and forth, and H changes its height. For this

reason, notwithstanding the pes varus, there is a possibility of change in value due to pes valgus. Thus, it is possible that in this method the H/X will be influenced by the form of the inside vertical arch. In full consideration of this phenomena, examination of both the normal adults and the patient group of the difference between left and right was made on the examination table, rather than just taking average values, making this examination more reliable.

For the stroke patient group, the H/X for the equinovarus of the orthotic group was lower than the values measured for the inversion of the normal adults. The H/X for the surgery group was lower still. This suggests that physical changes will occur such as aponeurosis, capsula articularis, and ligamentum, due to long term enforced pes varus. As with the normal adult group, there was some deviation in the data obtained, so that a definitive conclusion can not be made, but if the H/X is 0.3 or lower, this would seem to be a condition for either orthotic therapy, or surgery, while if 0.2 or lower, this would be a condition for surgery.

Treatment of the equinovarus of the orthotic group and the surgery group for the overall stroke patient group which was assessed by this examination, as the inversion values were greater than that of the normal adults, would require not only braces for the leg itself for correction, but also major attention to and examination of stability after correction.

At the same time as performing an assessment by examination of treatment, this three point measurement examination method of the ankle section is a supplemental examination which quantifies the level of disability, and helps to determine whether orthotic treatment or surgery is called for.

《CONCLUSION》

1. An attempt was made towards a simplified assessment method (lower leg three point measurement), of Equinovarus in Stroke Patients with Hemiparesis.
2. By this method, at the same time as analysis by examination on the examination table, we were able to quantify the degree of pes varus.
3. This test method was reproducible.
4. As the measured values were expressed as coordinates, we were able to limit as much as possible causes for deviation, such as leg size.
5. When pes varus exists in the lower leg portion, the H/X reduces, and can be used as the pes varus assessment parameter.
6. The inversion was significantly lower for the equinovarus of stroke patients in comparison with normal adults.
7. When the H/X is 0.3 or less, examination as to the suitability of surgery or orthotic therapy is necessary for ambulatory rehabilitation.
8. When H/X is 0.2 or less, examination of the suitability of surgery is necessary.
9. This is a supplemental assessment method which can determine the level of pes varus, and the suitability of orthotic therapy.
10. This method has a higher level of reliability than the original ROM test.

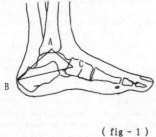
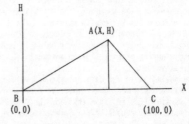

(fig - 1)

STRESS INCONTINENCE

PROSPECTIVE DOUBLE BLIND CONTROLLED TRIAL OF INTENSIVE PHYSIOTHERAPY WITH AND WITHOUT STIMULATION OF THE PELVIC FLOOR IN TREATMENT OF GENUINE STRESS INCONTINENCE

C Blowman, B.A. M.C.S.P., C Pickles, M.R.C.O.G, S Emery, V Creates, L Towell, N. Blackburn, N Doyle, B Walkden
Queens Medical Centre, Nottingham. NG7 2UH

INTRODUCTION

Urinary stress incontinence is a major problem and it is estimated that 33% of the female population at the age of 55 suffer from this disability. Mandelstam D. (1986)

Physiotherapy has been shown to increase the power of pelvic floor contractions and lead to improved continence. Karskov et al, (1986). However, many patients do not respond adequately to physiotherapy.

Full urinary continence requires a complex interplay between the urethral smooth muscle, the urethral and periurethral striated muscle with fast and slow twitch motor units, urethral vascular tone, the integrity of the pelvic floor and the relationship of the proximal urethra to the intra-abdominal pressure zone. Urinary incontinence may result from inadequacy of any combination of these functions. A number of factors could compromise the maintenance of continence, eg. neural damage in child-birth; Snooks et al, (1984) or atrophic changes associated with the climacteric.

Neurotrophic stimulation is a method of neuro-muscular electrical (N.M.E) stimulation which provides a waveform which is concomitant with normal neuronal physiology.

This type of stimulation differs from faradic and interferential treatments in that it allows for a recovery phase before the next stimulations.

The contractile properties of muscle fibres are determined in part by the neuronal input; Salmons et al, (1969). It has been established that muscle fibre properties can be modified by imposed electrical activity; Buller et al, (1960). When fast twitch muscles are stimulated at low frequencies they develop slow contracting, fatigue resistent properties. Not only can the contractile characteristics be altered within a muscle group, but also the capillary density; Scott et al, (1985). Furthermore, it has been shown that by using electrical stimulation E.M.G. activity can be recovered where previously there was none. Kidd, (1984).

This method of treatment therefore has several characteristics likely to assist with the return of the mechanics necessary for the maintenance of continence.

The objectives of this study were to assess the efficacy of neuromuscular stimulation (N.M.S) and pelvic floor exercises versus the treatment of genuine stress incontinence compared with pelvic floor exercises only.

PATIENTS AND METHODS

14 adult women were assessed in the urodynamic clinic at Queens Medical Centre, Nottingham as having G.S.I. without significant prolapse. All patients had bladder pressure studies performed using the Ormed 500 system.

Only patients diagnosed from these tests as suffering from G.S.I. were recruited for this study. They were referred to the physiotherapy department's gynaecology unit and gave informed written consent to take part in the trial. One member of the team assessed pelvic floor muscle power using a Bourne perineometer; Bourne Perineometer, (1986). The maximum pressure achieved by a pelvic floor contraction and the maximum pressure held for the count of 10 were recorded. (patients counted slowly aloud to 10 to prevent them holding their breath which can give a false reading on the perineometer). A further manual assessment of pelvic floor power was carried out using a scale devised by two of the physiotherapists. Appendix 1.

The patients were taught pelvic floor exercises by a second member of the team. (An obstetric physiotherapist) who gave individual instruction to each patient including visual bio feedback using the Bourne perineometer. All patients were instructed to practice their pelvic floor exercises at least 5 times a day. This training was reinforced and patients remotivated by the same physiotherapist at each of their fortnightly visits to the hospital.

The obstetric physiotherapist teaching the exercises was not involved in the assessments and was unaware of who had active or inactive stimulators; as was the assessor.

All patients took their stimulators (either active or placebo) home and used them for 60 minutes per day at a time convenient for the individual patient. Those with inactive-placebo stimulators were told to set the amplitude control to 3. The active group were instructed to turn up the amplitude control until they only just became aware of some electrical sensation. The stimulation sensation was minimal, not enough to cause a pelvic floor contraction and comfortable enough to be ingnored for the duration of treatment.

The patients were also asked to keep a daily diary of their frequency of micturition and number of incontinent episodes using continence charts.

The patients received stimulation for 60 minutes per day for four weeks at a frequency of 10Hz with a balanced contraction and relaxation time of four seconds each and a pulse width of 80 microsecs. Two weeks of further therapy using a higher frequency of 35Hz (all other parameters as before) was given for 15 minutes a day to try to augment the power of the muscle groups involved; Numsat et al (1976).

Our objective as stated earlier was to assess the efficacy of N.M.S. in the treatment of G.S.I. As clinicians with the knowledge of the usefulness of pelvic floor exercises in the treatment of G.S.I., we constructed the methodology in the manner outlined so as not to deny any patients this treatment.

RESULTS

The median age of the inactive group was 42.5 years range (38-64) and of the active group, 45.0 years range (33-68). The median number of years of incontinence of the inactive group was 3.5 years range (2-6) and of the active group 3 years range (1-50). Median parity of the inactive group was 2.7 (range (2-4) and of the active group 2.1 (range 1-3). Median gravidity of the inactive group was 3.3 and of the active group 2.1. Three of the 6 in the inactive group and 4 of the 7 in the active group had previous gynaecological surgery; no patients had previous surgery for G.S.I. One subject has not been included in the results as her compliance judged by interrogation of the N.T.4 unit by the N.T.16 was erratic.

The accident rate in the inactive group changed from a median weekly rate of 12.5 (range 1-31) at the beginning of the study to 6 (range 0-21) at the end of the study (p,n/s). In comparison the active group had a starting median accident rate of 5 (range 1-14) per week which by the end of the study had fallen to 0 (range 0-1) (P<0.05).

864

The perineometer maximum reading for the inactive group from the first to the final reading changed from a median of 6 (range 4-10) to a median of 9 (range 5-15). The active group also increased their perineometer maximum reading from a median of 5 (range 0-14) to 12 (range 5-16).

The maximum pressure held on the perineometer from the count of 10 showed a median change in the inactive group from 3.5 (range 1-5) to 5 (range 3-13) whilst in the active group the change was from 1 (range 0-8) to 5 (range 2-16).

On direct questioning none of the patients reported any discomfort or side-effects from the N.T.S.

The accident rate per week was reduced to 0 in the active group in 6 of the 7 patients. One of the patients in the inactive group achieved a zero score, ie. no accidents per week. None of the patients in the active group required further treatment. Four of the six patients in the inactive group required further treatment and have either since had surgery or are on the surgical waiting list. All the patients in the study were circulated with a confidential questionnaire 6 months after their treatment finished.

CONCLUSION

This study has demonstrated the combined effectiveness of neurotrophic stimulation and pelvic floor exericse. Patients treated with active neurotrophic stimulation improved their pelvic floor strength and endurance as measured by the perineometer reading and reduced their episodes of incontinence (as recorded on a daily diary) by a level which was statistically significant. This is supported by the finding that all patients so treated did not require further treatment, whereas 2/3rds in the inactive group did. These results are extremely encouraging and suggest that this safe and easy method of treatment could be offered as a first-line treatment to all patients with genuine stress incontinence severe enough to warrant surgery.

APPENDIX 1

MANUAL ASSESSMENT OF PELVIC FLOOR

Part 1   Objective

0 -   No contraction of the pelvic floor

1 -   Contraction of the pelvic floor but an inability to maintain for 2 seconds

2 -   Contraction held for >1 >5 seconds (patient audibly counting)

3 -   Contraction held for 4 to 9 seconds

4 -   Contraction held for 10 to 14 seconds

5 -   Contraction held for 15 or more seconds

Part 2   Subjective

1 -   No awareness   )
) Cannot stop mid-stream
2 -   Aware of pelvic floor contractions)

3 -   Can stop mid-stream, but still incontinent

4 -   Can stop mid-stream, no incontinence

Lowest score would be: 0/1
Highest score would be: 5/4

PELVIC FLOOR MUSCULATURE EXERCISES:
LONG-TERM EFFECTS IN THE TREATMENT OF URINARY STRESS INCONTINENCE

R Tuomi, H Leino-Kilpi
University of Turku, Department of Nursing
Turku, Finland

The purpose of this study was to evaluate the long-term effects of the pelvic floor musculature exercises (PFE) in the treatment of urinary stress incontinence in women. The assessment was based on the subjective evaluation of the participants in the study.

The research problems were:
1. How problematic have the women considered their urinary in-continence to be at the time of the questionnaire?
2. In what way have the women done the pelvic floor musculature exercises during the three months' PFE programme and during the 3 months to 3 years of continued PFE exercises at home?
3. What results have been obtained immediately after the three months' PFE programme and at the time of the questionnaire in urine loss in women?
4. What was the relationship between the continuation of PFE at home and any resulting incontinence, coupled with the general background of the patients?

For the collection of data, a questionnaire was mailed in February 1990 to 83 women with urinary incontinence who were re-ferred by gynaecologists for PFE in the Department of Physiat-rics in a university central hospital in Finland in 1986-89. The research data were collected by using a structured question-naire and from case records. The questions were divided into background information, PFE performance and the results of PFE in the treatment of urinary incontinence. The background inform-ation on the current living conditions of the study participants were asked, because they might have influenced their PFE pro-gramme performance and/or their urinary incontinence. The res-pondents were also asked to describe what kind of problems they had with the urinary incontinence.

74 (89%) women answered the questionnaire. All the subjects were instructed in PFE by a physiotherapist in five training sessions of 30 minutes for 3 consecutive months, and all the patients concerned had completed the programme with the physio-therapist 6 months before the study.

The physiotherapist instructed the patients to perform the PFE daily at home as many times as possible. At the end of the 3 months' PFE programme, the patients were advised to continue PFE at home daily for the rest of their life, or at least as long as they suffer from urinary incontinence.

The sample consists of 74 women, and their average age was 51 years (range 25-67); about 40% of them were under 50 years of age. Almost 80% of the respondents were married and lived in a city. Their basic education was comprehensive school, and 60% of them had physically heavy work. Three patients were nulliparous, 43 had given birth to one or two children and 28 had three or more children. The mean body height of the respondents was 164 cm (range 151-174) and the mean body weight 70 kg (range 55-120); 52 % were overweight.

The urodynamic examinations were measured by gynaecologists before the treatment in all the patients participating in the study. No measurements were made after the treatment; 52 (72%) patients had urodynamically proven stress incontinence, 16 (22%) stress and urge combined, and 4 (6%) urge. The degree of stress incontinence was graded as mild in 35, moderate in 18 and severe in 8 patients. 11 patients had previously had surgery to correct incontinence. 51% had suffered from incontinence for more than 5 years; the duration of symptoms ranged from 1 month to 40 years. The mean duration was 9 years.

The data was statistically analyzed by using the BMDP-program. The statistical methods employed included direct and percentage distributions, and means and cross tabulation. The relationships were tested by the x^2-test. This test was used to assess the influence of background information on the performance of the PFE programme, its continuation, and the results.

The first subjective assessment was made at the end of the 3 months' treatment period. The results showed that 45 (62%) of the patients improved and 28 (38%) failed to improve. The stress incontinence changed for the better between 2 weeks and 4 months after PFE; the changes were permanent in 20 (48%) and temporary in 22 (52%) of the patients. None of the patients found their urinary incontinence worse than before the exercises. 23 (31%) of the patients had had surgery for incontinence after the treatment.

Of the 74 women 63 continued PFE after the 3 months' treatment, 46 performed PFE further than that and 28 performed PFE daily at the time of the questionnaire. 35 patients (76%) did the exercise for less than 1 year, 9 (20%) for 1-2 years and 2 (4%) more than 2 years. According to the results of this study, there seems to be a significant relationship (P 0.05) between the continuation of the therapy and the following factors: sedentary work, physical training, duration of incontinence and how serious the problem was to the patient. Most of the women who had had sedentary work, done physical training, had had the incontinence for less than 5 years and had experienced a slight problem of incontinence, continued PFE after the 3 months' treatment. Satisfaction with the treatment encouraged the patients to do home exercises. Obesity also seems to have a connection with a reluctance to continue the exercises.

The second subjective assessment showed that neither the severity of the condition nor the patients' age, their education, marital status, parity and their current living conditions had a significant effect on the treatment results. At the time of the questionnaire, after 6-36 months of PFE, 53 (71%) of the patients had incontinence and 21 (29%) were cured. Of the 21 patients reported to have cured, 13 had opted for surgery after the 3 months' treatment. Of the 63 patients who continued the PFE at home, 8 were cured and decided against surgery. According to the results of the study, the effectiveness of the exercise programme seems to have an almost statistically significant relationship (p 0.05) with the seriousness of the problem and the ability to interrupt the urinary flow and the ability to perform the muscle contractions in an adequate way. Furthermore, there seems to be a conenciton between the physical heaviness of work and the effect of the treatment.

At the time of the questionnaire, 62% of the women considered their urinary incontinence to be a significant problem. They found the incontinence most problematic at work, and in daily life and hobbies. About one third have difficulty in talking about their incontinence with other people.

Based on the opinions of the patients, this PFE programme seems to be appropriate for the care of urinary incontinence. The results suggest that PFE relieves the symptoms of stress incontinence. The follow-up assessment showed that the improvements were not permanent.

The PFE programme requires good individual cooperation with the patient. The patient should have a high level of motivation to continue the exercises at home after the programme. About half of the patients performed the PFE daily after the programme, and half had stopped or reduced their home practice. The participants said thet they would like more 30 minute training sessions by a physiotherapist; about one programme every six months. Furthermore, they wished for more regular check-ups by a physiotherapist and by a physician. This represents a selected sample, and may not be representative of incontinent women in general. The findings should therefore be analyzed in that context and should not be interpreted for all incontinent women.

The results obtained from this study will be used for further development of the PFE method.

The effect of two pelvic floor muscle exercise regimens on female stress
urinary incontinence.

Bø, K., Hagen, P., Kvarstein P.
The Norwegian University of Sport and Physical Education,
P.O. Box 40, Kringsjå 0807. Oslo 8, Norway

INTRODUCTION
International Continence Society (ICS) has defined Incontinence as "a condition in which involuntary loss of urine is a social or hygenic problem
and is objectively demonstrable" (1). Genuine SUI is the type of incontinence most frequently affecting women, and is defined as: "the involuntary
loss of urine which occurs when, in absence of a detrusor contraction, the
intravesical pressure exceeds the maximum urethral pressure" (1).
Kegel (2) was the first to apply pelvic floor muscle (PFM) exercise to
treat female SUI and claimed that complete relief was obtained in 84% of
the women participating in the study. However, this study met a lot of
critisism and minimal research followed this first presentation. However
during the last decade, there has been a renewed interest in the effect
of PFM exercise in treatment of female SUI. Several studies have shown
positive effect of SUI (3,4). However, the results are difficult to inter-
prete because many researchers have not controlled for correct PFM contraction, the methods used to measure degree of SUI and PFM strength are
not reliable and /or valid and the strength training regimens applied vary
in duration, frequency of training and type of contraction. The purpose
of the present study was to construct reliable and valid methods to measure
SUI and PFM strength and to evaluate the effect of two PFM exercise regimens on female SUI.

MATERIALS AND METHODS
Fifty-two women; mean age 45.9 years (24-64) with clinically and urodynamically proven SUI participated in the study. Mean duration of the
SUI symptoms were 11 years (1-35). Fourty-nine were parous, fourteen
postmenopausal and 5 had previously been operatively treated for incontinence. The women were randomly assigned to one of two exercise regimens:

Home exercise (HE) consisting of:
- Individual instruction of anatomy and physiology of the lower urinary
  tract and function of the PFM.
- Control and feedback of PFM contraction by vaginal palpation and
  observation of movement of a vaginal catheter during PFM contraction.
- Measurement of PFM contraction by a vaginal balloon connected to a
  pressure transduser (4).
- Instruction to contract the PFM 8-12 repetitions three times a day for
  six months and to record training adherence in a training diary.
- Monthly meeting with the physiotherapist to measure PFM strength and for
  motivation to continue exercising.

Intensive exercise (IE) consisting of:
- The HE regimen
- Additional group exercise 45 minutes once a week. In this exercise group
  the emphasize was put on how to reach maximum contraction. The following
  principles were applied druing the exercise class:
- stimulation to maximum contraction by 6-8 sec. sustained hard contraction
  with 3-4 fast contractions at the end of each single contraction
- use of positions with legs in abduction to inhibit other muscle groups
  to contract simultaneously
- strong verbal encouragement by the physioterapist to stimulate to
  maximum contraction in every single attempt.

The IE group was encouraged to use the positions and same type of contractions during their three times a day home exercise. The main difference
between these two groups was that one group were told to contract as
hard ad possible while the other learned how to do it and had a close
follow up.

Degree of SUI was measured by urethra pressure profile, pad test with fixed
bladder volume, Leakage index (5 point scale conserning problems during
coughing, sneezing, laughing and several physical activities), Social
Activity Index (Visual analogue scale dealing with perceived problems
during participation in nine different social situations) (4) and personal
assessment. All instruments have been tested for reproducibility and been
found reliable.

RESULTS
Initially the two treatment groups were comparable with regards to all
measured parameters. Adherence to exercise was close to 100% for both
exercise groups.
Although they had had a thorough individual instruction, 32% of the
women did not perform correct PFM contraction at their first consultation.
The most commom errors were to contract gluteal muscles instead of the
PFM, or performing a valsalva. After 6 months treatment, still one woman in
the IE group and three in the HE group were unable to contract their PFM
muscles. Both groups significantly improved their PFM strength (p<0.01).
The IE group, however, significantly more (p<0.01) than the HE group
(HE from mean 7.9 cm H_2O (95% CI:5.5-10.3) to 15.3 (95% CI:12.0-18.6) and
IE from mean 7.0 cm H_2O (95% CI:4-10) to 22.5 (95% CI:17.7-27.3).
60% in the IE and 17% in the HE group reported to be continent or almost
continent after 6 months of PFM exercise (p<0.01).
The pad test demonstrated a significant (p<0.01) decrease from mean 27.0 g
(95% CI:8.8-45.1) to 7.1 g (95% CI:0.8-13.4) in the IE group. There was
no significant improvement in the HE group.
Sixty % in the IE converted a negative urethral closure pressure to
positive during cough. Only the IE group significantly increased
(p=0.02) the resting maximum urethral closure pressure from 38.8 cm H_2O
(95% CI:32.6-45.0) to 43.4 (95% CI:37.0-49.8). There was only significant
improvement (p<0.01) measured by the Social Activity Index in the IE group
(from mean 7.7 (95% CI:7.1-8.3) to 9.3 (95% CI:9-9.6). The overall cure
rate measured by the five instruments used in this study was 60% following
IE and 20% following HE regimen.

CONCLUSION
PFM contractions are difficult to perform. In clinical trials evaluating
effect of PFM exercise, control of correct contraction must be performed
to ensure valid data on effect. When measured by instruments tested for
reliability and validity, we found that only an intensive PFM exercise regimen stimulating to maximum contraction, proved to be effective in treatment of female SUI.

REFERENCES
1. Abrams, P., Blaivas, J.G., Stanton, S.L., Andersen, L.T. (1988), The
   standardisation of terminology of lower urinary tract function.
   Scand. J. Urol. Nephrol,, Supplementum 114:5-19.
2. Kegel, A.H. (1951) Physiologic therapy for urinary incontinence,
   JAMA, 146:915- 917.
3. Wells, I. (1990) Pelvic (floor) muscle exercise. JACS 38:333-337.
4. Bø, K. (1990) Pelvic floor muscle exercise for the treatment of
   female stress urinary incontinence. Methodological studies and clinical
   results. PhD thesis. The Norwegian University of Sport and Physical
   Education.

Effect of physiotherapy in Stress Incontinence (S.I.) and
Urge Incontinence (U.I.).

A. Devreese, W. De Weerdt, R. Lysens
University Hospital Gasthuisberg, 3000 LEUVEN, BELGIUM
University of Leuven, School of Physiotherapy

Incontinence imposes profound social and physical constraints on the
patient's life. This unpleasant handicap can arise at all ages and in all
social classes. The incidence of individuals suffering from this obvious
embarrassment is the highest in women and the elderly.
Kegel (1948) (1) introduced pelvic floor exercises as a treatment
procedure for female urinary incontinence. In the meantime a wide range of
ideas and methods have been developed to treat incontinence.

Aim of the study:

The aim of the present paper is to explain this initial part of the
evaluation and treatment procedure and to report if bladder drill and
pelvic floor exercises have a beneficial effect on S.I or U.I.

Subjects:

One hundred and twenty-nine incontinent women between 18 and 80 years old
received counselling and physiotherapy. Thirty-eight were postmenopausal,
22 underwent an hysterectomy and 11 had previously more than one
gynaecological intervention. Forty-four patients had had an average of
2.3 children with a mean birthweight of 3.3 kg. Twenty-eight patients
were overweight. 59 patients were clinically diagnosed as having stress
incontinence, 46 were found to suffer from urge incontinence and 15 had a
mixed incontinence. Six patients had enuresis and three pollakysuria.

Urodynamic diagnosis:

The initial urodynamic findings were : 66 patients with a stable bladder
(S.B.) and stable urethra (S.U.) ; 31 patients with a S.B. and unstable
urethra (U.U). Seven patients with unstable bladder (U.B) and S.U.
Fifteen patients with U.B. and U.U. For ten patients this information was
missing.

Voiding chart:

During a formal interview the physiotherapist documented the voiding
habits such as : volume, the habit to push, the jet, further urine loss
immediately after standing from the toilet and frequency during the day
and night. The voiding chart was analysed in cooperation with the patient
in order to detect inappropriate voiding habits. Some patients, as a
measure of prevention, would void before any major event such as leaving
home, or sudden changes in temperatures like walking into a cold room or
putting the hands in cold water.

Description of the evaluation and treatment procedure:

The physiotherapist performed a manual examination of the vagina in supine and side lying to identify weak muscles. She entered the vagina with the index or middle finger, the hand in pronation. She bended the last phalanx to palpate the diafragma pelvis and asked for a contraction of the m. pubovaginalis, m. puborectalis and m. pubococcygeus. If there is only a slight twitch the muscle score is one. If the finger is slightly elevated the muscle score is two. If the finger is elevated till the dorsal part touches os pubis the muscle score is three. If the three muscles can push the finger upwards against slight or full resistance the muscle score is 4 and 5.

The exercises during the physiotherapy sessions consist of two consecutive phases :

  (1) awareness of the muscles to be trained and
  (2) the perineal training itself.

Awareness of the muscles to be trained requires information about the anatomy of the bladder and urethra. The anatomy is shown by designs and pictures adapted to patient's level of comprehension. The function of the three different perineal muscle groups is explained. As a starting point, the physiotherapist will ask a general contraction of the vagina. Only then the therapist can feel which muscles contract and identify weak and inactive muscles. A slight stretch is given to the inactive muscles. If a good response is achieved, the patient is asked if she can feel some contraction. If not, the patient will herself palpate the muscle, until she perceives the activity. If the patient cannot not perform a clear contraction, further facilitation by means of stretching is needed. Furthermore, subtle alterations, simulating pushing and stopping of voiding and defecation are performed. All exercises learned in each session are repeated at home, three times a day. The patient must be able to perform the exercise for each muscle group faultless before progressions are built in the programme.

On the basis of the information from the voiding chart, the patient is strongly advised not to urinate as a conditioned reflex. The patient with urge incontinence is advised to wait sitting on the toilet during a few seconds (count till ten) before starting to void. The therapist will ask the patient never to push during voiding and to wait long enough till she has the impression of an empty bladder.

As soon as a conscious control of the pelvic floor muscles is achieved training sensu strictu can be started. If the patient looses urine by coughing or sneezing, mainly fast contractions are learned. Endurance training is more important for leakage during repetitive coughing and in sensory urge, where the contraction must be prolonged as long as the desire to void persists.

The exercises become gradually more difficult. They are performed in the supine position for muscle scores 1 and 2, in the upright and squat position for muscle stength score 3 and 4. Increased abdominal pressure is allowed from score 4. It is repeatedly stressed that the perineal muscles should contract before and throughout the contraction of the abdominal muscles, in order to stabilize the urethra. As soon as the pelvic floor musculature achieved a force score 3, individually adapted reflex conditioning exercises were given in order to incorporate the learned control in the Activities of Daily Living (A.D.L.). In a home training programme the patient is advised, to repeat each of the five exercises given ten times during every session and this three times a day. Speed and endurance were trained on seperate occasions. The exercises as described are initiated after a few sessions. Supervision of the maintenance programme lasts three months.

Results:

The mean frequency of therapy sessions was 3.5. Sixteen patients needed more than 5 treatment sessions to obtain their optimal effect. The mean pre-therapy muscle score was 1.1 and the mean post-therapy muscle score was 3.8. After a follow up period of three months forty-six (36%) patients were completely dry and 28 (22%) were better. Eleven (8%) patients did not improve. Thirty-three (26%) patients gave up and eleven (8%) were lost in follow up.

Discussion:

This study does not allow to differentiate between the treatment effect of pelvic excercises, bladder drill and counselling, because every patient regardless of the clinical diagnosis was offered the same concept of treatment.

Analysis of the data published in the annual congresses of the Société Internationale Fracophone d'Urodynamique (SIFUD)) and of our series underlines the problem of drop out. Indeed 26 % of the patients gave up and 8 % were lost during follow up. In other words 34 % of the patients were seemingly insufficient motivated to continue the treatment for three months. Several assumptions can be made. For some patients the vaginal region is still taboo and palpation or entering an instrument for perception of muscle force may have a negative psychological effect (3). For others training at a rate of three times a day at home is too much of an effort. Some seek a quick solution rather than a gradual control of the situation. Careful selection of patients is therefore mandatory to achieve success.

We prefer the personal (digital) perception of the vaginal contraction instead of the use of a perineometer. We agree with Chiarelli (2) that digital palpation is the best way to appreciate the contraction strength. The mean increase of muscle score in our series was 2.7 and these results were achieved without electrical stimulation. They compare well with the results of Grosse's study (3) in which he included a large number of postpartum cases. In our opinion electrotherapy should be reserved for patients with very weak muscles or very low awareness of their perineum.

References:

1. **Kegel AH**, (1948) Progressive resistance exercise in the functional resoration of the perineal muscles. Am. J. Gynecol. 56:238-248.
2. **Chiarelli PE, O'Keefe DR** (1981) Pysiotherapy for the pelvic floor. Austr. J. Physioth. 27:103-108.
3. **Grosse D, Sengler J, Jurascheck F** (1988) La rééducation périnéale. Annales Kinésither. 15:373-384.

A CLINICAL STUDY OF THE PELVIC FLOOR MUSCLES BY PERINEOMETRY

J. Laycock   D. Jerwood
Bradford Royal Infirmary, Bradford, England.

AIMS OF STUDY Weak pelvic floor muscles have been implicated in the aetiology of Genuine Stress Incontinence (GSI); however, the characteristics of the muscle fibres are part of an individual genetic endowment and wide variation is normal. This study uses perineometry to examine the pressures produced as a result of a Maximum Voluntary Contraction (MVC) in incontinent and asymptomatic i.e. continent women, using a new perineometer.

METHODS AND MATERIALS After a brief interview to establish details of medical history and to obtain informed consent, 233 women entered a prospective study to investigate the Pelvic Floor Muscles (PFM) and were classified as shown in Table 1.

AGE	GROUP 1 CONTINENT N = 86	GROUP 2 INCONTINENT N = 147	
			Group 1: no incontinence in the previous month.
MEAN	38.5	45.4	Group 2: one or more self-reported episodes of incontinence in the previous month.
RANGE	16 - 89	19 - 82	

Table 1   Classification by age and continence of 233 women in the study

Instruction in pelvic floor contraction was followed by a digital examination per vaginam to ascertain the correct muscle action. A new (water-filled) sensitive perineometer was then introduced into the vagina. This was attached to a pressure transducer (Gould P23XL) which was connected to a monitor and chart recorder (Datascope), and via an analogue to digital converter (ADC) to a computer, for data storage and analysis. Pressure measurements in mmHg were continuously recorded during a 10 second Maximum Voluntary Contraction (MVC). Constant encouragement and feedback were given during the test.

The following parameters were investigated:-
a)   The shape of the 10 - second MVC pressure profile.
b)   The maximum pressure recorded under MVC pressure profile = P.
c)   The area under the 10 - second MVC pressure profile = A.
d)   The MVC pressure gradient from base line to P = G.

RESULTS Four distinct types of pressure/time plot of the 10 second MVC pressure profile were identified and are illustrated below in Figure 1. The incidence rates of such profile types across the entire study group of 233 patients, together with the specific rates for subgroups of incontinent and continent patients are given in Table 2.

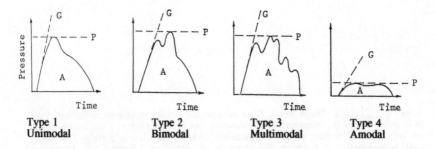

Type 1
Unimodal

Type 2
Bimodal

Type 3
Multimodal

Type 4
Amodal

Figure 1 Classification of perineometry pressure/time plots

PATIENT GROUP	TYPES OF PRESSURE / TIME PLOT				
	UNIMODAL	BIMODAL	MULTIMODAL	AMODAL	TOTAL
CONTINENTS	27 (32%)	0 (0%)	57 (66%)	2 (2%)	86(100%)
INCONTINENTS	38 (26%)	4 (3%)	59 (40%)	46 (31%)	147(100%)
COMBINED GROUPS	65 (28%)	4 (2%)	116 (50%)	48 (20%)	233(100%)

Table 2   Contingency Table of the distributions of perineometry plot types for continents and incontinents

Within the combined study group almost half of the patients exhibited a multimodal pressure/time response and with over a quarter of those patients tested the Type 1 (unimodal) response was observed. This rate was only slightly more prevalent within the study of the flat, featureless (amodal) profile, when the contractions of the perivaginal muscle fibres could barely register a response. It is not surprising to anticipate that these profiles are usually associated with incontinents (in a ratio observed at 24:1).

The Type 2 (bimodal) response was observed infrequently (less than 2%) and was found exclusively within the continent group. At least for the purposes of statistical analysis this bimodal response was deemed to be a limited manifestation of the popular multimodal response and these columns in Table 2 were annexed. Using a chi-squared test for association within this contingency table, the results ($\chi^2 = 28.43$ on 2 degrees of freedom, $P < 0.001$) indicate that there is strong evidence to conclude that the distributions of pressure/time profile types differ across the two groups of patients. In other words there is evidence of an association between incontinence and the pressure/time profile type. The nature of this association is (not surprisingly) generated in the main by the incidence of <u>amodal</u> profiles for continents and incontinents.

Generally however, knowledge of the profile type will be insufficient for accurate prognosis of incontinence, and more information may well be lodged with the profile parameters P, A and G. (See Table 3). Results indicate that for each of these parameters the incontinent group consistently shows a lower mean response. The relatively high standard errors (and the location of the mean values within their stated ranges) suggest that the distributions of P, A and G have long upper tails and that a non-parametric procedure (Mann-Whitney) should be preferred. The results of tests of significance reveal overwhelming evidence that incontinents produce lower mean responses for each of these profile parameters.

PATIENT GROUP	PRESSURE P (+/- S.E.) (RANGE)	AREA A (+/- S.E.) (RANGE)	GRADIENT G (+/- S.E.) (RANGE)
CONTINENTS (N = 86)	54 (+/- 22) (16 - 112)	362 (+/- 188) (45 - 908)	62 (+/- 31) (13 - 148)
INCONTINENTS (N = 147)	33 (+/- 20) (3 - 92)	224 (+/- 153) (24 - 713)	43 (+/- 35) (2 - 210)
COMBINED GROUPS	P < 0.00001	P < 0.00001	P < 0.00002

Table 3   Perineometry results for each pressure/time profile parameter. Mean values are stated together with standard errors (+/-S.E.) and observed ranges.

CONCLUSIONS The situation described here is clearly multivariate in its complex symptom structure where all the available information for any one patient should be considered simultaneously.   A more sophisticated statistical procedure (such as discriminant analysis) should be attempted in order to identify that combination of parameters, which will allow patients to be classified as continent or incontinent in some optimal sense. Such an analysis is currently being planned.

STUDY REPORT OF THE EVALUATION & CONSERVATIVE MANAGEMENT OF URINARY
STRESS IN THE OLDER FEMALE.

L. Wingate, Ph.D., P.T.
Massachusetts General Hospital, Boston, and Mount Auburn Hospital, Cambridge, Massachusetts, USA

Urinary stress incontinence is a distressing problem which adversely affects the quality of life
in the older woman. Every important aspect of life is affected by this condition--social,
psychological, and financial. It lowers self-esteem, adds to the cost of health care and may
result in loss of independence by virtue of the reluctance of women with this problem to leave
the house. Prevalence is difficult to estimate since it is underreported. At a consensus
conference it was determined that in industrialized nations stress incontinence occurs in 8%
to 51% of the population.[1] The reason for these wide estimate variations is that there are
differences in populations studied and definition of the condition. An estimated 10-12 million
adult Americans suffer with this problem annually at a cost of over $13.3 billion.[2] There is
a definitive difference in prevalence by gender with older women three times more likely to
have urinary tract problems as men. Genuine stress urinary incontinence is defined as the
involuntary loss of urine which occurs when, in the absence of a detrusor contraction, the
intravesical pressure exceeds the maximum urethral pressure.[3] The elements which maintain
higher intraurethral pressure at rest and during stress include the internal and external urethral
sphincters and support anatomically at the urethrovesical junction.[4] The presence of stress
incontinence was assessed by a history and physical examination, a pad test, the Q-tip test,
perianal sensory testing and urethroscopy. Uroflowmetry, water cystometry and urethral
pressure profiles were performed using Surgitek's UDS 1000, computerized urodynamic testing
equipment with microcatheters and multichannel recordings. In addition, patients were given
an extensive questionnaire that elicited information regarding the type of problem the patient
was experiencing as well as variables that have been hypothesized to be causally associated with
stress incontinence.

Data were collected relating to demographic characteristics including age, race, marital
status, education and height and weight so that Body Mass Index (BMI)[5] could be determined.
In addition, information was solicited regarding concomitant medical condition such as diabetes
mellitus or hypertension. The number of live births by vaginal delivery was determined as were
number of delivers in which the woman had an episiotomy, forceps were used, labor was
prolonged (more than 12 hours) and number of spontaneous births whether the infant weighed
over 8 lbs.

Uroflowmetry allowed the determination of peak flow rate, time to peak, volume
voided, flow time and mean flow rate. In order to determine the resting and stress pressures
simultaneously, within the urethra and bladder, a microcatheter was inserted into the urethra.
This catheter had a pressure-sensitive transducer distally (for recording bladder pressure) and
one proximally to measure urethral pressure. A second transducer was introduced into the
vagina; this measured intra-abdominal pressure. By subtracting abdominal pressure from
bladder pressure it was possible to determine the true vesical pressure. Water cystometry,
therefore, provided measurement of maximum true vesical pressure, volumes at first feeling
of fullness of the bladder and volume when feeling full, maximal urethral pressure when
coughing and total volume of water infused. Finally, with the bladder full and the patient

standing upright, intra-abdominal pressure was raised and the patient was observed for demonstration of stress incontinence. During the assessment of the urethral pressure profile, a puller or profilometer was attached to the microcatheter that had been inserted into the urethra and the microcatheter was mechanically withdrawn at a constant speed. This procedure allowed the measurement of the functional length of the urethra, defined as the length of the urethra along which the urethral pressure exceeds intravesical pressure. In addition, the Pressure Transmission Ratio was determined; the increase in urethral pressure expressed as a percentage of the simultaneously recorded increase in intravesical pressure when stress is placed on the system in terms of increased abdominal pressure.[3] It has been suggested that a short functional urethra and Transmission Pressure Ratios below 100% may be correlated with stress incontinence and that a quantitative relationship exists.[6,7]

A standardized pad test that had been modified for older patients was also used to assess the presence of stress incontinence. After voiding, patients were asked to don a preweighed pad and were then asked to drink 600 mls of water. Following one and a half hours of sitting, patients were asked to perform a number of provocative maneuvers designed to increase the intra-abdominal pressure. The pad was then reweighed to determine whether or not there had been any loss of urine. This test was repeated on a random basis on twenty patients to examine its reliability as a quantitative means of assessing stress incontinence.

Following their assessment, a number of patients were treated with intravaginal cream and some patients received oral estrogen also. In addition, patients with very poor urethral closure pressures were referred for physical therapy twice a week in order that they could receive interferential current therapy for pelvic floor musculature while those with some pelvic floor strength who were highly motivated were referred for pelvic floor exercises using the vaginal cones recently reported in the literature. Estrogen treatment, interferential therapy and vaginal cones have all been reported as effective treatments for stress incontinence but estrogens have been tried alone while the physical therapy treatments have been utilized with premenopausal women only.[8,9,10,11]

Analysis of the data from our initial patients has revealed no differences in demographic data between women who have stress incontinence and those who do not. A total of 56 patients were evaluated in the initial group. Six were referred for presurgical evaluation only. For the remaining 50 patients, 14 patients had a diagnosis of pure stress, 14 had urge incontinence, 21 patients had both stress and urge incontinence and one patient had overflow incontinence. The patients with the differing diagnoses had suffered these problems for a mean of 5.65 years (range 1-25), 8.21 years (range 1-40) and 7.14 years (range 1-20) and 2 years, respectively. Fifty-three patients were white and 3 were hispanic. The mean age of the group was 60.75 years (range 29-81); educationally, 42 (75%) were high school or college graduates, 8 (42%) had some high school, while 6 (10.8%) had 8th grade schooling or less. Using the Body Mass Index (BMI) it was determined that of the 53 patients on which these data were collected, 16 (30.18%) were at an "acceptable" weight, 24 (45.28%) were "overweight" and 13 (24.52%) were "obese." When the group was examined for the presence of specific concomitant conditions, of 56 patients, 4 (7.14%) had diabetes mellitus, 11 (19.64%) had hypertension and 3 (5.35%) had both diabetes mellitus and hypertension. It was interesting to note that 9 patients (16.07%) were smokers and 4 (7.14%) had a chronic cough, however none of the smokers complained of a chronic cough. Eighteen patients (32.14%) complained of constipation.

Twelve of the 56 patients were nulliparous. The mean number of spontaneous vaginal deliveries for the remaining 44 patients was 3.15 live births (range 1-11). Thirty-three (75%) women reported having undergone an episiotomy, 15 (34%) had prolonged labor (greater than twelve hours), 23 (52.27%) gave birth to at least one infant weighing more than 8 lbs., 18

(41%) patients indicated that forceps had been used during delivery of at least one infant and 6 women (11.36%) experienced stress incontinence during pregnancy.

Mean peak flow rates, time to peak, volume voided, flow time and mean flow rates assessed during water cystometry were found to be 35.46mls/sec, 6.96secs, 534 mls, 24.26 secs and 22 mls/sec, respectively. In the group of patients that has been examined to date, 5 of the women with stress incontinence had a functional urethral length of less than 2.5 cms, and 4 patients had Pressure Transmission Ratios of less than 100%. It was clearly evident from the reliability study of the pad test that this test may not be used to quantitatively assess the extent of stress incontinence since a statistically significant difference was found between the first and second pad weights ($p < .01$). These findings were somewhat surprising in view of the widespread use of this test and the fact that it had been standardized. The majority of patients using estrogen report an improvement in their incontinence problem and preliminary results with the cones are promising.

References

1. Consensus Development Conference on Urinary Incontinence in Adults (1990) Special Contribution. *Int Urogynecol J* 1:109-116

2. Norton PA (1990) Prevalence and social impact of urinary incontinence in women (1990) *Clin Ob & Gyn* 33(2):295-297

3. The standardization of terminology of lower urinary tract function recommended by the International Continence Society (1990) Special Contribution. *Int Urogynecol J* 1:45-48

4. Summitt RL, Bent AE, Ostergard DR (1990) The pathophysiology of genuine stress incontinence. *Int Urogynecol J* 1:12-18

5. Gray GA (1985) Obesity: definition, diagnosis and disadvantages. *Med J Australia* 142:S2-S8

6. Bump RC, Copeland WC, Hurt WG, Fantl JA (1988) Dynamic urethral pressure/profilometry pressure transmission ratio determinations in stress-incontinent and stress-continent subjects. *Am J Obstet Gynecol* 159(3):749-755

7. Hilton P, Stanton SL (1983) Urethral pressure measurement by micro-transducer: The results in symptom-free women and in those with genuine stress incontinence. *Br J Obstet Gynecol* 90:19-25

8. Olah KS, Bridges N, Denning J, Farrar DJ (1990) The conservative management of patients with symptoms of stress incontinence: A randomized, prospective study comparing weighted vaginal cones and interferential therapy. *Am J Obstet Gynecol* 162:87-92

9. Rudd T (1980) The effects of estrogens and gestagens on the urethral pressure profile in urinary continent and incontinent women. *Acta Obstet Gynecol Scand* 59:265-267

10. Hilton P, Stanton SL (1983) The use of intravaginal estrogen cream in genuine stress incontinence. *Br J Gynaecol* 90:940-946

11. Stanton S, Plevnick S, Peattie A et al (1986) A conservative method of treating genuine stress incontinence. In: *Proceedings of the 16th Annual Meeting of the International Continence Society*, Boston 227-229

THE PHYSIOTHERAPIST AS CONTINENCE ADVISER.

P.E. CHIARELLI.
HUNTER CONTINENCE ADVISORY SERVICE
10 SMITH ST.,CHARLESTOWN. 2290.N.S.W. AUSTRALIA.

AIM OF THE STUDY.

Incontinence is "the silent epidemic". The physiotherapist possesses skills unique to the profession which can be very effective in the management of incontinence.

Physiotherapists are now being called upon to treat signs of bladder dysfunction other than simple stress incontinence, such as urge incontinence and mixed stress/urge.

In order to maximise physiotherapeutic interventions, the averaged profile of all the women presenting for treatment was sought in order that it might be compared to the typical profile of a successfully treated patient. In this way, this clinical review might provide information for physiotherapists that will help them more confidently approach the treatment of incontinence.

METHODS.

Macintosh Plus computer with Foxbase and Excel 2.2 were used to examine the information taken from the case notes of patients seen between October 1988 and October 1990 suffering incontinence in various forms.

This study looked at 178 patients.21 women did not receive electrotherapy as part of their treatmentand, 10 were males.These 31 patients were not considered in this this review.

Patients filled in a time/volume chart before presenting for assesment, and were seen by a physiotherapist/continence adviser within a private, general physiotherapy clinic.

Pelvic Floor Muscle Assessment was done using the grading method described by Chiarelli and Laycock (Chiarelli and Laycock, 1989) and thus included a contraction grading from 0 -5, an assessment of length of hold and the number of repetitions possible.

Treatment Regime: This followed Laycocks "Algorithm for Physiotherapy Management of Incontinence" (Laycock,1989), and electrotherapy was delivered using a pre-modulated current from an Erbe1M interferential with a remote surge attachment(Scwellformer) via two, externally applied electrodes. The larger of the two(9 cms by 5.5cms) was placed over the anus, the smaller(5cms by 3cms), over the clitoral area. Vaginal stimulation became available in October1989 using a Medicon MS-105 personal stimulator and treatment using this stimulator was used, following the standard treatment protocols described by Bjarne Eriksen (Eriksen,1989).

Apart from the different application of the electrical current, other treatment parameters remained virtually the same. These included : pelvic floor exercise programmes, perineometer, weighted vaginal cones, inflated foleys catheter used within the vagina as a means of resistance and a bladder training programme where indicated.

RESULTS.

Referral Sources: | | | | |
|---|---|---|---|
| General Practitioner | - 44.06%. | Obstetrician/Gynaecologist | - 27.27% |
| Urologist | - 16.08%. | Self | - 12.59% |

Subjective assessment:

Subjective assessment was made using the patient's time/volume chart and a standardised assessment questionaire. Of the 147 patients the following information was recorded.

Age Range: from 23 yrs to 81 yrs, average 45.8 yrs.

Types of Incontinence: Regardless of any accompanying signs and symptoms, the patients were divided into 2 groups 120 (82%) were suffering urinary stress incontinence, 27 (18%) were suffering urgency and or urge incontinence without stress incontinence.

Length of Time Symptoms Had Been Present :

Less than 1 year - 14.2%	1-4 years - 28.5%,
5-9 years - 19.7%	longer than 10yrs - 30.6%.

Parity: Average parity was 2.6 and 10 of the women were non parous.

Obstetric Risk Factors: Those factors known to cause damage to innervation of the pelvic floor muscles were noted. 60 women(43.7%) reported no obstetric risk factors in 95 deliveries other than multiparity . Of the remaining 77 parous women, there were 281 deliveries. Some women reported up to 8 risk factors. There did not appear to be any correlation between types of risk factors and severity of symptoms or their response to treatment.

Previous Urogenital Surgery: 80 women(54.4%) reported no previous urogenital surgery. The number of surgical interventions on the remaining 67 women ranged from 1 to 7.

Need For Onward Referral: Covert contra-indications to treatment were not seen and therefore the need to refer on was minimal.. Of the total 147, 16 (10.8%) were referred thus:

7 referred to their General practitioner for review of medication
2 referred to G.P. for hormone replacement therapy for atrophic vaginitis.
5 referred back to referring specialist
1 referred to nurse continence adviser for testing of residual urine volume
1 referred to a psychologist specialising in sexual counselling

Other Factors That Might Be Contributing To The Incontinence :

None	53.99%
Chronic Airways Disease	10.43%
Recurent Infections	6.75%
Caffeine Intake	6.75%
Obesity	6.13%
Drugs	4.91%
Diabetes	4.29%
Surgery	3.68%
decreased fluid intake	3.07%

Stated Signs and Symptoms as Seen Against Actual Signs and Symptoms:

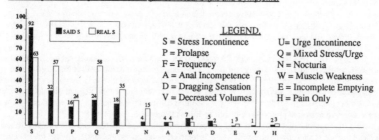

LEGEND.

S = Stress Incontinence   U= Urge Incontinence
P = Prolapse   Q = Mixed Stress/Urge
F = Frequency   N = Nocturia
A = Anal Incompetence   W = Muscle Weakness
D = Dragging Sensation   E = Incomplete Emptying
V = Decreased Volumes   H = Pain Only

Stress Incontinence: Of the 147 women in this study,120 had stress incontinence (81%).

88 described this as mild (73.9%)
25 described this as moderate (21%)
4 described this as severe (3.3%) and none of these were in the group of patients who were considered cured.

27 women (19%) were suffering urge incontinence without any stress incontinence.

Pad Protection: 70 women wore none at all, 33 wore pads only during certain activities, 17 wore panty liners and 15 wore pads.

Objective Assessment.

Urodynamic Assessment: Only 26 patients presented with the results of urodynamic testing.

Flow Stopping As A Test: Only 24 of the 120 stress incontinent women could stop their urine flow (20%), while 14 of the 27 urge/incontinent women could stop their urine flow (51.8%).

Pelvic Floor Muscle Assessment:

The average assessment was between Grades1 and 2 for stress incontinence and between Grades 2 and 3 for urge incontinence.

The average length of hold of the contraction was <3 seconds in the stress incontinent women and 3 seconds in the urgency/urge incontinent women.

The average number of contraction repetitions before fatigue was 5 in both types of incontinence.

TREATMENT RESPONSES.

The number of treatments received by each patient ranged from 3 to 24, the average being 7.5 treatments.

The timespan of these treatments in weeks was 1 to 28 with the average at 4 weeks.

Dropout rate was 14% (21 patients)

Of the 126 women who underwent treatment, 43 were cured (34%) , 54 were significantly improved(42.8%) and 26 were not helped at all (20.6%)

During a course of treatment, an increase in the assessed grade of muscle contraction was present in only 37% of all cases while increases in the "hold" ability and repetition of contractions improved more commonly.

A change in grade was noted in 44% of the "cured" group, 26% of the "improved " group but only 9% of the "no change" group.

Average age of each response group was

| CURE - 39.6yrs | IMPROVED - 50.57 yrs | NO CHANGE - 66.8yrs |

Electrostimulation Results

	CURE	IMPROVED	NO CHANGE
vaginal stimulation	56.7%	27%	16.3%
Interferential	28%	50%	22%

PROFILES: Taking the results of this clinical review, the typical profile of a woman most likely to respond to physiotherapy intervention for incontinence is as follows

	AVERAGE PRESENTED.	AVERAGE CURED.
AGE	45.8YRS	39.6
PARITY	2.6	2.4
HOW LONG SYMPTOMS	6-9YRS	1-5YRS
P.F.M. GRADE	1	2
GRADE IMPROVED	NO	YES
CONTRACTION HOLD	<3 SECS	5 SECS
CONTRACTION REPS.	5	5

DISCUSSION:

It would appear from this data that physiotherapy intervention is worthwhile in the treatment of incontinence. Incontinence appears to respond better to electrotherapy delivered vaginally than via the perineum It can also be seen that the age and the length of time the symptoms had been present of the patients successfully treated is lower than than thoseonly improved or not helped at all . This indicates that one of the most effective interventions that physiotherapists might undertake is more vigorous public promotion of pelvic floor muscle exercise programmes aimed at younger women, as soon after the onset of their symptoms as possible.

REFERENCES.

1. Laycock,J.(1989). Algorithm For The Physiotherapy Management of Incontinence. Neurourol and Urodyn. 8.4.353-354.

2. Chiarelli,P.,Laycock, J., (1989), Pelvic Floor Assessment and Re-education. I.C.S. Ljubljana. Papers read by title. 206-207.

3. Snooks,S.J.,Swash,M, M.,Henry,M.M.,Setchell,M.1985. Risk Factors In Childbirth Causing Damage to the Pelvic Floor Innervation. Br.J.Surg., Vol 72, Suppl.,Sept 1985

4. Eriksen.B.C. 1989. Electrostimulation of the Pelvic Floor in Female Urinary Incontinence. Tapir, Trondheim,Norway.

Stress incontinence : Physiotherapy Management in the U.K.

Jill Mantle, Physio Div, Polytechnic of E. London, London E15 4LZ.
Eboo Versi, Dept of Obstetrics & Gynaecology, The Royal London Hospital
London. E1 1BB.

INTRODUCTION

Over the last fifteen years Physiotherapists in the UK have
experienced a resurgence of interest in the conservative management
of patients with urinary incontinence, and particularly urinary
stress incontinence (S.I). Various physiotherapeutic modalities and
techniques are used in the treatment of S.I[1] but there is a lack of
efficacy data, and no reliable data even as to what constitutes the
concensus opinion as to 'best practice'.

METHOD

In February 1989 a postal survey was carried out using an eight paged
detailed questionnaire. This was sent to the District or Senior
Physiotherapist in each of the National Health Service District
Authorities/Boards/Units of management throughout the entire United
Kingdom. A concensus response was requested, via the physiotherapist
who most commonly treated SI in each area, regarding:-

1. seniority and qualifications of personnel commonly treating such
   patients,
2. agency and reason for referral,
3. modalities available and the two most frequently selected,
4. detailed treatment methodology,
5. rating of the efficacy of each available modality,
6. prognostic features.
7. current work load.

RESULTS

The response rate was 90%; 222 localities responded out of a total
of 246 (England 189 of 192, 98%; Wales 8 of 9, 89%, Scotland 18 of
25, 72%, Northern Ireland 7 of 20, 35%).

It was claimed by respondents that 58% of physiotherapist treating
SI were Senior 1 grade or above and that 65% of all physiotherapists
treating SI made a specialty of it. Gynaecologist were reported as
six times more likely to be the commonest agency for referral, and
the chief reason for referral for physiotherapy was as the first line
of treatment.

Table I to show modality availability and preceived efficacy

	Avalability	Efficacy.
Pelvic floor contractions	100%	73%
Interferential Therapy	93%	63%
General exercises	61%	37%
'Faradism'	52%	44%
Perineometer	27%	57%
Vaginal cones	16%	55%
Interupted D.C.	4%	23%

Table I shows the availability and perceived efficacy of each modality. Pelvic floor contractions (PFC) and Interferential Therapy (IT) were selected as the two modalities of choice (98% & 77% respectively) for SI and also considered to be the most effective.

Considerable variation was found in treatment methodology. Table II shows some of the data collected in relation to PFC as an example. However the greatest variation was shown with regard to Interferential Therapy. Technique was obviously dictated to some degree by the equipment available. A majority of respondents used 4000 H_z carrier wave and four electrodes. The frequency sweeps employed fell into two main groupings, 0-100 H_z (+ or - a narrower band) and 10-50 H_z (+ or - narrower band). There was a further small group which did not fit this division, and in all there were over 60 different permutations.

Table II mean data for pelvic floor contraction methodology.

Explain anatomy & condition	22 mins,	range 1 - 60
Teaching contractions	19 mins,	range 1 - 180
Hold each contraction	5 secs,	range 1 - 60
Repeat contraction per session	7 times,	range 1 - 50
Practice	Hourly, range every 15 mins	
		- 3 x per day.

General exercise consisted chiefly of trunk exercise often incorporating PFC; low frequency electrical stimulation of the levator ani muscle, available to 52% of respondents was usually applied with a sacral or abdominal indifferent electrode and an active vaginal or perineal electrode. A perineometer was available in 27% of localities but rarely was a patient able to take one home for practice. Vaginal cones were evidently gaining in popularity and in general were used according to the manufacturers' instructions.

Obesity, previous surgery, lack of motivation and a long history were considered pessimistic prognostic features, while positive motivation, recent onset of symptoms, being premenopausal and being able to produce a palpable pelvic floor contraction were judged as optomistic features. There was no correlation between the size of the population in a locality and the number of cases of SI being treated annually by physiotherapists.

CONCLUSION

These combined results for the four provinces of the United Kingdom agree with those already published for England[2]. Much variation in detailed methodologies was found, but PFC and IT were selected as the treatments of choice for urinary stress incontinence, and the patients' positive motivation was considered vital. There is an urgent need for well designed research to establish sound efficacy data.

REFERENCE

1. Polden, M., Mantle, J. (1990): Physiotherapy in Obstetrics and Gynaecology. Ch 11. Published by Butterworth Heinemann.

2. Mantle, J., Versi, E. (1991): Physiotherapy for stress urinary incontinence: a national survey. British Medical Journal (In press).

RESPIRATORY CARE

USE OF NASAL INTERMITTENT POSITIVE PRESSURE VENTILATION IN THE TREATMENT OF RESPIRATORY FAILURE DUE TO ACUTE EXACERBATIONS OF COPD.

J Bott, JH Conway, RA Hitchcock, SEJ Keilty, EM Ward, SH Mill, A Brown, M Carroll, MW Elliott, RC Godfrey, JA Wedzicha, ST Holgate, J Moxham. Department of Thoracic Medicine, King's College School of Medicine and Dentistry, London, Southampton General Hospital, Southampton and London Chest Hospital, London, England.

Nasal intermittent positive pressure ventilation (NIPPV) is now widely used in the treatment of chronic respiratory failure due to neuro-muscular or musculo-skeletal disease. Recent studies of NIPPV for episodes of acute on chronic respiratory failure have shown encouraging results.

We are conducting a randomised controlled trial of patients with acute respiratory failure ($PaCO_2$ > 6.0 kPa, PaO_2 < 7.5 kPa, breathing room air) due to exacerbations of COPD (chronic obstructive pulmonary disease: FEV_1/FVC < 50% predicted). The control group receive conventional therapy (any or all of: bronchodilators, steroids, antibiotics, diuretics, physiotherapy and respiratory stimulants), and the treatment group receive conventional therapy + NIPPV. Arterial blood gas tensions on air, spirometry, exercise tolerance and subjective measurements of breathlessness are recorded on admission, on days 3 and 7 and on discharge.

To date 22 patients have been studied and recruitment will continue until 60 have completed. This study will provide information on the place of NIPPV in the treatment of acute exacerbations of COPD.

INTERMITTENT POSITIVE EXPIRATORY PRESSURE BREATHING BY MASK IMPROVES
PULMONARY FUNCTION AFTER CORONARY-BYPASS SURGERY.

M. THORDÉN,S-E RICKSTEN,A.BENGTSSON,H.KVIST
Depatment of Physiotherapy,Anesthesia and Intencive Care and Radiology,
Sahlgrenska Hospital, Gothenburg, Sweden.

INTRODUCTION: Patients undergoing coronary-bypass surgery frequently develops severe
pulmonary dysfunction after the operation. Different breathing apparatus has been
used as an aid to chest physiotherapy. The aim was to study the effect of two
different breathing devices on patientundergoing elective coronary bypass surgery.
TREATMENT AND METHODS: Thirty-three patients were preoperatively stratified according
to pulmonary function, age, body weight, smoking history and sex and randomized to one
of two groups: (1) Control group, reciving postoperatively incentive spirometry(Triflo)
for 30 breaths every awake hour for five postoperativ days. (2) PEP-group, with the
postoperative application of PEP (Positive Expiratory Pressure) on a face mask with
a one-way valve and a peak expiratory pressure of 10-15 cm H2O, for 30 breaths every
awake hour for five postoperative days. The (A-a)O2-difference (50% oxygen), chest
x-ray and FRC (Functional Residual Capacity) Were recorded preopeatively and on the
first, third and fifth postoperative day. FVC (Forced Vital Capacity) and FEV.1 were
measure preoperatively and on the fifth postoperativ day.
RESULTS: There were no significant difference between the two groups concerning the
above mentioned parameters preoperatively and immediatly after the operation and on
the first postoperative day. However on the third and fifth postoperative day the
(A-a)O2-difference were significantly lower in the PEP-group compared to the control
group. There were no significant differences between the two groups as referring to
preoperative and postoperative values of chest x-ray, FRC, FVC or FEV.1 .
CONCLUSION:After coronary bypass surgery, chest physiotherapy using intermittent
application of postoperative expiratory pressure significantly improves postoperative
(A-a)O2-difference compared to incentive spirometry.

THE EFFECT OF INCENTIVE SPIROMETRY IN POST-OPERATIVE BREATHING EXERCISE

G. I. ODIA
DEPARTMENT OF PHYSIOTHERAPY, COLLEGE OF MEDICINE, UNIVERSITY OF LAGOS,
SURULERE, LAGOS, NIGERIA.

Post-operative pulmonary complications (PPC) make up the largest single cause of morbidity and prolonged hospitalization after major surgical procedures[1]. Atelectasis is the commonest of such complications[2]. The aetiology of PPC is presumed to be a decrease in lung volumes[3]. The physiotherapist therefore spends a lot of time in improving lung volumes both pre- and post-operatively. The regimen involved includes deep breathing exercises, regional expansion of the lung, and expectoration of sputum. In this paper, this regimen is termed conventional chest physiotherapy (CCP). Several reports on the effectiveness of CCP have appeared in the literature. The results of these reports are mixed. This led Kigin[4] to conclude that there is need for further studies that carefully define breathing exercises and their benefits to post-operative patients. CCP is essentially an educational process. The fact that the value of such a training is in doubt necessitates the introduction of better and more objective techniques. The importance of feedback in the learning process is well recognised[5]. In biofeedback therapy, audiovisual displays are used to shape the patient's response towards a desired goal. Incentive spirometry (ISP) presents such a feedback. In this paper, a trainer which produces a simple audio-visual feedback for Forced Vital Capacity (FVC) and Peak Expiratory Flow Rate (PEFR) is described, the effectiveness of CPP and training using ISP are evaluated, and a comparison of the therapeutic advantage offered by ISP over CPP is clinically studied. INSTRUMENTATION: The spiro Trainer used in this study is a pocket spirometer (M.S. Krausz Harari Ltd., 87 Ravensdale Road, London, England) modified by removing its outer dial ring and replacing it with a nylon dial ring which carries a metal pin connected to the negative end of the battery supply. The calibration on the nylon dial ring is a replica of that on the clock arm of the positive end of the battery, the terminal which is split to end in the door bell and torch-light bulb, both of which are fixed to the wooden box. The circuit is closed only when the needle pointer of the spirometer makes contact with the metal pin of the nylon dial ring, and when this happens the door bell rings, and the torch-light bulb is lit simultaneously. The patient sets a new target each time during practice.

For the Peak Flow Trainer, the Mini-Wright Peak Flow Meter (Mini-Wright Peak Flow Meter, Clement Clarke International Ltd., 15 Wigmore Street, London, England) is used. A nylon ring which can be slided up and down is fixed round the Mini-Wright casing. Two metal strips are mounted on the nylon ring. The lower strip is attached to the positive terminal from the battery supply, and the top metal strip is attached to the negative terminal of the power supply. These terminals are split to end in the door bell and the torch-light bulb, both of which are fixed to the wooden box. The circuit is closed when the pointer of the peak flow meter makes contact with the top metal strip mounted on the nylon strip. When this happens the bell rings, and the light bulb is lit. These two instruments were then calibrated in the Chemical Engineering Department of the University of Lagos.

METHOD: Operation lists from three firms in the Department of Surgery of the Lagos University Teaching Hospital viz: Orthopaedics, General Surgery and Thoracic Surgery were collected weekly pre-operatively. From the Orthopaedics lists all patients undergoing sequestrectomy of the humerus, ulnar, radius tibia and femur were classified as operations to the limbs. In the General Surgery list, all patients undergoing laparatomy, and cholecystectomy were classified as upper abdominal operations. In the thoracic surgery group, patients undergoing thoracotomy without removal of lung tissue were chosen. After categorizing them, each patient was allocated by random sample of 1 in 2 into either Group A or Group B. Group A was taught to improve FVC and PEFR using CCP while Group B was taught using both CCP and ISP. For ethical reasons, a group receiving no training was ruled out. The patients then carried out the training post-operatively for 5 minutes every hour between 9.00 a.m. and 12.00 noon, and 2.00 to 4.00 p.m. The FVC and PEFR of each patient were measured daily until pre-operative levels were reached or until discharged, using a spirometer (Vitalograph Ltd., Buckingham, England) and a Wright's peak flow meter respectively. Allocation of patients for each operation was stopped whenever 10 patients had been allocated to each group.

ANALYSIS OF DATA: The mean values of FVC, and PEFR for each day for each group of patients was calculated and used to plot a graph which shows the percentage of the pre-operative value of FVC (Fig. I) and PEFR (Fig. II) for 10 days after the operation. The paired ('t') test was used to compare the lung function values, FVC, and PEFR for both CCP and ISP groups: A confidence expressed as (P) was set at P 0.5. In all figures all 10 patients in each group were considered together for any significant changes.

RESULT: Fig. I shows the mean FVC expressed in percentage of pre-operative value for up to ten days after the operation in both groups. There is reduction in FVC on Day I which varies according to the operation. Sequestrectomy being least affected (5%), low abdominal operations by 12 to 20%, and high abdominal operations by 46 to 68%. FVC readings improved and reached pre-operative values within a day in limb operations, two to four days in lower abdominal operations, and did not reach 100% in the ten days in upper abdominal operations. When 't' test was used to compare the CCP and ISP groups, there was no statistically significant difference between them in operations to the limb (t = 1 n.s.).

Fig. II shows values for PEFR. The figures are similar to those of FVC except that the percent drop in PEFR in the first post-operative day for upper abdominal and thoracic operations was more than that of FVC.

There is a statistically significant difference of varying degrees between groups A and B in all other operations (Table I).

DISCUSSION: Both FVC and PEFR are adversely affected by operations. The fact that limb operations are less affected, than abdominal operations suggest that incisions are of greater importance in bringing about these changes than anaesthesia. This impression is confirmed by Anscombe[6]. PEFR values in Fig. II are less than those of FVC. PEFR may therefore be

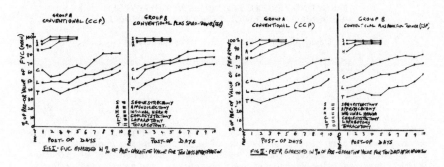

FIG.I. FVC EXPRESSED IN % OF PRE-OPERATIVE VALUE FOR TEN DAYS AFTER OPERATION

FIG.II. PEFR EXPRESSED IN % OF PRE-OPERATIVE VALUE FOR TEN DAYS AFTER OPERATION

OPERATION	DEGREE OF SIGNIFICANCE FVC	DEGREE OF SIGNIFICANCE PEFR
Sequestrectomy	N.S.	N.S.
Appendicectomy	P < 0.5	P < 0.5
Hernia	P < .05	P < .05
Cholecystectomy	P < .01	P < .01
Laparotomy	P < .01	P < .01
Thoracotomy	P < .01	P < .01

TABLE I: P VALUE WHEN CPP AND ISP GROUPS WERE COMPARED

be a more sensitive indicator of chest complications than FVC.

A pilot study carried out before this study was embarked on indicated that it is not possible to use the trainers without first explaining the desired goal to the patients. This in effect was CCP. Hence the grouping ISP is actually CCP plus ISP. Therefore, although the spiro and peak flow trainers are shown here to provide better results, they do not replace but complement CCP.

REFERENCES

1. Barlet RH et al (1973) Studies on the pathogenesis and prevention of post-operative pulmonary complications. Surg. Gynae. and Obst. 137: 925 - 933.
2. Tisi GM (1979) Pre-operative evaluation of pulmonary function. Am. Rev. Respir. Dis. 122: 147 - 154.
3. Peters RM, Turnier E (19) Physical Therapy: Indications for and Effects in Surgical patients. Am. Respir. Dis 122: 147 - 154.
4. Kigin CM (1981) Chest Physical Therapy for the post-operative or traumatic injury patient. Physical Therapy 61: 1224 - 1736.
5. Basmajian JV (1981) Biofeedback in Rehabilitation: A Review of principles and practices. Arch. Phys. Med. Rehabil. 62: 969-975.
6. Anscombe AR (1957) Pulmonary Complications of Abdominal Surgery. Lloyd-Luke (Medical Books) Ltd., 49 Newman St., London.

TARGETING AEROSOLISED DRUGS AT THE ALVEOLI
- DESIGNING A PROTOCOL & CHOOSING EQUIPMENT.

David Lester.   B.App. Sci. (Physiotherapy)

The delivery of medication via a nebuliser has the advantage of targeting a relatively small dose directly to the site of action, enabling a more rapid onset of action, while reducing systemic side effects. Disadvantages of nebuliser therapy may include dependance on appropriate equipment and effective technique, reduced effectiveness where airway obstruction and/or alveolar filling are present, and ability to contain systemic conditions (2).

Physiotherapists are involved in the administration of nebulised therapeutic aerosols in a variety of treatment situations. While some nebulised aerosols are targeted at the conducting airways, eg bronchodilators, others need to reach the bronchioles and alveoli. These include Pentamidine for PCP in AIDS, Antibiotics for Cystic Fibrosis, antivirals for conditions such as bronchiolitis, cortico steriods for asthma, COAD and inflammatory conditions, as well as diagnostic applications such as lung function testing and differential diagnosis of pulmonary emboli.

By improved targeting of aerosols to the lower airways and alveoli, the effectiveness of most aerosol therapies can be enhanced, drug utilisation improved, and side effects, both systemic and in the upper airways, reduced (2).

Aerosol particles deposit themselves be either inertial impaction on the airways, especially at bifurcations, or by gravitational sedimentation in the small airways and alveoli. As a guide, particles with a diameter of > 8 μm. will primarily deposit in the orophorynx, for $5 - 8\mu$m. in the larger airways (generations $1 - 8$), $2 - 5\mu$m. in the larger airways (gen. $9 - 16$), $0.5 - 2\mu$m. in the bronchioles and alveoli (gen. $17 - 23$), & those $< 0.5\mu$m. will be exhaled (2,3).

The goal of aerosol therapy is the delivery of an adequate dose of a drug to the appropriate sites in the lungs. The effectiveness of aerosol therapy using a nebuliser will depend on the equipment and how it is used, the characteristics and actions of the person, and the environment in which therapy in given.

The Equipment.
The major factor which determines the site of deposition is the particle size profile. Particle size is primarily determined by the characteristics of the nebuliser, the design of the system delivering the aerosol to the person, plus the flow rate of the driving gas.

<u>Nebulisers</u> Most clinical nebulisers will produce a cloud of particles which vary in size. The best measure of such a heterodispersed cloud is its Mass Median Aerodynic Diameter (MMAD), which tells us that 50% of the total mass of the aerosol will be contained in particles smaller than the value indicated.

The Mass Median Diameter (MMD) and Volume Median Diameter (VMD) are also useful measures. The MMAD is the product of the MMD and the square root of the liquids density. The Geometric Standard Deviation (GSD or σ_g) is sometimes quoted. It is the ratio of the 84% to 50% points on the cumulative mass distribution. It indicates the degree of spread of particle sizes. Its value should be between 1.5 and 2.5. Measures such as % of particles smaller than a given size, say 5 µm., are misleading as the bulk of the total mass could be in a few relatively large droplets.

The volume of fluid in the nebuliser will not greatly affect the MMAD. Larger volumes will increase the time to completion, possibly effecting compliance. The smaller the fill volume the greater the proportion of drug either not nebulised, or trapped in the system (ie. the dead volume). A volume in the range of 4-6 ml is recommended (2).

Delivery Systems. A variety of configurations are available. Convoluted tubing may excessively trap aerosol and reduce output. Storage reservoirs, in combination with valves redirecting exhaled air, reduce aerosol loss and optimise output. A purpose designed baffle valve downstream of the nebuliser will reduce the MMAD by blocking mainly large particles (4).

Gas Sources. The higher the flow rate of the gas passing through the nebuliser the smaller the particle size it produces. This effect will vary in degree between nebulisers. Most nebulisers will need flow rates in excess of 6 l.min[-1] and may need up to 10 l.min[-1] to produce an MMAD of 1.5 - 2µm. for alveolar targeting. Bottled gas allows greater flexibility in flow rate selection, but tends to be inconvenient and expensive. Hospital ducted gas often has too low a flow rate. Compressors are more convenient but less flexible and tend to be more unreliable, often with no gauge to check output pressures and therefore flow rates. Pressure and flow rate are inversely related. Manufacturers usually quote 'static' pressures and maximum 'free flow' rates. These measures are usually twice the more representative 'dynamic' pressures and flow rates that occur when a nebuliser is placed in line(2,3).

The Person.
Aerosol deposition is reliant on the distribution of ventilation, which may be effected by anatomical variation, previous surgery/trauma, lung disease (alveolar filling and airway obstruction), posture, breathing pattern and psychological response to treatment.

If indicated secretion removal stratagies should be implemented ahead of therapy. Bronchodilators should be used where previous use has been necessary or if the person experiences excessive coughing during therapy. Possible benefits from blanket use of bronchodilators must be weighed against side effects. Do not use the same apparatus for different drugs.

In sitting, while breathing from FRC, ventilation goes to dependent zones (5). Changing to supine creates a more even distribution but reduces the FRC, risking small airway closure. Breathing from residual volume produces even distribution in either posture.

A more significant factor is the inspiratory flow rate (IFR). At high IFR (80 l. min^{-1}) impaction on upper airways accounts for most of the aerosol. Lower IFR (25 l.min^{-1}) gives deeper penetration and sedimentation in small airways and alveoli, though preferentially to dependent zones (5).

Increasing the inspired volume favours increased peripheral deposition. Holding the inspired breath favours peripheral sedimentation (2,3). Preferably a nose clip should be worn to prevent nasal breathing, including exhalation.

The Environment. The humidity of the driving and diluting gases will affect particle size, dry gas tending to reduce MMAD. The humidity within the persons airways will tend to increase particle sizes.
The therapy room should be well ventilated. Exposure of staff to toxic drugs via released aerosol will be very low if the room is ventilated, the exhalation port on the system has a filter, the person wears a nose clip and turns off the nebuliser when removing if from their mouth (1).
N.B. Equipment should be cleaned with warm soapy water, rinsed, dried and then left to dry thoroughly before storage. Education of staff and patients is vital to avoid potentially lethal infections.

Summary.
When choosing equipment for alveolar targeting of aerosols it is essential that the equipment is evaluated as a unit. Manufacturers claims are often misleading and interchange of component parts can vary aerosol characteristics by as much as a factor of 5 (2).
The aerosol produced at the mouth piece should have an MMAD of 1.5 - 2μm. and GSD of approx. 2. This will probably need a purpose designed nebuliser, driven by a dynamic flow of 8 l.min^{-1}, and delivered via a system which includes an in line baffle valve as well as an exhalation phase reservoir.
The person should be comfortably seated perferably in a reclining chair. After bronchodilator therapy and a 10-15 minute break, the person will inhale normally from the mouth piece, nose clip in position. They should be instructed to inhale slowly, holding the breath for 3-4 seconds every 5 breaths. Every minute they should exhale fully followed by a slow deep inhalation. The person should recline to approx. 45 degrees halfway through treatment.
Excessive coughing may be helped by reducing the driving gas flow rate if it is >10 l.min^{-1}, or by reducing the persons IFR.

References:
(1)-Montgomery AB, Corkery KJ, Brunette H, Leoung GS, Waskin H & Debs RJ (1990) Occupational exposure to aerosolised Pentamidine. Chest, 98: 386-388.
(2)-Newman S.P. (1989) Nebuliser Therapy: Scientific and technical Aspects. Astra, Lund.
(3)-Phipps P, Borham P, Gonda I, Bailey D, Bautovich G & Anderson S (1989) Eur. J Nuc. Med., 13: 183-186.
(4)-Simonds A.K., Newman S.P., Johnson M.A., Talace N., Lee C.A., Clarke S.W. (1989), Simple Nebuliser modification to enhance alveolar deposition of Pentamidine. Lancet: Oct 89, 953.
(5)-Stahlhofen W., Gebhart J., Heyder J., Scheuch G., (1983) Deposition pattern of droplets from medical nebulisers in the human respiratory tract. Bull. Europ. Physiopath. resp. 19: 459-463.

CHEST WALL STRUCTURE AND BIOMECHANICS: SOMETHING OLD AND SOMETHING NEW

L.D. Crane
University of Miami; Dept. of Orthopaedics and Rehabilitation, Division
of Physical Therapy, Coral Gables, Florida, U.S.A.

Optimal ventilation of the lungs is essential to the overall function of
the human body and is dependent on the musculoskeletal framework which
encloses the lungs, mediastinal structures and abdominal cavity. The
three components of the chest wall (CW) include the rib cage (and
associated muscles), the diaphragm and the abdomen.[1] Ventilation of the
lungs is only one of the many functions of the chest wall which also
include but are not limited to speech, singing, movements of the trunk,
maintaining posture and coughing.[2] The respiratory muscles are unique
compared to other skeletal muscles because they must contract
rhythmically and intermittently throughout life, their control is both
voluntary and involuntary and they work against resistive (airway) and
elastic (CW and lungs) loads rather than gravitational forces.[3]

The skeletal framework of the ventilatory pump includes the
manubriosternum, twelve pairs of ribs, costal cartilages and twelve
thoracic vertebrae and their intervertebral discs. Ribs 1-10 articulate
with the bodies and transverse processes of the thoracic vertebrae and
anteriorly join the sternum via their own costal cartilage (ribs 1-7) or
a common "network" of costal cartilages (ribs 8-10). The costovertebral
and costotransverse, costochondral and chondrosternal joints form a
closed kinematic chain. The orientation of the axes of motion of the
ribs for the interdependent costovertebral and costotransverse joints
generally occurs nearly in the frontal plane for the upper ribs and
approaching the sagittal plane for the lowermost ribs resulting in the
classic "pump-handle" and "bucket-handle" motions.[4,5] A controversy
regarding rib motion involves the types of motion which occur at costo-
vertebral articulations and the elasticity of the ribs. Do the ribs
rotate around a single axis or successive rotations around a shifting
axis? [5,6]

Any muscle which attaches to the chest wall and many which attach
to the shoulder girdle and thoracic vertebrae contribute to ventilation.
There is no evidence that anatomic arrangements or recruitment of the
respiratory muscles differs between males and females.[1] The diaphragm
is the primary muscle of inspiration and is really two muscles (costal
and crural) which are embryologically derived differently and function
differently.[7] The costal portion functions in "series" and the crural
diaphragm in "parallel" with each other and the intercostal and
accessory muscles. The net result of contraction of either portion of
the diaphragm depend on intercostal muscle activity, abdominal and
pelvic floor muscle activity, lung volumes, load, posture and other
influences.[8]

The intercostal muscles are traditionally classified according to
their anatomical orientation (layered external to internal in the
intercostal spaces). It is widely reported that the external
intercostals have an inspiratory action and the internal intercostals
are expiratory although the functions of the intercostal muscles are
very controversial and still not well understood. It has more recently
been conclusively shown that the interchondral part of the internal
intercostals, or parasternals, are inspiratory agonists.[9] Hamberger, in

1727, described his theory that the orientations of the insertions of the intercostal muscle fibers determine their action on the ribs. Recent studies using electromyographic (EMG) and electrical stimulation techniques show that both interosseous intercostals have similar effects on the ribs to which they attach.[10] The differences in motion during inspiration and expiration are believed to be associated with differences in compliance of the ribs between conditions of high and low lung volumes. Technological advances including EMG, radiologic and computerized motion analyses have improved the analyses of actions of the respiratory muscles but are limited because they do not provide answers regarding when these muscles function as agonists, antagonists, synergists and stabilizers.

Other muscles active during quiet inspiration include the scalenes which essentially counteract the tendency of the parasternals to pull the sternum downward. Accessory muscles such as the sternocleidomastoid, pectoralis and trapezius muscles are extremely important during exercise, disease, forced ventilation and any unsupported upper extremity activity.[11]

Expiration in quiet breathing is usually felt to be passive with elastic recoil of the lungs and chest wall. In actuality, certain muscles (such as the triangularis sterni and abdominals) may be active during expiration, especially in the upright position and end-expiration during exercise, in certain disease states (e.g. COPD) and during active or forced expiratory activities (e.g. laughing, coughing).[2,8] The abdominals can also assist with inspiration by increasing intraabdominal pressure which acts on the appositional lower ribs and pushing the diaphragm cranially with resulting upward pull on the ribs. The net effect of the abdominals on the rib cage probably depends on the balance between the muscle insertional forces (favoring expiration) and increasing intra-abdominal pressure (favoring inspiration).[8]

Integration and coordination of respiratory muscle activity becomes more complex as body position changes, during exercise, when respiratory muscles are recruited for activities other than ventilation and in chest wall and lung deformity and disease states. The complexity of the respiratory control system is related to the fact that breathing is under both voluntary and automatic control, a variety of peripheral receptors are involved and because many different combinations of muscles can be recruited for ventilation in different conditions.[12] Activation of muscles not normally active during quiet breathing is affected by habit, posture and activities being carried on simultaneously. Precise modulation of respiratory and nonrespiratory muscles via mechanoreceptor feedback is necessary in order to breathe while sustaining contraction in respiratory muscles involved in nonrespiratory activities.[13] The actions of the ventilatory pump are designed to meet the metabolic demands of the body.

Normal development and aging and pathologic conditions necessarily affect and change the biomechanics of chest wall motion and actions of the various muscles involved with ventilation.[14] The shape and compliance of the rib cage and its' articulations change significantly from the neonate to old age. Individual ribs and many articulations become less compliant with aging due to ossification of cartilage, fibrosis and fusion of anterior rib cage joints and wear and tear on costo-vertebral articulations. Various obstructive and restrictive pulmonary diseases and deformities alter normal kinematics of the chest wall and result in various forms of compensation and dysfunction.
Physical therapists, no matter what type of patients they treat, should be aware of the structure and function of the chest wall and the effects of the various perturbations they impose on patients have on ventilatory function.

REFERENCES

1. Derenne JP, Macklem PT, Roussos CH (1978) Respiratory muscles:Mechanics, control and pathophysiology (Parts I & II). Am Rev Respir Dis 118:119-133, 373-390
2. Celli BR (1989) Clinical and physiologic evaluation of respiratory muscle function. Clin Chest Med 10:199-214
3. Rochester DF, Braun NM (1978) The respiratory muscles. Basics Resp Dis 6:1-6
4. Crane LD (to be published Fall 1991) The Chest Wall, In Norkin C, Levangie P Joint Structure and Function (2nd ed), F.A. Davis, Philadelphia
5. Kapandji IA (1974) The physiology of the joints (2nd ed) Churchill Livingstone, New York, pp 130-163
6. Saumerez RC (1986) An analysis of possible movements of upper rib cage. J Appl Physiol 60:678-689
7. DeTroyer A, Sampson M, Sigrist S et al (1981) The diaphragm: Two muscles. Science 213:237-238
8. DeTroyer A, Estenne M (1988) Functional anatomy of the respiratory muscles. Clin Chest Med 9:175-193
9. DeTroyer A, Kelly S, Zin WA (1983) Mechanical action of the intercostal muscles on the ribs. Science 220:87-88
10. DeTroyer A, Kelly S, Macklem R et al (1985) Mechanics of intercostal space and actions of external and internal intercostal muscles. J Clin Invest 75:850-857
11. Macklem PT, Macklem DM, DeTroyer A (1983) A model of inspiratory muscle mechanics. J Appl Physiol 55:547-557
12. Cherniack NS (1990) The CNS and respiratory muscle coordination. Chest 97:52S-57S
13. Barnas GM, Mills PJ, MacKenzie CF et al (1991) Regional chest wall impedance during nonrespiratory maneuvers. J Appl Physiol 70:92-96
14. Estenne M, Yernault JC, DeTroyer A (1985) Rib cage and diaphragm-abdomen compliance in humans:Effects of age and posture. J Appl Physiol 59:1842-1848

CLINICAL EVALUATION OF DIAPHRAGMATIC MOVEMENT IN HEALTHY HUMAN SUBJECTS

Margaret Waterhouse
School Of Physiotherapy, Curtin University Of Technology
Selby Street, Shenton Park, Western Australia, 6008

Introduction: The diaphragm is the main muscle of respiration[1]. Accordingly, objective evaluation of the cardiopulmonary patient traditionally includes assessment of diaphragmatic excursion(DE), as it is important to have an indication of the amount of diaphragm movement in order to be able to appropriately plan a treatment programme.

Various methods exist to test DE in the chest. These include clinical evaluation, x-ray (during inspiration and expiration), kymography, fluoroscopy and ultrasonography. Chest wall percussion is commonly used, although it has been shown to be subject to significant intra-observer variation[2].

In order to determine diaphragmatic movement in the clinical situation, it has been suggested that simple observation will show whether the patient is using the diaphragm or accessory muscles of respiration[3]. Alternatively, observation of the movement of the costal margin may be used to determine diaphragmatic movement. The observation of costal margin movement, should be performed with the patient placed in either the supine position[4,5,6] or the semi-recumbent position[7]. It is also believed that observation of displacement of abdominal contents infers diaphragmatic movement. Whilst observation of costal margin movement is commonly used in the clinical situation as an indicator of DE, there is no published research establishing the relationship. Nor is there any objective measure made of either abdominal wall or costal margin movements, which are usually "subjectively" rated as "good", "fair" or "poor". Barrascout[8] discusses the importance of assessing the contribution of the diaphragm and intercostal muscles to the inspiratory phase of breathing, stating that these should be observed and recorded, but gives no indication of how this should be done.

Similarly, there is no reference in the literature to the effect of age on subcostal angle(SCA) or DE. Indeed, Zadai[9] states "Nowhere in the traditional literature could I find references to the normal resting positionof the thorax" (p.370). There is a paucity of accurate information available on SCA. Gardiner, Gray and O'Rahilly[10] state that "The subcostal angle is commonly between 70 and 110 degrees" (p.339), whilst Moore[11] gives the basic detail that "the infrasternal angle also varies in size from person to person and increases during inspiration" (p.62).

There were, therefore, three main objectives for this study.
1. To investigate the relationship between DE and (a) SCA change, and (b) abdominal girth change, through inspiratory capacity(IC).
2. To obtain normative data for (a) SCA at Functional Residual Capacity(FRC) and Total Lung Capacity(TLC), (b) change in SCA through IC, and (c) DE, in the half lying posture.
FRC and TLC were chosen as this is a range of breathing that is commonly used in the clinical situation. The half lying posture was chosen as this is one of the most functional for respiratory patients.
3. To provide a valid, simple method of measuring diaphragm function in the clinical setting.

Methods: The sixty subjects who participated in the study were healthy adult volunteers who were naive to the study hypotheses. Subjects were excluded from the study if they:
(a)   had a history of chronic lung disease;
(b)   had a recent history (within the last six weeks) of severe acute upper respiratory tract infection;

(c) had a significant neurological or musculo-skeletal disorder involving the trunk;
(d) smoked more than five cigarettes per day;
(e) were more than 20% heavier than predicted body weight;
(f) had communication difficulties;
(g) were pregnant;
(h) had been exposed to a radiation dose in the past twelve months.

The latter two were important because subjects were to be exposed to a radiation dose during the measurement of DE.

Prelimininary testing using a Collin's Survey Spirometer was required to determine consistency of interrupted measures of FRC and TLC.This was necessary because it was not possible to measure DE, SCA and abdominal girth during the same breath, as this would have exposed the researchers measuring SCA and abdominal girth to excessive amounts of radiation. Of the subjects tested, only 28 were deemed valid, with an equal number of Males and Females.

Results showed that for three interrupted measures of FRC there was a variation of -73.2 to +67.8 mls of overall mean of FRC. For three interupted measures of TLC there was a variation of -50 to +50 mls of overall mean of TLC. It was considered that these variations were acceptable, and could be explained by the effects of spirometer loading , and mouthpiece and noseclip effect. Based on these results, it was deemed appropriate to proceed with the main part of the study.

There were two independent variables used in the study: (a) age; and (b) gender. Age was a continuous variable from 18 to 65 years inclusive. Gender consisted of two groups, with an equal number of males and females. Working with subjects of only one gender may have created an experimental bias.

The dependent variables, SCA at TLC, SCA at FRC, range of movement of SCA (ROM SCA), abdominal girth change (ROM ABDO) and DE were measured using a variety of apparatus. In particular, DE was measured using a fluoroscopy screen and image intensifier on a modified tilting radiology table. Excursion of right and left hemidiaphragms was measured in centimetres and the mean taken for use in data analysis. This was deemed to be a valid method of measuring DE as it has been extensively reported in the literature.

The experimental procedure was pilot tested prior to the actual testing to ensure that the procedures were appropriate. On the day of testing, informed consent was obtained and demographic data was collected. During the testing, the same operators were used to obtain each measure. The chest was exposed and landmarked, and a magnification marker was positioned at the anterior axillary line. To ensure protection it from ionising radiation, protection aprons for the thyroid and abdominal regions were worn by all subjects.Standard instructions were given to all subjects. The radiology table was tilted to 45^0 from the horizontal. The subject was given a practice of the breathing technique to be used during the testing, and then the data was collected. Firstly, SCA and abdominal girth were measured during the same breath at FRC and TLC. Then, the distance of each diaphragm from a fixed point was obtained at FRC and TLC. In this way DE was then able to be determined.

The data were analysed using the Pearson product-moment correlation to test for any correlation between DE and ROM SCA, and DE and ROM ABDO. Statistical evaluation of the effect of age and gender on SCA TLC, SCA FRC, ROM SCA and DE was done using a generalised linear model, with multiple and simple regression procedures, as well as non-linear regression.

Results: In the posture studied, it was found that there was no correlation between DE and ROM SCA (power=.58). A significant, moderate positive correlation (r=.548) was found to exist between DE and ROM ABDO (power=1.0). SCA TLC, SCA FRC and DE were all shown to increase significantly with increasing age. Interestingly, ROM SCA did not change with age. There was a significant gender difference in the values for SCA TLC only. In this case, the pattern of change through the age range studied was different for males and females. In males, the relationship was linear, whereas for females it was quadratic. For descriptive purposes, SCA FRC was also separated into the two gender groups. The same pattern was seen to occur. It was concluded that whilst there is a difference between the starting and ending points (SCA TLC and SCA FRC), the actual range through which each individual's SCA moves during an IC is the same.

Discussion: The lack of correlation between DE and ROM SCA, and the positive correlation between DE and ROM ABDO through IC was surprising. The effect of diaphragm contraction on the abdomen and the costal margin of the chest is widely reported in the literature. During a tidal breath, protrusion of the abdomen occurs. With increasing depth of inspiration, however, the costal fibres of the diaphragm develop a force on the rib cage which moves it upwards and outwards[4,12,13]. It therefore could be expected that abdominal wall movement would reflect DE during a tidal breath, and costal margin movement would reflect DE during a maximal breath.

The increase in SCA TLC and SCA FRC that was found to occur with increasing age can , in part, be explained by the fact that with increasing age, an increase in residual volume occurs[14]. It could, in turn, be expected that SCA TLC and SCA FRC will increase with age. The increase in DE is more difficult to explain. It is important to note, however, that whilst a statistically significant increase in DE was found to occur with age, the increase is of doubtful clinical significance, as the regression coefficient for the slope was only .022.

Conclusion: Normative values for SCA TLC, SCA FRC, ROM SCA and DE have been determined. Commonly used methods of inferring DE in the clinical setting have been shown to be either inappropriate or of only moderate value.

References:

1. Shaffer TH, Wolfson MR, Bhutani VK (1981) Respiratory muscle function, assessment and training. Physical Therapy 61(12): 1711-1723.
2. Williams TJ, Ahmad D, Morgan WK (1981) A clinical and roentgenographic correlation of diaphragmatic movement. Archives of Internal Medicine 141: 878-880.
3. Downie P (Ed.) (1987) Cash's chest, heart and vascular disorders for physiotherapists (4th ed.) London: Faber.
4. Cherniack RM, Cherniack L (1983) Respiration in health and disease. Philadelphia: W.B. Saunders and Co.
5. Frownfelter D (1987) Chest physical therapy and pulmonary rehabilitation (2nd ed.) Chicago: Year Book Medical.
6. Irwin S, Tecklin JS (Eds.) (1985) Cardiopulmonary physical therapy. St. Louis: C.V. Mosby Co.
7. Brewis RAL (1985) Lecture notes on respiratory disease. Oxford: Blackwell Scientific Publications.
8. Barrascout JR (1984) Chest physical therapy and related procedures. In Burton G.G. and Hodgkin JE (Eds.) Respiratory care: a guide to clinical practice (2nd ed.) (p.656-677). Philadelphia: Lippincott.
9. Zadai C !1986) Pathokinesiology:The clinical implications from a cardiopulmonary perspective. Physical Therapy 66(3): 368-371.
10. Gardiner E, Gray D,.O'Rahilly, R. (1975) Anatomy - A regional study of human structure (4th ed.) Philadelphia: W.B. Saunders.
11. Moore KL (1985) Clinically oriented anatomy. Baltimore: Williams and Wilkins.
12. Dail DH (1982) Anatomy of the respiratory system. In Spearman CE, Sheldon RL (Eds). Egan's Fundamentals Of Respiratory Therapy (4th Ed) (p.81-114) St. Louis: Mosby.
13. Roussos C, MacKlem P (1982) The respiratory muscles. The New England Journal of Medicine 303(13): 786-799.
14. Beeckman P, Demedts M, Clarysse I, Vanclooster R (1983) Radiographic Evaluation Of the Influence of age and smoking on thoracic and regional pulmonary dimensions. Lung 161: 39-46.

EVALUATION OF DIAPHRAGMATIC FORCE AND FATIGUE IN PRACTICAL SITUATIONS

Christer Sinderby, Lars Sullivan and Lars Lindström
Spinal Injuries Unit, Inst. of Neurosurgery and Dept. of Clinical Data Processing, Sahlgrenska Hospital, Göteborg, Sweden.

Physiotherapy treatment in respiratory disorders affecting the balance between the force demand and the force available frequently involve physical training and specific respiratory muscle training. However, there are poor knowledge of the effects on respiratory muscles of such intervention. In this paper we will give a brief presentation of a method for evalution of diaphragmatic function in practical situations.

METHOD PRESENTATION AND DISCUSSION
A schematic test description is presented in Figure 1.

Flow
Ventilatory flow at the mouth was measured by means of a pneumotachograph (Jaeger Screenmate, 1/E 0586, resistance 36 Pa/l/s, Erich Jaeger GmbH & Co.KG). Volume was calculated in the computer by time integration of flow. Tidal volume (Vt) divided by time of inspiratory flow (Ti) represented mean inspiratory flow (Vt/Ti).

Esophageal and gastric pressures
Two latex balloons were glued to a modified quadruple-lumen Swan Ganz Pacing-TD catheter (93-200H-7F, American Edwards Laboratories) 110 cm in length (1) and registered gastric (Pga) and esophageal (Pes) pressures. Each balloon was 10 cm in length, 3.5 cm in circumference and 0.12-0.15 mm in thickness (AE Medical Corporation). Each balloon on the catheter was connected to a differential pressure transducer (SCM-Screenmate-spezial, Erich Jaeger GmbH & Co.KG) with the reference side open to atmospheric pressure. The thin lumen catheter used has a filtering effect on the recorded pressure signal. The dominating influence is that of a low-pass filter. The influence of the catheter was compensated for by adding to the pressure signal a portion of its time differential. In order to suppress the increased influence of noise due to this process, a low-pass filter was added. The cut-off frequencies of the two compensating filters were determined by minimising the difference between the modified pressure signal and a "true" pressure signal obtained at the same time through a wide lumen catheter. The

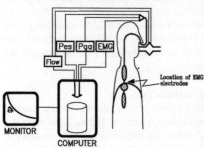

Figure 1. The test set-up

characteristic frequencies obtained were 1.4 Hz for the differentiating filter and 8.7 Hz for the noise-suppressing filter.

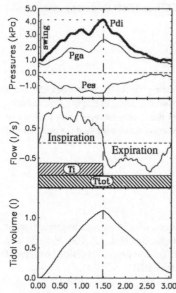

Figure 2. The upper panel illustrate the swing in Pdi and the contribution of Pes and Pga to Pdi. Middle panel depicts how Ti/Ttot is calculated from flow during one tidal breath (lower panel).

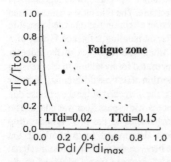

Figure 3. The contribution of Pdi/Pdi$_{max}$ and Ti/Ttot to TTdi for one breath calculated from the data obtained in Figure 2.

Transdiaphragmatic pressure was calculated as the difference between Pga and Pes (Pga-Pes). To represent the diaphragmatic force, the transdiaphragmatic pressure swing (Pdi) was used (Figure 1). Inspiratory Pdi as a fraction of maximal Pdi (Pdi/Pdi$_{max}$) was then calculated to represent the relative force of contraction during each breath. Flow and pressure signals were sampled at 125 Hz.

Tension time index

During each breath, the ratio between the force demand and the force available during periodic loading was assessed by the tension time index of the diaphragm (TTdi). TTdi was calculated as the product of Pdi/Pdi$_{max}$ and Ti/Ttot (2,3). Ttot was defined as the time passed when the pressure-volume curve closed with maximum area. Within Ttot, Ti was defined as the period of inspiratory flow. Further details are given in Figure 2 and 3.

Diaphragmatic electromyogram

Diaphragmatic EMG-signals (EMGdi) were obtained by means of two 2 mm long cobalt electrodes (Elgiloy™) situated 15 mm apart on the balloon catheter. The signals were amplified (Medelec AA6 Mk III EMG machine with preamplifier), band pass filtered with cut-off frequencies at 8 and 800 Hz respectively and sampled at 2 kHz. An anchoring balloon, 3 cm in length and 3.5 cm in circumference, was attached 15 cm distally of the most distal EMG electrode on the catheter in a way that would place one balloon in the middle third of the esophagus, and the other in the abdomen.

EMG off line analysis

The EMGdi signals were visualised on a video monitor and continuous sequences of 255 ms were manually gathered where clear EMGdi signals were present and no cardiac QRS complex was observed. For each sequence, EMGdi signal strength was calculated as the root mean square value (RMS). Also, the centre frequency of the EMGdi (CFdi) and the mean Pdi over 255 ms was calculated. The EMG centre frequency was obtained by analysing the EMG power spectrum (4). Changes in CFdi is related to changes in the action potential propagation velocity in the muscle fibre mainly influenced by the metabolic conditions in the muscle. Decrease in CFdi was also shown to be an early indication of diaphragmatic fatigue (3). The propagation velocity also depends on the longitudinal resistance of the muscle fibres and therefore changes with the fibre diameter, in turn dependent on the muscle length (5). However, in most applications involving cyclic movement patterns, the mean value of the centre frequency over the movement cycle well describes the development of the muscle ischaemia and has become the basis for the use of the EMG spectral method in ergonomics and sports physiology. In measurements on muscles performing cyclic work around mean muscle lengths that may vary, as is the case with the diaphragm (Figure 4). Therefore, care has to be taken in the interpretation of the EMG findings (Figure 5). The change in CFdi was verified by linear regression and correlation analysis.

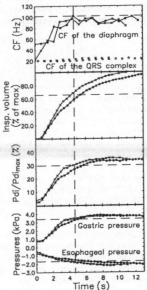

Figure 4. Illustration of two maximal inspirations in a patient with cervical cord injury and no intercostal muscle function. Increase in volume and pressures, assumed to reflect diaphragmatic length, were associated with increase in CFdi until the Pdi/Pdi$_{max}$ reached 30%. At contraction levels above 30% CFdi did not correspond to volume or pressure probably indicating a progressive development of ischaemia. CF of the QRS complex of the heart was not affected.

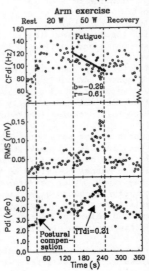

Figure 5. Arm cranking test in one cervical cord injured (C5-6) wheelchair marathon runner. The rapid shift in Pdi and CFdi at start of exercise probably reflects shortening of the muscle in order to maintain posture. After increase to 50 W RMS and Pdi was clearly increasing and CFdi decreasing significantly until end of exercise indicating ischaemic conditions in the diaphragm.

REFERENCES

1. Javaheri S., A. Vinegar, J. Smith and E. Donovan. Use of a modified Swan-Ganz Pacing catheter for measuring Pdi and diaphragmatic EMG. *Phlügers Arch.* 408: 642-645, 1987.
2. Bellemare F. and A. Grassino. Effect of pressure and timing of contraction on human diaphragm fatigue. *J. Appl. Physiol.* 53: 1190-1195, 1982.
3. Bellemare F. and A. Grassino. Evaluation of human diaphragm fatigue. *J. Appl. Physiol.* 53: 1196-1206, 1982.
4. Lindström L., R. Kadefors and I. Petersén. An electromyographic index for localized muscle fatigue. *J. Appl. Physiol.* 43: 750-754, 1977.
5. Walsh J. M., S. Romano and A. Grassino. The effect of force, length and velocity on the center frequency. *J. Appl. Physiol.* (in press).

ACUTE LOBAR ATELECTASIS: A COMPARISON OF TWO CHEST PHYSIOTHERAPY REGIMENS

K Stiller, R Grant, T Geake, J Taylor, B Hall
Department of Physiotherapy, Royal Adelaide Hospital, North Terrace,
Adelaide, South Australia, Australia

Introduction: Acute lobar atelectasis is frequently encountered in the critically ill patient. Because of the potential complications of persistent atelectasis which include hypoxaemia, bronchopulmonary infection and pulmonary fibrosis, an aggressive approach towards its treatment has been advocated.[1,2] Although a number of studies have shown multimodality chest physiotherapy to be effective in the treatment of this condition, there has been little research evaluating which components of this therapy are effective.[1-4] The aim of the present study was to compare the effect of a multimodality physiotherapy treatment with that of a more simple physiotherapy treatment on the rate of resolution of acute lobar atelectasis over a six hour treatment period.[5]

Method: Any patient who developed acute lobar atelectasis while in the Intensive Care Unit of the Royal Adelaide Hospital was included in the study and allocated in an alternate fashion to one of two treatment groups. Acute lobar atelectasis was diagnosed on chest x-ray findings. Treatment in group 1 comprised:
. positioning - with the patient in flat side lying with the involved lung uppermost
. vibrations to the chest wall
. hyperinflation (or deep breathing in the non-intubated patient)
. suction (or coughing and huffing in the non-intubated patient).
Group 2 involved:
. hyperinflation (or deep breathing) and
. suction (or coughing and huffing)
These techniques were performed in a similar manner to those for group 1. Intensive treatment was given hourly for six hours in both treatment groups. Following this, routine treatment every two hours was resumed.

Measurements: Chest x-rays were obtained following the first treatment intervention, the six hour intensive treatment period and, whenever possible, at 24 and 48 hours. X-rays were evaluated independently by two radiologists in the manner described by Marini et al.[1] Both radiologists were blind to the study. Other measurements taken during the study period included arterial blood gases, the maximal lung volume achieved during hyperinflation or deep breathing, patient temperature, white blood cell count and volume of sputum obtained. All statistical analyses were made using the analysis of variance.

Examiner reliability study: The two radiologists independently assigned scores to a series of 30 chest x-rays with evidence of complete or

resolving acute lobar atelectasis and repeated this procedure two weeks
later with the same films. Acceptable intra-examiner agreement (within
10% of each other) was found on 89% of occasions for radiologist 1 and
87% of occasions for radiologist 2. Inter-examiner agreement was 88%.

Results: Fourteen patients were included in the study, seven in each
treatment group. The two groups were similar with respect to age, sex
and intubation/ventilation status. The left lower lobe was involved in
seven cases, the right lower lobe in four cases and the left lung, right
upper lobe and right lung in one case each.

Figure 1 compares the mean
percentage of resolution of
patients allocated to groups 1
and 2. Patients in group 1 had
a significantly greater
resolution of atelectasis
(mean value 60.1%) than
patients in group 2 (mean
value 7.6%) after one
treatment intervention (p <
.006). After the intensive six
hour treatment period the
difference between the two
groups was marginally
statistically significant (p<
.055), favouring group 1 over
group 2. The difference
between the groups became less
apparent at 24 and 48 hours (p>
.10 and > .20 respectively).

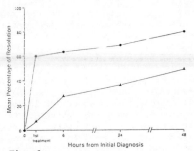

Fig. 1
Percentage resolution of acute lobar
atelectasis, comparing groups 1 and 2
   ● Group 1 - mean value
   ▲ Group 2 - mean value

Arterial blood gas levels did not show a consistent change in either
treatment group over the six hour treatment period, although a trend in
PaO_2 was evident (mean change in PaO_2 for group 1: +25 mm Hg, group 2: -
31 mm Hg, p > .07; mean change in $PaCO_2$ for group 1: -2 mm Hg, group 2:
-3 mm Hg, p > .70). Lung volume measured during hyperinflation (or deep
breathing) increased significantly from the first treatment intervention
to the end of the six hour treatment period when all patients were
considered together (p < .01; mean increase 230 mls). There was no
significant difference between groups in this measurement. Although
patient temperature was not significantly different between the two
groups at entry into the study (group 1 mean 37.9° C, group 2 mean 37.6°
C; p > .40), the change in patient temperature from the first to last
treatment in the six hour period did differ significantly between group
1 and 2 (-.18°C and +.37°C respectively; p < .05). For all the other
data collected, no significant differences were detected either for the
patients as a whole or between the two treatment groups.

Discussion: The present study, although restricted in patient numbers,
demonstrated a significantly better rate of resolution of acute lobar
atelectasis after one treatment intervention in patients who received
positioning, vibrations, hyperinflation and suction (group 1) than

patients who received hyperinflation and suction alone (group 2). At the conclusion of the six hours of intensive treatment this difference was marginally statistically significant. Although the two groups were not significantly different at 24 and 48 hours, it can be seen that their mean percentage of resolution differed by approximately 25% from the six hour treatment period onwards (Fig. 1). Clinicians involved in the treatment of acute lobar atelectasis generally advocate a vigorous treatment regimen to achieve prompt results. On this basis the differences between groups 1 and 2 after the initial treatment, and perhaps also after the six hours of treatment would be considered to be clinically significant. However, if clinicians are content to achieve a satisfactory resolution of the atelectasis over 24 or 48 hours, it may well be that this might be achieved regardless of whether a basic or more involved treatment was given initially. Whether this alters associated morbidity or justifies the use of a basic treatment regimen throughout is a point that cannot be answered with certainty from the results of the present study.

A number of questions still require investigation. Firstly, was the positioning or the vibrations (or the combination) the effective additional component? Would the inclusion of traditional postural drainage positions further enhance the response to treatment? Do patients receiving positioning, vibrations, hyperinflation and suction require hourly treatment for six hours or could the same result be achieved and sustained with only one treatment? Do patients with persistent lobar atelectasis for more than 48 hours have an increased mortality or morbidity? These questions are being addressed by the current authors, but further investigation to verify the results of this study is still required with larger patient samples, perhaps by the use of multicentred trials.

References:

1. Marini JJ, Pierson DJ, Hudson LD (1979) Acute lobar atelectasis: a prospective comparison of fiberoptic bronchoscopy and respiratory therapy. Am Rev Respir Dis 119:971-8

2. Johnson NT, Marini JJ, Pierson DJ, Hudson LD (1987) Acute lobar atelectasis: effect of chest percussion and postural drainage (CPPD) on resolution. Am Rev Respir Dis 135:A433

3. Mackenzie CF, Shin B, McAslan TC (1978) Chest physiotherapy: the effect on arterial oxygenation. Anesth Analg 57:28-30

4. Hammon WE, Martin RJ (1981) Chest physical therapy for acute atelectasis. A report on its effectiveness. Phys Ther 61:217-20

5. Stiller K, Geake T, Taylor J, Grant R, Hall B (1990) Acute lobar atelectasis. A comparison of two chest physiotherapy regimens. Chest 98:1336-40

MODIFICATION OF OXYGEN SATURATION, OXYGEN CONSUMPTION AND VENTILATORY VOLUME WITH BREATHING ASSIST ON HYPOBARIC HYPOXIA

C Yamamoto*,   T Fujiwara**,   K Yanagisawa,   G Ueda,   A Sakai,
Y Yanagidaira,   K Maruta,   *   Rehab.   Centre, Kanazawa
Neurosurg. Hosp. Ishikawa JAPAN ** Shinsu Univ., Matsumoto JAPAN

INTRODUCTION

One of the purpose of chest physical therapy was to increase ventilatory volume(VE).   Increase of VE carried out increasing oxygen saturation(SaO2).   Kryger reported the drug effect on SaO2 in the patients in sleep[1]. Hudgel reported the change of breathing pattern in sleep[2], on the other hand, Hanson reported the change in respiratory rate. SaO2 and VE during hypoxic state[3].   There are many studies in SaO2 although, there is no report that SaO2 change due to operate breathing pattern.   Five healthy subjects, with experimental hypoxia due to high altitude, as simulation models for clinical hypoxia, were used in this investigation.   And modification of oxygen saturation were observed before and after breathing assist.

METHOD

This study was performed on Mt. Animaqing,   4660 meter above sea level, at Qinghai plateau in China.
1) Subject
Five   healthy   subjects,   no medical history of cardio-respiratory disease,   32.6 years as a mean(range between from 22 to 47 years), usually live around Matsumoto city(ca. 610 meter).
2) Acclimate to high altitude
Subjects acclimated to high altitude circumstance subacuetly. They had to spend 23 days to achieve 4660 meter high, because of prevention for unexpected influence and acute mountain sickness.
3) Method of breathing assist
Respiratory rate showed increase and VE showed decrease on hypoxic hypoxia.   There is similar to patients with chronic obstructive pulmonary disease(COPD).   The main purpose of breathing assist was to maintain adequate VE.   Emphasis breathing, both abdominal and thoracic pattern, was introduced by physical therapist.   Subjects were added certain resistance toward perpendicular direction just above the abdomen on ab-dominal pattern.   The respiration was maintain against that resistance(procedure 1).   On the other hand, on thoracic breathing pattern, subjects were introduced to expand their chest toward lateral direction(procedure 2).   All subjects

received some verbal command to emphasis their breathing. This experiment was arranged by only one physical therapist to avoid inter-individual variation.

4) Procedure

First of all, subjects kept resting states on supine position with knee and hip joints flexed slightly. Then, SaO2, pulse rate(PR), VE and oxygen consumption(VO2) were observed during procedure 1 and 2 using pulseoxymeter(Co. CSI type 502) and expiratory gas analyzer(oxylog Co. MORGAN). SaO2 and PR were detected every ten seconds and VO2 and VE were detected every sixty seconds. (see Fig. 1)

RESULTS

At 4660 meter above sea level, the mean of SaO2 showed 82 ± 6.0 percent, PR showed 93.2 ± 11.9 beats/min., VE showed 15.8 ± 3.1 L/min., and VO2 showed 0.39 ± 0.1 L/min. at rest. SaO2 increased 10.2% on abdominal breathing($p < 0.01$) and 6.2% on thoracic breathing(n. s.)(see Fig. 2). PR was decreasing just after the starting point of breathing assist on abdominal pattern. VO2 was showed with a minimum fluctuation and VE was showed transiently increase, on both abdominal and thoracic pattern.

DISCUSSION

Respiratory rate was decreasing and V̇E was increasing after both procedures. Increment of V̇E was induced by increase of tidal volume and decrease of physiological dead space. It was suggested that above mentioned results were induced by improvement of effectiveness of respiration. Generally speaking, diaphragm muscle was mainly used in abdominal breathing, and it charged from 60 to 70 percent at resting state. Oxygen consumption remained lower level in abdominal breathing compared with thoracic one. Abdominal breathing was used as successive breathing pattern for patients with pulmonary disease. There has been a few study established that abdominal breathing was effective method for improvement of VE definitely. It indicated that SaO2 was increasing and PR was decreasing by abdominal breathing assist. Based on the results of this investigation,
it suggested that such kind of study should be continued to search patients with hypoxia at the sea level.

CONCLUSION

Simulation models of hypoxia were made by acclimatization on high altitude condition with hypobaric hypoxia experiment.
It was clarified that SaO2 and VE were increasing by manual breathing assist.

REFERENCES

1. Kryger M, Glas R, Jackson D, McCullough R E, Scoggin C, Grover R F, Weil J V, (1978) Impaired oxygen druring in excessive polycythemia of high altitude:improvement with respiratory stimulation. Sleep 1(1):3-17
2. Hudgel D W, Martin R J, Capehart M, Johnson B, Hill P, (1983) Contribution of hypoventilation to sleep oxygen desaturation in chronic obstructive pulmonary disease. JOURNAL OF APPLIED PHYSIOLOGY 55(3):669-77
3. Hanson P G, Lin K H, McIlroy M B, (1975) Influence of breathing pattern on oxygen exchange during hypoxia and exercise. JOURNAL OF APPLIED PHYSIOLOGY 38(6):1062-6

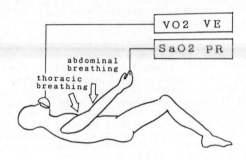

Fig. 1   Diagram

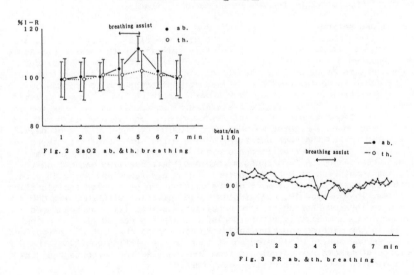

Fig. 2 SaO2 ab. &th. breathing

Fig. 3 PR ab. &th. breathing

MUCUS CLEARANCE IN CYSTIC FIBROSIS - A COMPARISON BETWEEN POSTURAL DRAINAGE, POSITIVE EXPIRATORY PRESSURE (PEP) AND PHYSICAL EXERCISE

L. Lannefors, P. Wollmer
Depts. of Lung Medicine, Depts. of Clinical Physiology
University Hospital of Lund, 221 85 Lund, Sweden

Introduction

Getting the excess bronchial secretion out of the lungs is one important part of the every day treatment that patients with Cystic Fibrosis (CF) are asked to do (1, 2). The patients are nowadays also recommended to perform physical exercises, in order to keep or increase both cardio pulmonary fitness (3), mobility of the chest and muscle strength (4) as well as clearing the mucus from their lungs. Performing a comprehensive exercise program daily or several times a week in addition to the ordinary chest physiotherapy requires a lot of time. A combination of physical exercise and mucus clearing is used in some CF-centres (5) to save time.

Different chest physiotherapy techniques have been developed at different CF centres throughout the world and many studies have been carried out where two or more techniques have been compared in order to find out wich is the most efficient (6). Most studies have been based on measurements of the amounts of expectorated sputum and/or lung function measurements over varying periods of time (5, 6, 7, 8, 9, 10, 11).

The purpose of this study was to measure the acute effects of three different chest physiotherapy techniques on mucus clearance.

Material and method

9 clinically stable CF patients with the mean age of 25 (12-36) participated in the study. All patients were chronically colonized with Pseudomonas Aeruginosa and had daily sputum production. In four patients the daily production was estimated to be less than 30 ml and in five patients more thab 30 ml. The patients performed 1)the active cycle of breathing techniques in one postural drainage position, 2) PEP-mask breathing and 3) physical exercise on a bicycle ergometer. The postural drainage position used was the one to clear the right middle lobe: left side-lying, slightly backwards rotated and 15° head down. The three methods were studied on three different days. All treatments had the same duration, included the same number of pauses for FET with the same number of forced expirations. Spontaneous coughing was allowed when needed. All patients maintained their baseline medications, including inhalation of beta 2 agonists. Mucus clearance was assessed with a technique based on measurement of the elimination of inhaled radiolabelled particles. Tc-99m-labelled colloidal albumin particles with the size MMD = 4.9 µm were inhaled from an air jet nebulizer. Radioactivity was measured over the lungs immediately after inhalation, after a period of 15 minutes of rest in the sitting position, after 20 minutes of chest physiotherapy and after a second period of 15 minutes of rest in the sitting position. The clearance of tracer was calculated from the lungs as the percentage of tracer eliminated between successive measurements.

Results and discussion

The radioactive particles were observed to be deposited mainly in the central airways. Mucus clearance during the first 15 minutes of rest in the sitting position before treatment was biggest from the right lung at 21 of the 27 study occasions (9 patients x 3 study occasions). Mucus clearance from both lungs during postural drainage, PEP and physical exercise was 19% (range 11-26), 17% (12-28) and 15% (9-20), (Fig. 1).

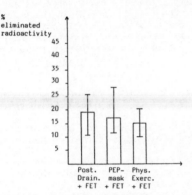

When clearance is measured over both lungs the PEP treatment and physical exercise are directly comparable, while the postural drainage treatment was aimed at improving clearance from the right lung only. We therefore analyzed the right and left lungs separately.

Fig. 1   Mean effect from both lungs in all subjects.
The vertical lines represent range.

Mucus clearance from the right lungs showed similar pattern with respect to treatment in six subjects; PEP was most efficient followed by postural drainage and physical exercise was the least efficient technique (Fig. 2). The remaining three subjects showed a more variable response. Mucus clearance from the left lung was biggest during postural drainage in seven subjects even though the position used was meant to clear the right lung, especially the right middle lobe (Fig. 3). Also in the left lung PEP treatment tended to be more efficient than physical exercise.

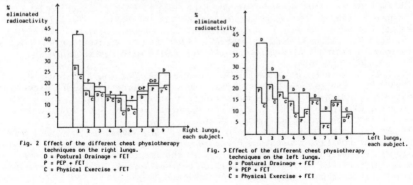

Fig. 2 Effect of the different chest physiotherapy
techniques on the right lungs.
D = Postural Drainage + FET
P = PEP + FET
C = Physical Exercise + FET

Fig. 3 Effect of the different chest physiotherapy
techniques on the left lungs.
D = Postural Drainage + FET
P = PEP + FET
C = Physical Exercise + FET

The differences in mucus clearance between the three different chest physiotherapy techniques used in this study were small. Physical exercise combined with FET was the least efficient technique. This may indicate that physical exercise although having many beneficial effects in patients with CF can not be regarded an effective method for mucus mobilisation in most patients.

The finding that postural drainage was more effective in the left (dependent) lung than in the rigt lung was surprising. The result does not reflect a better clearance from the left lung lung in general in these patients, since clearance during the first period of rest was biggest from the right lung. The finding may indicate that the effect of gravity is not directly on the mucus in the airways but possibly mediated by its influence on the distribution of ventilation.

References
1. Goodchild M & Dodge J. (1985) Cystic Fibrosis: Manual of Diagnosis and Management. 2nd Edition. Bailliére Tindall, 1 St Anne´s Road, Eastborne, East Sussex, Bn21 3 UN, England.
2. Desmond KJ, Schwenk WF, Thomas E. (1983) Immediate and long term effects of chest physiotherapy in patients with cysti fibrosis. J Pediatr, 103, 538.
3. Orenstein DM, Franklin BA, Doershuk CF, Hellerstein HK, German KJ, Horowitz JG, Stern RC. (1981) Exercise Conditioning and Cardiopulmonary Fitness in Cystic Fibrosis. Chest, 80:4, October, 392-398.
4. Rose J, Sandy J. (1986) A Comprehensive Exercise Program for Persons With Cystic Fibrosis. Journal of Pediatric Nursing, Vol 1, No 5 (october), 323-333.
5. Andreasson B, Jonsson B, Kornfält R, Nordmark R, Sandström S. (1987) Long term effects of physical exercise on working capacity and pulmonary function in Cystic Fibrosis. Acta Paediatr Scand, 76, 70-75.
6. Schöni MH. (1989) Autogenic Drainage: a modern approach to physiotherapy in cystic fibrosis. Journal of the Royal Society of Medicine, Suppl No 166, Vol 82, 32-37.
7. Hofmeyr JL, Webber BA, Hodson ME. (1986) Evaluation of positive expiratory pressure as an adjunct to chest physiotherapy in the treatment of cystic fibrosis. Thorax, 41, 951-954.
8. Falk M, Kelstrup M, Andersen JB, Kinoshita T, Falk P, Stövring S, Göthgen I. (1984) Improving the ketchup bottle metehod with Positive Expiratory Pressure (PEP) in Cystic Fibrosis. Eur J Respir Dis. 65, 423-432.
9. Salh W, Bilton D, Dodd M, Webb AK. (1989) Effect of exercise and physiotherapy in aiding sputum expectoration in adults with Cystic Fibrosis. Thorax, 44, 1006-1008.
10. Falk M, Kelstrup M, Andersen JB, Pedersen SS, Rossing I, Dirksen H. (1988) PEP treatment or physical exercise - Effects on secretions expectorated and indices of central and peripheral airway function. Congress Abstracts, Excerpta Medica, Asia Pacific Congress Series, 10th International Cystic Fibrosis Congress, Sydney, Australia, 35.
11. McIlwaine M, Davison AGF, Wong LTK, Pirie GE, Nakielna EM. (1988) Comparison of Positive Expiratory Pressure and Autogenic Drainage with Conventional Percussion and Drainage Therapy in the treatment of CF. Congress Abstracts, Excerpta Medica, Asia Pacific Congress Series, 10th International Cystic Fibrosis Congress, Sydney, Australia, 120.

MUCOCILIARY CLEARANCE AT REST AND DURING EXERCISE IN HEALTHY MEN AND IN PATIENTS WITH BRONCHIAL HYPERSECRETION

Olséni L, Midgren B & Wollmer P.
Departements of Physical Therapy, Lung Medicine and Clinical Physiology. University of Lund.

INTRODUCTION
Inhaled particles which are deposited on cilated airways are cleared by mucociliary transport or cough. The rate of mucociliary transport can be measured by external monitoring of the clearance of inhaled radiolabelled particles (1).
Mucociliary clearance is affected by autonomic stimuli. In view of the suspectibility to autonomic stimuli, mucociliary clearance may be expected to be related to general physical activity.
Patients with bronchial hypersecretion often have reduced mucociliary clearance, and various forms of chest physiotherapy are used to increase the elimination of secretions.
In recent years, increasing emphasis has been placed on techniques for physical therapy which include physical activity and active participation of the patient. Various forms of exercise have thus been introduced in the physical therapy of patients with chronic lung disease and have been shown to improve exercise tolerance and gas exchange (2, 3). Physical exercise has therefore been suggested to improve the quality of life in patients with chronic lung diseases.
Little is known about the effect of exercise on mucus clearance in patients with bronchial hypersecretion.
The purpose of this study was to measure the effects on mucus clearance of a simple exercise program.

MATERIAL AND METHODS
We studied eleven healthy nonsmoking men with a mean age of 48 ±7(SD) years and eleven patients with a mean age of 52±12 with bronchial hypersecretion.
Spirometry including vital capacity (VC) and forced expiratory volume in one second (FEV$_1$)was performed with a dry spirometer.

The subject was positioned in front of a gamma camera. A transmission scintigram of the chest was obtained using a flood source. This scintigram was used in the data analysis to delineate the lungs. The subject then inhaled a radiolabelled aerosol. An air jet nebulizer was used to nebulize a suspension of ^{99m}Tc-labelled millimicrospheres.The subject was instructed to inhale the aerosol by somewhat forced, deep inhalations. The administration of the aerosol was stopped when a count rate of 1500-2000 s^{-1} had been reached.
Four sets of scintigraphic images were obtained with exactly 15 minute intervals. Each set of scintigrams consisted of images in the anterior and posterior view.
The first set of images was obtained immediately after the inhalation of the aerosol. The subject was allowed to rest in the sitting posture for 15 minutes before the second set of images was obtained. The subject then exercised on a bicycle ergometer with a work load corresponding to approximately 80% of the predicted maximum capacity. The third set of images was obtained after 15 minutes. A second period of 15 minutes of rest in the sitting posture was followed by the final set of images.
Heart rate, breathing frequency and minute ventilation were measured immediately before

and at the end of exercise.

Regions of interest were delineated in the transmission scintigram and subsequently projected onto the aerosol scintigrams. Three regions of interest were selected for each lung; total lung, central part and peripherial part. The clearance of inhaled particles was measured as the decrease in count rate between successive sets of scintigrams for each of the three regions.

RESULTS

VC and FEV_1 were within or slightly above the normal range in the normal subjects. VC and FEV_1 were slightly to moderate reduced in most patients.

The scintigrams obtained immediately after the inhalation of aerosol showed prominent deposition of particles in the central airways. On average, 37 % of the aerosol was deposited in the central region and 63 % in the peripheral region in the normal subjects. In the patients 46% and 54% of the aerosol was deposited in the central and peipheral region, respectively. The heart rate during exercise corresponded to about 75% of the predicted maximum heart rate in both groups. Minute ventilation increased by a factor of approximately 3 .

All patients but one coughed during the measurement but none of the normal subjects coughed. Clearance rate did not differ substantially between periods of rest and exercise in either group.

DISCUSSION

The purpose of this study was to evaluate the effects of moderate exercise on mucociliary clearance.

The technique we used for assessing mucus clearance relies on measurement of the clearance of inhaled radiolabelled particles. We measured clearance during different periods after a single inhalation of tracer rather than on different occasions. This design was selected because of the well known difficulty to achieve reproducible aerosol deposition (4).

The use of exercise, as a means of self-administered physical therapy in patients with chronic lung disease, is limited to exercise at moderate work load for a relatively short time. We therefore chose to study the subjects at sub-maximal work load for appoximately 15 minutes. We did not find any substantial difference in mucus clearance between the periods.

In a previous study (5), Oldenburg et al. measured mucus clearance in subjects with chronic bronchitis during intermittent exercise (5x4 min with 4 min intervals). They found clearance to be slightly, but significantly faster during exercise than at rest. They also found, however, that directed coughing alone improved mucus clearance much more than exercise. The patient material in the study by Oldenburg et al. differs from our material by having greater sputum production and greater lung function impairment. Furthermore the patients in the study by Oldenburg were instructed not to cough during exercise, whereas our patients were allowed to cough during the whole study. These differences may explain the different results of the stuies. We are aware of only one previous study of the effect of exercise on mucociliary clearance in normal subjects (6). Wolff et al. measured mucociliary clearance during 0.5 h of intermittent exercise (5x4 min with 2 min intervals) and for a 1.5 h resting period after exercise.The authors found clearance to be similar at rest prior to exercise and during exercise, which is in agreement with our findings.

We thus found no evidence that moderate exercise increases mucus clearance in normal subjects nor in patients with bronchial hypersecretion. With the experimental design used in this study, small effects of exercise on mucus clearance may have been overlooked. We feel confident, however, that any clinically relevant beneficial effect of exercise on mucus clearance would be detectable.

Exercise appears to have small, if any, effects on mucus clearance in normal subjects and in patients with mild to moderate bronchial hypersecretion. Exercise may have many beneficial effects in patients with chronic bronchitis, but should not be regarded a replacement for chest physiotherapy as a means of promoting sputum mobilization and expectoration in all patients.

REFERENCES

1   Newman S.P., Agnew J.E.,Pavia D. & Clarke S.W. (1982) Inhaled aerosols: lung deposition and clinical applications. Clin Phys Physiol Meas, 3, 1-20.
2   Kirilloff L H, Owens G R, Rogers R M & Mazzocco M C (1985) Does chest physical therapy work? Chest 88: 436-444.
3   Sutton P P.: Chest physiotherapy: time for reappraisal (1988) Br J Dis Chest 82: 127-137.
4   Del Donno M., Pavia D., Agnew J.E., Lopez-Vidriero M.T. & Clarke S.W. (1988) Variability and reproducibility in the measurement of tracheobronchial clearance in healthy subjects and patients with different obstructive lung diseases. Eur Respir J, 1, 613-620.
5   Oldenburg F A, Dolovich M B, Montgomery J M & Newhouse M T (1979) Effects of postural drainage, exercise and cough on mucus clearance in chronic bronchitis. Am Rev Respir Dis 120: 739-758.
6   Wolff R.K., Dolovich M.B., Obminski G. & Newhouse M.T. (1977) Effects of exercise and eucapnic hyperventilation on bronchial clearance in man.
    J Appl Physiol, 43, 46-50.

PHYSIOTHERAPY REGIMEN FOR TUBERCULOSIS PATIENTS AT
RIETFONTEIN HOSPITAL, SOUTH AFRICA.

B Baise
Rietfontein Hospital
South Africa

"There is a dread disease - a disease in which death and life
are so strongly blended, that death takes a glow and hue of life,
and life the gaunt and grisly form of death - a disease which
medicine never cured, wealth warded off, or poverty could boast
exemption from, which sometimes moves in giant strides, and
sometimes at a tardy, sluggish pace, but slow or quick, is ever
sure and certain." From Nicholas Nickleby, (Charles Dickens).

Tuberculosis is one of the most widespread infections known to
man. It is the largest single cause of death in the world.
1.7 Billion people or 33% of the world harbour the causative
organism. Every year 8 million individuals develop new clinical
disease. In South Africa 50 000 new cases are notified annually.

The epidemic began at the end of the last century. Tuberculosis
only became notifiable after 1920 and the graph of the incidence
rates shows that the disease progressed slowly until the middle
of the century when an upsurge occurred which almost certainly
was related to South Africa's own industrial revolution. The
Aids pandemic has compounded the TB problem and there is an
increased incidence in patients infected with the HIV virus. The
heaviest toll of both diseases is in young adults - the parents,
workers and leaders of society and this is an impediment to
social and economic development.

Pathogenesis: TB is caused by an organism, Mycobacterium Tuberculosis. Infection is by droplet spread. A patient usually becomes
infected by inhalation causing the primary infection. In a small
proportion the infection is not controlled and progressive
disease occurs. In the vast majority the body overcomes the
infection and some immunity to re-infection is developed. Most of the
bacilli are destroyed by the immune mechanism but a few always
remain. These are inactive and do not metabolize. However, at
any stage during the patients life should the immunity be
depressed by stress, malnutrition, alcohol or immuno-suppressive
treatment the bacilli will again start multiplying and cause TB.
It is important that one differentiates very clearly between
patients who have been infected with the tubercle bacillis and
those with tuberculosis disease.

Signs and symptoms: The typical patient presents with

(1) Productive cough (2) weight loss (3) Night sweats
(4) Haemoptysis (5) Chest pain (6) Dyspnoea. These symptoms have
most often been present for a number of weeks.

Diagnosis: Confirmation of disease is with a positive sputum test.
Acid fast bacilli on direct microscopy are very suggestive of TB
and diagnosis is confirmed with a positive culture. The chest
Xray of a TB patient is very typical. Note the cavity and
infiltration. Upper lobe involvement tends to be the rule. The
tuberculin test is an important diagnostic tool especially in
children.

Treatment: This is either ambulatory or in hospital depending
on the clinical or social circumstances of the patient. Standard
treatment consists of a combination of drugs viz. Isoniazid,
Rifampicin and Pyrazinamide for a minimum of 6 months. A number
of other effective drugs are available but reserved for selected
problem cases. After one week's treatment most patients are not
contagious. One can virtually guarantee a complete cure with
modern drug therapy provided the disease isn't very extensive
and the patient is compliant.

Rietfontein is a referral hospital for complicated tuberculosis.
Further investigations such as bronchoscopy and bronchography,
lung and plural biopsies are undertaken. Resection of lobes and
lungs damaged by TB is regularly performed.

Physiotherapy: In the critically ill patient physiotherapy is not
given. Recovering patients receive exercises within their
capabilities. Dyspnoea is treated with controlled breathing
exercises, nebulization and oxygen where indicated. Ambulant
patients are introduced to a graduated scale of exercises
including distance walking and classes to improve exercise
tolerance. An additional advantage is that the classes alleviate
the side effects of boredom and depression due to the prolonged
hospitalization period.

Pulmonary complications: The most common are (1) Pleural effusion
(2) Empyema (3) Pneumothorax. Intercostal drains are inserted
which may remain in situ for months arising to further
complications viz. frozen shoulders, atelectasis and postural
defects due to diminished respiratory excursion. Breathing
exercises are given and mobilization where required. (4) Pyogenic
lung infections including lung abscesses. (5) Bronchiectasis.
Gentamicin nebulization, postural drainage and exercises are used
in the treatment program.   (6) Associated asthma and bronchitis
are commonly found and treated medically and by the usual
physiotherapy procedures.

 Extra-Pulmonary complications:
(1) Severe debilitation resulting from TB leads to muscle weakness
joint stiffness and decreased function. In the geriatric sufferer
rapid deterioration of mobility occurs.

Mobilization and general exercises are given. (2) Arthritic
conditions are exacerbated by the presence of TB and treated by
conventional physiotherapy. (3) Peripheral neuritis results from
neurotoxic drugs administered either by doctors or traditional
medicine men and is also exacerbated when there is a history of
alcohol abuse. Loss of funciton expecially in the lower limbs
varies from total flaccid paralysis to slight muscle weakness.
Relevant treatment is given with rewarding results. (4) TB
Meningitis affects any age and is common in children despite BCG
immunisation and is responsible for significant mortality and
morbidity. Patients can present with gross spasticity,
unconsciousness, aspiration pneumonia and pressure sores. These
symptoms are treated along the usual physiotherapy lines. (5) TB
of the Spine was described by Percival Pott in 1779. The greatest
incidence occurs in the lower dorsal spine. The initial focus of
infection is most commonly the vertebral bodies, which are
gradually destroyed and ultimately collapse. The neural arch
and intervertebral joints remain intact and therefore angulate
sharply forwards forming a kyphus. The grave complication is
paraplegia. Treatment is rest, anti TB drugs and operative
fusion when indicated. Rehabilitation is commenced early.
(6) Lung Surgery: Bronchograms, bronchoscopies and lung function
tests are diagnostic procedures undertaken as a pre-requisite to
surgery.

Lobectomies are performed for localised areas of bronchiectasis,
destroyed lobes, and haemoptysis.
Pneumonectomies are indicated for destroyed lungs due to
destructive cavitating disease, fibrosis and gross pyogenic lung
infections.

Thoracoplasty is indicated where resectional surgery is contraindicated in (1) A non-resolving pneumothorax with empyema and
broncho-pleural fistula and where an intercostal drain has been
present for several months. (2) A massive cavity, usually
apical, is present and the patient is having severe haemoptysis.
A thoracoplasty is usually performed in 2 stages. In the first
stage the 1st and 2nd ribs are excised and the back ends of the 3rd
and 4th. In the 2nd stage the front ends of the 3rd and 4th and
back ends of the 5th, 6th and 7th are excised and the scapula is
embedded to close the cavity. Pre and post operative chest physiotherapy is given with special attention to preventing shoulder
stiffness and scoliosis.

Physiotherapy has proved its value in the treatment of patients
with Tuberculosis.

References:
1. W.H.O. Tuberculosis Control and Research Strategies for the
    1990's. Addressing the problem of Tuberculosis 2 - 4.
2. Collins T.F.B., Tuberculosis 4 - 12.
3. Glattlaar E: Tuberculosis: Basic Prespectives
4. Epidemiological Comments. Vol 17 No 1 Jan 1990 3 - 13

RESPIRATORY MANAGEMENT IN A.I.D.S.

R.J.Savage

Special Care (A.I.D.S.) Unit,
Prince Henry Hospital,
Sydney   Australia

The lung is the organ most frequently affected in Acquired Immunodeficiency Syndrome(AIDS). For up to 60% of patients, respiratory symptoms will be their first presentation and 85% will have respiratory involvement at some stage.

At present there are an estimated $\frac{1}{2}$ million AIDS cases and 7 million HIV positive individuals worldwide. As the epidemic continues it is thus inevitable that increasing numbers of physiotherapists will be involved in the management of respiratory problems related to AIDS.

This paper will address the main issues related to physiotherapy management for this patient group -
1.Knowledge of the common respiratory conditions - pneumocystis carinii pneumonia,cytomeglavirus and lymphoid interstitial pneumonitis,tuberculosis and kaposis sarcoma effecting lung tissue.
2.Appropriate physiotherapy interventions -
 a)Education of patient and carers
 b)Diagnostic tests - sputum inductions,exercise oximetry and lung function tests
 c)Treatment strategies
 d)Prophylaxis - aerosolised pentamidine therapy
3.Infection control guidelines relevant to physiotherapists
4.Research initiatives -delivery of drugs to the alveoli, exercise prescription

THE RESTRICTIVE VENTILATION DISORDER OF SCOLIOSIS PATIENTS UNDER THE INFLUENCE OF A PHYSIOTHERAPY REHABILITATION PROGRAM

H.R. Weiss, MD, P. Minnick, PT
Katharina Schroth Clinic, Spinal Deformities Rehabilitation Center, Leinenbornerweg 44,
D-6553 Sobernheim, Germany

Even adolescent scoliosis patients with Cobb angles of less than 60 degrees show marked impairment of breathing mechanics and cardiopulmonary performance[1,2,3]. It is assumed, that the scoliotic breathing pattern leads to an increase in curvature and rotation[4,5] as well as to restricted rib mobility[5,6]. So here we find the starting points for prevention and rehabilitation in the management of patients with idiopathic scoliosis. Vital capacity(VC) is a suitable index for characterisation of the restrictive ventilatory disturbance[7,8]. It decreases with an increasing angle of curvature[9]. The greater the impairment of VC the greater the right ventricular work[6]. On the other hand we can expect an improvement of right ventricular funktion with increasing VC.

Material and Methods

All scoliosis patients with a first time in-patient treatment between 1988 and beginning of 1990 at Katharina Schroth Rehabilitation Center have been included. There were 1466 patients with an average age of 24,2 years (SD 12,.95) and and average Cobb angle of 48 degrees (SD 24). Changes of vital capacity (VC), forced expiratory volume (FEV), maximal flow (MF) and changes of exspiration time (ET) have been reviewed. Only the highest of three VC's have been evaluated. Chest expansion was determined on the basis of the difference between the trunk circumference at maximum expiration and maximum inspiration. The measurements were taken under the armpits, at the junction between the xiphoid process and the body of the sternum and at the waist. Sagittal chest expansion was measured by use of a measuring circle at two levels (sternal corpus/manuprium and sternal corpus/xiphoid process). Measurement of lung volumes at Katharina Schroth Clinic is performed routinely using a resistance free Pulmonary Funktion Analyser (Hospal). The values were automatically converted to BTPS. Measurement of trunk circumference differences was done using a conventional tape measure marked in millimetres. All measurements have been performed by the same trained members of staff who have been familiar with the procedure since the end of the 70's.

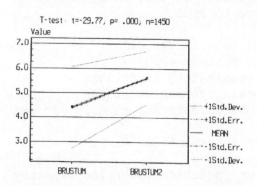

T-test: t=-29.77, p= .000, n=1450

Value

+1Std.Dev.
+1Std.Err.
MEAN
-1Std.Err.
-1Std.Dev.

BRUSTUM   BRUSTUM2

Fig.1. High significant increase of chest expansion measured at middle level (corpus sterni/xiphoid process) in the described sample

The in-patient rehabilitation program according to Schroth[10]

The rehabilitation program lasts 4-6 weeks with an exercise intensity of 6-7 houres daily. The method of treatment is based on sensomotor and kinesthetic principles and therefore uses different feedback models and certain asymmetric exercise postures. The patient learns his individual postural correction routine supported by "Rotational Breathing" witch is integrated into the postural exercises. The treatment program consists of correction of the scoliotic posture and correction of the scoliotic breathing pattern with the help of proprioceptive and exteroceptive stimulation as well as mirror control. First the postural correction of the pelvis and lower limbs is worked out before the spinal curves are corrected one after the other from the lumbar up to the cervical spine. Secondly the patient assumes his asymmetric exercise position. The adjustment of this position depends on whether there is a lumbosacral curve or not.

At the end of such a course of in-patient treatment the patient is capable of independently assuming his personal corrected postural stereotype without the assistance of the therapist and without mirror control and is able to maintain this position in his daily activities.

After an intensive course of in-patient treatment lasting several weeks the scoliosis patient is discharged with a short daily exercise routine to perform on his own under the regular supervision of a physiotherapist in the community.

Results

For the sake of clarity the value changes are presented in tabular form (Tab.1). All values show increases at a significance level of p<0,001.

The increases in VC, FEV, MF and ET amounted to 13,5%, 13,1%, 21,6% and 22,8% respectively. The increase in sagittal chest expansion was 17,8% at the upper and 19% at the lower level whereas the increases in trunk circumference differences amounted to more than 25% at all measuring levels.

Discussion

Bjure[11] and Götze[12] were not able to show increases in VC after several weeks of other physical training. However significant increases of cardiopulmonary performance and VC in a small sample of adolescent scoliosis patients treated in the Katharina Schroth Clinic have been found by Götze[7]. We ourselves have reported on increases in VC between 13% in adult scoliosis patients[13] and over 20% in adolescents[14]. Actually there were increases in VC of 13,5% in the present study in accordance with the relatively high age of patients. However there was a slight negative correlation (r=-0,143/p<0,001) between patient age and VC increases. In view of the fact, that in scoliosis patients the right ventricular work increases with increasing impairment of VC[6] a course of in-patient treatment according to Schroth[10] can be expected to be beneficial to scoliosis patients at cardiac risk. Changes of chest expansion show increases of rib mobility in frontal and in sagittal plane witch is important considering scoliosis to be a flatback deformity. Breathing seems to be more economic after the

	mean before treatment	mean after treatment	t-Test
FVK	2.920ccm (SD 864)	3.255ccm (SD 908)	p<0,001
FEV	2.343ccm (SD 719)	2.591ccm (SD 744)	p<0,001
MF	.266ccm (SD 104)	.317ccm (SD 107)	p<0,001
ET	19,5 sec. (SD 11,6)	36,3 sec. (SD 12,0)	p<0,001
Chest expansion(Trunk circumference differences)			
Armpits	4,55 cm (SD 1,01)	5,78 cm (SD 1,05)	p<0,001
Xiphoid	4,39 cm (SD 1,67)	5,61 cm (SD 1,09)	p<0,001
Waist	4,06 cm (SD 1,91)	5,26 cm (SD 1,18)	p<0,001
Saggital Expansion			
Upper	1,25 cm (SD 0,47)	1,77 cm (SD 0,51)	p<0,001
Lower	1,32 cm (SD 0,46)	1,90 cm (SD 0,58)	p<0,001

Tab.1: Changes in lung volumes, exspiration time and breathing excursions after in-patient rehabilitation program in 1466 scoliosis patients

in-patient rehabilitation program in view of the increases in FEV, MF and expiration time.

Conclusions

The physiotherapy program as developed by Schroth[10] can be regarded as highly effective for prevention or treatment of secondary functional impairment of ventilation. A beneficial effect on scoliosis related pain has been shown[14] as well as a reduced progression rate compared to natural history[15]. Decreasing scoliometer values measured on a special designed device show, that physiotherapy can , at least in part, correct the scoliotic breathing pattern (Unpublished data). An in-patient treatment according to Schroth seems to be indicated in scoliosis patients with actual deterioraton of the physical state before orthosis treatment is initiated. In case orthotic treatment is necessary, the exercise program is beneficial as an additional mode of therapy because of similiar correction principles.

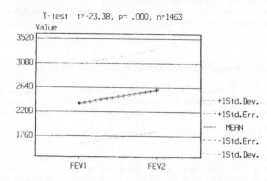

Fig.2. High significant increase of FEV in the described sample. This showes, that even the parameters for obstructive ventilation disorders, often following long-lasting restrictive impairment can be influenced.

(Missing values = 3)

References:

1. SMYTH RJ et al (1986) Ventilatory Patterns During Hypoxia, Hypercapnia and Exercise in Adolescents with mild scoliosis. Pediatrics 77:692-297.
2. DIROCCO PJ, VACCARO P (1988) Cardiopulmonary function in adolescent patients with mild idiopathic scoliosis. Arch Pys Med Rehabil 69:198-2o1.
3. WEBER B et al (1975) Pulmonary function in asymptomatic adolescents with idiopathic scoliosis. Am Rev Respir Dis 111:389-397.
4. HENKE G (1982) Rückenverkrümmungen bei Jugendlichen. Bern, Huber-Verlag, pp 90-91.
5. JORDANOGLOU J (1969) Rib movement in health, kyphoscoliosis and ankylosing spondylitis. Thorax 24: 407-414.
6. MEISTER R (1980) Atemfunktion und Lungenkreislauf bei thorakaler Skoliose. Stuttgart, Thieme Verlag, pp 82-96.
7. GÖTZE HG, SEIBT G, GÜNTHER U (1978) Metrische Befunddokumentation pulmonaler Funktionswerte von jugendlichen und erwachsenen Skoliosepatienten unter einer vierwöchigen Kurbehandlung. Z. Krankengymnastik 3o:333-338.
8. HEINE J, MEISTER R (1972) Quantitative Untersuchungen der Lungenfunktion und der arteriellen Blutgase bei jugendlichen Skoliotikern mit Hilfe eines funktionsdiagnostischen Minimalprogrammes. Z Orthop 11o:56-62.
9. BJURE J, GRIMBY G, NACHEMSON A (1968) Correction of body height in predicting spirometric values in scoliotic patients. Scand J clin Lab Invest 21:190-192.
1o. LEHNERT-SCHROTH Ch (1986) Die dreidimensionale Skoliosebehandlung Third edition, Stuttgart, Gustav-Fischer-Verlag, p 194.
11. BJURE J, GRIMBY G, NACHEMSON A (1969) The effect of physical training in girls with idiopathic scoliosis. Acta orthop scand 4o:325-333.
12. GÖTZE HG (1976) Die Rehabilitation jugendlicher Skoliosepatienten. Untersuchungen zur cardiopulmonalen Leistungsfähigkeit und zum Einfluß von Krankengymnastik und Sport. Habilitation thesis, Münster.
13. WEISS HR (1991) The effect of an exercise programme on vital capacity and rib mobility in patients with idiopathic scoliosis, Spine 16 in press.
14. WEISS HR (1989) Ein Modell klinischer Rehabilitation von Kindern und Jugendlichen mit idiopathischer Skoliose. Orthop Praxis 25:93-97.
15. WEISS HR (1990) Krümmungsverläufe idiopathischer Skoliose unter dem Einfluß eines krankengymnastischen Rehabil-

A REVIEW OF THE OCCURRENCE OF POST-OPERATIVE RESPIRATORY
COMPLICATIONS AFTER SURGERY FOR MORBID OBESITY.

J.C. Nosworthy, C.J. Martin
St. Vincent's Hospital, Melbourne, Victoria, Australia

For over 20 years, bariatric surgery has been used to assist
the morbidly obese patient with weight control. It has been
refined gradually to eliminate longer term metabolic problems
and now is a very effective management approach for weight
reduction in this patient group.

In reviewing the incidence of postoperative respiratory
complications, consideration must be given to the effects of
obesity and surgery on the respiratory system.

Morbid obesity is a relatively common condition. Patients
are considered to be potentially suitable for surgery, when
they reach 100% above their ideal body weight or have a body
mass index (BMI) of greater than 39. Such excessive weight
is associated with significant morbidity and mortality. In
particular, it is a known risk factor in the development of
cardiovascular diseases, osteoarthritis in the weight bearing
joints, diabetes, cholelithiasis, cirrhosis and malignant
neoplasms (Hubert et al, 1983). There is a higher mortality
rate associated with these diagnoses in the presence of
morbid obesity (Strauss and Wise, 1978).

The influence of excessive weight on the respiratory system
is varied. In some patients exertional dyspnoea is the only
evidence of respiratory distress. Others have significant
symptoms such as daytime somnolence and sleep apnoea,
hypoxaemia, polycythaemia and cor pulmonale. Pulmonary
function testing usually reveals a reduction in functional
residual capacity (FRC), total lung capacity (TLC), residual
volume (RV) and expiratory reserve volume (ERV) whilst the
forced expiratory volumes remain unaffected. Many patients
are heavy smokers and all the potential pathophysiological
changes associated with smoking may further complicate the
picture (Thomas et al, 1989).

Surgical and anaesthetic factors independently affect the
respiratory system in bariatric surgery. The use of a
vertical incision has been shown to contribute to the
development of atelectasis and hypoxaemia in the obese
patient (Halasz, 1964; Vaughan and Wise, 1975).

The induction of anaesthesia alters the level of activation of both the diaphragm and the pharyngeal muscles leading to a reduction in FRC and thus airway closure, collapse of the dependent parts of the lung, arterial hypoxaemia, reduction in the ERV, the TLC and the thoracic compliance (Nunn, 1990).

In the immediate postoperative period, pain control is of critical importance. Pain provokes a physiological response which affects many of the body's systems. In the respiratory system it may create the effect of an acute restrictive condition, namely increased respiratory rate and a reduction of tidal volume, vital capacity, FRC and RV. The proportionate contribution to the reduction of FRC from anaesthesia and pain is not well established, but its lowest point occurs between 24 to 48 hours and it returns to normal levels by Day 10. It is the reduced FRC which is most critical as at normal FRC, ventilation and perfusion are optimised (Brown and Carpenter, 1990). Thus the combination of the effects of obesity, surgery, anaesthesia and post-operative pain place patients undergoing bariatric surgery at considerable risk.

The most commonly seen approach is the vertical banded gastroplasty - Mason type. The stomach is partitioned by a double vertical staple line and the outlet of the resulting pouch is formed by an inelastic band. The volume of the pouch should measure between 10 and 25 ml (Mason, 1987).

A common approach to this patient group involves a multidisciplinary team, usually a combination of medical and nutritional staff. At St. Vincent's, such an approach was instituted in 1983 but included a psychiatrist, a physiotherapist and a social worker. All patients are assessed by each team member. The physiotherapist's role is to assess simply the patients' fitness and to set a program of exercise to accustom them to complying with a routine in the post recovery period. Once the patient is accepted for surgery, then a preoperative education program is commenced. This emphasises the need for independent mobility of the patient in and out of bed but also includes teaching deep breathing exercises, the forced expiration technique and an effective cough. In the postoperative phase the patients are sat out of bed within 1 to 2 hours of returning to the ward. Each patient is expected to get up with stand-by assistance and to stay sitting out for half an hour. This procedure is repeated 2 to 3 times on the day of surgery and thereafter all patients are rapidly mobilised to walking around their beds and or rooms. All patients have intravenous pethidine infusions or epidural analgesia which provides effective pain relief.

In the seven year period since 1983, only 18 operations of this type have been performed, of which two were repeat operations. The average BMI was 48 ± 6 (range 39 - 62). Two patients (11%) developed symptomatic respiratory infections (elevated temperature, chest Xray and auscultatory signs and productive cough). Two patients developed asymptomatic Xray changes. There have been no patient deaths. This outcome is supported by a number of much larger studies where a slightly higher incidence of symptomatic chest infections (16%) is noted but these do not appear to have any longer term consequences (Carr et al, 1989; Owen et al, 1989).

These results indicate there is a surprisingly low incidence of respiratory complications despite the enormous potential for such problems. These very large patients present a difficult challenge, but attention to preoperative education and an aggressive approach to the immediate postoperative period can reduce the incidence of chest infections.

1. Hubert HB, Feinleib, MD, MnNamara, PM and Castelli WP (1983) Obesity as an Independent Risk Factor for Cardiovascular Disease: A 26 Year Follow-up of Participants in the Framingham Heart Study. Circulation 67:968-977
2. Strauss, RJ and Wise L (1978) Operative Risks of Obesity. Surgery Gynecology and Obstetrics 146:286-291
3. Thomas PS, Owen ERTC, Hulands G and Milledge JS (1989) Respiratory Function in the Morbidly Obese before and after weight loss. Thorax 44:382-386
4. Halasz NA (1964) Vertical vs Horizontal Laparotomies 1. Early Postoperative comparisons. Archives of Surgery 88:911-914
5. Vaughan RW and Wise L (1975) Chice of abdominal operative incision in the obese patient: a study using blood gas measurements. Annals of Surgery 181:829-835
6. Nunn JF (1990) Effects of Anaesthesia on Respiration. British Journal of Anaesthesia 65:54-62
7. Brown DL and Carpenter RL (1990) Perioperative Analgesia: A Review of Risks and Benefits. Journal of Cardiothoracic Anesthesia 4:368-383
8. Mason EE (1987) Morbid Obesity: Use of Vertical Banded Gastroplasty. Surgical Clinics of North America 67:521-537
9. Carr ND, Harrison RA, Tomkins A, Baughen R, Demmer S, Godfrey J and Clark C (1989) Vertical banded gastroplasty in the treatment of morbid obesity: results of three year follow-up. Gut 30:1048-1053
10. Owen ERTC, Abraham R and Kark AE (1989) Gastroplasty for morbid obesity: technique, complications and results in 60 cases. British Journal of Surgery 76:131-135

EXERCISE TESTING SOON AFTER MYOCARDIAL INFARCTION

Hislop HJ, Blessey RL, Chambers DW, Thomas SD
Department of Physical Therapy, University of Southern California
Los Angeles, California, 90033, USA

Coronary artery disease is the leading cause of death in industrialized societies.[1] Hundreds of thousands survive a myocardial infarct (MI) each year. Early assessment of degree of risk for further cardiac events can most effectively guide a rehabilitation program.[2,3] Traditionally, for this purpose, the post-MI exercise stress test has been at submaximal effort with a workload limit of four METS, administered 4 to 6 weeks after the MI. The maximal effort stress test, however, yields greater and more accurate information.[4] The clinical questions raised about submaximal vs maximal testing, therefore, are: what specific patients, how soon and at what intensity can maximal stress testing be used as a prognostic tool?[2,3] The purposes of this study were to: (1) assess the safety of maximal level stress testing soon after MI, and (2) to describe the profile of the patient who can safely undergo early maximal stress testing.

Fifty-eight MI patients were tested to a maximal or near-maximal symptom-limited endpoint prior to hospital discharge using the Sheffield modification of the Bruce treadmill protocol. The 48 men and 10 women were a mean of 59 years of age and were tested between 4 and 11 days post MI. The group included patients with both complicated and uncomplicated hospital courses as described by McNeer.[5] The complications included congestive heart failure, complex arrhythmias and persistent ischemia or extension of the infarct. Such complications occurred within the first four days after infarct if they occurred at all.

Medical records, admission data, hospital course and predischarge stress test results were the source of 64 variables which were analyzed to construct profiles of the tested subjects.

The stress tests were conducted by physical therapists with advanced competency in cardiopulmonary care. The Sheffield treadmill protocol allowed two warm-up stages prior to the first stage of the Bruce test procedure. Patients were tested at the time of discharge. If there were complications, the stress test was not performed until 24 hours after resolution. The attending cardiologist was consulted about potential problems when such were detected.

Patients were encouraged to continue the test until they completed the protocol or until a limiting symptom was reached: dyspnea, fatigue, angina, systolic or diastolic hypertension, systolic hypotension, a 2mm drop in ST segment, a sustained complex arrhythmia, equipment failure, or if they reached 75% of age-adjusted maximal heart rate. All tests were completed with a multi-lead continuous ECG recorder using standard lead placements.

There was no mortality and no morbidity among the 58 subjects tested to a symptom-limited maximum. Patients were divided into two groups based on the level of tolerance to the stress test: the high-level performance group (n=31) were those who continued to exercise into stage 2 of the Bruce protocol (> 4 METS) or beyond; the low-level performers (n=27) were those who could not progress into stage 2.

The high-level group was tested at a mean of three days earlier (6th day) than the low-level performers (9th day) after their infarct. The high-level performers were younger, had fewer complications, stabilized earlier and were less often on anti-arrhythmic drugs. The high-level group also achieved greater heart rates during testing, higher blood pressures and greater RPP (rate pressure products).

MEAN BLOOD PRESSURE RESPONSES

	Low Performers	High Performers
Resting BP	102/76mm.Hg.	126/78 *
Maximum BP	147/76	164/80 *
Max. RPP	15,101	19,682 *

Adaptive response	n = 7		n = 17
Blunted/flat	13		12
Hypotensive	4		0 *
Hypertensive	3		2

* $p < .05$

Only one test (in a low performer) was terminated for cardiac arrhythmia. Fatigue was the most common limiting factor in both groups and 11 (35%) subjects in the high-performance group reached target heart rates. Three low performers had testing terminated because of hypotension. Two patients in each group experienced anginal symptoms. Mean rate pressure products (RPP) between the two groups at the onset of angina were significantly different: 13,303 for the high-level group and 19,626 for the low performers ($p < .05$).

ST segment depression greater than 1.0 mm during the first stage of the Bruce protocol occurred in 41% of the low performers but in only 10% of the high performers. The time at onset of the ST changes also were significant: at 281 sec. into the test for the low performers and at 549 seconds for the higher-level group.

Significantly, total treamill time in the low-level group was 355 sec. in contrast to 663 sec. among high performers (p <.05). Maximum heart rates in the high group were 120 bpm in contrast to a mean of 102 bpm in the low group. Delta heart rates also were significantly different, 33 vs 69 in the low and high level groups respectively.

Despite significant differences between the two levels of treadmill performance, no consistent predictive profiles emerged from pretest data. Maximal testing for the MI patient early after infarct appears to be safe except when there are persistent resting complications. Prediction of stress test performance based on hospital course only resulted in an incorrect prognosis in 1/3 of the patients in this study. Four persons predicted to be at low risk for future cardiac events based on hospital course (no complications) showed evidence of severe CAD but only after testing had continued beyond the traditional limit of 4 METS. One-third of the low-level performers had no complications after infarct, yet the stress test yielded a high-risk prognosis for a future cardiac event.

1. Pasternak RC, Braunwald E, Sobel BE (1988) Acute myocardial infarction. In: Braunwald E. (ed.) Heart Disease. Philadelphia WB Saunders Co.

2. Baron DB, Licht JR, Ellestad MH, (1984) Status of stress testing after myocardial infarction Arch Intern Med 144: 595-601

3. Amer Coll Cardiology/Amer Heart Assoc (2986) Task force on assessment of cardiovascular procedures (subcommittee on Exercise Testing) J Am Coll Cardiol: 725-738

4. Irwin S, Blessey RL (1985) Patient evaluation. In: Irwin S, Tecklin JS (eds) Cardiopulmonary Physical Therapy. St Louis, CV Mosby Co.

5. McNeer JF, Wallace AG, Wagner GS, et al. (1975) The course of acute myocardial infarction: feasibility of early discharge of the uncomplicated patient. Circulation 51: 410-413

CLINICAL JUDGEMENT OF FITNESS IN THE POST MYOCARDIAL INFARCT POPULATION

H McBurney
Department of Physiotherapy, LaTrobe University, Melbourne, Victoria,
Australia

After a Myocardial Infarct (MI), patients often ask questions about their
prognosis especially with respect to mortality and functional ability.
A 1956 paper written by Bruce[1] for the American Heart Association outlines
the importance of accurate assessment of functional capacity in order to
advise the patient on major lifestyle decisions, for example return to
work. Bruce defines functional capacity as 'an estimate of what the
patient's heart will allow him to do' that is, a relationship of the
stresses of the patients ordinary activities to his symptoms of cardiac
impairment.

In the past 25 years a large number of studies investigating prognosis
post MI have appeared in the literature. The exercise electrocardiogram
or exercise test has become a favoured method for evaluation of patients
after a recent MI. Miller and Borer[2] reviewed the risks and benefits of
exercise testing early after MI and question the value of this against
other methods of obtaining the same information and the use to which the
information is put. DeBusk[3] in a 1989 review clearly points out the many
variables involved in exercise testing which make the results of many
tests unable to be directly compared. Exclusion from exercise testing on
medical grounds related to cardiac dysfunction has been found to be an
independent indicator of high risk for a further cardiac event.

The clinical judgement of physicians regarding the capacity of patients to
safely resume their usual activities after acute MI is regarded as
generally correct,[4] but this assertion is not backed by any evidence.

The aim of this study was to assess the accuracy of clinicians as judges of
physical work capacity for post MI patients.

Method
Ten case histories were randomly selected from a group of 93 patients
exercise tested at a cardiac rehabilitation centre in the preceding year.
All histories were from patients entering a cardiac rehabilitation program
within 4 weeks of their first MI, not having undergone any form of
exercise test. Diagnosis of MI was based on World Health Organistaion
criteria. Information collected from the history for each case is
indicated in Table 1.

Clinician working in the cardiac rehabilitation field were given these
case summaries and asked to state for each case, on the day given for the
exercise test: 1. for how long would the patient exercise (duration of
exercise test) in minutes? 2. Would the patient have angina pectoris

during the test? (Yes/No) For the purpose of this study angina pectoris was defined as a lesser intensity of that pain previously associated with ischaemic events or with MI. All patients had symptom limited exercise tests on a treadmill using the standard Bruce protocol[5], between 4 and 10 weeks post MI. (mean 7.4)

Table 1. Case History Information

age	body mass index
sex	cardiac risk factors
date of infarct	occupation
site of infarct	recreational activities
peak enzyme level	current exercise level, with heart rate
past medical history	responses and any signs/symptoms
medications	exercise test date

Six clinicians volunteered to make the judgements, 4 physiotherapists, 1 nurse and 1 occupational therapist. Clinicians were encouraged to make their decisions quickly. Each clinician read the 10 case summaries and made their judgements on all within a twenty minute time span.

Results
Actual exercise test results were then compared with predictions from each clinician for each case. Pearsons correlation of actual results with predictions from each clinician are given in Table 2. All results were found to be statistically significant at the .05 level. Of the 60 exercise duration predictions made, 30 were 1 minute or less from the actual result.

Table 2. Pearsons correlation of predicted with actual result

	Exercise Duration $r=$	Occurrence of Angina $r=$
Clinician 1	.602	1
Clinician 2	.724	1
Clinician 3	.877	.667
Clinician 4	.904	1
Clinician 5	.708	.667
Clinician 6	.864	.509

Discussion
The data indicate that the clinicians who participated in this study are accurate judges of patient physical work capacity, as measured by the exercise test. Whilst the results obtained are statistically significant their clinical utility must be considered.

This study may be criticised for its presentation of clinical data in paper and pencil form, rather than the use of live patients. This approach was used as it had several advantages. Firstly the judgements were isolated from the actual process of information gathering; in fact none of the patients were known to the clinicians. Exactly the same information was available to each of the clinicians. This allowed comparisons to be made between the clinicians and allows repeated judgements to be made at a later date. Studies[6] have found correlation of clinical judgements made on real interviewed patients to be high, when compared to judgements made for the same patients presented using paper and pencil techniques. These studies concluded that paper patients are a valid representation of real patients and provide a useful tool for investigation of actual clinical judgement.

Further analysis of discrepancies between actual and predicted results for cases presented here indicated that the clinicians erred on the side of caution and underestimated work capacity. The largest errors were made by the 2 clinicians usually working in an acute care setting who did not expect the patients to perform as well as they actually did.

In the prediction of occurrence of angina clinicians again erred on the side of caution. All errors were in predicting angina when in fact this did not occur. There were no cases where angina occurred and was not predicted.

Conclusion
These results suggest that clinicians are accurate in assessment of physical work capacity for post MI patients. Errors occurred on the side of caution, making the clinicians safe, but perhaps not optimally effective in setting exercise programs for this group of patients.

References

1. Bruce RA (1956) Evaluation of functional capacity and exercise tolerance of cardiac patients. Modern Concepts of Cardiovascular Disease 25:321-326

2. Miller DH, Borer JS (1982) Exercise testing early after myocardial infarction: risks and benefits. The American Journal of Medicine 72:427-438

3. DeBusk RF (1989) Specialised testing after recent acute myocardial infarction. Annals of Internal Medicine 110:470-481

4. DeBusk RF, Blomqvist CG, Kouchoukos NT, Leupeker RV, Miller HS, Moss AJ, Pollock ML, Reeves TJ, Selvester RH, Stason WB, Wagner GS, Willman VL (1986) Identification and treatment of low risk patients after acute myocardial infarction and coronary artery bypass graft surgery. The New England Journal of Medicine 314:161-166

5. American College of Sports Medicine (1986) Guidelines for exercise testing and prescription 3rd edn Lea & Febiger Philadelphia p20

6. Kirwan JR, Chaput DeSaintonge DM, Joyce CRB, Currey HLF (1983) Clinical judgement in rheumatoid arthritis. Annals of the Rheumatic Diseases 42:644-647, 42:648-651, 43:686-694, 45:156-161

Housework-adapted exercise testing in female patients after myocardial infarction. Description of a method.

A.S. Norlen *, B. Aronsson*, J. Perk**, O. Torstensson**
* Department of Physiotherapy and Occupational Therapy
** Department of Internal Medicine, Oskarshamn Hospital, Oskarshamn, Sweden

Introduction:

During the past years the incidence of myocardial infarction (MI) among women has increased, in contrast to the male population.

Cardiac rehabilitation programmes (CRP) after MI or coronary artery bypass grafting (CABG) are nowadays available in many hospitals. A beneficial effect of CRP on risk-factors, e.g. blood pressure, lipids and smoking habits, has been reported. Even quality of life and return to work may be improved by CRP (1,2).

Women and men seem to benefit from CRP in a similar way: the effect on exercise test parameters, i.e. exercise capacity, heart rates and blood pressure, does not differ (3).

Women tend to participate less in CRP: several reports show a low rate of attendence of female MI patients and a high number of drop-outs (4).

Female MI patients in the Oskarshamn CRP.

Since the start of our programme in 1977 all women < 65 years have been encouraged to participate. The programme consists of post-MI information for groups of patients and their families, standardised follow-up at a post-MI clinic, and physical training in out-patients groups at the department of physiotherapy (5).

A recent evaluation showed that less women participated in physical training especially during the first years of the programme: women 50.8% vs men 80.3%. When we compared the non-participating women with the training female patients, we observed a tendency to higher blood pressure, less return to work among the non participants. These women even reported anxiety, depression, a considerable fear of physically demanding housework and a sense of beeing insufficient at home, which has been confirmed by other studies (6, 7).

In order to design a rehabilitation programme that would better meet the needs of our female patients we then interviewed patients recently discharged from the hospital . A group of female MI-patients was invited to a further discusson on an adapted type of CRP. In both the questionnaire and the discussion group we were confronted with questions about cardiac risks during everyday household activities. It seemed that fear for and preoccupation with household tasks limited part of our population to participate in CRP.

Although there are in the literature numurous studies on work capacity in healthy people, data on adequate advice are lacking for female MI-patients, who wish to resume their previous housekeeping activities (8,9).

Our patients demanded answers on questions like:

-How much do different housework activities strain the heart?

-What type of housework can be recommended to MI-patients after
 discharge from hospital without major risk of hazardous arrythmia,
 angina pectoris or cardiac failure?

Thus, the aim of our study is to develope a safe and reliable type of exercise test, based on common housework activities. It should be able to perform outside a laboratory setting, and easy to conduct by physio- or occupational therapists.

The study consists of four phases:
1. Defining relevant housekeeping activities
2. Developing a test model in a pilot group of female volunteers
3 . Performing the test in a group of low risk female patients
4. Using the final test design in a prospective group of female
MI-patients at discharge from hospital.
In this report we will describe the development of the first three stages.

Stage 1. Defining housekeeping activities.

The occupational therapists and physiotherapists of the CRP team studied heart rate (HR) and estimations of exertion according to the Borg scale in a wide variety of common housekeeping activities in five healthy female volunteers (10,11). HR at start, peak and end of the activity were measured with a Holter ECG monitor. Among the activities the following were chosen for further study in a standardised manner:

I. Making a bed   III. Cleaning a bathroom   V. Laundry
II. Vacuum cleaning   IV. Cleaning a staircase   VI. Shopping

I-IV Dynamic activities; V-VI Combination of static and dynamic labour.

Stage 2. Developing the test in a pilot group

In order to relate the cardiac response of the six housework activities the five volunteers performed a standardised leg-exercise test on a bicycle ergometer using a starting at 30 W with a 10 W increase per minute, and a standardised arm-exercise test on a bicycle ergometer starting at 10 W with a similar increase per minute.
HR, blood pressure (BP), estimations of perceived exertion and dyspnoe according to the Borg scale were measured at one minute intervals.
In the housework exercise test (HET) the volunteers were asked to perform the above-mentioned six tasks in the department of occupational therapy. Each activity lasted six minutes; a five minute rest between the strenuous moments was given. HR and rates of exertion were studied at two minute intervals during each of the six household tasks.
Due to practical difficulties no BP could be measured during HET. The occurence of serious arrhythmias (ventricular tachycardia, AV block grade III) or ST-segment depression (exceeding 1 mm) were studied with continuous Holter ECG monitoring.

We found that HR during all six activities remained well within the limits of the arm- or leg ET. However, the pilot group tended to overestimate the level of perceived exertion during household activities V and VI, when compared with estimates at corresponding HR during arm- or leg ET. No adverse events occurred during HET.

Stage 3. Performing the test in low risk cardiac patients

The study group consisted of 12 women < 70 yrs; 6 post-CABG and 6 post-first MI patients, retrospectively collected from the register of the Department of Internal Medicine. Patients with signs of cardiac failure, unstable angina pectoris or recent MI (<1 yr) were excluded.
All patients performed a maximal arm- and leg ET. The HET was performed in an identical manner as in the pilot study. Resuscitation equipment was available during testing.

No serious adverse events during testing occurred. One patient developed mild angina pectoris when carrying shopping bags. No arrhythmias were found on the Holter ECG.

Discussion

There appears to be a need for rehabilitation programmes designed to meet the demands of female cardiac patients. These programmes may include psychosocial support, early ~dvice by a dietician and physical training with larger emphasis on reducing fear of job- and household activities.

On discharge from the hospital women (and men!) often need vocational advice before resuming their household tasks. Predischarge exercise testing could therefore focus in a greater extent on these issues, as complement to conventional ET.

We have found that household exercise testing can be performed in a low risk group of female cardiac patients. The test was safely conducted outside the setting of a laboratory of clinical physiology, under supervision of a physiotherapist or occupational therapist.

The results of phase 4, a prospective study using HET in a group of female MI patients at discharge from hospital, will be presented in a forthcoming report.

References

1. Cannistra LB, Balady GJ et al. Women in cardiac rehabilitation: Clinical profile, compliance and outcome. J Cardiopulm Rehab 1990;10:352.
2. Ben-Ari E, Kellerman JJ et al. Benefits of long term physical training in patients after coronary artery bypass grafting. J Cardiopulm Rehab 1986;6:165-170.
3. Griffo R, Vecchio C, et al. Rehab of women with recent MI. Results and comparison with men. Arch Mal Coeur 1983;3:285-293.
4. O'Callaghan WG, Teo KK, et al. Comparative response of male and female patients with coronary artery disease of exercise rehabilitation. Eur Heart J 1984;5:649-651.
5. Hedbäck B, Perk J. Five year results of a comprehensive rehabilitation programme after MI. Eur Heart J 1987;8:234-242.
6. Boogaard MA. Rehabilitation of the female patient after myocardial infarction. Nursing Clin North Am 1984;19:no 3.
7. Mickus D. Activities of daily living in women after MI. Heart and Lung 1986;15 (4):376-381.
8. Kilbom Å. Physical training with submaximal intensities in women. Reaction to exercise and orthostasis. Scand J Clin Lab Invest 1971;28:141-161.
9. Åstrand I. Estimating the energy expenditure of housekeeping activities. Am J Clin Nutr 1971 (b);24:1471-1475.
10. Borg G. Perceived exertion as an indicator of somatic stress. Scand J Rehab Med 1970;2-3:92-98.
11. Borg G. Psychophysical basis of perceived exertion. Med and Science in Sports and Exercise 1982;14:377-381.

HEMODYNAMIC RESPONSES AND RECOVERY PERIODS FOR DIFFERENT ACTIVITIES IN
CARDIAC PATIENTS

A. Dossa D. Helman
Spaulding Rehabilitation Hospital, 125 Nashua Street, Boston, MA 02114.
America

Introduction:
Research on the cardiac patient has focused on early exercise
post coronary artery bypass graft surgery and myocardial
infarction (MI)(1,2). Although the compromised myocardium is in need
of adequate rest(recovery) periods after exercise to maximize its
function, little emphasis has been placed on investigating adequate
rest periods (3).
Recommendations regarding rest prescriptions and methods of conserving
energy, thus far unsubstantiated by scientific research, are often
made by clinical staff prior to discharge of the cardiac patient. The
purpose of this study was to develop guidelines to validate
recommendations regarding rest prescriptions following four functional
activities - sit shower, stand shower, ambulation and stair climbing,
in the geriatric cardiac patient.

Methods:
The sample consisted of eight medical and surgical patients from the
in-patient Cardiac Rehabilitation program. Subjects had documented
evidence of coronary artery disease with ejection fractions ranging
from 12%-58% and mean age of 76 years; those on beta blockers were
excluded from the study. All subjects met pre-determined functional
criteria.
Testing took place at the same time each day for three consecutive
days; activities were randomly ordered, each one on a different day,
with the exception of ambulation and stair climbing which were
performed in random order on the same day.
Subjects rested in sitting for 30 minutes prior to testing. Baseline
measurements of blood pressure (BP), heart rate (HR)/EKG (using a V2
or V5 lead), and Borg's rating of perceived exertion (RPE) scale were
obtained. Pressure-Rate product (PRP),i.e. systolic blood pressure X
HR was also calculated as an estimation of myocardial oxygen
consumption. (4) Following all activities, peak measurements of all
variables were obtained within 15 seconds of task completion.
Subjects were then monitored in sitting, for one minute recovery
measurements of all variables, until resting baseline of BP $\pm$ 6 mm Hg.
and HR $\pm$ 4 beats/minute were reached.
Data analysis: Data was analyzed by a general linear model using
analysis of variance.

Results:

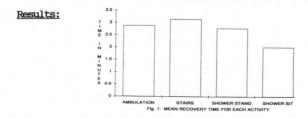

Fig. 1: MEAN RECOVERY TIME FOR EACH ACTIVITY

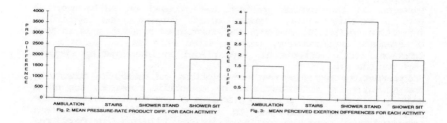

Fig. 2: MEAN PRESSURE-RATE PRODUCT DIFF. FOR EACH ACTIVITY

Fig. 3: MEAN PERCEIVED EXERTION DIFFERENCES FOR EACH ACTIVITY

There were no significant differences between the four activities for the variables measured. Trends showed the following order for mean baseline-peak differences of variables measured: 1) Recovery time: Stairs > ambulation > stand shower > sit shower (Fig.1).2) PRP: Stand shower > stairs > ambulation > sit shower (Fig.2).3) Perceived exertion: Stand shower > shower sit > stairs > ambulation (Fig.3).

Discussion and Clinical Implications:

Although there were no significant differences between the four activities for the variables measured, trends showed that recovery time was the greatest for stair climbing and ambulation; however the mean recovery time for stair-climbing was 3.1 minutes(m),(range: 1-5 m.),and for ambulation, 2.8 m.,(range:1-6 m.). These recovery times are much shorter than those in Alteri's study where mean recovery times were 20m. for stand shower, 7.5m. for ambulation and 5 m. for stair climbing; in this study, recovery times for stand shower, walking and stair climbing were investigated for 10 MI patients, mean age 57.6 years. (3) Our patients took less time to recover; perhaps these patients perform activities of daily living at a slower pace, being older and more deconditioned than the younger cardiac patient and may not need rest prescriptions as extensive as those in Alteri's study. Patients took the longest time to recover from stair climbing; this may be the most tiring activity for these patients and physical therapists may validly have patients perform this activity late during their rehabilitation stay.

938

Trends showed that stand shower produced the greatest PRP differences during peak. This is similar to Alteri's study where showering produced the greatest cardiovascular alterations. Other studies have also found that HR and BP were higher for arm activity vs leg activity. (5,6) Shower sitting produced the least mean PRP difference and had the lowest recovery time; this may indicate that sitting activity produces less stress on the cardiovascular system than standing activity. Thus, recommendations made to cardiac patients to sit while showering or doing other activities may be valid.

Replication of this study with a larger sample is needed to be done to determine whether recovery periods vary for different activities. Further study on the 1) effects of medical vs. surgical patients and 2) varying ejection fractions on recovery periods could be done.

Summary:

Hemodynamic responses and recovery periods for sit shower, stand shower, ambulation, and stair climbing were tested for eight cardiac patients.

Due to the short recovery periods, we were unable to obtain guidelines to validate recommendations for rest prescriptions; trends showed that stair climbing had the longest recovery time for this patient population. Due to the small sample size of eight patients and no significant differences between activities for the variables measured, no conclusions could be made as to which activity produced the highest cardiovascular stress, although trends showed that shower standing had the highest PRP difference.

References:

1. Dion WF (1982) Medical problems and physiologic responses during supervised inpatient cardiac rehabilitation: the patient after coronary artery bypass grafting. Heart and Lung, 11:3,248-255.

2. Wenger NK (1971) Cardiac conditioning after MI - an early intervention program. Cardiac Rehabilitation Quarterly 2:17.

3. Alteri CA (1984) The patient with MI: rest prescriptions for activities of daily living. Heart and Lung 13:4 355-360.

4. Nelson RR et al (1974) Hemodynamic predictors of myocardial oxygen consumption during static and dynamic exercise. Circulation 50.

5. Johnston BL (1981) Oxygen consumption and hemodynamic and electro-cardiographic responses to bathing in recent post MI patients. Heart and Lung 10:4 666-671.

6. Astrand P et al (1968) Circulatory responses to arm exercise for different arm positions. Journal of Applied Physiology 25:5 528-532.

TRAINING AFTER REHABILITATION AND RETURN TO WORK OF CARDIAC
SURGERY PATIENTS

V. Gunnarsdóttir Schram, B. Baldursdóttir, I. Ingvarsdóttir
National Hospital, Cardiac Rehab Unit, Rehabilitation Dept.
101 Reykjavík, Iceland

Introduction:
 Adjustment to normal life after a coronary artery sugery is a multidimensional
phenomenon that is influenced by psychosocial aspects as well as medical factors.
These factors influence both compliance to exercise and return to work. Some of the
most important ones are symptoms, preoperative work status, age, sex and educational
level. The variation in compliance and return to work is great, drop out rate of exercise
programs is generally 40 - 50% at 6 - 12 months after coronary surgery (1). The return
to work rate for cardiac surgery patients has been reported to range from 38% to 81%
and a significant portion (22%) of previously employed patients do not return to work
after a cardiac event (2,3,4,5). Relief of symptoms and good functional status does not
always reflect into a greater participation in work after the cardiac surgery but structured teaching post-operatively seems to enhance compliance with health behavior (6).
 Open heart surgery started in Iceland in June 1986. We studied the functional capacity
of 44 of the first surgery patients (7). The patients went though a structured in-hospital
rehabilitation program, with low level exercise and educational classes about life style
changes, risk factors, diet and exercise. Approximately 6-8 weeks post op all the patients went to a rehabilitation clinic where they underwent intensive , comphrehensive
cardiac rehabilition for 4 weeks. At the end of this period (approx. 3 months post. op)
they had a maximal graded exercise test (GXT) at our hospital (test 1). After that they
were on their own with regard to exercise since there was no cardiac program for phase
3 patients in existence at that time. There has so far been no study that shows the compliance with prescribed exercise and the return to work of Icelandic cardiac surgery
patients.
 Our purpose with this study was therefore:
1. To evaluate the functional capacity of cardiac surgery patients 17-33 months after the
operation and to find out if they continued exercise on their own after the rehabilitation
period ended.
2. To measure the return to work rate and the amount of work these patients do.

Method and measurement: 34 of the 44 returned for a second GXT (test 2) and to
answer a questionnaire. Five of the 44 could not be reached and 5 declined participation
for various medical reasons. The group consisted of 32 men and 2 women, mean age
60,5 years (49 -74ys.) mean weight 83.5 kg (68 - 125 kg). The GXT´s were performed
on a treadmill by a modified Bruce protocol. Heart rate (HR) and EKG were continuously monitored and blood pressure (BP) was monitored every minute with auscultation
using a mercury manometer. The patient was asked to rate the perceived exertion
(RPE) on the Borgs scale (8). Each patient was familiar with this scale from previous
tests. The oxygen uptake (VO2) was estimated by using the standard ACSM formulas
(9). 17 of the patients were on Beta blocking drugs at the time of test 1 and 14 at test 2.

All the patients had received exercise prescription at the end of their cardiac rehab program. They were told to exercise 2-3 times a week for 20 to 60 minutes at a time. The statistical analysis for the variables measured on the GXT was done with a t- test. P-values ≤ 0.05 were considered significant.
At the time of test 2 the patients answered the following questions:
1. Did you exercise regularly before the operation?
2. Do you exercise regularly now?
3. Did you continue regular exercise after the end of your rehabilitaion program?
   If yes : for how long? If no: reasons for stopping.
4. Are you employed?
5. Do you work the same number of hours as before the operation ?
6. If changed, what was the reason for changing the number of hours?
7. Have you been hospitalized since your operation?

Results:

Table 1 Results from the GXT´s . (mean values)

	Test 1	Test 2	P-value
HR beats/min.	134.2	144.2	0.05
SBP mmHg	184.5	201.5	0.001
VO2 ml/min/kg	32.9	37.3	0.01
RPE	16.8	17.8	0.05

On test 1, 26 patients (76.5%) reached max intensity without symptoms and at test 2, 25 pts. (73.5%) reached max.

Table 2 Exercise time/wk, before surgery and after 17-33 months.

	Before operation	17-33 mths.later
< 1 hr/week	15 (44.1%)	2 (5.4%)
1 - 2 hrs/week	9 (26.5%)	5 (14.7%)
2 - 4 hrs/week	8 (23.5%)	12 (35.3%)
> 4 hrs/week	2 (5.9%)	15 (44.1%)

21 patient (61.8%) said they had exercised continuously since the rehab program and 13 (38.2%) had quit. The time for quitting was from 1 month after finishing the rehabilitaiton up to 1 year, with a mean of 4.7 months. The reasons given were lack of time (53.9%) lack of facilites (15.3%) and illness (30.8%).
All the patients, save one, were employed. The one that was not was retired. All had resumed work after the rehab period ended. 27 (81.8%) worked 30 hrs/week or more and of those 16 or 48.5% worked 40 hrs/week or more. 9 (26.5%) had changed the number of hours put in after the operation. Of those 2 (5.9%) had increased the number of hours and 7 (20.6%) had decreased the hours.
The reasons for decreasing were: 1.Too stressful physically = 4 patients (pts) or 44.4%, 2. Too stressful psychologically = 1 pt. or 11.1% 3. Other reasons = 4 pts. or 44.4%.
Seven of the patients had been hospitalized during this period but only two of them because of heart problems.

Conclusion: The functional capacity of this group of patients has improved significantly since the time of rehabilitation. The mean capacity is over 10 Mets (35 ml/min/ kg) and is above the average of cardiac rehab patients in the USA which is 6 - 9 Mets. 61.8% of the patients have exercised ever since the rehab period and 79.4% exercise more than 2 hrs/week. Both the exercise compliance and the return to work rate is excellent and above the average rate found in other countries. The number of patients is not great but these results give us an indication that is encouraging.

References:

1. Oldridge N.B.: Compliance with Exercise Programs . Heart Disease and Rehabilita
tion, Pollock, Schmidt (eds). Wiley &Sons 1988.
2 Allen J.K.: Physical and psychosocial outcomes after coronary artery bypass graft
surgery: Review of the literature. Heart & Lung 1990;19:49-55
3. Walter P.J.: Return to work after coronary artery bypass surgery. European Heart
Journal 1988 9 (Suppl. L), 58-66
4. Gehring J. et al.: The influence of the type of occupation on return to work after
myocardial infarction, coronary angioplasty and coronary bypass surgery. European
Heart Journal, 1988, 9 (Suppl. L), 109-114
5. Knapp D. et al.: Returning the Patient to Work. Heart Disease and Rehabilitation,
Pollock, Schmid (eds), Wiley&Sons 1988.
6..Marshall J. et al.: Structured postopertive teaching and knowledge and compliance of
patients who had coronary artery bypass surgery.
Heart & Lung 1986;15:76-82.
7. Gunnarsdóttir V.: Könnun á starfsgetu og sjúkdómseinkennum við áreynslu hjá
hjartasjúklingum. Læknablaðið/Icel.Med.J. 1989:75(1 47 (abstr.)
8. Borg G.: Perceived exertion as an indicator of somatic stress. Scand J Rehab Med
1970;2:92-98
9. American College of Sports Medicine: Guidelines for Exercise Testing and Prescription. Lea & Febiger, 1986.

A CONDITIONING-REHABILITATION PROGRAMME FOR POTENTIAL HEART-LUNG AND
SINGLE LUNG TRANSPLANT RECIPIENTS.

CE Bray, A Lui, PS Macdonald, SZ Newell and P Spratt
Cardiopulmonary Transplant Unit, St Vincent's Hospital,
Victoria Street, Darlinghurst, Sydney, Australia

Our work in the area of transplantation has illustrated a unique
rehabilitation need in potential heart-lung (HLT) and single lung (SLT)
transplant recipients.

In the pre-operative period our patients have experienced physical and
psychological problems which result in a poor quality of life for the
potential recipients and their support people. Most patients can
anticipate a wait of 1-2 years for suitable donor organs to become
available. This time can be both depressing and stressful for these
patients.

Post-operatively we have seen a range of problems including: fear of
intubation/ventilation; poor patient awareness/control of breathing;
general and specific fatigueability; and weakness.

The usefulness of pre-operative rehabilitation for prospective transplant
candidates has been demonstrated and well supported by both the Stanford[1]
and Toronto[2] groups. In reviewing our experience of heart-lung transplantation, it was apparent that physiotherapy had much to offer in the
prevention and management of the problems identified. It was considered
that any pre-operative rehabilitation should provide potential recipients
with:-

    - constructive use of their time
    - achievable and on going physical goals
    - an improved physical status

Furthermore, the inclusion of specific upper limb, trunk and respiratory
muscle conditioning in this pre-operative training should assist post-
operatively in the:-

    - rapid weaning of patients from mechanical ventilation
    - early increase in physical activity
    - early implementation of nutritional and rehabilitation programmes

Our aim then, was to develop an intervention strategy to better prepare
potential HLT and SLT recipients for surgery and to improve their quality
of life while awaiting transplant.

We have developed a Conditioning-Rehabilitation Programme (CRP) for
potential HLT and SLT recipients. The CRP involves five treatment/train-
ing components: Patient Education, 'Aerobic' Training, Specific Muscle
Training, Thoracic Mobility Techniques and Relaxation and Stress
Management Techniques. Each of the five components specifically address
one or more of the identified problems and involves a number of
techniques.

The CRP is summarised in Table 1.

TABLE 1

CONDITIONING-REHABILITATION PROGRAMME

COMPONENT 1: Patient Education

Problem/s Addressed — Management/Techniques

- Poor quality of life while awaiting transplant
  - ADL advice
  - Alternative strategies for recreational time
  - Instruct family in massage and relaxation techniques

- Fear of intubation/ventilation
  - Explanation of surgical and intensive care procedures
  - Visit to Critical Care Area
  - Talk with (selected) recipients

- Poor awareness of patterns of breathing
  - Review of chest anatomy, muscles of breathing, normal and abnormal breathing patterns
  - Practice in isolating specific muscles and patterns of breathing

COMPONENT 2: 'Aerobic' Training

- Poor endurance
  - Treadmill and bike ergometer programmes
  - Home walking programme

COMPONENT 3: Specific Muscle Training

- Muscle Weakness
  - Weight programme
  - Abdominal programme
  - Quadriceps programme
  - Home programme

COMPONENT 4: Thoracic Mobility Techniques

- Pre-operative musculoskeletal discomfort and
- Post-operative pain
  - Soft tissue techniques
  - Joint mobilisation for cervical, thoracic, costal and sternal articulations

COMPONENT 5: Relaxation and Stress Management

- Pre-operative respiratory crisis and
- Post-operative pain
  - Relaxation techniques

We have trialed the CRP with a group of 8 potential HLT and SLT recipients, all with well advanced respiratory disease [bronchiectasis (1), Eisenmenger's complex (1), emphysema (3), fibrosing alveolitis (1), lymphangiomatosis (1), pulmonary interstitial disease (1)].

Subjects were selected from the active waiting list and considering their access to our centre (that is, they were resident within the Sydney metropolitan area). Following familiarisation with the aims of the CRP and walking on the treadmill, baseline testing was commenced. Throughout a six minute treadmill-walk test, oxygen saturation, pulse and respiratory rates, number of rests required and total distance covered were recorded. Specific muscle strength in the upper limb and trunk was graded[3] and patients were asked to subjectively assess their performance in a range of activities (using a scale of perceived exertion) and any musculoskeletal discomfort. Patient training was then commenced and involved 2 to 5 times weekly visits to the outpatients department and a home programme. After three months participation in the CRP, the same testing and questioning was applied. Our results are summarised in Table 2.

TABLE 2

SIX MINUTE WALK TEST	BASELINE		3 MONTHS	
	MEAN	RANGE	MEAN	RANGE
Resting O_2 Saturation (%)	93	88-98	95	92-98
Desaturation from Rest (%)	12.5	4-19	6.8	1-14
Distance (metres)	102.5	15-180	180.1	90-400
Respiratory Rate: breaths/ minute:-				
Resting	24.3	16-40	22.4	16-34
Maximum	31.9	23-44	27.1	23-35
Number of Rests	1.1	0-5	0.1	0-1

The three month trial has also seen improved specific muscle strength in the upper limb and trunk musculature, in all patients. Subjectively, all patients have reported an increased ease of activity in a range of tasks, a decrease in musculoskeletal discomfort and improved self esteem. It is anticipated that such a programme will be useful to most potential recipients and may have application to the more broad area of Pulmonary Rehabilitation.

References

1. Marshall S, Kramer M, Lewiston N, Starnes V, Theodore J. (1990) Selection and Evaluation of Recipients for Heart-Lung and Lung Transplantation. Chest 98:6:1488-1494.

2. Toronto Lung Transplantation Group (1988). Experience with Single Lung Transplantation for Pulmonary Fibrosis. JAMA 259:2258-2258.

3. Daniels L, Worthington C. Muscle Testing Techniques of Manual Examination. 4th Edition (1980) W.B. Saunders Company.

POSTER PRESENTATIONS

PHYSICAL FACTORS IN HIGH-ALTITUDE SPELEO-THERAPY OF CHILDREN WITH BRONCHIAL ASTHMA

F M Toichieva, A A Madraimova,
T M Bektursunov, D K Smanova
Kirghiz Research Institute of Ecology
Frunze
U S S R

The effect of combined use of sinusoidal modulated currents (SMC) and high-altitude speleotherapy (HS) on clinical and functional manifestation of bronchial asthma was studied in 96 children aged from 7 to 14. The research was done in the "Chon-Tooz" high-altitude speleoclinic located at 2100 m above sea level.

It was found that the overwhelming majority of the patients (96.8%) showed beneficial changes in clinical status, values of extrarespiratory function and cardiohemodynamics. The degree of beneficial changes in clinical functional status was more pronounced in patients who underwent a combined exposure of SMC and HS. It was revealed that a marked decrease of bronchial obstruction phenomena is associated with beneficial changes in pulmonary blood flow, a decrease in pulmonary hypertension and changes in central hemodynamics.

The use of SMC course in combination with speleotherapy promotes an increase in high-altitude speleotherapy efficiency, which is proved by a decrease in complication incidence of extrapulmonary nidi of chronic infection, by a decrease in markedness of disadaptation disorders and an increase in stability of therapeutic effect.

PHYSICAL FACTORS IN TREATMENT OF CHRONIC OBSTRUCTIVE BRONCHITIS

V.M.Bykhovsky, T.S.Simonenko, L.S.Sokurenko, S.G.Gosselbakh
Kirghiz Research Institute of Ecology
Sovetskaya 34, Frunze 720451, U S S R

The purpose of the present work was to study the all-round effect of non-medication treatment and short-term adaptation to medium altitude on low altitude residents with chronic obstructive bronchitis (COB).

124 residents of low altitude (Frunze, 760 m above sea level) with various degrees of ventilation insufficiency (VI) were observed in a pulmonary clinic at an altitude of 1340 m above sea level. 83 of them were males and 41 females aged from 20 to 55 years, mainly with disease history from 5 to 10 years. All the patients were on the rehabilitation treatment used for exacerbation-free period in the phase of incomplete remission.

Ventilation function (VF) was studied by spirography methods to determine pulmonary vital capacity (VC), forced expiratory volume in 1 sec. (FEV_1), maximum expiratory flow at 25, 50 and 75% FVC ($FEF_{25-75\%}$). The intensity of ventilation impairments was graded by the Kanaev classification: moderate (VI-1), considerable (VI-2) and sharp (VI-3) / 1 /. 51 patients demonstrated moderate obstructive changes in the bronchi, 40 patients had considerable VI through the whole bronchial tree, and 33 patients showed sharp VI.

For the analysis of immunological changes all the COB patients were divided into two groups: Group 1 with VI-1 and Group 2 with VI-2 and VI-3. In Group 2 the VF values were studied separately in patients with VI-2 and VI-3.

During VF studies at baseline it was found out that VC (in %% predicted) was in patients with VI-1 97.4+3.0; VI-2 - 83.8+2.7; VI-3 - 62.6+2.8; FEV_1 was 90.0+3.1; 66+2.9 and 40.1+2.3; FEF_{25} was 55.0+1.9; 36.0+1.5 and 20.5+1.0; FEF_{50} was 55.2+2.8; 37.2+1.5; 16.7+1.2 and FEF_{75} was 48.5+3.1; 40.0+2.9 and 14.8+1.1 respectively.

As it is seen, the patients with COB demonstrated changes both in VC and bronchial patency as the intensity of ventilation insufficiency was increasing.

The main subjective and objective symptoms corelated with the character and severity of the disease.

The overwhelming majority of the patients complained of cough with sputum. Dispnea during physical load (rapid walk, uphill climbing) was observed in 93.2% of the subjects, but in 24 (72.7%) COB patients with VI-3 it emerged during minor load (1st floor acsent). The majority of the patients showed pulmonary sound percussion with wooden resonance in some of them. Most of patients demonstrated harsh breathing, and weak breathing testifying to emphysema development was in 33.3% of patients with VI-3. Dry rale of various pitch and intensity were heard in practically all the patients.

The following immunological tests were used: quantitative assays of T-lymphocytes (E-RFC), B-lymphocytes (EAC-RFC), "active" T-lymphocytes (AE-RFC), teophilline resistant and teophilline sensitive T-lymphocytes (T_r-RFC and T_s-RFC), determination of T-lymphocyte mitogen-induced activity by the reaction of blast transformation with "Serva" FGA (RBT), serum A, M, G immunoglobulin concentration determination.

The study of immune homeostasis at medium altitude before treatment revealed statistically significant decrease of T- and B-lymphocyte number in practically all the patients. Marked changes were also observed in T-lymphocyte blast-forming capacity. RBT in Group 1 was 19.69±1.89%, in Group 2 - 16.7±2.02% in contrast to 55.34±2.67% in control (P < 0.001). At the same time, T_r-RFC content in both groups was significantly higher than the control data which reflects the state of activation in the given cell subpopulation.

In patients with VI-1 we observed stimulating teophilline effect on E-receptor modification manifested by negative values of T_s-RFC (-67.86±42.1•10⁷/L). In Group 2 this value was practically normal.

An increase of "active" T-lymphocyte cell affinity to sheep erythrocytes in Group 1 was observed in contrast to Group 2 (639.13±65.03•10⁶/L and 429.3±65.9•10⁶/L respectively).

An increase of IgA synthesis was found in immunoglobulin studies in patients of both groups. Besides, hyperproduction of IgG was observed in patients with VI-1.

The treatment included decimetre-wave (DW) therapy in the intercapular region for 10 to 15 min, a course of 10 applications every second day. On the days free from DW therapy the patients were given autotransfusion of ultra-violet irradiated blood (AUVIB): 1 mL of blood per 1 kg of weight, 5 to 7 times a course on the background of therapeutic exercises and salt-alkaline inhalations. In case of inflammatory process in bronchi in the course of treatment, adequate medication therapy was given.

As a result of the treatment favourable changes in the subjective and objective COB symptoms were marked in both groups, primarily with higher pulmonary function indices. The study of VF revealed significant improvement in VC (up to 70.0±2.2%, P<0.05) and FEV_1(up to 55.5±4.4, P<0.05) only in patients with VI-3 as well as an increase in bronchial patency. FEV_{25} was increased from 20.5±1.0 to 30.2±1.7% (P<0.05), FEF_{50} - from 16.7±1.0 to 24.2±1.5% (P<0.05), FEF_{75} - from 14.8±1.1 to 24.3±1.0% (P<0.05). In patients with the baseline moderate and considerable VI the treatment significantly increased the patency of peripheral bronchi only: FEF_{50} in Group 2 was increased to 42.8±2.4% whereas FEF_{75} in Group 1 was 62.6±3.8%, in Group 2 - 52.5±2.3% (P<0.05).

As a result of the treatment the absolute content of T- and B-lymphocytes has reliably increased and reached normal values in patients with VI-1 and was $1005.46±67.5\cdot10^6$/L and $328.21±23.85\cdot10^6$/L respectively.

The number of T_S-RFC was also normalised ($138.69±60.27\cdot10^6$/L). The rest of the values had positive changes, but they did not reach the normal readings by the end of the treatment.

A significant increase of B-lymphocytes and mitogen-induced T-lymphocyte activity was marked in patients with severe VI. However, normalization of these values was not observed.

As it is seen from the data above, the treatment which was out is effective for patients with various degree of airway obstruction and results in VF improvement and correction in several links of cell immunity.

Reference:
Kanaev NN (1976) Respiration indices assessment criteria. In: Respiratory functional studies in pulmonological practice. Leningrad, pp. 17-23.

THE RELATIVE EFFICACY OF A REHABILITATION-PROGRAMME
IN COPD PATIENTS.

Gosselink*,H., A.van Keimpema**, R.Wagenaar*,
R.Chadwick-Straver*.

Depts of Physical Therapy* and Pulmonary Diseases**,
Free University Hospital, Amsterdam/NL.

In 31 COPD patients (age $57.5\pm9Y$; FEV_1/IVC $55\pm18\%$), the effects
of a rehabilitation programme (RP) and medication treatment
(MP) were compared. The RP lasted 3 months and comprised exercise training, breathing exercises, education and medication.
In a randomised controlled cross-over study, Group 1 received
inially RP for 3 months and, subsequently, MT for another 3
months. Group 2 started with the RP after an initial MT-period
of 3 months. The following tests were used: 6-min. walking test
(WT), maximal (MCT) and submaximal cycle ergonometer test
(SMCT), endurance cycling test (ECT), questionnaire for Well-
being and the Chronic Respiratory Questionnaire (Gyuatt, G.H.
et al. Thorax 1987; 42:773). Both between-group differences and
within-group differences were analyzed, using non-parametric
statistics. There were significant improvements in WT, ECT and
maximal work. load. The items Well-being, Invalidity, Dyspnea
during ADL, Emotion and Mastery in the questionnaires also
improved significantly. The physiological parameters (VO2, fH,
Ve) during the MCT and SMCT did not change significantly. It
is concluded that this programme is effective in terms of ADL,
and Well-being.

UPPER LIMB MOVEMENT ANALYSIS

Characteristics of Normal Reaching Movements

P.M. van Vliet
School of Physiotherapy, Coventry Polytechnic
Coventry CV1 5FB, England

Introduction

At the last World Congress (1987), Roberta Shepherd discussed the need for deriving clinical implications from current scientific knowledge rather than continuing to use therapeutic approaches not well-supported by scientific findings. Where analyses of functional activities in neurological patients is concerned, a normal model of movement with which to compare abnormal movement can be derived from areas of science such as biomechanics, motor control, neurophysiology, neuroanatomy and muscle biology. Activities such as walking, and more recently, standing from a chair, have been studied in some detail. Until recently information on the motor control and biomechanical characteristics of purposeful upper limb movements, such as reaching, has been scarce. This has changed, however, and this paper reviews findings on reaching and discusses some clinical implications of these findings.

Movement organisation and Biomechanics

Considerable interest has arisen in the nature of the programming of reaching within the CNS. Through examination of biomechanical data, insight has been gained into programming. Schmidt's (in Kelso, 1982) idea of a schema for movement, '...an abstract memory structure planned in anticipation of movement...', or something similar to this, is now widely accepted. Feedforward mechanisms as well as feedback are thought to control movement (Kelso, 1982). Some insight into reaching is particularly given by Jeannerod's experiments (1981; 1984). He has performed high-speed film analyses of reaching for objects, examining hand opening and closing as well as transport of the hand. In these experiments he identified events which were temporally synchronised in the reaching movement. First, that the transport of the hand towards the object and the opening of the hands began together, and then later in the movement the closing of the hand (called maximum grip aperture) coincided with a low-velocity phase, as the hand neared the target.

Marteniuk et al. (1987) and others have verified these findings. Jeannerod hypothesised that synchronising these events would require less information processing by the CNS. This is an important point, as other psychologists, particularly Bernstein (in Kelso, 1982), have demonstrated that the CNS must have methods of linking events together into functional coordinative structures, in order to control them. For example, it is pointed out that if one were to control each of the major muscles in the arm as a separate unit, there would be 26 items to monitor; if each motor unit were controlled separately, the number would be several thousand. Indeed, work by Buys et al. (1986) suggests that some muscles are organised into a synergy (e.g. those concerned with a pincer grip) that is supplied by one cortico-spinal neurone.

From his studies Jeannerod suggested that there are two independent visuomotor channels for reaching, one controlling transport of the hand, the other the opening and closing of the hand, and that these are loosely linked by temporal events at various points. He also describes these components by their relationship to the object - the transport channel for processing the extrinsic characteristics of objects (e.g. their spatial location) and the grasp channel for their intrinsic characteristics (e.g. the size and shape of the object). Interestingly, in observations of two-handed tasks, Jeannerod (1984) found that the two hands began moving at the same time.

Another possibility is that events within transport and grasp are spatially rather than temporally linked. Wing et al (1986) have found evidence for this in that the size of the maximum grip aperture increased as a response to increasing the speed of the reaching movement, and to reaching with eyes closed, presumably to account for the increased possibility of making an error. This spatial compensation, with maintenance of the temporal link which Jeannerod described, raises the possibility of organisation of reaching being organised in spatial, as well as temporal terms. Further support for this idea comes from a study on curved reaching movements. Haggard and Wing (1989) found that subjects delayed their maximum grip aperture until they were at approximately the same position along the transport axis as in the straight movement.

With regard to thumb movement, an interesting findiong of Wing et al. (1986) was that the thumb remains fairly static during reaching while the fingers do most of the opening and closing.

Information processing

The CNS receives a variety of information about movement from muscle spindles, Golgi tendon organs, cutaneous receptors, vision, hearing and the vestibular system. The parameters used by the CNS to generate and monitor motor patterns are being investigated. Soechting and Lacquaniti (1981) have found some evidence for movement being represented by a coordinate system based on joint angles. In a pointing task they observed a linear relationship between the angular velocities of the elbow and shoulder that occurred towards the end of the movement. In a later study (1986) Lacquaniti and Soechting found that the pattern of EMG responses to perturbation of the arm could be correlated with net joint torque. Alternatively, Hinton (1984) has proposed that movement is computed by expressing the positions, orientations, and motions of parts of the body in terms of a single world-based frame of reference rather than in terms of joint angles or an ego-centric frame based on the body itself. Alderson and Sully (1976) present some evidence for this idea in their study on ball-catching, where the fingers were closed at an appropriate time based on time to contact with the ball. The computation of movement is still unresolved, but there is pertinent information here for understanding patients' movement problems.

Environmental effects

The task in which the reaching movement is performed seems to significantly influence the movement organisation and biomechanics. Marteniuk et al. (1987) compared reaching trajectories when grasping different objects In a series of movements, subjects grasped discs of different sizes, and grasped a fragile object (a light bulb) and a soft resilient object (a tennis ball). In the tasks where more precision was required the peak velocity occurred earlier in the trajectory, allowing for a longer deceleration phase (perhaps to make better use of visual feedback).

Different subsequent tasks also affect trajectory. Van Vliet (1990) compared grasping the same object either to move it, or to move and rotate it (a more complex task). The latter caused a wider maximum aperture to be used, and a larger proportion of time to be spent in the initial transport phase. Marteniuk et al. (1987) found subjects who were grasping a disc either to throw it into a large box or to place it in a tight-fitting well, had an earlier peak velocity allowing for a longer deceleration phase when dong the latter task, which required more precision. Rosenbaum (1988) describes an experiment where subjects chose different ways (pronated or supinated) of grasping a horizontal dowel in order to place it upright depending on which end it was to be placed.

Implications for treatment

These comments will be confined to neurological patients, thought the information above undoubtedly has wider application than this. Whatever approach one takes to the training of upper limb function, these findings from motor control and biomechanics can be used to improve the accuracy of our analyses. Many findings here give insight into the coordination of separate components in reaching. Temporal and spatial features of normal reaching can be used to compare with abnormal reaching. Normally transport and hand opening appear to be synchronised in time at the beginning of the movement and more loosely when maximum grip aperture occurs. These could be considered to be invariant features of reaching and in part be a basis for analysing reaching. Training methods could be devised to effect a more normal movement pattern, with regard to the temporal and spatial features of a movement. As movement in neurological patients tends to be characterised by prolonged recruitment of motor units, with underactivation of some muscle groups and overactivation of others, the temporal relationship between components seems a key factor. A holistic analysis, including timing and amount of muscle activity, joint range movement, and neural control of events could result in more effective training.

As individual biomechanical features emerge from the literature, such as the greater contribution of finger than thumb movement in grasping an object at the front, these findings can be used to ascertain the patient's main problem in grasping, something emphasised by Carr and Shepherd (1987) in their problem-solving approach to training.

The literature offers some guidance to training as well as analysis. It is evident that the two phases of reaching appear to be organised in a coordinated manner. In instructing patients to practice part of the reaching task, they probably lose the opportunity to organise the movement in the normal way. Several authors, including Gentile (1987), have stressed the need for the patient to attempt to perform the whole movement in the normal manner, with appropriate timing, even if they are unsuccessful at doing so. There is some evidence that this does improve task performance (e.g. Gentile 1987). Perhaps performing the whole movement is more likely to activate the appropriate motor program(s) for reaching.

The author, from a previous study (1989) can shed some light on this aspect of training. The reaching movements of a stroke patient were recorded by an optical tracking system as an addendum to an experiment with normal subjects. Interestingly, the patient demonstrated an increased ability to open the hand when performing the actual task of grasping a mug compared to opening the hand with the arm at rest. The maximum grip aperture obtained from several attempts when the hand was opened as an isolated movement was 7 cm. When reaching for the mug the aperture was consistently between 9 and 11.5 cm.

Lastly, the task-specific training approach advocated by Carr and Shepherd (1987) has increasing support in the literature. The experiments relating to effect of the object and task on movement organisation indicates that they are used in planning a movement. Perhaps, patients will not perform as well without specific task and environmental information being present.

It is hoped that this discussion illustrates the value of applying motor control research to the treatment of upper limb function in neurological patients. The issues discussed here have applications to both the analysis and training of reaching movements.

References

Shepherd RB (1987) Movement science and physiotherapy: deriving implications for the clinic. Proceedings of the tenth international congress for the World Confederation of Physiotherapy, pp. 6-11.

Kelso JAS (1982) Human Motor Behaviour: an introduction. Lawrence Erlbaum Associates, Hillsdale, New Jersey, pp. 239-282.

Jeannerod M. (1981) Intersegmental coordination during reaching at natural visual objects. In Attention and Performance IX (ed. J.Long and A. Baddeley), pp.153-169, Erlbaum Associates, Hillsdale, New Jersey.

Jeannerod M (1984) The timing of natural prehension movements. Journal of Motor Behaviour, 16, 235-254.

Marteniuk RG, MacKenzie CL, Jeannerod M, Athenes S, Dugas C. (1987) Constraints on human arm trajectories. Canadian Journal of Psychology, 41, 3, 365-378.

Buys EJ, Lemon RN, Mantel GWH, Muir RB.(1986) Selective facilitation of different hand muscles by single corticospinal neurones in the conscious monkey. Journal of Physiology, 381,529-549.

Wing AM, Turton A, Fraser C. (1986) Grasp size and accuracy of approach in reaching. Journal of Motor Behaviour, 18, 3, 245-260.

Haggard P, Wing AM (1989) Phases of control: trajectory formation during reaching. Experimental Psychology meeting, Cambridge.

Rosenbaum DA, Marchak F, Barnes HJ, Vaughan J, Slotta JD, Jorgensen MJ (1988) Constraints for action selection. Proceedings of Attention and Performance XIII. Saline Royale, France.

Soechting JF, Lacquaniti P F (1981) Invariant characteristics of a pointing movement in man. Journal of Neuroscience, 1, 710-720.

Lacquaniti F, Soechting JF (1986) EMG responses to load perturbations of the upper limb: effect of dynamic coupling between shoulder and elbow motion. Experimental Brain Research, 61, 482-496.

Hinton G. (1984) Parallel computations for controlling an arm. Journal of Motor Behaviour, 16, 2, 171-194.

Alderson GJK, Sully DJ (1974) An operational analysis of a one-handed catching task using high speed photography. Journal of Motor Behaviour, 6, 4, 217-226.

Van Vliet P (1990) The role of environmental context in the planning and control of reaching movements. Proceedings of the Third International Physiotherapy Congress, Hong Kong.

Carr JH, Shepherd RB (1987) A Motor Relearning Programme for Stroke. 2nd ed., Rockville, Aspen.

RELIABILITY OF ISOKINETIC MEASUREMENTS OF ELBOW FLEXION AND EXTENSION

Nitschke JE, McMeeken JM & Burry HC
Department of Medicine (Royal Melbourne Hospital), University of Melbourne, Victoria, Australia.

Fundamental to the use of isokinetic measurements of elbow muscle performance obtained from the Kinetic Communicator III Exercise System (KIN/COM) is the determination of a test protocol that will produce reliable measurements when repeated within the same test session and on separate days. Two factors that must be ascertained to establish reliability are first that the measurements are a true representation of muscle performance and not representative of variance due to measurement error, and second that any instability in the initial measurements which may be attributed to motor learning, muscle warm-up or other factors should be excluded from the test protocol.

Therefore the aim of this investigation was twofold. One, to to establish a test protocol that will produce test-retest reliability of single muscle actions of isokinetic concentric and eccentric elbow flexion and extension at 60°/s, and two to identify the number of trials required to obtain stable data.

EXPERIMENTAL DESIGN
29 subjects (19 females, 10 males) between the ages of 18 and 33 participated in this investigation. All subjects were tested once and 18 (14 females, 4 males) were retested between 7-14 days later. Exclusion criteria were previous pathology in the shoulder elbow or wrist in the last 12 months, current training for any sport that involved only the upper limbs, and familiarity with the use of isokinetic exercise for the upper limb.

The KIN/COM III was used. Subjects were seated in the customized chair with trunk and upper arms were firmly secured to the chair with straps. The lever arm of the KIN/COM was attached proximal to the wrist with the forearm in full supination. The axis of the lever arm was aligned with the lateral epicondyle of the elbow. Isokinetic concentric and eccentric elbow flexion and extension at 60°/s were examined on their dominant arm. The elbow was tested through a range of 80 degrees, from 30-110. Each subject performed 12 maximal trials of both concentric and eccentric elbow flexion, each separated by a 30 second rest interval.

Each series of 12 trials was separated by at least two
minutes. The order of testing was randomized to avoid the
possible effect of always performing in the same sequence.
No verbal encouragement was given except for an explanation
prior to commencement of the exercise that maximum effort
would be required throughout. Nò knowledge of results was
given.

Gravity corrected values of peak (PT) and average torque (AT)
were obtained for concentric and eccentric flexion and
extension.

RESULTS
Correlation coefficients were calculated for adjacent trials
in session 1 (S1) and session 2 (S2) as well as an overall
intra-session reliability coefficient for each movement.
Table 1 shows this coefficient with corresponding standard
error of measurements (SEM) and 95% confidence intervals
(95%CI), demonstrating high intra-session test-retest
reliability for flexion and extension.

Movt	Session 1			Session 2			Inter-session		
	r	SEM	95%CI	r	SEM	95%CI	r	SEM	95%CI
FcAT	0.99	1.82	3.72	0.99	1.25	2.64	0.99	2.35	4.96
FcPT	0.99	2.14	4.39	0.99	1.33	2.81	0.99	2.53	5.34
FeAT	0.99	2.48	5.09	0.98	2.48	5.22	0.99	2.77	5.84
FePT	0.99	2.8	5.73	0.99	1.84	3.88	0.98	3.16	6.68
EcAT	0.98	2.14	4.39	0.98	1.99	4.19	0.99	2.39	5.03
EcPT	0.96	3.49	7.16	0.97	3.12	6.59	0.99	3.72	7.85
EeAT	0.98	3.49	7.15	0.96	3.87	8.17	0.97	5.58	11.78
EePT	0.97	6.17	12.66	0.96	6.76	12.15	0.97	8.27	17.45

Table 1. Reliability coefficients, SEM & 95%CI(NewtonMeters).
         (F-flexion, E-extension, c-concentric, e-eccentric)

Inter-session reliability coefficients were calculated
comparing the mean values of all trials in both sessions.
Table 1 shows the inter-session reliability coefficients for
the means on each day and corresponding SEM and 95%CI.

The mean absolute deviation (MAD) of all trials and their
means and standard deviations were calculated to identify any
systematic error across trials and the most stable trials.
Concentric movements demomstrated a larger deviation in
torque score on the first trial only and no systematic error
over trials. Eccentric movements showed a greater deviation
over the first two trials and a systmatic decrease in torque

scores (particularly for eccentric extension) over each session which was within the 95%CI for both eccentric flexion and extension.

DISCUSSION
The results from this investigation have demonstrated high intra- and inter-session test-retest reliability for isokinetic concentric and eccentric elbow flexion and extension with this test protocol at an angular velocity of 60°/s. Measures of both peak and average torque were highly reliable.

The intra-session SEM and 95%CI indicate the magnitude of the variation in torque scores that could be expected within each test session. This may be used to identify actual differences in the muscle performance between subjects for each muscle action.

The inter-session SEM and 95%CI indicate the variability in torque scores that could be expected between test sessions with this protocol such that if torque scores fall outside the 95%CI for a particular muscle action at the second test session, then a change in muscle performance has occurred. The SEM and 95%CI for EeAT and EePT are double those for the other muscle actions, which although highly reliable renders these muscle actions less sensitive to a change in muscle performance with this test protocol than the other muscle actions. The variability of the torque scores between sessions was only slightly greater than within each session except for EePT in which the inter-session 95%CI was 5Nm higher than the intra-session 95%CI.

The results of this study revealed that concentric muscle actions required only one maximal warm-up trial for the first test session, and that eccentric muscle actions required two maximal warm-up trials.

CONCLUSION
A reliable test protocol for peak and average torque measurements of isokinetic concentric and eccentric elbow flexion and extension has been established at 60°/s. This consists of one maximal warm-up trial for concentric muscle actions and two maximal warm-up trials for eccentric muscle actions at the initial test session, followed by three maximal trials of concentric or eccentric elbow flexion or extension. Each trial should be separated by a 30 second rest interval including the interval between the warm-up and trial repetitions.

MECHANICAL CHARACTERISTICS OF KINETIC "MUSCLE CHAINS" IN THE UPPER LIMB.

G. PIERRON, B. LANDJERIT.

ECK BOIS LARRIS BP 12 60260 LAMORLAYE FRANCE

ENKRE 12 rue du Val d'Osne 94410 ST-MAURICE FRANCE

ENSAM 151bd.de l'Hôpital 75013 PARIS FRANCE

The organization of muscles in the upper limb in the kinetic "muscle chains" can be classified into : serial chains devoted to speed and amplitude, parallel chains maximizing available power. The assesment of mechanical parameters for speed and amplitude was done with an infra-red Motion Analyser of the "SAGA3". Power assesment of mecanichal parameter was studied with a "MERAC" isometric dynamometer. The datas validates our theorical model.
The repercussions on stress applied to the humerus by the "Speed" and the "power" muscle chain were studied by two and three-dimensional photoelastometry and by numerical analog conversion for each type of load. This allowed us to classify various degrees of stress as, in order of increment : (1) elbow extension + shoulder flexion, (2) elbow flexion + shoulder flexion, (3) elbow flexion + shoulder extension, (4) elbow extension + shoulder extension.
Measurements of stress and strain on the humerus make it possible to schedule timely rehabilitation exercises.

THE ABDUCTION OF THE SHOULDERGIRDLE
from osteokinematics to arthrokinematics

J.H.C.Vuurmans, manual therapist, lecturer.
School for Manual Therapy, Utrecht, the Netherlands.

From earlier studies on the abduction movement of the shouldergirdle we
have learned that it is an articulatio composita.
The abduction movement can be described in 4 phases in which all participants have their specific contribution to complete abduction.
This is an osteokinematic description. The description of the participation of each bone to the movement.

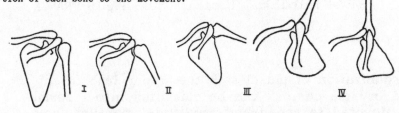

I II III IV

Phase I: Humeral abduction, at 30° the movement is inhibited by the
              ligamentum conoideum of the acromioclavicular joint because
              the scapula will follow the humeral abduction.

Phase II: Raising of the clavi-scapular fork, its axis passes through
              the sternoclavicular joint and the medial root of the spina
              scapula. This movement is inhibited by the costo-clavicular
              ligament at 30° of abduction.

Phase III: Scapula abduction, the axis passes through the acromioclavi-
              cular joint. Simultaneously there is a backward turning over
              of the clavicula and scapula across the thorax which results
              in even more spatial abduction of the humerus.

Phase IV: Internal rotation of the humerus over the forward-facing
              glenoid cavity of the scapula, resulting in abduction.

Because this is a bone description of a movement it is called osteokinematics. A model of the abduction movement.
There is, of course, an individual variety in which this movement can
take place and this is important when we have to treat this joint in case
of complaints.
Abduction of the scapula is a clear movement, if we want to mobilise it
we must look at the gleno-humeral joint and the acromio-clavicular joint.
In the gleno-humeral joint the abduction of the scapula is a downward and
lateral movement. In the acromioclavicular joint abduction is an upward

and lateral movement. In the same way claviular abduction in the sterno-clavicular joint is an upward movement and in the acromio-clavicular joint a downward movement.
Rotation in the transversal plane can be seen as an internal rotation from the clavicula in the sterno-clavicular joint as a movement forwards, in the acromio-clavicular joint as a movement backwards and this is identicle for the scapula.
Variation in the form of the bones, joint surfaces, development of muscular proportions and ligaments (as a result of function) will give an individual position from which the abduction movement is starting. This position gives the direct relation of the shouldergirdle to the cervical-, thoracic- and lumbar spine, ribs and pelvis.

Joint surfaces show a curvature, from the shape the evolute of the joint-profile can be found. And if we make the evolute from that part where there is cartilage we can find the places where there is possible contact with the other joint-partner. The difference in curvation of the 2 articular-bones that form the joint gives 2 evolutes, the evolute of concave lies further from the joint-surface than the evolute of convex. The rotationcentres can be found on the perpendicular from the point of contact. Because of the 3-dimensional shape of joint profiles we must add the 3rd dimension to this 2 dimensional explanation.
There can never be one axis when we describe the movement in a joint.

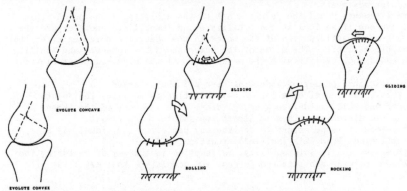

There is always more cartilage on the convex part of the joint than on the concave part.
This means that the angular movement in a joint has a great variety of displacement of the cartilage surfaces to eachother.
By looking at the gleno-humeral joint we see the convex humerus head and the concave glenoid. The collection of rotation centres can be found between the joint surface and the evolute of concave.
Abduction is a roll lateral and upwards, with the rotation centre in the jointsurface, equal displacement on convex and concave will give an angular abduction. It will be stopped very soon because the end of the cartilage of the glenoid is reached.
If the rotationcentre is located in the convexity we will get the possibility to slide downward during this roll and a greater abduction is

965

reached.
Describing the scapula to the humerus, abduction is a rocking movement
downward with its rotationcentre in the jointsurface again little
spatial abduction is possible, when the rotationcentre is located in the
humerushead a glide in the same direction will lead to a greater angular
abduction.
In the same way every other joint can be described and in 3-dimensional
view.
Thus mobilisation must always be done with angular, 3-dimensional movements, gentle movements and it must always stay within the fysiological
boundries of the joint.
Traction and translation are movements that are biomechanically incorrect
as far as the joints are concerned. They are a-fysiological and can not
be produced by any tissue in the body. And if present we intent to speak
of instability of the joint.
The arthro-kinematical description is fysiological and it can be achieved
by human activities of several tissues.
Collagen is the steering tissue, passively, in the joint mobility and
muscular activity is able to provide varieties in the angular movement.
The m.deltoideus abducts the humerus by rolling it lateral/upwards, the
m.supraspinatus provides the slide downwards during this abduction.

And this may well be the function of the rotator-cuff muscles in all
shouldermovements.
The ligaments round the joints adapt to the mobility of the joint. This
we can see if we look at the mobility of an immobilised shoulder and the
changes in participation of the bones in the abduction movement after the
immobilisation. The slide of the humerushead has lessened and mobility
is ended much earlier with the early start of the clavi-scapular elevation.
The described phases of abduction have all been changed.
Arthrokinematics gives a lot of possibilities to mobilise the joint,
more/less roll, slide, rocking, gliding, spin in every of the three
possible directions. This is almost impossible to carry-out.
Therefore it is necessary to analyse our patient's individual way of
functioning. From this individual functioning model
optimalisation in jointmobility, in function is the way of restoring the
balance between mobility and forces, and complaints that may arise with
that.

Literature:
1.Osteo- en arthro-kinematika: Harry H.N.Oonk
  Uitg.Henric Graaff van IJssel.
2.De schoudergordel, biomechanische aspekten:
  H.v.d.Linden,J.H.C.Vuurmans,School voor Manuele Therapie,Utrecht.
3.De abductiebeweging van de schoudergordel,H.v.d.Linden,
  J.H.C.Vuurmans,Ned.Tijdschrift v.Manuele Therapie.no.1,1984.
4.The abduction movement in the shouldergirdle, J.H.C.Vuurmans,
  proceedings 3rd.int.phys.congress Hong Kong, 1990.and
  U.T.M.T.no.2,1990.

THE WRIST,A THREE DIMENSIONAL ARTHROKINEMATIC MODEL

J.J.M. Pool
School for Manual Therapy, Utrecht, the Netherlands

INTRODUCTION

Allthough it has always been seen as a single joint complex,the wrist should be seen in a kinematic system of joints including the elbow,shoulder, cervical and thoracic spine. This holistic vision is common at the Utrecht school. Treatment should therefore always enclose this total view.To get a proper view of the wrist I shall limit myself to the wrist alone.An arthrokinematic study(1) of the movements of the jointsurfaces shows us the following descriptions. Moving a convex surface over a concave surface there is a roll accompanied with a slide and a spin (fig.1)
Moving a concave surface over a convex surface there is a rocking accompanied with a gliding and a spin (fig.2).The centre of rotation is always sited in the area between the evolute of convex and the surface of the concavity.(fig 3 constructing an evolute and fig 4).All the centres of rotation in a joint during a movement are called the centrode.
To move one part of a joint towards another is only possible when an angular movement occurs.That means a translation without a rotation never occurs!.

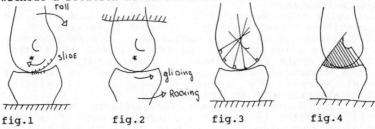

fig.1   fig.2   fig.3   fig.4

ANATOMY

Art. Radio-carpea;egg-shaped joints,between radius and discus articularis as proximal concave part and ossae scaphoideum, lunatum and triquetrum as distal convex part.
Art. Medio-carpea;two egg-shaped joints, between scaphoid as concave proximal part and trapezium and trapezoideum as convex distal parts,and lunatum and scaphoideum as proximal concave parts and capitatum as distal convex part.

And a saddle-shaped joint between triquetrum and hamatum.
In the frontal plane the triquetrum bone is concave and the hamatum is convex, in the sagittal plane the triquetrum is convex and hamatum is concave.
Art.intercarpea proximale these are saddle-shaped joints in the frontal plane, the lunatum is bi-concave.
The os pisiforme has an egg-shaped joint with the os triquetrum and is bi-concave.
Art.intercarpea distales, also saddle-shaped joints, capitatum is bi-concave and trapezoideum is bi-convex, both in the frontal plane.

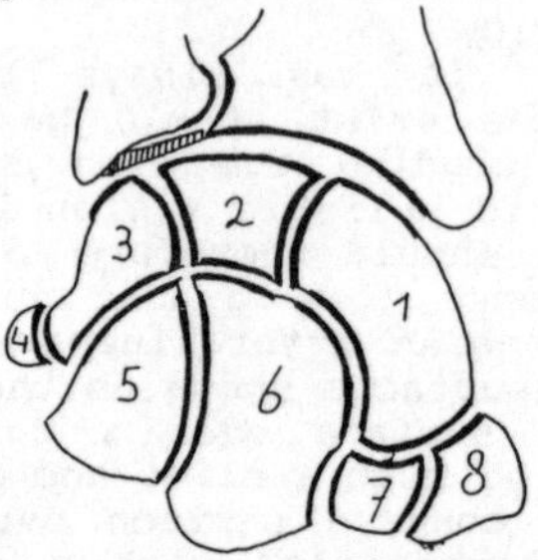

fig.5. 1;Os Scaphoideum
       2;Os Lunatum
       3;Os Triquetrum
       4;Os Pisiforme
       5;Os Hamatum
       6;Os Capitatum
       7;Os Trapezoideum
       8;Os Trapezium
       Frontal section

KINESIOLOGY
Palmair-flexion is mostly combined with ulnair abduction and external-rotation(1). The quality and quantity of those movements in terms of roll,slide,rocking and gliding vary per individual.Different authors propose a system of three longitudinal chains,others a proximal and a distal row.
longitudinal chains;radial chain consists of radius-scaphoideum-trapezium/trapezoideum. Central chain consists of radius/discus-lunatum-capitatum. Ulnar , chain consists of triquetrum-hamatum.
The following arthrokinematic remarks can be made when the above mentioned three-dimensional movement is carried out.
radial chain; scaphoid versus radius makes a roll ventrally and medially,a slide dorsally and laterally and an external spin.In this chain the scaphoid is the fastest bone(2) so that the trapezium and trapezoideum makes an opposite movement versus the scaphoid; rocking and gliding dorsally/laterally with an internal spin.
central chain; lunatum versus radius/discus simular to scaphoid. Capitatum is the fastest bone, because it is more curved(2),so capitatum makes a roll ventrally/medially, a slide dorsally/laterally and an external spin.
Ulnar chain; consists of a saddle shaped joint between triquetrum and hamatum which maens it is more "stable" than an egg-shaped joint.
Triquetrum versus discus simular to lunatum,hamatum versus triquetrum the opposite movement; rocking and gliding dorsally(concave surface), roll laterally and a slide medially(convex surface) and a internal spin.

Looking at the proximal row the investigations of Kauer(2) showes a linking movement between scaphoideum and lunatum. Because of the different curvatures of the bones, scaphoid is more curved, and the shape of the ligament interosseus, which is tight dorsally and somewhat loosened ventrally there is an internal spin of the scaphoid versus lunatum during palmair flexion;in arthrokinematic terms;rocking and gliding ventrally(concave surface), roll proximally and slide distally(convex surface) and a flexion spin!

Pisiform, the pisiforme bone is to be considered as a sesamoid bone, but it shows a lot of connections in the wrist itself and has to be considered as an important structure.In vitro the surface seems to be bi-concave so it is rocking and gliding over the triquetrum(3). Failure of the movement has direct consequence on for example the scaphoid-lunatum movement and therefore on the stability of the wrist.

PRACTICAL CONSEQUENSES

When a limitation of movement is found arthrokinematically it means there is a change in positioning of the centrodes of a joint.Centrode is the total of all rotationcentres of that joint with no change in form of the jointsurfaces.

The centrode is positioned towards the jointsurface which means there is more roll than slide,or more rocking than gliding compared with the normal joint-movement.

To restore the"normal" movement a force has to be made, very gentle and percise,to move the centrode away from the joint surface . It is established by stimulating a slide for a convexity and a glide for a concavity.(1,3)

Literature;
1. Oonk HN,Osteo- en Arthrokinematica (1988) Uitg. Henric Graaff van IJssel
2. Kauer MG,(1986) The mechanism of the Carpal Joint. Clinical Orthopaedics and related research 202
3. Syllabus extremiteiten (1990)School voor Manuele Therapie

A BIOMECHANICAL ANALYSIS OF THE UPPER EXTREMITY DURING PITCHING

Y Hatanaka, H Tsuneoka, Y Hirasawa
Department of Rehabilitation, Kyoto Prefectural University of Medicine
Kawaramachi-hirokoji, Kamigyo-ku, Kyoto, Japan

INTRODUCTION
Upper extremity problems, such as baseball elbow or rotator cuff injury, are commonly encountered in the sports physical therapy field. Many investigators have advanced our knowledge of the mechanisms underlying injuries sustained in pitching, and have developed special techniques employing EMG system or isokinetic machine. In this study we used a video processing system to analyze the forces on the upper extremity during pitching.

MATERIALS AND METHODS
Twenty normal male subjects without upper extremity problems were studied at Kyoto Prefectural University of Medicine. Five subjects were currently active college league pitchers, and fifteen had various experiences in organized baseball ranging from " sandlot " baseball to high school competition. The difference between these two groups in level of technical skill was obvious. The college pitchers ranged in age from 20 to 22 years, with a mean of 21.0 years; the amateurs ranged in age from 20 to 27 years, with the average age being 23.7 years. Each subject was instructed to pitch as fast as he could. Two video cameras with high-speed shutters (500 frames/sec) were used to record motion; the one camera was placed behind the catcher to record motion in the frontal plane, and the other was placed directly to the side of the pitching rubber to record motion in the sagittal plane. The cameras were placed exactly 10 m apart for precise analysis.
The Ariel Performance Analysis System was used to process data. This system consists of an AST premium 286 computer, graphic monitors, video cameras, video playback unit, and a mouse. The two video sequences from the VCR were captured, and the video images were then converted into digitalized body joint locations using the mouse. The digitized joint locations were saved for the transformation module, which converted them into true three-dimensional images. The transformation process consisted of two distinct phases: (1) time synchronization of the two video sequences used to record the activity, and (2) computation of the true image coordinates for the body joints in each frame from the multiple sets of digitized coordinates. Generally speaking, digitized data contain random errors or noise due to imprecision in locating the position of body joints. We used the smoothing module to eliminate such errors and noise from the computed image coordinates. The smoothing module employed the cubic spline method. Smoothed data were imaged as graphs of displacement, velocity, acceleration, energy, and momentum. The wave forms and amplitudes of graphs for college pitchers were compared with those for amateurs.

The motion of pitching was divided into the four stages Gowan has described,as follows:

1) Wind-up: preliminary activity dominated by upper extremity flexion while the ball is held in both hands.

2) Cocking:the period of shoulder abduction and external rotation that begins as the ball is released from the non-dominant hand and ends when maximal external rotation of the shoulder is attained;contact of the forward foot with the ground divides this stage into early and late phases.

3) Acceleration: starts with the posture of maximal abduction and external rotation of the shoulder and continues until ball release, i.e., as the ball leaves the fingers.

4) Follow-through: the final stage of arm motion : this stage is further subdivided by the point of maximal humeral internal rotation into early and late phases.

RESULTS

Linear movement
The wave forms of graphs of displacement,velocity and acceleration for each joint for each group resembled that for the other group.Amplitude of displacement,velocity and acceleration for each joint increased quickly during the acceleration stage until ball release. However, the amplitudes of velocity and acceleration for the college league pitchers were greater than those for the amateurs.

Joint angle
Among active college league pitchers, the wave forms of graphs of displacement for all joint were characteristically synchronized at the moment of ball release. By contrast,time lags were observed among the wave forms of graphs of displacement for the amateurs.Furthermore,the wave forms of graphs of velocity and acceleration for each group showed patterns similar to those graphs of displacement.

Energy
Amplitude of rotational energy of the joints in the upper arm increased quickly during the acceleration phase,and those for joints in the forearm and hand were slight by comparison. In both groups,the wave forms of graphs of linear energy for joints in all segments of the arm were similar to those for velocity.

Moment
Although the wave forms of graphs of linear moment in each segments for the college league pitchers were also similar to those for amateurs,the wave forms of the rotational moment of joints in the upper arm showed quite different patterns in each group.

DISCUSSION

Although the use of EMG is the most precise method of observing muscle activities during pitching, the use of wire electrodes is not common in a clinical setting. Furthermore, although an electrical goniometer is the most precise instrument for measurement of joint angle, Natural pitching pattern may be altered by attachment of the instrument. The two-dimensional data obtained in this study are mere projected images,which on account of the rotation of various body segments, do not necessarily provide true values. We therefore used only the three-dimensional data during pitching.

Regarding differences between skilled pitchers and amateurs in pitching mechanics. Gowan reports that professional pitchers use the subscapularis muscle, while amateurs use other rotator cuff muscles and the biceps brachii muscle. He also reports that professional pitchers use the pectralis major, the serratus anterior, and the latissimus dorsi more extensively than other muscles. He further reports that during acceleration trunk rotation and the activities of the muscles which project the scapula forward generate the rotational momentum of the upperarm. Our results support this finding.

CONCLUSIONS

When pitching,throwing the ball in a well-coordinated manner is important for prevention of injuries of the shoulder and elbow. Skilled pitchers are able to transfer their entire energy to the ball accurately and quickly. In the early stages of pitching, the movement pattern of each joint was similar in college league pitchers and in amateurs. During acceleration, the patterns of rotational moment of the upper arm shown by the two groups diverged. Efficient transfer of momentum is needed to prevent injuries, as any residual momentum that is not transfered to the ball can be absorbed by the joints and muscles. The purpose of this study was to analyze the forces acting on the upper extremity during pitching. This knowledge can be helpfull in instruction on methods of preventing injuries.

REFERENCES

1. Pappas AM, Zawacki RM, Sullivan TJ: Biomechanics of baseball pitching. A Preliminary report. Am J Sports Med 13: 216-222,1985
2. Gowan ID, Jove FW, Tibone JE, Perry J, Moynes DR: A comparative electromyographic analysis of the shoulder during pitching. Professional varsus amateur pitchers. Am J Sports Med 15: 586-590,1987
3. Braatz JH, Gogia PP: The mechanics of pitching. J Orthop Sports Phys Ther 9:56-69,1987
4. Jove FW, Tibone JE, Perry J, Moynes DR: An EMG analysis of the shoulder in throwing and pitching. A preliminary report. Am J Sports Med 11: 3-5,1983
5. Tullos HS, King JW: Throwing mechanism in Sports. Orthop Clin North Am 4: 709-720,1973
6. Pedegana LR, Elsner RC, Roberts D, Lang J, Farewell V: The relationship of upper extremity strength to throwing speed. Am J Sports Med 10:352-354,1982
7. Tippett SR: Lower extremity strength and active range of motion in college. A comparison between stance leg and kick leg. J Orthop Sports Phys Ther 8: 10-14,1986
8. Bartlett LR, Storey MD, Simons BD: Measurement of upper extremity torque production and its relationship to throwing speed in the competitive athlete. Am J Sports Med 17: 89-91,1989
9. Wilson FD, Amdrews JR, Blackburn TA, Mccluskey G. Valgus extension overload in the pitching elbow. Am J Sports Med 11: 83-88,1983

THERAPY IN PSYCHIATRY

EFFECTS OF DIFFERENT FORMS OF EXERCISE ON THE FITNESS, MOOD AND MEMORY OF A SAMPLE OF PROBLEM DRINKERS

M Donaghy   Department of Physiotherapy, Queen Margaret College, Edinburgh
G E Ralston Department of Psychological Medicine Southern General, Glasgow
N Mutrie   Department of Physical Education, University of Glasgow.

Introduction
Alcohol abuse can damage most of the tissues of the body and the problem drinker can be affected by physical, mental and social disabilities (WHO 1977). There is evidence to indicate that aerobic exercise may be beneficial in the treatment of problem drinkers in terms of improved fitness and lowered anxiety and depression. (Sinyor et al 1982, Palmer et al 1988) Although few controlled studies have been conducted to date and none which look at the effects of non-aerobic exercise.

Method
The subjects in this study were 45 male new referrals to the Alcohol Problem Clinical (APC) at Dykebar Hospital, Paisley. The subjects met three times per week for a 30 minute exercise session.   Subjects were placed in three groups:
A   an aerobic group (16 subjects) (13 completed);
B   non-aerobic weight training group (15 subjects) (12 completed); and
C   relaxation attention placebo control group   (14 subjects) (12 completed)

The total number of subjects who failed to complete the programme was 7, they left the unit, with 1 further subject, failing to be re-tested on any parameters.

Apparatus
The Monarch bicycle ergometer, a PE 3000 heart rate monitor, a platform scale sit and reach boards, a multi-gym and standardised exercise log (Glasgow University Department of Physical Education and Sports Science 1988) and a Hartz standard sphygmomanometer were also used.

Procedure
The study was a randomised three group design with pre- and post-measures of physical fitness and psychological measures taken at the beginning and end of a 8 week programme.   New referrals to the APC who had given informed consent and had received medical clearance to participate were interviewed by a clinical psychologist and were assessed on the following measures: the Beck Depression Inventory; the Leeds scale for Anxiety and Depression; the Weschler memory scale.

Subjects were then referred to the physiotherapist where they were randomly allocated to one of the three groups. Some patients were on antabuse medication, to counterbalance for this variable two randomised lists with equal numbers for each condition were used.

The clinical psychologist was blind to the group allocation of participants. Fitness measures were undertaken by the physiotherapist as follows: an Astrand Rhyming Bicycle Ergometer Test (Astrand and Rodahl 1977); a standardised sit-up test to measure abdominal muscle endurance; and a standardised sit and reach test to measure flexibility.

The procedure followed the guidelines detailed by the American College of Sports Medicine. Body weight, blood pressure, and resting heart rate were recorded.

The aerobic group maintained continuous aerobic activity for at least 20 minutes at an average intensity of training of 70-75% of maximum heart rate reserve. Heart rate was monitored at regular intervals to ensure intensity. The programme consisted of taped graded exercise.

The non-aerobic weight training group undertook a 6 station programme which was paced to allow heart rate of the subjects to remain at or below 50-60% of the estimated maximum heart rate reserve.

The relaxation attention placebo control group were instructed in an autogenic relaxation programme which included some gentle stretching exercises of the trunk and limbs. All groups had the same amount of time and attention from the physiotherapist throughout the programme.

Results
Preliminary findings are detailed below, further analysis is currently being undertaken.
Using the SPSS-X computer package: dependent t-tests by group were carried out on the pre- and post- test scores for all dependent measures.

The Beck Depression Inventory
There was significant reduction in depression scores over time for both group A, and group B. Group C had shown some reduction in this depression score but it was not significant.

Other variables
The group differences in depression scores were confirmed by analysis of the individual Leeds sub-scales.

Anxiety both general and specific as measured by the Leeds scale was significantly reduced in group A and B, while group C showed a slight increase in anxiety over time. The Memory tests showed no significant change over time.

Measures of fitness
There was improved fitness Submaximal Vo2 ML/KG/MIN over the 8 weeks in group A only, with group B showing some improvement and group C showing no change.

Group A and C improved in abdominal endurance and also in flexibility. Group B improved in abdominal endurance, but not in flexibility.

There was no change in resting heart rate or blood pressure for any of the groups.

Discussion

After 8 weeks of either aerobic or non-aerobic exercise the depression scores of problem drinkers significantly reduced on the BDI (confirmed by the Leeds scale). While the control group carrying out relaxation showed no such difference in depression scores.

The reduction in anxiety was also significant in the two exercise groups on the Leeds scales, while the control group showed slight increase in anxiety.

Thus the findings indicate that exercise would appear to have an important part to play in the treatment of the problem drinker in the improvement of mood. The significant improvement in the fitness found in the aerobic group but not in the weights group indicates that the psychological improvement is not dependent on improved physiological change. This is important as it indicated that greater choice can be used in planning exercise programmes taking into account the preferences and needs of individuals.

It is important to note that the three groups had the same attention from the physiotherapist and the same amount of time allocated to the exercise programme. The differences are therefore less likely to be caused by peripheral effects of the experimental situation, e.g. interaction and motivation of the therapist.

Conclusion

The findings of this study indicate that exercise can reduce depression and anxiety levels in the treatment of problem drinkers.

The cost effectiveness of exercise compared to other treatments for depression and anxiety amongst problem drinkers make thus area of work worthy of further research and application within psychiatric hospitals where day-patients and in-patients with alcohol related problems are treated.

Thus the following conclusions can be drawn from this study:
(i)   aerobic and non-aerobic exercise can reduce depression and anxiety levels in the treatment of problem drinkers;
(ii)   aerobic exercise over an eight week programme can improve fitness as measured by estimated Vo2 max. with problem drinkers;
(iii)   the interaction of the therapist and the patient accounting for the outcome of treatment can be discounted; and
(iv)   there is no clear indication that an exercise programme improves the memory of problem drinkers.

REFERENCES

Sinyor, D. Brown, T. and Rostant, L. and Seraganian, P. The role of physical program in the treatment of alcoholism. J. Stud, Alcohol 43: 380-386, 1982.
Palmer, J. Vacc, N. Epstein, J. Physical Exercise as a Treatment Intervention Journal of Studies on Alcohol Vol 49, No 5 1988.

EFFECT OF A PHYSICAL EXERCISE PROGRAM ON BODY IMAGE AND PHYSICAL ACTIVITY OF PATIENTS WITH BULIMIA AND ANOREXIA NERVOSA

M. MacKay-Lyons, MSc (P.T.), D. MacDonald, M.D., M. Mahoney, BSc(P.T.)
Departments of Physiotherapy and Psychiatry, Victoria General Hospital,
Halifax, Nova Scotia, Canada, B3H 2Y9

Anorexia nervosa and bulimia are eating disorders characterized by an intense fear of fatness, an obsessive desire for thinness, a distorted body image, and denial of illness or of weight loss.[1] Patients pursue weight loss by either severe restriction of caloric intake (anorexia nervosa) or by restriction of food alternating with periods of binge eating that terminate in self-induced vomiting and/or in the use of laxatives and diuretics (bulimia). Excessive physical activity is a common method of achieving weight loss in both types and may be the earliest sign of an incipient eating disorder.

There is a growing population of patients with eating disorders whose condition appears refractory to traditional therapeutic strategies. Clinicians agree that a multidimensional treatment approach with active patient participation is necessary. Bruch[2,] a leading theorist in the study of eating disorders, considers the correction of the patient's body image disturbance to be a precondition to recovery. The difficulty lies in ascertaining *how* to change disturbed self-perceptions.

At our general hospital the eating disorder treatment team traditionally consisted of psychiatrists, psychiatric nurses, occupational therapists, dieticians, and psychologists. Four years ago, the psychiatrists began referring patients to physiotherapy. The physiotherapist's role was to design an exercise program for each patient and to educate the patient in the relation between exercise and eating disorders. The premise was that through this intervention cognitive restructuring would be facilitated and that alterations, not only in physical activity, but also in body image would ensue.

No studies have been cited that deal with the effects of therapeutic exercise programs for patients with anorexia nervosa or bulimia. Despite the abundance of information on body image disturbances and excessive physical activity few authors suggest intervention to specifically address these problems. While Davison[3] describes a physiotherapy program to improve the body image and physical well-being of the anorexic patient, she fails to document the effectiveness of this program.

This study was undertaken to determine if participation in a physiotherapy program would 1) normalize the body image of patients with body image disturbances, 2) reduce cognitive distortions regarding the relationship between exercise and health, 3) alter the nature of physical activity.

METHOD
Subjects
Female volunteers (n = 26) with the diagnosis of bulimia or anorexia nervosa were referred for participation by a psychiatrist The subjects were randomly assigned to either the Exercise or Control Group Nine Exercise subjects (56%) and five Control subjects (50%) had anorexia nervosa (Tab.).

TABLE: Subject Characteristics

Parameters	Experimental Group (n = 16)		Control Group (n = 10)		t^a
	$\overline{X}$	s	$\overline{X}$	s	
Age (yr)	25.9	5.0	26.0	3.0	-.04
Age at Diagnosis (yr)	23.2	6.2	23.5	3.7	-.13
Body Mass Index [b]	13.00	3.77	11.41	3.45	-1.06
Wrist circumference (cm)	14.58	0.53	14.24	0.79	1.31
Elbow circumference (cm)	59.94	3.82	59.00	5.27	.53

[a] non-significant/ df = 24   [b] Body Mass Index = (body weight/height)/2 x 100

Procedure

Pretest. During a single session a week prior to the initiation of the exercise program data was collected on demographics; history of eating disorder; and a physical activity inventory (including nature and frequency of activity). Measurements were taken of weight, height, and wrist and elbow circumference. The Body Image Assessment (**BIA**) was performed, the details of which are provided elsewhere.[4] Briefly, the subject stands in front of a sheet of paper (1.5 x 1 m) fixed fixed to the wall.. The subject indicates on the paper points which correspond to her estimate of the width of her shoulders, waist, and hips. Body width indices are calculated for each of the body width estimates (estimated width - actual width x 100). The Body Self Relations Questionnaire-Short Form (**BSRQ**) was used as a measure of body image.[6] This questionnaire assesses three domains of body image (physical appearance, physical fitness and physical health) in terms of three dimensions (evaluation, attention/importance and activity). A multiple choice questionnaire (**MCQ**) provided a gross assessment of knowledge of basic anatomy and the relation between exercise and health.

Exercise Program. The Exercise subjects attended physiotherapy sessions while the Control subjects did not participate in a formal physiotherapy program. The latter subjects were instructed not to change their customary life style and activity level. Both groups were requested to keep a log of their physical activity over the course of the study. In addition, they were requested to continue with their other therapies (e.g.psychiatric counselling, occupational therapy, and nutritional counselling). Any modifications to these therapies were postponed until the completion of the study. The physiotherapy program consisted of two one-hour sessions weekly for four weeks. There were two groups of five participants and a third group of six. The educational component involved a 30-minute group discussion in a relaxed, comfortable environment. Topics for the sessions included: the classification of exercise (aerobic vs non-aerobic); exercise and caloric expenditure; bones and joints; muscles; postural correction; stress reduction; and positive and negative effects of exercise. The second half of each session involved a 30-minute period of individually tailored exercises. Essentially, those parts of the body about which the subject expressed dissatisfaction were addressed through the appropriate exercises. The emphasis was on non-aerobic exercises, i.e. exercises that involve strengthening and isometric 'toning' of muscles and stretching of soft tissue. A home program of exercises was designed for use after completion of the last session.

Posttest and Followup. The protocol used in the pretest was followed at posttest for all subjects. Also, the subjects in the Exercise Group were asked to complete a program evaluation form. Followup testing of all subjects was conducted six months after entry into the study. One subject in each group did not return for the followup assessment.

Data Analysis. Subject characteristics were compared by group using independent samples t-tests. A group by trial analysis of variance (ANOVA) for repeated measures was used to determine statistically if differential effects were obtained between the two groups on each of the dependent variables.We used a significance level of .05 for all hypothesis testing.

RESULTS

Attendance and Physical Activity Inventory. The attendance at the physiotherapy sessions was 85%. The reported frequency of physical activity did not change significantly over the course of the study and ranged between 0-10 hours per week for Exercise subjects and between 0-14 hours per week for Control subjects. Examination of the activity logs revealed that the nature of exercise changed in the case of the Exercise subjects. Initially, nine (56%) participated in aerobic exercise program while by posttest this was reduced to four (25%). By the six month followup eight (53%) had resumed their original participation in aerobic exercise. Six (60%) Control subjects maintained participation in aerobic programs throughout the study.

Body Image. The ANOVA results for the waist index of the BIA showed a significant change over time but the interaction of time with group was not statistically significant. Similarly, while a time effect was evident for three of six BSRQ subsections the interaction of time with group was not significant.

Background Knowledge. Twelve (75%) Exercise subjects and nine(90%) Control subjects had post-secondary education. The ANOVA results of the MCQ did not reveal statistically significant differences in the scores By way of example, in response to:"*What are the tissues that normally account for most of the girth (thickness) of the thigh?*" 13 (81%) Exercise subjects responded incorrectly "bone and fat" at pretest. Eight (50%) responded similarly at posttest and followup.

Program Evaluation. The 12 (75%) subjects who completed the evaluation form were positive about the program and felt that they could recommend it to other people with eating disorders. The majority responded that the educational component was the most important part of the program.

DISCUSSION

Being aware of the reluctance of patients with anorexia nervosa and bulimia to receive treatment, we were not anticipating high compliance with the program.Thus, the high attendance rate and favorable feedback from the program evaluation form were gratifying. Possibly the program's non-threatening orientation to exercise and education (as opposed to the more common orientation to body weight and eating habits) was a factor in generating this enthusiasm. The endorsement of the program led us to expect significant changes in the parameters under study. In general, this was not the case.

The reported frequency of physical activity at pretest was lower than anticipated for both groups of subjects. However, reliance on self-reporting for this patient population is problematic. Patients with anorexia nervosa or bulimia have the reputation of being highly manipulative.[1] One subject in the Exercise Group stated at pretest that she engaged in an average of eight hours of physical activity per week. Yet, during an exercise session, she reported performing three hours of aerobic exercises, 20 miles of stationary bicycling and 500 'sit-up' exercises on a *daily* basis. A desirable change in the nature of physical activity from aerobic to non-aerobic exercise was apparent from the activity logs of Exercise subjects but by the six month followup this effect was no longer evident. If these self-reports are indeed accurate, the pattern of change in this behavior suggests that the program may have had a temporary effect on some of the subjects.

The BIA results, which assess the perceptual or schematic representation of body parts, and the BSRQ results, which assess the affective reaction to one's body, indicated that the program did not contribute to changes in body image. The fact that several subsections of the BSRQ and the waist index of the BIA changed over time for subjects in *both* groups is difficult to explain. Possibly, the repetition of the testing procedure at pretest, posttest, and followup influenced the results. Szmukler[6] suggested that responses of the anorexic patients may actually "bear a closer relationship to their attitudes to treatment or to the experimenter than to their perception of their bodies."(p.553)

Possibly the most perplexing finding of the study was the fact that the physiotherapy program did not affect performance on the MCQ. Despite the high proportion of subjects with post-secondary education and the deliberate repetition of information pertinent to the MCQ during the educational sessions, the subjects in the Exercise Group failed to improve their performance. In other words, the cognitive restructuring that we hoped to achieve was not evident. This result underlines not only the extent of cognitive distortions, but also, the degree of resistance to change these distortions.

That our hypotheses were not supported in this study is disheartening. However, the findings may be limited by a number of factors. First, the sample size was small rendering attainment of significant results difficult. Second, intragroup differences in subject characteristics were apparent. More restrictive inclusion criteria would lead to more homogeneity which, in turn, might enhance the effectiveness of the program. Third, the program duration was only four weeks. A longer program may be necessary to elicit the desired changes. Last, the limitations of self-reporting and body image assessments as objective findings preclude generalizing from the results of this study.

CONCLUSIONS

This study represents an initial attempt to assess the effectiveness of a physiotherapy program for patients with anorexia nervosa and bulimia.While program participation was high and subjective feedback positive, objective changes in the parameters under study were not forthcoming.and the participants exhibited resistance to adjusting their cognitive distortions. Further research is warranted if the role of physical therapy with this patient population is to be developed.

References

1. A Canadian Medical Association Review (1989) Eating disorders: Anorexia and bulimia
2. Bruch H (1973) *Eating Disorders.* New York,NY Basic Books
3. Davison K (1988) Physiotherapy in the treatment of anorexia nervosa. Physiother 74:62-64
4. Pierloot RA, Houben ME(1978) Estimation of body dimensions in anorexia nervosa. Psychol Med 8: 317-324
5. Winstead BA, Cash TF(1984) Reliability and validity of the Body-Self Relations Questionnaire: A new measure of body image. Paper presented at Southeastern Psychological Association Meetings, New Orleans, LA
6. Szmukler G (1984) Body image disturbances in anorexia nervosa. Brit J of Psychiatry 144:553

The BAS - a Reliable Way to Measure Changes in Body Awareness.

Author: A. Winberg
Adress: Dep.of Physiotherapy, St.Sigfrids sjukhus, Box 1223
S-351 12 Växjö, Sweden

This project is one part of an evaluation of a psychiatric hospital ward for psychotherapeutic treatment of schizophrenia. The whole project is led by Professor Alf Nilsson at the Dep. of Applied Psychology, Univ. of Lund, Sweden, and can be described as a combination of basic and applied research. The group of researchers consist of a psychiatrist, psychotherapists, psychologists, psychiatric social workers, a physiotherapist and a psychiatric nurse. Young schizophrenic patients are to be treated for three years (approx) on a newly-opened (1988) psychiatric ward in Växjö. The treatment approach on the ward is mileu-oriented and psychotherapeutic. The whole project consists of three parts called 1) structure evaluation, 2) process evaluation, 3) effect evaluation.

1. Within the framework of the structure evaluation it is the ward's "assets" that are studied - these contain the ward environment, the staff on the ward and all others connected to the ward.

2. The process evaluation studies the processes taking place on the ward, in the individual therapy sessions and in the supervision.

3. The effect evaluation covers:
a) psychological testing including cognitive function tests and perceptgenetic personality tests
   b) clinical psychiatric testing based on CPRS and an interview-based life quality scale (Kajandi)
   c) study of body consciousness, body management and general movement pattern and their eventual changes, based on Body Awareness Scale (BAS) by Dr. Gertrud Roxendal
   d) evaluation of the work, conducted by staff connected to the ward, with the patients' closest relations.

Even though we started working on this project in 1988 , it is still in it's infancy. So far, 4 patients and their controls have been assessed once (before treatment). The entire project will consist of 8 patients and 8 controls, who will be tested 3 times: before treatment, after treatment and one year after treatment. That means, there are no results yet. I am therefore going to concentrate the rest of my speech on how the assessment is made.

Though it is well known that schizophrenic patients have changes in their body experience, both during their psychotic period and afterwards, it is not so easy to describe it in scientific terms. My experiance is, that the patients themselves do not talk spontaneously about these phenomena, perhaps it is because the experiences are frightening and strange that they don't want to talk about them. Whereas I believe there must also be unconscious factors involved: What you don't quite realise, you cannot express.

These difficulties demand a special method of assessment, which includes both psychological and physical mechanisms. Apart from the mechanical aspect which is in all movements, you also have to deal with mental aspects, such as cognitive thought processes and experiences concerning the body. It is also relevant to look upon the body as an instrument of self-expression.

The BAS, which I am using, has got this dynamic, multifactoral way of looking at movements, in order to, among other things, measure body awareness as a whole. The scale has been tested in different studies and has shown good inter-rater reliability, which makes it able to assess changes over time. All items in the scale have the scale-steps 0-3, with operational definitions of each scale-step. The scale is well-structured and not too difficult to learn.

In addition to the BAS, I also use video-recording during the whole session.

BAS gives us different kinds of information:
On one hand : The patients own report, via an interview, which contains items concerning emotional symptoms as well as bodily reactions.
    eg: Inner tension, hostile feelings, hypochondriasis, muscular tension report, depersonalisation, attitude to physical ability, attitude to own apparance, etc.

On the other hand: The rater's observation during the interview and during a structured movement test. This consists of common movements, adapted to the needs of everyday life, such as different types of walking exercises, jumping, arm swinging. The exercises are well known to most physiotherapists, but in the BAS you look at them in a different way. In gait, eg. you consider walking as a result of both mechanical and mental aspects and focus on motor behaviour as a whole, not on the movement in each single joint, as in gait analysis.
    eg.of items: Relation to the ground, relation to the center line, associated movements in walking, personal space, open or closed body posture, isolated movements, muscular tension, etc.

When you then compare these two different sources of information, there might be incongruence between the patient's report and the rater's observation. That is of course important to notice and is thus a source of more information.
    eg.the patient denys hostile feelings, but he does it in a hostile way or show hostility against the rater.

In order to give a better idea of how a movement test is done, a sequence from a demonstration video will be shown.

Ref: Roxendal G, Body Awareness Therapy and the Body Awareness Scale, Treatment and Evaluation in psyciatric Physiotherapy, Thesis Göteborg 1986

NEUROLOGICAL SYSTEM / NEUROLOGY

COMPENSATORY AND SUBSTITUTION MOVEMENTS FOLLOWING ACUTE BRAIN LESIONS: USEFUL OR NOT.

J.H.Carr, Dip.Phty., M.Ed. (Columbia), F.A.C.P., R.B.Shepherd, Dip.Phty., Ed.D. (Columbia), F.A.C.P.
School of Physiotherapy, Cumberland College, The University of Sydney.

It is almost certain that rearrangement of neuronal connections does occur following CNS trauma in humans. Moreover, animal evidence is compelling in demonstrating that connections that form are physiologically operational and are likely to contribute in some way to function (Steward, 1989). Any growth responses, therefore, that do occur in humans following CNS injury are likely to play a role in outcome for the individual.

What is potentially of considerable importance to rehabilitation of brain-damaged individuals is the concept that the process of reorganisation of remaining circuitry as well as sprouting within the CNS may be influenced directly by certain factors. The recently suggested linkage between external stimulation and the process of reorganisation (Marshall, 1990) compels us to look closely at both the intervention strategies utilised in rehabilitation and the environment in which rehabilitation occurs, since rehabilitation itself must have a significant effect on what motor behaviours emerge and become learned.

The perspective that rehabilitation needs to address the "emergent" motor behaviours following lesion is congruent with the dynamical systems viewpoint of contemporary action theorists. These theorists consider that motor behaviour shares fundamental principles of organisation with a general class of non-linear complex, open systems (Abraham and Shaw, 1982). Rather than considering functional activity as the result of a set of neuronal commands generated hierarchically as part of an a priori motor program, a dynamical systems approach views motor activity as resulting from the co-operation of many sub-systems. The information provided by the context is considered an active contributor to the emergence of the behaviours (Ulrich, 1989). This theory has its origins in terms of motor control in the work of Bernstein (1967) and more recently Kelso, Kugler, Turvey and others (e.g., Kugler & Turvey, 1987; Saltzman & Kelso, 1987). As well as the many theoretical papers on the subject, several authors have utilised a dynamical systems approach in studies of motor behaviours which are directly relevant for clinical physiotherapy (e.g., Clark & Phillips, 1987; Winstein & Garfinkel, 1989).

Taking this viewpoint ourselves, Roberta Shepherd and I have increasingly emphasised the importance of an understanding of biomechanics, muscle biology and kinesiology, in addition to cognitive psychology and neuroscience, in the analysis of motor dysfunction and in the development of training methods.

One mechanism which may limit recovery following brain damage is the practice of compensatory and substitution movements. People with motor dysfunction spontaneously utilize compensatory movements in order to accomplish a particular goal. That is, they perform the required action in the most biomechanically effective manner they can given the state of the system. Furthermore, many rehabilitation settings actively encourage the learning of substitution behaviours by providing one-arm-operated wheelchairs and broad-based walking sticks with the aim of providing early independence.

Le Vere (1980) suggests that compensation is incompatible with recovery of function. That is, if compensation is successful and the individual is able to achieve goals by compensating for the disrupted behaviour, then obviously there is no stimulus to the partially damaged neuronal system to recover. Indeed, Le Vere suggests that not only does compensation interfere with recovery but also that recovery can occur only by utilising those motor, sensory and cognitive systems that were directly affected by the neural injury.

Compensatory movements are adaptive movements which illustrate the ability of the lesioned system to put together an action out of what remains of the various sub-systems (whether neural, muscular or skeletal) with the emergent movement isomorphic with the demands of the environment. That is, actions are performed in the most advantageous way given the effects of the lesion, the nature of the musculo-skeletal system and the environment in which the action is performed. Such compensations are often effective in a limited way, enabling the individual to "get by" given that assistance will be provided by others and that the environment will be less demanding than usual.

There is another consideration apart from the therapeutic encouragement of compensation, If as seems likely, motor behaviour emerges as a result of the context, that is, the "pattern" of standing up emerges as a result of what the individual is sitting on, the sitting posture, or how strong or well controlled the leg muscles are, then it may not be enough to practise the action of standing up itself, since the individual will find the task so difficult that only a rough approximation of it can be practised. The task or the environment may need to be modified or adapted (e.g., standing up practised from a higher seat until the leg muscles are able to generate sufficient extensor force from a lower seat). The individual may possess the necessary neural substrates and the mechanical ability to sequence joint actions but lack sufficient muscle strength and postural control to demonstrate it under the normal environmental conditions. Modification is, therefore, necessary to deter the individual from using compensatory strategies, the early learning of which would interfere with the eventual ability to learn more effective patterns of movement (Carr & Shepherd, 1989).

REFERENCES

Abraham RH, Shaw CD (1982) Dynamics-The Geometry of Behaviour. Santa Cruz, CA: Aerial Press.
Bernstein NA (1967) The Co-ordination and Regulation of Movements. London: Pergamon Press.
Carr JH, Shepherd RB (1989) A motor learning model for stroke rehabilitation. Physiotherapy, 75, 372-380.
Clark JE, Phillips SJ (1987) The step cycle organization of infant walkers. Journal of Motor Behaviour 19:421-433.
Kugler PN, Turvey MT (1987) Information, Natural Law and the Self-assembly of Rhythmic Movement. Hillsdale, NJ:Erlbaum.
LeVere TE (1980) Recovery of function after brain damage. A theory of the behavioural deficit. Physiological Psychology, 8:297-308.
Marshall LF (1990) Current head injury research. Current Opinion in Neurology and Neurosurgery 3:4-9.
Saltzman E, Kelso JAS (1987) Skilled actions: a task dynamic approach. Psychological Review 94:84-106.
Steward O Reorganization of neuronal connections following CNS trauma: principles and experimental paradigms. Journal of Neurotrauma 6:99-152.
Ulrich BD (1989) Development of stepping patterns in human infants: a dynamical systems perspective. Journal of Motor Behaviour 21:392-408.
Winstein CJ, Garfinkel A (1989) Qualitative dynamics of disordered human locomotion: a preliminary investigation. Journal of Motor Behaviour 21:373-391.

HEAD INJURY - WATER AND MOVEMENT REHABILITATION

Margaret J. Reid Campion
School of Physiotherapy,   Curtin University of Technology and
Royal Perth Rehabilitation Hospital, Western Australia

Movement rehabilitation is the major aim of treatment for the neurosurgical patient and water offers unique ways in which such rehabilitation may be achieved.

The conventional techniques[1] are of limited value a specific approach comprising the essential components of movement rehabilitation is required.

Why use hydrotherapy?

Hydrotherapy can be fun. It should be. Hydrotherapy is probably the most enjoyable form of physiotherapy for most patients, largely due to the pleasure to the freedom of movement and independence it provides.

Dimensions of movement not possible on land as there are two forces - gravity and buoyancy, act simultaneously. Body weight is relieved; the buoyancy of water reduces the effects of gravity[2]. The patient is warm throughout the treatment and is easily manoeuvred. Extremes of posture can be achieved easily. The variability of the environment ensures no one body surface being stimulated at any time. There is increased body awareness due to all round sensation of the water on the body.[3]

Aims for hydrotherapy for the neurosurgical patient.

The aims may be divided into: 1. Physical aims. 2. Psychological aims.

Physical Aims

1. Reduce tone	6. Retrain reciprocal patterns of movement
2. Stimulate movement	7. Redevelop functional movement
3. Provoke and retrain righting reactions	8. Improve respiratory function
4. Strengthen weak movement patterns	9. Improve & maintain cario-vascular fitness
5. Encourage rotational patterns of movement	10. Treat any orthopaedic complications

Psychological Aims
1. Provide relaxation and enjoyable recreation
2. Provide motivation
3. Provide opportunities for socialization

PHYSICAL AIMS

Reduction of Tone

The reduction of tone may the warmth and support of the water and the all round stimulation. Decreased spinal excitability has been found due to diminution of gamma fibre activity as a result of warmth stimulation of the exteroceptors in the skin of the neck.[4,5]

A pool temperature of 35 C causes a general hyperthermia which has its effects on tone but above this may lead to dissipation of the beneficial effects of immersion[6,7,8]

On land when movement in space is required tone increases in proportion to be 'perceived effort' as seen by the patient. In water the hydrodynamical principles of relative density and metacentre can bring about a reduction in 'perceived effort' thus decreasing tone.[9,14]

Techniques to reduce tone such as vestibular stimulation require that the physiotherapist provides appropriate support whilst carrying out an effective treatment. Minimum support is required to allow the patient maximum control over the body. Such control comes from the head and whilst head injured patients may require a neck float initially, head control can still be developed. Slow rhythmical swinging, rocking and rolling movements will reduce tone and bring about relaxation. Rotational movements around the longitudinal axis of the body diminish spasticity[10] We 'tow' the patients in supine lying in straight lines, 'S' shaped paths, progressing to swaying from side to side, incorporate rotation and encourage head turning - the patient being told to 'eyeball' the physiotherapist.

The patient becomes aware of the warmth and pressure of the water, as well as the movement of the hips and lower limbs on the trunk, trunk rotation and head movement.

Stimulating Movement

The neuro-surgical patient may have little voluntary movement and not know how to move. Thermal regulation of the body is centred in the hypothalamic area. The reticular formation is involved not only with temperature regulation but also with the maintenance of alertness in the patient. The vestibular system has connections with the reticular formation, the cerebellum and with the thalamus and midbrain control of muscle tone. This forms the basis for movement rehabilitation in the hydrotherapy programme.

In supported supine lying; small rotations allow the water to touch the cheeks the patient being instructed to turn the head away. Blowing the water away from the mouth aids respiratory function. Swaying the patient from side to side, developing lateral flexion by reaching to the ipsilateral knee develops an appreciation of vestibular stimulation and voluntary and assisted lateral flexion. Using drag effects and bow wave appropriately movement can be increased. The judicious use of floats on the unaffected or least affected leg; the affected or more affected leg will sink further may be used to implement movement.

Retraining righting and rotational patterns

It is difficult to retrain righting and rotational patterns on land where tone, either increased or decreased make movement more difficult. It is easier with the support and security provided by water and the physiotherapist; the patient can learn to react to the destabilizing effects of limb movements on the body and develop strategies to obtain stability. Metacentric effects on the changed shape and density of the patient due to disability and deliberate changes of shape, are utilized to develop righting and rotational reactions. The patient must learn to react to any changes of shape, voluntary or involuntary and return to the original position or maintain it against any disturbing forces to maintain balance.

Lateral and vertical rotation patterns are utilized to stimulate and retrain righting reactions and develop and/or control rotational effects. Progression is by forward and backward side to side displacement, head turning, arm movements in all directions and altering shape by changing the symmetry of the lower limbs.

Both rotations help the patient to become aware of the role of head control in initiating and controlling movement. Total flexion and extension may be achieved body image and awareness of body parts are enhanced and the rotational component of movement aided.

Strengthening Weak Movements

From a stable positions, positioning of the limbs appropriately can augment and increase weak movements. Buoyancy is used to assist movement and the patient is encouraged assist the upward movement. Starting positions may be varied and flotation equipment applied to enhance the movements

Reciprocal Pattern Movement

Reciprocal patterns of movement begin in supine lying with the patient supported by neck and pelvic floats. The physiotherapist gives maximum assistance to the movement patterns. Slow, rhythmic alternate flexion/abduction/external rotation and extension of the lower limbs should be mastered first, abduction/adduction of the arms following; eventually the patient can propel the body through the water, becoming aware of the co-ordination of limbs, learns concentration and movement disassociation and gains independent movement in the water.

'Straight' kicks are developed in prone and extension of the head, neck, trunk and limbs are developed combined with lower limb co-ordination.

Functional Movement Patterns

Exercises practiced as functional patterns are more likely to produced the desired movements. Reciprocal arm swinging in walking may be difficult, co-ordination of the limbs in swimming can usefully lead to achieving the arm swing.

Maintaining the 'sitting' position demands precise balance of the head on the neck and control of the arms and hands. The judicious placing of turbulence around the patient increases the demand for balance control.

Walking and getting from lying to sitting in the water helps the patient appreciate functional movement patterns and may carry over on to land.

Improve Respiratory Function

Good breathing patterns essential for speech, are encouraged from the beginning by instructions to 'blow' whenever water is near the face. Total relaxation is essential as tone in the abdominal musculature interferes with its proper use in respiration. The co-operation and participation of the speech pathologist, preferably in the pool, is vital if speech is to be re-established appropriately.

Hydrotherapy encourages movement and play and these can be used to produce voice and speech as part of the programme improvising and maintaining cardio-vascular fitness.

Cardio-vascular fitness is promoted by exercise in water and swimming since energy requirements are greater in water than air. [11]

Treating Orthopaedic Complications

Fractures to the limbs and/or spine may be treated by surgery and plastering. The joint stiffness and pain that follow removal of the plaster cast may be effectively treated in the pool where the warmth and support bring about relaxation, a decrease in pain and allow freer movement. Walking may be commenced earlier in water at the appropriate depths.

PSYCHOLOGICAL AIMS

Relaxation and Enjoyable Recreation, Motivation and Socialization

This type of relaxation comes through enjoyment of the medium and the recreation it provides. Independent movement through the water provides an enormous sense of achievement and freedom and leads to a more positive approach to long term rehabilitation. Hydrotherapy is a change in the treatment programme and is enjoyable and motivating and provides opportunities for socialization in recreational type programmes and group activities.

Contra-indications

Contra-indications for hydrotherapy are concerned with incontinence of bowel and bladder, fractures of the base of the skull and the effect of heat on the patient. [4]

Where a patient has 'dry periods' the time can be used for hydrotherapy; urinary incontinence in the male patient is manageable.

Adverse Reactions

Some patients may demonstrate adverse reactions following hydrotherapy such as an increase in tone; a 'hot-flushed' look; extreme lethargy and tiredness; low blood pressure; and persistent ear infections. Hydrotherapy should be temporarily discontinued in the instances of an increase in tone and the 'hot flushed' look.

Sedative drugs may be the culprit for the extreme lethargy and tiredness. If blood pressure changes occur blood pressure should be monitored before and after the hydrotherapy sessions. Retention of water in the ears may cause persistent ear infections, careful drying of the ears is indicated.

Guidelines for Successful Treatment

The treatment of the neuro-surgical patient by hydrotherapy has not been encouraged in the past. However, in Western Australia we find hydrotherapy invaluable. Work is on a one-to-one basis for specific hydrotherapy and in group activities the one-to-one basis is maintained within the group.

Good handling is vital. Associated reactions are usually brought about by poor handling, rapid and arhythmical movements.

Treatments are goal orientated based on careful and detailed assessment with hydrotherapy in mind.

Family members are often called on to train as assistants. Such participation helps the family come to terms with the patient's trauma and makes them feel useful and games and group activities introduced at the end of a treatment session increase the enjoyment and fun of hydrotherapy.

REFERENCES

1. Davis, B.D., Harrison, R.A. 1988. "Hydrotherapy in Practice", Edinburgh : Churchill Livingstone.

2. Harrison, R. Bulstrode, S. 1987. "Percentage Weight Bearing during Partial Immersion in the Hydrotherapy Pool". Physiotherapy Practice, Vol. 3, pp. 60-63.

3. Palmer, R.P. 1978. "Guidelines to Neurological Rehabilitation, 2nd Ed. Queensland : Multiple Sclerosis Society

4. Jegasothy, G. 1990. "Hydrotherapy in the Treatment of the Neurosurgical Patient". In "Adult Hydrotherapy. A Practical Approach" M. Reid Campion (ed) Oxford : Heinemann Medical Books.

5. Fisher, E. & Solomon, S. 1965. "Physiological Response to Heed and Cold". In (Lichts, S. Kamenetz, H.L. eds) Therapeutic Heat and Cold, pp 126-169. Baltimore : Waverley Press.

6. Franchimont, P.,Juchmes, J., Leconte, J. 1983. "Hydrotherapy - Mechanisms and Indications". Pharmacology Therapeutic 20,pp 79-93.

7. Harris, S.R. 1978. "Neurodevelopmental Treatment approach for teaching swimming to cerebral palsied children". Physical Therapy, 58, pp 979-983.

8. Skinner, A. & Thomson A. 1983. "Duffield's Exercise in Water". London : Bailliere Tindal.

9. Reid Campion, M. 1990. "Adult Hydrotherapy - A Practical Approach". Oxford : Heinemann Medical Books.

10. Sullivan, P.E., Markos, P.D., Minor, M.A.D. 1982. "An Integrated Approach to Therapeutic Exercise : Theory and Clinical Application". Reston, Va : Reston Publication Co.

11. Reid Campion, M. 1985. "Hydrotherapy in Paediatrics". London : William Heinemann Medical Books.

RECOVERY OF MOVEMENT PATTERNS FOLLOWING TRAUMATIC HEAD
INJURY

A F VanSant
Department of Physical Therapy, College of Allied Health
Professions, Temple University, Philadelphia, PA, USA

The recovery of motor behavior has been described by
Brunnstrom[1] and Bobath[2] for those who have sustained a brain
insult due to stroke. Their classic descriptions serve as
guides for the neurologic evaluation and treatment by
providing indicators of the level of recovery and a guide
for therapy objectives and procedures. The motor behavior
of individuals with traumatic head injury is less well
described. Although hemiplegias, ataxias and other general
neurologic diagnostic descriptors have been applied to the
residual motor deficits, little more than annecdotal
information is available concerning the motor behavior and
motor recovery of individuals following closed head injury.
The study reported here represents a description of the
righting ability in adults with moderate and severe head
trauma, and the recovery of movement patterns within a
righting task. It was proposed that individuals with more
severe injuries would demonstrate behaviors analagous to
earlier appearing developmental steps when compared to
those with less severe injuries. Further it was proposed
that the recovery would be characterized by change from
earlier appearing movement patterns to patterns that
predominate later in development.   Subjects and Methods
The subjects of this study were 29 adults with head injury
(HI), with a mean age of 29.5 years. Five subjects were
women; the remainder were men. The subjects were classified
as having a moderate or severe HI based on results of the
Glassgow Coma Scale, administered at the time of admission
to the Neurosciences Intensive Care Unit at the Medical
College of Virginia Hospitals. Eighteen subjects were
classified as having a moderate HI and 11 were classified
as severe HI. When the subjects attained a score of 70 on
the Galveston Orientation and Amnesia Test,[3] and if they
were without orthopedic or other medical or surgical
complications, they were admitted to the study. After the
initial data collection session subjects were then followed
at 3, 6, and 12 months following injury.

Subjects were asked to lie supine on a floor exercise
mat and on request to rise to standing as quickly as
possible. With the exception of one subject who performed
just two trials, and three subjects who performed 5 trials,
all subjects performed 10 consecutive trials of rising. The
interval between trials was self-paced by the subject.

The movement patterns of each subject on each trial

were classified using movement pattern descriptions developed in previous studies of healthy individuals performing the same task.[4,5] This method of movement pattern description focuses on the action of three body regions: the upper extremities (UEs), the axial region (AX) and the lower extremities (LEs). There were four patterns of UE action, four patterns of AX action, and six patterns of LE action used to describe the subjects' movements. The movement pattern descriptions for each body region have been proposed to represent developmental steps for the action of that region within this rising task.[5]

Results The incidence of UE, AX, and LE movement patterns differed between the moderate and severe HI groups. While the most common UE pattern, an asymmetrical push and reach pattern, was observed on approximately 50% of the trials of both groups, the remaining trials of the severe HI subjects tended to be at a earlier apppearing developmental steps, while the majority of trials of the moderate group were classified at more advanced developmental steps. In the AX region the most common pattern differed between the groups: the moderate group most commonly demonstrated step three of the AX developmental sequence while the severe HI group demonstrated step 1 or 3, with relatively equal frequency. The severe group demonstrated the lowest developmental step as their most common LE action while the moderate group demonstrated step 3 as their most common pattern.

There were differences in the recovery patterns of the two groups. The 10 subjects with moderate HI who were followed across time demonstrated a pattern of change from developmentally less advanced toward more advanced patterns. This trend was most apparent in the LEs although it was consistent across all three body regions. For the 7 subjects with severe HI who were followed across time, the movement patterns of the AX region demonstrated little change. In the UEs and LEs there was a trend toward using developmentally more advanced patterns with time. This tendency was found to be strongest for the LE region.

Discussion The results of this study indicate that individuals with lower as compared to higher GCS scores on admission to a neuroscience intensive care unit are more likely to demonstrate developmentally primitive righting movements during the course of recovery from HI. Further, those with lower as compared to higher GCS scores are likely to make slower progress in attaining developmentally advanced movement patterns following HI.

The method of classifying movement patterns that was developed through studies of healthy subjects was found to be adequate as a beginning method of description of motor recovery following HI. The finding that individuals with HI are recovering their righting ability in the order proposed to represent developmental sequences for this rising task is likely a reflection of the tendency for the task to reflect dynamic balance abilities. The developmental steps reflect a trend toward using fewer transitional postures in the process of rising and a less circuitous, more direct route from supine to standing. The tendency for severe HI subjects to fractionate the task of rising from supine into a series of movements from one transitional posture to the next with pauses in each posture is a finding worthy of further investigation, particulary if done in concert with studies of balance abilities.

Supported by NIDRR Grant # G0087C0219

References

1. Brunnstrom S (1970) Movement Therapy in Hemiplegia. New York: Harper & Row

2. Bobath B (1990) Adult Hemiplegia Evaluation and Treatment, 3rd Edition. London: Heinemann

3. Levin H S, O'Donnell V M, Grrossman R G (1979) The Galveston orientation and amnesia test: A practical scale to assess cognition after head injury. Journal of Nervous and Mental Disorders 167:675-684

4. VanSant AF (1988) Rising from a supine position to erect stance: Description of adult movement and a developmental hypothesis. Physical Therapy 68:185-192

5. VanSant AF (1988b) Age differences in movement patterns used by children to rise from a supine position to erect stance. Physical Therapy 68:1130-1138

STANDING BALANCE ABILITIES IN PATIENTS WITH TRAUMATIC BRAIN
INJURY

R A Newton
Dept Physical Therapy, Temple University, Philadelphia, PA

To maintain standing balance an individual needs to receive
appropriate sensory information and exhibit appropriate motor
behavior. Input from the visual and somatosensory system
provide information relative to the external environment;
whereas the vestibular system, an internal reference,
provides information relative to gravitational orientation
and resolves conflicts between the other two systems. A
finite number of motor responses for balance are available;
ankle, hip, and step strategy.[1] Each strategy has defined
borders. When the limits of one strategy are surpassed the
person switches to another to maintain standing balance.
Individuals with traumatic brain injury (TBI) have varying
degrees of balance instability. Deficits in balance responses
(BRs) include: limited repertoire of movement strategies,
delay in the onset of the balance response, an increase in
the amount of sway excursion, and the inability to ignore
inappropriate or conflicting sensory information.[1] With the
advent of computerized dynamic posturography, the ability to
quantify these characteristics of the balance response has
improved.

The purpose of this study was to quantify BRs of adults
with TBI when exposed to unexpected linear perturbations and
different sensory conditions in which somatosensory and
visual input were altered or eliminated.

Method. Twenty-three moderate (mean age = 34.2 years) and
23 severe (mean age = 31.2 years) TBI patients were tested
after scoring 70 on the Galveston Orientation and Amnesia
Test. Moderate TBI patients had a Glasgow Coma Score of 11.6
(s $\pm$ 2.1) and the GSC for the severe group was 6.4 (s $\pm$ 1.6).
Moderate TBI patients were tested 3.2 (s $\pm$ 2) weeks post
injury and severe TBI patients were tested 8.8 (s $\pm$ 4.7)
weeks post injury. Patients were excluded if they were under
16 years of age; received gun shot wounds to the head; had
neurologic, musculoskeletal or behavioral problems that
precluded standing for more than one minute.

Patients stood barefoot on a moveable force platform facing
a visual surround with their medial malleoli aligned over a
center strip. Patients wore a safety harness to prevent
falls, but it did not interfere with movement. Patients first
were exposed to brief medium and large amplitude linear
translations in the forward or backward direction. Each

linear translation was repeated 5 times. Next, patients received 6 different Sensory Organization Test (SOT) conditions whereby visual and somatosensory input was systematically altered or eliminated. During the first 3 SOT conditions the subject stood on the stationary force plate with 1) eyes open, 2) eyes closed, and 3) the visual surround moving in concert with forward and backward sway movements. During the last three conditions, the platform moved in concert with the subject's forward and backward sway movements while the eyes were 4) open, 5) closed, and when 6) the visual surround moving in concert with sway movements. Each SOT condition lasted 20 sec and was repeated 3 times. If the subject took a step or fell, the trial was stopped and recorded as a fall. The subject's feet were repositioned and the next trial in the test sequence began.

Load cells in the platform sampled torque and shear forces generated during each BR at a rate of 100 Hz. For the linear translations latency, symmetry, and amplitude of the balance response was determined. Symmetry was also examined prior to perturbation. For the SOT conditions, balance scores were obtained by comparing the amplitude of the sway response to the theoretical maximum sway response of 12°. All calculations used the NeuroCom Inc software program. The number of individuals with latency or symmetry values below the 5th percentile was determined.

Results. By visual inspection all TBI patients had at least one value below the 5th percentile in the perturbation tests. Prior to and following perturbation approximately one-third of the individuals stood asymmetrically with vertical forces generated predominately thorough one leg. The amplitude of sway excursion occurring in response to the linear perturbation was within age appropriate ranges.

Although not statistically significant, latencies of onset of the balance response for the medium and large forward and backward perturbations tended to be high when compared to age appropriate norms. Age appropriate norms ranged from 130-160 msec and latencies for TBI patients averaged between 170 and 193 msec.

Balance scores on the SOT were analyzed in age groups by decade. Because of the small number of subjects per decade, statistical analysis was not conducted. Although some moderate TBI patients had low scores (in the 5th percentile), they were spread across all conditions. In the severe TBI group, patients tended to score low on test conditions 5 and 6. During test condition 5, vision is eliminated and the support surface provides altered input, i.e. the platform moves in concert with the person's sway. In condition 6, both the visual and somatosensory systems monitor altered sensory inputs, i.e, both the platform and visual surround move in concert with the person's sway movements. The vestibular system is the only system providing a true reference point in test conditions 5 and 6. Based on these data, it is apparent that TBI patients have balance problems due in part to vestibular dysfunction as well as a decrease in the individual's ability to compensate with the other two senses.

<u>Discussion</u> Based upon the results of the study patients with traumatic brain injury have decreased balance responses due in part to sensory selection problems, delay in onset of the balance response or a combination of the two. It appears that TBI patients have difficulty ignoring inappropriate sensory information and relying on appropriate input to generate a motor response to maintain balance. The fact that the balance response may be evoked later than normal contributes to balance instability.

By early identification of the sensory systems preferentially used by the patient and an indication of the status of the vestibular system, the therapist can more readily develop appropriate rehabilitative strategies. Quantification of the balance response during perturbation determines what characteristic(s) of the balance response are altered. In the case of the TBI patient a longer latency is expected. This knowledge is extremely useful in developing programs for balance retraining. The individual may have an appropriate repertoire of balance responses, but the response appears too late to maintain balance. Lastly, and most important, dynamic posturography provides quantitative documentation, useful to document recovery and the effectiveness of rehabilitation. (funded by NIDRR Grant No G0087C0219)

1. Newton RA: Recovery of Balance
   Abilities in Individuals with
   Traumatic Brain Injuries. In
   Balance, APTA, Fairfax VA, USA,
   1990, pp 69-72

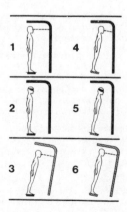

Fig 1. Sensory Organization Test

THE EFFECT OF SERIAL CASTING ON CALF MUSCLE LENGTH: A CONTROLLED TRIAL

A M Moseley
Department of Physiotherapy, Lidcombe Hospital, Joseph Street,
Lidcombe NSW 2141, Australia

Calf muscle shortening is a common and significant secondary problem following traumatic head injury (1). It restricts the range of ankle dorsiflexion movement, which interferes with the performance of functional tasks (for example, standing-up and walking) and motor training. Serial casting has been used to prevent or reverse calf muscle shortening in the traumatic head injured population.

Previous studies have suggested that serial casting increases calf muscle length in acute management (2) and later-stage rehabilitation (1,3). Sullivan et al report a mean increase in passive ankle dorsiflexion of 20 degrees with serial casting in an unconscious group (2), while increases in passive ankle dorsiflexion of 19 to 24 degrees (3) and 11 degrees (1) have been reported in later-stage rehabilitation. These existing studies may be criticised for a lack of appropriate control groups (1-3), variation in casting duration (2,3), failure to document the measurement procedure and reliability (2,3) and lack of statistical analysis (2,3).

The purpose of this study is to examine the effect of serial casting on calf muscle length, compared to no stretching intervention, in the traumatic head injured population. It is hypothesised that serial casting will be associated with an increase in calf muscle length.

Method

SUBJECTS: Seven patients who had sustained a traumatic closed head injury and were admitted to Lidcombe Hospital Head Injury Unit for rehabilitation participated in the study. Subjects were selected using the following criteria:

1. sustained a traumatic closed head injury
2. presence of calf muscle shortening
3. no dermatological conditions (shank and foot)
4. no peripheral vascular problems
5. able to lie prone for cast application, and
6. written informed consent from subject or legal guardian.

The seven subjects were 6 males and 1 female with a mean age of 24.3 years (range 16 to 32 years). Four of the subjects had serial casts applied bilaterally, giving a total of 11 casted limbs. The mean time between injury and casting was 76 days (range 36 to 106 days).

PROCEDURE: A cross-over design in which each subject underwent both experimental and control conditions was used. The experimental condition involved the application of a serial cast for 7 days. The control period involved 7 days with no stretching intervention for the calf muscle group.

The experimental and control conditions occurred in random order.

During both the experimental and control conditions all motor training and stretching intervention for other muscle groups was standardised within subjects. All training was based on the principals of motor learning and biomechanical analysis (4).

The serial casts were applied using the protocol described by Ada and Scott (5). The skin was protected with a layer of stockingette and minimal padding was placed over bony and tendinous prominences. The subject was positioned in prone with their knee flexed 90 degrees, the soleus component of the calf muscle was stretched into maximal obtainable dorsiflexion using a board placed on the foot. The ankle was immobilised in this position using fibreglass casting materials. While the cast was on, the gastrocnemius component of the calf muscle group was stretched by positioning the subject's knee in extension for prolonged periods of time.

Passive ankle dorsiflexion, which reflects calf muscle length, was measured on days 0 (commencement), 7 (cross-over) and 14 (conclusion) using a standardised testing procedure (6). The skin was marked with long-lasting skin marking dye over the head of fibula, lateral maleolus and head of fifth metatarsal. These skin markers remained intact throughout the measurement period. The subject was positioned in supine with their knee extended, and a known torque was applied to dorsiflex the ankle. A polaroid photograph was taken to record ankle angle, which was measured later using a protractor. The reliability of this procedure is .97 for the head injured population (6).

DATA ANALYSIS: T-tests were used to analyse all data (7).

Results

The mean increase in passive ankle dorsiflexion associated with serial casting was 15 degrees (SD=11.12). This increase was statistically significant (t=4.42, p<0.0013). During the control period the mean decrease in passive ankle dorsiflexion was 4.5 degrees (SD=9.44), which was non-significant (t=-1.57, p<0.15). The difference between the serial cast and control conditions was highly significant (t=4.38, p<0.0003).

Discussion

The main finding of this study was that a single cast applied to stretch the calf muscles was associated with a significant increase in passive ankle dorsiflexion, compared to a control period of no stretching intervention. In other words, serial casting is an effective method of increasing calf muscle length. This result is consistent with previous reports (1-3).

Several factors may influence the effectiveness of serial casting, including cast duration, degree of stretch, the use of pre-medication and the casting materials/techniques used. Future studies are required to determine the optimum parameters of serial cast application.

In this study, increased calf muscle length has not been correlated with changes in the performance of functional activities. Future research is required to correlate changes in calf muscle length with changes in performance of functional tasks.

Conclusion

It is suggested that serial casting is an effective method of increasing calf muscle length, and thereby facilitates the training of functional activities.

References

1. Moseley A (1989) An evaluation of serial casting to correct calf muscle contractures. Recovery from Brain Injury: Expectations, Needs and Processes International Conference -- Conference Abstracts:55

2. Sullivan T, Conine TA, Goodman M, Mackie T (1988) Serial casting to prevent equinus in acute traumatic head injury. Physiotherapy Canada 40(6):346-350

3. Booth P, Doyle M, Montgomery J (1983) Serial casting for management of spasticity in the head injured adult. Physical Therapy 63(12):1960-66

4. Carr JH, Shepherd RB (1987) A Motor Relearning Programme for Stroke (2nd Ed). London: Heinemann

5. Ada L, Scott D (1980) Use of inhibitory, weight-bearing plasters to increase movement in the presence of spasticity. The Australian Journal of Physiotherapy 26(2):57-61

6. Moseley A, Adams R (1991) Measurement of passive ankle dorsiflexion: Procedure and reliability. Submitted to The Australian Journal of Physiotherapy

7. Minitab Statistical Software (1989). Minitab Inc.

THE SYMPATHETIC NERVOUS SYSTEM IN NEUROMOTOR FUNCTION AND DYSFUNCTION

David M. Selkowitz

4920 Coronado Ave., Oakland, CA, 94618, USA

Sympathetic nervous system (SNS) involvement in neuromotor dysfunction and pain is poorly understood, and the clinical manifestations continue to go largely unrecognized in medicine and rehabilitation. Reflex sympathetic dystrophy (RSD) is one of many terms associated with these problems, which, in addition to involving the extremities, may develop after musculoskeletal spine injuries and manifest on the trunk. Chronic frozen shoulder and thoracic outlet problems also may include SNS involvement. Pain problems involving the SNS are usually characterized by one or more of the following: hyperpathia, allodynia, pain lasting beyond the normal expected time of healing, pain that appears to be out of proportion to the extent of the original injury, pain referral in a nonsegmental distribution, complaints of burning, aching, and tightness, and poor tolerance of palpation and movement of the affected areas. Often, there is objective evidence of vascular, trophic, and sudomotor changes, and neuromotor problems such as spasm, tremor, weakness, atrophy, dyscoordination, and difficulty initiating movement. Difficulties worsen with disuse and the progression of other concurrent somatic dysfunctions. People may suffer a devastating psychological impact due to severe and prolonged physical problems, and their frequently being mislabeled as malingerers or psychogenic problem cases. Motor problems may appear suddenly and precede pain by weeks or months, and may be mirrored on the other side of the body.[1] Aggressive sympathetic blockade may be effective early on but usually not in stage 3 disease.[1]

One possible explanation for the presence of neuromotor dysfunction concerns the apparent interaction of the SNS and the muscle spindle. Anatomic evidence of a direct SNS innervation of the spindle has been discovered in animals.[2-5] Axons and nerve endings with morphological and histochemical characteristics of noradrenergic SNS fibers have been located equatorially within the spindle capsule[2-5] and at the polar regions.[2,4] SNS innervation of extrafusal fibers (EFFs) has also been found.[4,5] The extent of SNS innervation of the intrafusal fibers (IFFs) and EFFs appears to vary depending on the muscle studied.

Physiological and functional evidence of a direct SNS influence on the spindle has been reported by Passatore and colleagues.[6,7] Summarizing their results and conclusions: electrical stimulation of the SNS supply to certain muscles in animals caused a marked increase in tension (i.e., isometric force) produced by these muscles, mainly due to SNS action on IFFs and, to a small extent, on EFFs.[6,7] The tension response was due to SNS stimulation of the spindle because, during the administration of electrical stimulation of the SNS supply to a muscle: 1) the animals were deeply anesthetized and paralyzed to block the somatosensory and motor nerves to the muscles; 2) there was no change in tension (i.e., no further decrease) after further administration of paralyzing agents, or cutting the somatosensory nerve supply to the muscles, or serially removing other SNS-innervated structures in the region; 3) the tension response was abolished by a-adrenergic blockers[9]. Also, it was not due to vasoconstriction because the tension was unchanged by occlusion of the arterial supply, and the time for development of the tension response was much less than that which occurs with vasoconstriction.[6] The authors concluded that the tension response was due mainly to SNS stimulation of IFFs rather than EFFs because, after serially disconnecting each jaw elevator muscle, they found that: 1) the tension contributed by each muscle to the total response was better correlated with the number of spindles it contained than its mass; 2) the tension would have been of greater magnitude, with the peak force occurring at higher frequencies than the 10-15 Hz in their study, if it was due to EFF contraction from alpha or gamma motor neuron stimulation.[6] However, they concluded that some SNS-induced EFF contraction probably occurred because the tension response was greater than what was expected for IFF contractions.[6] Stimulation of the SNS supply to rabbit digastric muscles, which were reported to have no spindles, also resulted in increased tension.[8] This may have been due to SNS stimulation of EFFs. SNS stimulation may overcome muscle fatigue, as shown by the resultant increases in tension of fatigued, SNS-stimulated rabbit digastric muscles.[9]

A spontaneous tonic action of the SNS on IFFs (i.e., a baseline SNS activity controlling a baseline IFF contraction) has been discovered: after cutting the SNS supply to the muscle (prior to electrical stimulation), the baseline muscle tension decreased; it was restored to the previous level upon electrical stimulation of the distal stump of the SNS supply at the normal low operating frequency of the SNS, and decreased again upon cessation of the stimulation.[6]

SNS stimulation of IFFs also resulted in an increase in activity of spindle afferents, mainly of the secondary endings; the characteristics of the increased afferent activity paralleled those of the increase in tension.[6,7] This was found mainly for the secondary endings probably because the stimulated contractions were isometric. This finding by one of the methods used to measure the afferent activity has been challenged.[10]

In a live human with simultaneously functioning SNS and somatic nerve supplies, the mechanisms and relationships may change. Possibly, both systems would modify each other. There may be dual control of the spindle via the gamma and sympathetic efferent systems, and of the EFFs via the alpha and SNS efferents; i.e., there may be sympathetic biasing as well as gamma biasing of the spindle.

Possible mechanisms for the activation and perpetuation of neuromotor dysfunction by the SNS may involve some initial (nerve) injury, which activates slow- and fast-conducting somatic afferents, which send pain and proprioceptive messages to the spinal cord - and might then go to higher centers (including the diencephalon and the brain stem) and return to the cord - and activate the somatic motor neurons and sympathetic neurons (directly or via interneurons) to the spindles of a region. Then, the IFFs contract and activate the fast-conducting spindle afferents, which return to the cord and perpetuate the cycle of activation; slow-conducting fibers need not be involved. This cycle of activation may also result in hyperactivity of the interneuron pool which can spread activation up, down, and across the cord. Wide-dynamic-range neurons in the cord may mediate the spread of activation resulting in the perpetuation of pain by the SNS without pain-fiber transmission.[11] This may also be operative in neuromotor dysfunction. Enhanced SNS activity may be a normal consequence in the early stages of injury; it is its failure to decrease that can result in debilitating problems. The apparent unpredictability of this failure may be related to some individual variation in the pathways, excitation mechanisms, number of sympathetic endings in a spindle, or number of SNS-innervated spindles in a muscle.

The best strategy for dealing with these problems is probably early recognition and referral to an anesthesiologist skilled in performing and interpreting diagnostic sympathetic blocks. This may be necessary before physical therapy can be tolerated; then, treatment of the structural and functional musculoskeletal problems can proceed. Some physiotherapeutic interventions may assist in reducing the sympathetic outflow and interrupting the cycle of hyperactivity. The clinical presentations typically involve chronic neuromuscular tightness that can be painful. Stretching to lengthen the affected area is usually not tolerated well. Neuromuscular relaxation techniques that are gentle, and avoid extremes of sensation and handling of the symptomatic areas seem to work best. For example, techniques based on the principles and applications of strain and counterstrain[12] may affect the spindle apparatus (via prolonged hypershortening of the affected muscle), and handling of the affected region is limited. Connective tissue massage[13] need not involve such handling either, but its mechanism of action is less apparent, and may actually involve a vascular component. Areas remote to the symptomatic region that may provoke or perpetuate the symptoms and signs, may benefit from more vigorous treatment; e.g., mobilization of the cervical or thoracic spine to treat signs and symptoms in the upper extremities. In contrast to sympathetic-maintained syndromes, where there is hyperactivity of the SNS which perpetuates neuromotor dysfunction and pain after the somatic problem has resolved (i.e., tissues have healed and normalized) somatic-maintained SNS hyperactivity may also occur, where a structural or somatic problem is responsible for the SNS hyperactivity. In the latter instance, the hyperactivity will return after temporary interruptions by treatments (including sympathetic block injections) that are directed at the SNS; such problems include scar tissue investing the neural tissue in the thoracic outlet region, and a variant anatomical relationship of the anterior and middle scalenes causing compression of the associated nerve trunks, leading to the signs and symptoms of thoracic outlet syndrome which are also characteristic of SNS dysfunction. As with other problems, no one strategy will always work well with all people or all presentations of SNS problems.

Despite the laboratory findings, the theoretical considerations for which they formed the basis, and the clinical experience presented, the actual mechanisms occurring and the clinical significance of the data are yet to be firmly established, and are in a state of evolution. My intention has been to increase the awareness of the clinical problems involving the SNS so that people presenting with these problems might not be misunderstood as merely hysterical or faking; and, to present hypotheses based on the current body of information to assist in the logical investigation and effective treatment of these difficult problems.

I respectfully acknowledge Franklin J. Day, M.D., and Dahlis M. Day, M.D., of the Pain Relief Center, Walnut Creek, CA, for their invaluable contributions to clinical practice and problem-solving in this field; and I am grateful for our long-term collaboration and friendship. I also thank Professor Magda Passatore for her generous communication.

References

1. Schwartzman RJ, Kerrigan J (1990) The movement disorder of reflex sympathetic dystrophy. Neurology 40:57-61
2. Santini M, Ibata Y (1971) The fine structure of thin unmyelinated axons within muscle spindles. Brain Res 33:289-302
3. Ballard KJ (1978) Typical sympathetic noradrenergic endings in a muscle spindle of the cat. J Physiol (Lond) 285:61P
4. Barker D, Saito M (1981) Autonomic innervation of receptors and muscle fibres in cat skeletal muscle. Proc R Soc Lond B 212:317-332
5. Barker D, Saed HH (1987) Adrenergic innervation of rat jaw muscles. J Physiol (Lond) 391:114P
6. Passatore M, Grassi C, Filippi GM (1985) Sympathetically-induced development of tension in jaw muscles: the possible contraction of intrafusal muscle fibres. Pflugers Arch 405:297-304
7. Grassi C, Filippi GM, Passatore M (1987) Tension development in lumbrical muscles and concomitant increase of activity in Aa and Ab afferents during sympathetic stimulation in the cat. Brain Res 435:15-23
8. Lund JP, Matthews B (1987) Tension produced in the jaw muscles of the rabbit by sympathetic stimulation. J Physiol (Lond) 386:86P
9. Grassi C, Passatore M (1990) Sympathetic nerve stimulation at physiological frequencies can modify the contraction of fatigued and nonfatigued digastric muscle in the rabbit. J Physiol (Lond) 422:14P
10. Petit J, Filippi G-M, Gioux M, Laporte Y (1989) Does stimulation of sympathetic axons elicit an increase in cat spindle afferent discharge detectable by the antidromic collision technique? Brain Res 503:181-184
11. Roberts WJ (1986) A hypothesis on the physiological basis for causalgia and related pains. Pain 24:297-311
12. Jones LH (1981) Strain and Counterstrain. Newark, OH, American Academy of Osteopathy
13. Ebner M (1985) Connective Tissue Manipulations: Theory and Therapeutic Application. Malabar, FL Robert E. Krieger Publishing Co., Inc.

THE RE-EDUCATION OF NORMAL MOVEMENT USING PROPRIOCEPTIVE INPUT VIA KEY POINT CONTROL.

M.E.Lynch

The Bobath Centre 5,Netherhall Gardens
London N.W.3 5R.N. Great Britain.

Introduction ; Proprioceptive information or afferent input is a powerful control on directing Neuroplastic Adaptation within the Central Nervous System,and in particular the Spinal Cord.Key Points of Control are defined as particular parts of the body whereby postural tone,and therefore selective movement is modified, adapted and changed because of there specific relationship to proprioceptive input.

Treatment : The use of Key Points of Control in relation to many different aspects of proprioceptive input is analysed in patients with Stroke,Head Injury and Multiple Sclerosis.The following aspects are examined in detail.The use of Gravity vs Base of Support in the Postural Set.The choice of the Motor Goal,Pattern and selective movement to be re-educated. The use of information via the specific receptors of Muscle Spindles,Golgi Organs and Joint Receptors. Speed and Repetition of movement is also examined in respect of differing aspects of tone i.e. Hypertonus vs Hypotonus.

Conclusion : It is suggested that the selective and appropriate use of differing aspects of proprioceptive information related to the individual problems of the patient gives a neurophysiological basis for experiential re-learning of Normal Movement.

QUANTITATIVE EVALUATION OF MOVEMENT SMOOTHNESS
BY A MINIMUM JERK COST CRITERION

H Ito, H Nagasaki
Department of Kinesiology, Tokyo Metropolitan Institute of Gerontology,
Tokyo, Japan

Introduction
    Recently, the optimal control theory is applied to the trajectory
formation in human limb motion. The minimum-jerk model, among others, has
been tested empirically in which mean-squared jerk ("jerk cost") is to be
minimized and jerk is the rate of change of acceleration (e.g., Flash and
Hogan 1985; Nagasaki 1989). The minimum-jerk model is appealing since it
provides an criterion for the optimally smooth trajectory that is an
indicator of skilled motor performance. The cost actually consumed could
be easily measured by the kinematics of the trajectory, and thereby
contrasted with the optimal criterion predicted by the model. Although
its potential significance, however, the measure of jerk cost has been
rarely applied to evaluating a motor disability or a motor skill
acquisition (Wann 1987; Schneider and Zernicke 1989). We measured here
jerk cost of the trajectory formation in a two-joint leg movement of
hemiplegic patients, and compared it with the cost for normal subjects
under the optimal criterion given by the minimum-jerk model.
Methods
    Five healthy subjects (male, 20-40 years old) and 7 hemiplegic patients
(5 males and 2 females, 58-76 years old) due to cerebrovascular accidents
participated in this experiment. Each subject lying in a supine position
with the knee and hip joints extended was required to move the ankle of
one leg to the knee of the opposite leg and place the heel on the patella
(Fig.1). Light emitting diodes (LEDs) were attached to the lateral side
of the ankle, knee and hip joints, and also to the costal part of the
trunk. Using an infrared photoelectric tracking system (SELSPOT), each
LED position was measured in a Cartesian coordinate system on the sagittal
plane as defined in Fig.1. Each LED position was sampled with the rate of
312.5Hz and a resolution of about 0.5mm and stored in a digital computer
for later analysis.
    The trajectory of the ankle was displayed on a monitor placed beside
the subject. A circular target with 0.8cm diameter was also displayed
on the monitor. The position of the target was adjusted for each subject

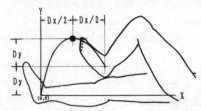

Fig.1 The trajectory of the ankle
joint in the two-leg movement.
(● :Target)

so that it located at the middle between the ankle and knee joints and at the height of two times the final ankle position (Fig.1). Seeing the trajectory displayed on the monitor, the subject was asked to move the ankle joint through the target onto the opposite patella as smoothly as possible at preferred speed. The leg examined was right side for the normal subjects and affected side for the patients. After practice, the subject performed 10 to 15 trials for the experimental session.

Displacement data were smoothed digitally using a low-pass filter with a cut-off frequency of 3Hz. This frequency was determined as an optimal frequency to satisfy the contradictory requirements to remove noise and to prevent information loss up to the third derivative(jerk) of the trajectory. Using displacement data of the ankle joint, velocity, acceleration and jerk in each direction were calculated. Movement time, denoted by Tx in X- and Ty in Y-direction, was defined as an interval between two points of zero-crossing of the velocity curve at the start and the end of the movement. Jerk cost defined by $1/2 \int_0^T J^2$ dt was calculated using jerk data (J) and movement time (T=Tx or Ty). In order to visualize smoothness of the trajectory, the acceleration vector (Schneider and Zernicke 1989) was computed on the trajectory every 32msec (Fig.2). By use of the equations of the optimally smooth trajectory given by Flash and Hogan(1985) for a via-point movement, the minimum jerk cost for the ankle trajectory was calculated to be $Cx=494.3(Dx^2/Tx^5)$ for X-direction and $Cy=21591.6(Dy^2/Tx^5)$ for Y-direction, where Dx and Dy were defined in Fig.1. The cost measured was also normalized by Dx^2/Tx^5 or Dy^2/Ty^5 in each direction. Thus a cost-performance in terms of smoothness was evaluated by the ratio of the measured cost to the optimal cost independently from movement time and extent.

Results

In Fig.2a, the ankle trajectory and the acceleration vectors predicted by the minimum jerk model are illustrated. The acceleration vector changes regularly from start to end of the trajectory showing the smoothest movement. Figure 2b shows an exemplar ankle path and the acceleration vectors for one normal subject; The path was smooth crossing the center of the target circle and the acceleration vectors changed regularly through the movement. The path and the acceleration vectors in Fig.2b were very similar to those of the model in Fig.2a and, in fact, the cost-ratio was 1.64 in X- and 1.53 in Y-direction. The hemiplegic patients exhibited clearly the less smooth trajectories (Fig.2c). In Fig.2c, the path deviated from the target and the acceleration vector

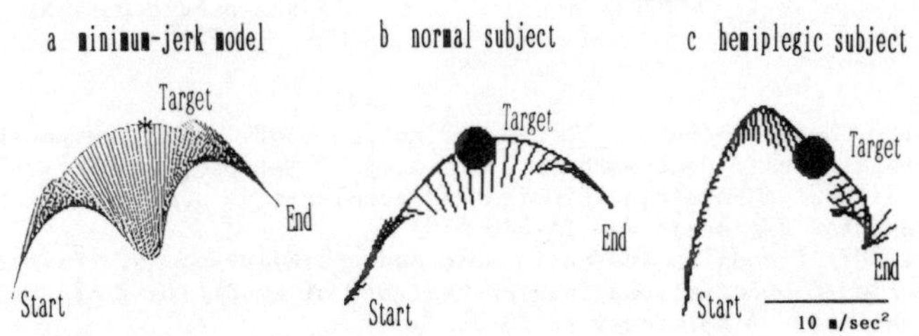

Fig.2 The trajectory and acceleration vectors of the ankle joint.

changed irregularly, especially during initial and final phases of the movement; The cost-ratio was 197.90 in X- and 34.15 in Y-direction.

In Fig.3, the averaged cost-ratio in each direction was plotted against movement time for the normal (N) and hemiplegic (A) subjects. Each shaded zone in the figure shows 95%-confidence intervals of the second-order regression applied to the data from a pilot experiment in which the normal subjects performed the leg movements at various speeds. As seen in Fig.3, the leg movement of the patients was not only slower than the normal subjects, but also less smooth than the normal movement of the same speed. The mean cost-ratio for the normal subjects was 3.3 in X- and 1.6 in Y-direction, whereas 48.5 and 13.5 for the patients.

Discussion

The present study quantified motor performance in terms of jerk cost or smoothness of the trajectory formation in a two-joint leg movement. The results showed that the movement of the hemiplegic patients consumed jerk cost more than that of the normal movement of the same speed. Wann(1987) measured jerk cost of handwriting for primary school children providing evidence that the cost may be reduced during development. Schneider and Zernicke(1989) examined the change in jerk cost during practice of a hand movement and showed a reduction in the cost after practice. Their studies, however, did not consider the optimal criterion of jerk cost which can be predicted by the minimum-jerk model. The minimum-jerk model showed that the minimum cost remains invariant in the leg movements if the cost is normalized by D^2/T^5, thereby providing an optimal criterion to be contrasted with jerk cost actually consumed. The present study thus confirmed that smoothness of the leg movement deteriorated for hemiplegic patients as compared with normal subjects. The results suggest that the method to measure jerk cost for the trajectory formation by contrast with its optimal criterion may be useful in evaluating quantitatively a loss or an acquisition of motor skill.

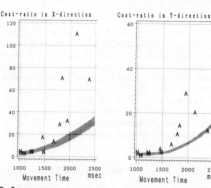

Fig.3 The ratio of measured jerk cost to optimal cost.
N:normal subject
A:hemiplegic patient

References

1. Flash T, Hogan N(1985) The coordination of arm movements:an experimentally confirmed mathematical model. J Neurosci 5:1688-1703
2. Nagasaki H(1989) Asymmetric velocity and acceleration profiles of human arm movements. Exp Brain Res 74:319-326
3. Wann JP(1987) Trends in the refinement and optimization of fine-motor trajectories: observations from an analysis of handwriting of primary school children. J Mot Behav 19:13-37
4. Schneider K, Zernicke RF(1989) Jerk-cost modulations during the practice of rapid arm movements. Biol Cybern 60:221-230

THE EFFECT OF MOVEMENT, GAIT AND RESISTANCE TO STRETCH OF SPASTIC MUSCLE FOLLOWING AN ISOKINETIC STRENGTHENING PROGRAMME

Patricia Baker, Dr. Barry Rawicki
Caulfield General Medical Centre/Alfred Group of Hospitals
294 Kooyong Road, South Caulfield. Victoria. Australia

INTRODUCTION:
    Objective measurement is the key to treatment evaluation. Recent advances in computer operated hydraulic dynamometers allows accurate measurement of muscle resistance to passive movement (RPM), at constant selected speeds. These capabilities enable the assessment of spasticity which is defined as an increased resistance to passive muscle stretch which is velocity dependent. Physiotherapists are primarily concerned with movement and function. Assessment of spasticity when used for treatment evaluation must therefore take into account the ability of patients with spasticity to generate voluntary muscle action. When normal muscle is strengthened a corresponding increase in functional ability is expected. Physiotherapists are hesitant to resist spastic muscle if any increase in muscle tone is observed. While open chain, (non weight bearing), resisted strengthening techniques are not used with patients with spasticity many of the other forms of treatment commonly used when treating patients with spasticity are in fact closed chain, (weight bearing) strengthening techniques, e.g. sit to stand. In this functional activity the spastic quadriceps, resisted by body weight is strengthened both concentrically when standing up and eccentrically when sitting down. The aims of this study are to determine (i) if strengthening spastic muscle, (quadriceps), results in an increase in RPM, (spasticity) of that muscle. (ii) If an increase in muscle strength of the spastic muscle, (quadriceps), would show a corresponding increase in function.

METHODOLOGY:
Subjects:
Twelve subjects (9 male and 3 female), with an average age of 68.8 years and average length of time post CVA, (6 = R, 6 = L) of 5.3 years (range 1 - 14.7 years) completed the experimental procedure. Five subjects walked unaided, 4 used a single stick, 2 used 4 point sticks and one used a frame. Four subjects has ankle foot orthoses. Subjects were referred from local Day Hospitals and Community Health Centres and were accepted into the study if they satisfied the following criteria: first CVA, minimum length of time since CVA of 12 months, clinical evidence of spasticity as measured by hyperreflexia of quadriceps and passive resistance to manual knee flexion/extension, not receiving individual physiotherapy.
Ten normal subjects not matched for sex or age participated in the initial muscle testing procedure but not in the muscle strengthening programme.

Apparatus:
(i)   A computer controlled dynamometer, (Kin-Com)
(ii)   EMG: Designed to be used in conjunction with KinCom.
(iii) A micro-computer stride analyser, (B.L. Engineering), was used to determine the temporal distance parameters of gait.
(iv)   Computer based video analysis was used to determine knee angle at mid stance.

Procedure:
Muscle Testing:
(i)   Resistance to passive movement, (knee flexion/extension) of quadriceps muscle group at velocities of 250°, 150°, 90°, 40°, and 6° per second were performed through the available knee range of movement. Subjects were seated for the assessment with the hips stabilised at 90° of flexion. Hip and thigh stabilising straps were in place. Subjects who presented with an orthosis were tested with the orthosis in situ. (The head was maintained in the mid-line position and the arms rested on the thighs.) Simultaneous EMG was recorded for both agonist and antagonist. Before the test commenced the lower limb was weighed at a 45° angle and the data automatically corrected for gravity. The sequence of testing was from highest to lowest speeds.
(ii)   Voluntary torque generation both concentrically and eccentrically of the quadriceps muscle group at velocities of 90° and 40° per second through the available knee range of movement. Simultaneous EMG was recorded for both agonist and antagonist muscles. The resistance to passive movement at each velocity was recorded three times. A three second pause was allowed between the reciprocal movements. Voluntary torque generation of the quadriceps muscle both concentrically and eccentrically was recorded

Gait Analysis:

Insoles were fitted within the subjects shoes, a micro computer attached to their waist and subjects walked a set 9 metre pathway. Subjects walked at their own comfortable speed with their usual ambulatory aid and orthosis. An initial walk to familiarise the subject with the apparatus was performed. Velocity and symmetry, (duration in seconds of single limb stance), were the measures selected for analysis.

Video Analysis:

A lateral view of the subject walking the 9 metre pathway without gait analysis equipment was recorded for video analysis. The knee angle in mid stance was the measure selected for analysis.

Following the initial testing the 12 subjects with spasticity participated in a concentric/eccentric quadriceps strengthening programme. This consisted of three sessions per week for four weeks. The subjects were positioned as for the initial testing. Continuous concentric/eccentric contractions of the quadriceps were performed at a velocity of $40o^{s-1}$. On the first visit three sets of three maximum contractions were performed. The sets and repetition were progressively increased to suit individual performance with the last session usually containing six sets of six repetitions.

Statistical Analysis:

Several paired and unpaired t-tests were used to test for statistical significance. To guard against testing multiple hypothesis tests involving torque and EMG outputs both concentrically and eccentrically at five selected velocities were deemed to be significant at $p<.005$. The pair t-tests used in the pre and post strengthening analysis and functional evaluations were deemed significant at $p<.01$.

Results:

There is a significant difference in the RPM of spastic and normal muscle when stretched at velocities of $250o^{s-1}$ ($p<.001$), $150o^{s-1}$ ($p<.000$), $90o^{s-1}$ ($p<.004$). There was no significant difference at the lower speeds of $40o^{s-1}$ and $60o^{s-1}$. There was no significant difference between RPM resulting from an eccentric quadriceps stretch, (velocities 250°, 150°, 90°, 40°, 6°) pre and post strengthening of spastic muscle. Spastic muscle strengthened significantly, ($p<.008$) when exercised concentrically at $40o^{s-1}$. No significant change was noted eccentrically at $40o^{s-1}$ or at the concentric or eccentric readings at $90o^{s-1}$. No significant differences were found in the functional measures of gait speed, symmetry or the knee angle in mid-stance.

DISCUSSION:

The major finding of this study was the lack of significant difference in RPM of spastic muscle across a wide range of velocities, before and after an isokinetic strengthening programme which resulted in significant ($p<.008$) improvement in concentric muscle strength at a velocity of $40o^{s-1}$. Strengthening spastic muscle did not result in an increase in spasticity. The strengthening programme selected consisted on an isokinetic concentric/eccentric programme for quadriceps, (spastic muscle) at an angular velocity of $40o^{s-1}$. Chapman and Wiesendanger[1] in their review of the physiological and anatomical basis of spasticity conclude that while the literature abounds with attempts to explain the phenomenon of spasticity the anatomical and physiological basis is far from being clearly defined.

Spasticity is attributed to an imbalance between excess in excitatory mechanisms, (increased phasic stretch reflexes), and deficits in inhibiting control by higher centres. The co-activation of the quadriceps, (agonist) and hamstrings, (antagonist) in voluntary movements of spastic patients illustrates the imbalance of excitatory and inhibitory processes[2].

Knutsson[3] notes it is not possible to decide whether the activation of the antagonists in voluntary movement of spastic muscle is due to facilitation of stretch reflexes or to misdirected descending commands. The antagonist activation results in restraint to the voluntary movement thus making it weaker. Sahimann and Norton[4] when evaluating relationships between stretch reflexes and voluntary movement concluded the impairment of movement is not due to antagonist stretch reflexes but rather to limited and prolonged recruitment of agonist contraction and delayed cessation of agonist contraction at the termination of movement.

Tang and Rymer[5] acknowledge the loss of descending excitation as an important component of the weakness of voluntary spastic muscle contraction but highlight observations suggesting disorganisation of the motor output at the segmental level and that this disorganisation may also contribute to muscle weakness. Motor unit discharge rates are abnormally low in spastic muscles. The style of strength training for spastic muscle is discussed by Furness and Strauss[7] who suggest an increase in strength gained by an eccentric training programme for the spastic agonist may not be compromised by an increase in tone. With eccentric training of the spastic angonist, (quadriceps), the antagonist is not stretched, there is no resistance to movement and therefore such training may result in reduced tone in the antagonist. Concentric training on the other hand would result in a lengthening of the antagonist. This lengthening of the antagonist causes stimulation of the stretch reflex with resultant activation and resistance to the voluntary movement. Knutsson[3] advocates that assessments of spasticity include amongst other requirements estimations of the voluntary muscle strength and how it is influenced by abnormal stretch reflexes both when they oppose the voluntary effort in concentric work and when they support the voluntary effort in eccentric work. As both styles of muscle action are necessary for normal function and both styles of strengthening used in functional activities, (sit-stand) in physiotherapy clinics it was decided to incorporate both concentric and eccentric muscle work in the strengthening programme.

Whilst significant gains were obtained at $40^\circ s^{-1}$ concentrically this gain was not reproduced eccentrically at the same speed or either concentrically or eccentrically at the higher $90^\circ s^{-1}$. Huge inter-individual variation and small subject numbers combined to reduce the likelihood of significant findings. The standard deviations for the eccentric movements were twice the range of the concentric standard deviations. As $40^\circ s^{-1}$ was the training speed the strength gain recorded may reflect specificity of training response. During their training period subjects displayed a greater ability to overlay their concentric muscle contractions in contrast to their eccentric contractions. The eccentric contractions appeared to fatigue towards the end of each set of repetitions. This characteristic has been previously noted[7]. Most subjects were familiar with the concentric version of muscle strengthening through past life experiences but all were basically learning a new motor skill to perform the required eccentric muscle strengthening component. Smaller standard deviation for concentric muscle action pre-strengthening, practice at $40^\circ s^{-1}$ and familiarity with the concentric concept of muscle strengthening may be factors explaining the specific strength gain in the concentric $40^\circ s^{-1}$ programme.

Whilst strengthening spastic muscle resulted in an increase in motor unit recruitment of the agonist muscle group there was also a corresponding increase in motor unit recruitment of the antagonist. This additional motor unit activation did not however result in any significant increase in resistance when the post strengthened muscle was stretched passively. These results support Sahimann-Norton[4] findings who concluded the impairment of movement with spasticity is not due to the restraint generated by antagonist stretch reflexes but rather to limited recruitment of motor unit activity in the agonist. The average torque generated by spastic muscle was far below that of normal muscle when contacting concentrically at $40^\circ s^{-1}$. There was minimal overlay between the groups. (N.M. range quadriceps 383 - 1442 N.M., SM 85-280 N.M.; N.M. Hamstrings 118 - 362 N.M.; S.M. 22 138 N.M.) Did the increase in strength of spastic muscle have any functional benefits? No significant differences were found. Again the small subject numbers and high inter individual differences would retard the likelihood of statistically significant findings. Lack of functional improvement cannot be sustained however if each subject is evaluated individually. Seventy-three per cent of subjects improved in speed and symmetry of gait and 70% experienced a move towards the normal 13o of knee flexion at mid stance. It was stressed to the subjects upon entry to the program that the aim of the research was to gain a better understanding of muscle function. The connotation of "treatment" was discouraged. Many subjects however commented on how much better they felt. Two remarked that they were no longer dragging their foot, one stated he could now squat, and another she now felt confident enough to walk in a crowded situation.

Spastic muscle can be strengthened concentrically without fear of a corresponding increase in the RPM of that muscle. Strengthening spastic muscle will result in increased motor unit requirement of both the agonist and antagonist. Whilst increasing motor unit recruitment of the spastic agonist may enhance a component of the movement problem, recent advances in the motor sciences would not support isolated muscle work as a method of improving function. Movement is reviewed on a wider basis than neurophysiological with a greater emphasis on biomedical behavioural influences.

Further studies involving a much larger subject group need to be undertaken to determine the functional contribution resulting from better torque production in spastic muscle.

REFERENCES:

Chapman C.E. and Wiesendanger M. (1982) The Physiological and Anatomical Basis of Spasticity: Arena. Physiotherapy Canada. 34:125 - 136.

Rosenfalk A., Andreassen S. (1980) Impaired Regulation of Force and Firing Pattern of Single Motor Units in Patients with Spasticity. J. Neurology, Neurosurgery and Psychiatry. 43 907-16.

Knutsson E., 1987 The Measurement and Treatment of Spasticity Post Conference Symposium of the Tenth W.C.P.T. Conference Western Australia 29 and 30 May 98-102.

Sahrmann S.A., Norton B.J. (1977) The Relationship of Voluntary Movement to Spasticity in the Upper Motor Neuron Syndrome. Ann. Neurol 2: 460 - 65.

Tang A., Rymer W., (1981) Abnormal Free EMG Relations in Paretic Limbs of Hemiparetic Human Subjects. J. Neurology, Neurosurgery and Psychiatry 44: 690 - 698.

Furness A. and Strauss G.R. (1987) Characteristics of Concentric and Eccentric Muscle Actions in CNS Dysfunctions Post Conference Symposium of the Tenth W.C.P.T. Conference Western Australia 29 and 30 May. 103 - 110

A PROPOSED MODEL FOR THE CONCEPTUALIZATION OF MOTOR CONTROL

M J Majsak
Program in Physical Therapy, Hahnemann University,
Vine and Broad Streets, Philadelphia, PA, USA 19102-1192

Motor control is a complex phenomenon which involves a variety of numerous components. A physical therapist must understand these components to comprehensively study or teach motor control and to treat patients with motor control deficits. The purpose of this presentation is to share a model for the conceptualization of motor control, and to describe how this model can be used as a teaching device, an assessment tool, and a treatment guide.

The Model - The Motor Control Pyramid

Motor control can be described as the ability of an individual to move into, maintain, and move out of postures and positions, as well as select and perform postures and movements appropriate for functional goals within a specific environment. The basic elements which affect motor control fall into three categories: Biomechanical Elements, Neuromuscular Elements, and Psychological Elements (see Figure 1). Biomechanical elements are the components of an individual's physical structure and the physical properties of the surrounding environment. Neuromuscular elements are the components of an individual's ability to generate and integrate sensorimotor activity. Psychological elements are the cognitive, perceptual, and emotional components of an individual.

BIOMECHANICAL	NEUROMUSCULAR	PSYCHOLOGICAL
Posture	Reflexes	Cognition
Alignment	Motor Tone	Perception
Muscle Length	Timing	Emotion
Soft Tissue	Recruitment	Spatial Awareness
Conformation	Coordination	Motivation
Center of Gravity	Selective Control	Ability to Attend
Base of Support	Movement	Ability to Learn
	Initiation	Alertness
	Endurance	Readiness
	Sensorimotor	Knowledge of
	Integration	Movement
		Knowledge of
		Results
		Pain

Figure 1. The Basic Elements of Motor Control

Motor control is determined by more than the summation of these basic motor control elements. To a greater degree motor control is determined by the combination and integration of these basic elements as expressed in three types of motor activity: Unskilled Automatic motor activity, Deliberate motor activity, and Skilled motor activity (see Figure 2).

Unskilled Automatic motor activity provides the center core for motor control, and is comprised of Reflexive and Reactive motor activity. Reflexive activity occurs at the spinal cord level, is generally not susceptible to prior instruction, and is not adaptive to task. Examples of this type of activity are stretch and flexor withdrawal reflexes. Reactive activity occurs at spinal and supraspinal levels,

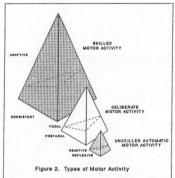

Figure 2. Types of Motor Activity

is susceptible to prior instruction, and is adaptive to task. This activity, which occurs in stereotypical patterns, is the product of motor programs. Examples of this type of activity are righting, equilibrium, and functional postural reactions. These two types of Unskilled Automatic motor activity are critical components of Deliberate and Skilled motor activty.

Deliberate motor activity intentional and calculated motor activity. This activity involves a decision to maintain a position, to move, or a combination of the two, and how to perform these activities. Deliberate activity is comprised of Postural and Focal activity which each occur at spinal, supraspinal, and cortical levels. Postural activity is the way an individual orients and stabilizes the body in the external world for an intended task. Postural activity can be further delineated into Postural Set (the postural orientation an individual assumes in preparation for a task), and Postural Drive (any and all of the postural adaptations whic occur during the performance of a task). Examples of Postural activity are: ´intentionally correcting from a postural displacement, assuming a particular posture for a task, changing postures during a task, and altering posture in response to a change in Focal activity. Focal activity is the way an individual moves or manipulates parts of the body, objects, or both, in respect to oneself and the environment. Focal activity can be further delineated into Ballistic, Discontinuous, and Continuous movement. Ballistic movement is fast and explosive programmed movement which occurs without the use of internal feedback. An example of Ballistic movement is when one quickly swings a limb at a moving object. Discontinuous movement is variable speed, non-programmed movement which occurs with the use of internal feedback. An example of Discontinuous movement is when one changes movement direction and speed while learning to reach for an object. Continuous movement is variable speed, well-learned movement which occurs with or without the use of internal feedback. An example of Continuous movement is when one gently throws an object. Constant interactions occur between Postural and Focal activity, not only at a Deliberate level, but often between Deliberate and Ubskilled Automatic levels. Unskilled Automatic and Deliberate motor activity are critical components of Skilled motor activity.

Skilled motor activity is comprised of patterns of movement which are either highly Consistent or Adaptive and which may occur with relatively little effort or conscious attention. This type of activity develops through a motor learning process from the creation and matching of specific holding and movement patterns to specific tasks. These activity patterns occur at spinal, supraspinal, and cortical levels. Consistent movement is important for unchanging or "closed" environments, while Adaptive movement is important for changing or "open" environments. A "feel" for the movement develops which can be referred to as either a perceptual trace or a recognition schema. An "idea" of the movement also develops which can be referred to as either a memory trace or a recall schema.

A strict division does not separate these three types of motor activity. All three work together closely, and the transition from one type of motor activity to another is not always easily discernable. These three types of motor activity framed within the three types of basic motor control elements form a Motor Control Pyramid (see Figure 3).

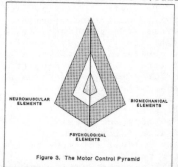

NEUROMUSCULAR ELEMENTS

BIOMECHANICAL ELEMENTS

PSYCHOLOGICAL ELEMENTS

Figure 3. The Motor Control Pyramid

Educational and Clinical Application

This model acts as a guide to assist one in the organization of concepts of motor control. It can be used with a wide range of individuals regardless of age or degree of motor function. The model can be applied to numerous cases in both the classroom and the clinic.

As a teaching device, this model can be used to define, describe, and help one to remember the numerous components of motor control. This model can also be used as a tool with which one can critically analyze the concepts and principles of different approaches of rehabilitation to evaluate how well those approaches confront the elements and types of motor activity necessary for the production of motor control.

This model can be used in the clinic to assist in the assessment and treatment of a patient's motor control deficits. A therapist can use this model to decipher which components of motor control have been altered or lost, and to plan suitable treatment strategies to address those components. This model guides a therapist to design treatment plans which address not only reflexes and reactions, but also the types of postural activity and the ballistic, continuous, and discontinuous focal movements which are a part of normal motor control. A therapist is guided to consider the consistency and adaptability of skilled task performance. A therapist is reminded that the biomechanical, neuromuscular, and psychological elements of motor control must always be considered, and that various types of motor activity as well as these elements must be addressed simultaneously to promote the highest degree of motor control within a patient.

THE EFFECT OF REPEATED ECCENTRIC CONTRACTIONS OF THE SPASTIC QUADRICEPS ON RANGE OF
MOVEMENT AT THE KNEE JOINT

Margaret Hoessly, Anne Recordon, Susan Coutts
School of Physiotherapy, Auckland Institute of Technology, Auckland, New Zealand

The restriction imposed upon active movement in patients with upper motor neuron lesions
has two major components. The first is the abnormality of neural function itself (Knutsson
1987, Sahrmann 1977, Tanaka 1983, Burke 1988) while the second comprises shortening changes
which occur in muscle and connective tissue (Dietz, Quintern & Berger 1981, Grossman,
Sahrmann & Rose 1982). The latter may eventually contribute significantly to muscle
stiffness which constitutes a mechanical load against which the weak antagonist must work.
There is an additional element which also contributes to the stiffness of both spastic and
normal muscle, namely its thixotropic properties which fluctuate with the kind of muscle
contraction performed. This consistency change taking place in muscle is similar to that
occurring when by a thixotropic process a gel becomes temporarily liquid when shaken and
returns to its original state at rest (Lakie, Walsh & Wright 1984).

Limitation of movement imposed by spastic stiffness can frequently be overcome to some extent
by the use of repeated eccentric contractions of the spastic muscle. This subsequently
decreases stiffness enhancing performance of the restricted antagonist and increasing active
range of movement. Former levels of stiffness can be restored by repeated shortening
contractions (Hoessly 1991). These two effects, a decrease or increase in stiffness, appear
to be related to the thixotropic after effects which occur following lengthening or
shortening contractions. Changes in both the thixotropic properties of normal muscle and
stretch reflex sensitivity have been demonstrated following active and passive large
amplitude finger flexion and extension movements. Increased stiffness and an enhanced
stretch reflex followed active and passive shortening while decreased stiffness and
depression of the stretch reflex followed active and passive lengthening and isometric
contraction. (Hagbarth, Hagglund, Nordin & Wallin 1985). This thixotropic element is
thought to be the same in both normal and spastic muscle (Brown, van Rensburg, Walsh, Lakie
& Wright 1987). It is considered that during muscle contraction stable cross bridges between
actin and myosin filaments in both intra and extrafusal muscle become detached and will
reform at whatever length the muscle is held. If it is held in the lengthened position
(as occurs following lengthening contractions) cross bridges will reform so that both extra
and intra fusal fibres are slack producing a loosening effect on the muscle. The Ia spindle
fibre response decreases, thus depressing the stretch reflex. (Morgan Prochazka & Proske
1984).

A recent study to further identify the effect on movement of repeated eccentric contractions
was carried out with the co-operation of three patients with multiple sclerosis, all women
between the ages of 40 and 50 whose condition was stable and who were receiving no other
treatment. All three had spasticity of the quadriceps and difficulty bending one knee when
walking.

Method
An ABAB design was used and carried out over a six week period. A pre-treatment baseline

(A) was established over four consecutive days. Each subject from a prone position performed 10 knee flexion movements in two sets of five with a two minute rest in between each set. Over four days a total of 40 knee flexion movements were recorded. The treatment procedure (B) was also carried out in prone. Each subject performed five sets of 10 eccentric (lengthening) contractions of moderate degree with a two minute rest in between each set. Over four days a total of 200 contractions were performed. This was followed by three days' rest after which the four days of treatment was repeated. Measurement of active knee flexion in prone was taken following each set of 10 eccentric contractions making a total of 40 measurements over the whole treatment period.

A standard universal goniometer was used to measure knee flexion. Measurements were taken at the same time of day for each subject and in a consistent environment. The same non professional but trained tester with no knowledge of the study carried out all measurements. On day four of each week walking was recorded on video. No attempt was made to show each patient how best to use their increased flexibility by retraining gait as would routinely be done in a clinical situation.

RESULTS

Table 1 shows means, ranges and standard deviations for degrees of active knee flexion across all three subjects:

TABLE 1   DEGREES OF KNEE FLEXION
MEANS, RANGES AND STANDARD DEVIATIONS   N = 40

SUBJECT		PRE TREATMENT BASELINE	TREATMENT 1	POST TREATMENT BASELINE	TREATMENT 2
CB X	=	18.575	75.325	19.675	93.225
Range	=	7-41	23-115	13-27	38-119
SD	=	6.059	28.477	3.689	22.150
NH X		70.800	115.05	96.775	115.85
Range		55-92	98-125	70-108	103-125
SD		11.789	5.905	8.601	4.342
HS X		76.5	124.7	115.85	132.625
Range		15-130	17-137	113-125	55-145
SD		47.021	23.76	4.342	18.79

An independent samples t test was used to compare sets of data. In all subjects comparison of pre treatment baseline with first and second treatments, post treatment baseline and second treatment showed a high level of significance (p=.000). One subject (CB) showed a significant increase between first and second treatments (p=.002) having returned to a post treatment baseline which was not significantly different from her pre treatment one. The remaining two subjects (NH & HS) showed no significant improvement between the first and second treatments. However, their post treatment baselines did not revert to pre treatment levels, (NH p = .000, HS p= .025).

Computer analysis of two steps in each gait video series using a Flextrac Expert Vision Video Motion Analysis system indicated a trend towards an improvement in speed of gait, knee flexion angles (two subjects) and linear velocity of knee flexion (three subjects) when pre treatment baseline and second treatment averages were studied.

CONCLUSION

The excessive stiffness of muscle in spasticity appears to be due to a number of factors;

the increased stretch reflex, changes in connective tissue and visco elastic properties of muscle together with the inherent thixotropic properties which in turn influence the state of the stretch reflex. It would appear that of all these factors the one most likely to be influenced by repeated eccentric contractions is the thixotropic element especially in view of the restoration of stiffness which occurs following shortening contractions. The temporary loosening effect on both intra and extrafusal muscle appears also to result in depression of the stretch reflex and this in turn may contribute to the decrease in resistance to active movement which becomes apparent following this procedure. It is the view of some investigators however, that the increased stretch reflex is little if any impediment to voluntary movement in spasticity (Landau 1980, Sahrmann 1977). This factor may therefore be of minor importance in terms of function.

From a practical point of view any positive change in freedom of movement is a welcome one for many patients. It also enables facilitation of the antagonist to proceed with greater ease than would otherwise be the case.

REFERENCES

1. Knuttson E (1987) Analysis of spastic paresis. Proc. Tenth Int. Cong. W.C.P.T. Sydney, Australia.
2. Sahrmman SA (1977) The relationship of voluntary movement to spasticity in the upper motor neurone syndrome Ann. Neurol. 2: 460-465.
3. Tanaka R (1983) Reciprocal Ia inhibitory pathway in normal man and in patients with motor disorders in Motor Control Mechanisms in Health & Disease. Desmedt JE (Ed) Raven Press, New York.
4. Burke D (1988) Spasticity as an adaptation to pyramidal tract injury. Advances in Neurology 47: Functional Recovery in Neurological Disease. S G Waxman (ed) Raven Press, New York.
5. Dietz V Quintern J Berger W (1981) Electrophysiological studies of gait in spasticity and rigidity. Brain 104:431 - 439.
6. Grossman MR Sahrmman SA Rose SJ (1982) Review of length associated changes in muscle: experimental evidence and clinical implications. Physical Therapy 62: 1799 - 1807.
7. Lakie M Walsh EC Wright CW (1984) Resonance at the wrist demonstrated by the use of a torque motor: an instrument of analysis of muscle tone in man. J Physiol. 353: 265-285.
8. Hoessly M (1991) The use of eccentric contraction of muscle to increase range of movement in the upper motor neurone syndrome. Accepted for publication in Physiotherapy Theory and Practice.
9. Habgarth KE Hagglund JV Nordin M Wallin EU (1985) Thixotropic behaviour of human finger flexor muscles with accompanying changes in spindle and reflex responses to stretch. J. Physiol. 368: 323-342
10 Morgan Dl Prochazka A Proske U (1984) The after effects of stretch and fusimotor stimulation on the responses of primary endings of cat muscle spindles. J. Physiol. 356: 465 - 477
11 Brown JK van Rensburg F Walsh G Lakie M Wright GW (1987) A neurological study of hand function in hemiplegic children. Dev. Med and Child Neurol. 29: 287-304.
12 Landau WM (1980) Spasticity: what is it what is it not? in Spasticity. Disordered Motor Control. Feldman RG, Young RR, Koella WP. Chicago Year Book Publications.

The authors wish to acknowledge the assistance of Dr B Wilson, University of Otago for the video analysis.

REINFORCEMENT OF RECIPROCAL INHIBITION (RI) BY CONTRALATERAL PROPRIOCEPTIVE INPUT IN LOWER LIMB IN MAN

TREMBLAY L.E., GIRARD P. AND DELWAIDE P.J.

UNIVERSITY OF LIEGE BELGIUM AND LAVAL (QUEBEC) AND OTTAWA UNIVERSITY (ONTARIO) CANADA

All physiotherapists know RI. It is a basic concept incorporated into procedures of therapeutic exercises. RI is believed to play a crucial functional role in motor control and is a spinal "inhibitory interneuron" known as "la" and is clearly involved in it. In this study we looked at whether or not contralateral proprioceptive "influences" were able to modify RI. Fifteen normal volunteers (24.8 $\pm$ 4 years) were studied in measuring on homolateral limbs, the soleus H-reflex at rest and during a synchronized electrical stimulion (ES) on the nerve supplying antagonist muscle (common peroneal nerve (CPN)) or during a standardized isometric voluntary contraction (SIVC) of tibialis anterior muscle (TA). The conditioning contralateral maneuvers consisting either on ES on tibial nerve or CPN or ES on tibial nerve plus SIVC of soleus muscle(s) or ES of CPN plus SIVC of TA. RI at rest or during TA contraction is not modified by either ES on contralateral tibial nerve and CPN. But, during TA contraction situation, the contralateral ES of tibial nerve or CPN respectively associated with the muscle contraction, increase significantly RI by 11.5% (P<0.05) for S and 17% (P<0.01) for TA. We clearly demonstrated that the contralateral proprioceptive input change the excitability of "la" interneuron. These results suggest that the therapist should use the contralateral appropriate muscle contraction in order to reduce the spasticity by increasing homolateral RI.

FACILITATION OF NORMAL FUNCTIONAL MOVEMENTS IS MORE THAN STRUGGLE WITH PATTERNS

Inge Berlin
Instructor for PNF - Am Heidehof 18D - D-1000 Berlin 37 - Germany

The aim of this paper is to bridge the gulf between Western and Eastern thinking for the reason of getting more harmony into the treatments of our patients. While PNF is a product of Western thinking, acupressure techniques have developed in the tradition of the East. Having worked with PNF for 30 years and with acupressure for a period of ten years now, I have come to the conclusion that a combination of the two conceptions can be put into a working reality.

The two systems

The techniques of PNF may be defined as a method of promoting and hastening the response of the neuromuscular mechanism through stimulation of the proprioceptors.

The acupressure methods SHIATSU and YIN SHIN DO are defined as a therapy administrated by the thumbs, fingers and palms, sometimes even by means of elbows, knees and feet. Both methods avoid the use of any instruments to apply pressure to the human body. The overriding principle is to bring into balance the patients's life force and to maintain and strengthen the reliance on his or her natural healing power. This is done within the framework of the *yin-yang* philosophy of ancient oriental health art.

Yin and *yang* can be seen as opposites, where *yin* respresents the passive principle and *yang* its active counterpart. Accid muscletone and low blood pressure is related to *yin* and hypertone muscles as well as high blood pressure is related to *yang*. Like positive and negative, which very rarely exist without their counterpart, there is never a sole state of either *yin* or *yang*. Both occur together in the same person in the form of more *yin* and less *yang* or vice versa. For physical and emotional health a balance of *yin* and *yang* is required in the same person.

The philosophy of PNF is a philosophy of total patient treatment. The goal is optimum function of the person as a whole. PNF incorporates a number of basic principles and techniques which have a stimulating or relaxing effect on the patient's neuromuscular mechanism, making receptors more or less sensitive to facilitation and inhibition.

Working with PNF means the training of body awareness for a functioning everyday life. It is here that important aspects of *yin-yang* philosophy can be made use of. I strongly believe that the principles of *yin-yang* offer sound ways of helping to improve the patient's physical condition.

The Breathing Activity

Breathing supplies energy for all movements. The comparison of our own breathing movements and the patient's breathing rhythm can be a keystone for an effective treatment. It is well-known that emotions and will-power influence the way of breathing. The classical works of Japanese medicine are unanimous in stating that lower abdominal breathing, called "hara" or "tandem" breathing is the center of harmony between *yin* and *yang*, called "ki". Over-activity in breathing should be inhibited and passiveness in breathing should be changed and turned into more active breathing during treatment.

While breathing the patient should feel relaxed and comfortable. While giving pressure, the therapist's body weight can support the treatment and at the same time give feedback to the therapist. When the patient rests on the mats, lying on his side, the therapist who prefers a kneeling position can place his hands vertically on the patient's thorax. His arms outstretched, the therapist applies pressure to the patient by shifting his own body forward as the patient breathes in and backward as the patient breathes out. The closer the therapist kneels next to the patient, the easier it is to highten the pressure. The groove of the pressure is downwards to the center of the belly.

While breathing, the patient should be asked to place the centre of his thinking behind and slightly below his belly-button. Long lasting pressure will help to exhale and provides a sedation effect. If the patient's breath frequency has to be slowed down, the therapist should take his own respiration rythm for giving the commands "Breath in and out!". Poor and weak breathing activity needs stimulation. Shifting the body wheight more quickly causes stimulation of the sympathetic nervous system. This procedure is identical with the "PNF quick-stretch".

Total movements

For diagnosis in PNF we have the patient roll on the mat and watch out whether he prefers flexion or extension patterns. Then we act according to *yin-yang* theory: "Take the present condition as it is and work from that point to relieve it". If, for example, the patient is not able to turn his head to the right you gently turn it to the left for a couple of times. This corresponds to the PNF practice of starting with the best movements and not forcing the patient into the opposite.

Diagnosis

The Western touching diagnosis looks at the condition of the skin, the muscles, the joints and ligaments. Quite often this procedure results in a strong reaction on the part of the patient. Oriental touching diagnosis is performed with instinctive compassion and without any scare. The therapist passes the hand along the spine, the abdomen and along the meridian lines. These meridian lines cover the whole body. They are defined as channels of living magnetic energy. Sometimes these twelve channels can be associated with the functioning of certain well-defined internal organs.

Each meridian line is made up of a pair of *yin* and *yang*. The *yin* part of the meridian lines covers more or less the adduction components of PNF, whereas the *yang* part of the meridian lines covers the abduction patterns of PNF. By experience I have found out that you can either tonify or sedate the energy within the twelve meridian lines by varying the degree of resistance which you set against rotation movements while working with PNF patterns.

When you have found the maximum point of elongation before you move through the range of the pattern the meridian will surface in the skin enabling you to diagnose whether the meridian energy is more *yin* or *kyo* or *yang* or *yitsu*. The *kyo* quality feels flabby and weak, the *jitsu* condition will appear as hard but elastic. According to oriental medicine *kyo* areas are treated with long-lasting pressure for up to five seconds. For this reason the movements of the PNF patterns within a *kyo* area need longer-lasting elongation. In addition, a soft adequate initial stretch will help to start the movement.

The *jitsu* area needs less and short pressure. Here, work with the PNF patterns should have a sedation effect. We move through the range of motion up to the point of tightness. Here we ask for a prolonged hold. While giving adequate resistance we make sure that the patient breathes in a relaxed way in the lower part of his stomach before we ask him to move further through the range of motion.

Trunk movement

A coordinated and well-balanced gait depends to a large degree upon the mobility and underlying stability of the trunk. The spine needs a certain amount of flexibility in order to create a response in the synergistic muscle activity.

Patients with tightness along the spine do not develop the functional timing for the control of motion. Instead of achieving effective trunk movements, they will fight with neck, arms and legs. Again, pressure may be used to help the patient understand the direction of the anticipated movement. This pressure will be placed paravertebrally. In these areas there are a number of association points which correspond segmentally to the internal organs and also have a relationship to the meridian lines. Again, with the proximal hand the therapist applies light pressure combined with traction or approximation and rotation resistance. In addition, the improvement of breathing patterns will have a positive effect upon the development of trunk movement.

Self care

In order to achieve long-standing success and independence, self-care is an important goal of our treatment. The ability within the patient's potential is the guideline to develop skilled daily activities. Meridian stretching exercises supported by breathing awareness help the patient to feel the flow of energy in the meridian lines involved.

The patient is requested to remain in the same position when he has reached his own maximum stretching point without bouncing, breathing in and out for about three times. The variety of selected exercises is very much related to the pattern of facilitation. The exercises have to be performed gently and without any force or power. Their overall success depends on daily practice in a calm and relaxed state of mind.

Final remarks

The combination of PNF and accupressure techniques in a unified treatment helps to overcome the separation of psyche and soma. Its application may lead us one step further to the general aim which is to treat the human being as a whole and not only the patient's body. A well-balanced combination of the two approaches might be the secret of modern physiotherapy.

FACILITATION BY CUTANEOUS STIMULATION OF MUSCLE RESPONSES TO TRANSCRANIAL MAGNETIC STIMULATION

D.W. Maskill, N.J. Davey, P.H. Ellaway. Department of Physiology, Charing Cross and Westminster Medical School, Fulham Palace Road, LONDON W6 8RF.

Introduction: Cutaneous stimulation is employed in physiotherapy to facilitate contraction in weakened muscle or during recovery from central nerve lesions. It has been employed as direct mechanical brushing or icing over the muscle (1). To understand the mechanisms of the cutaneous component of these therapeutic practices and to investigate their physiological basis, the effect of localised cutaneous stimulation on the response of skeletal muscle to stimulation of the motor cortex in man has been investigated using using transcranial magnetic stimulation (TMS). This relatively new technique (2) allows the motor cortex to be stimulated to evoke a response in skeletal muscle without the considerable discomfort associated with electrical stimulation.

It is well known that changes in motoneurone excitability and reflex responses to cutaneous stimulation vary with the location of the skin stimuli (3,4). In particular, electrical stimulation of the digital nerve of the index finger has been shown to inhibit the response of the first dorsal interosseous muscle to TMS (5). Our preliminary work has revealed that cutaneous stimulation facilitates the response of the adductor pollicis muscle to TMS of the motor cortex (6).

Methods: With the approval of the local ethical committee 10 male and female subjects aged 22 to 64 years with no history of neurological disease were studied.

Subjects were seated with a forearm semipronated, resting on a padded arm support, and the elbow flexed to approximately 100°. Electromyographic (EMG) activity from the adductor pollicis muscle was recorded using surface electrodes placed over the belly of the muscle and the interphalangeal joint of the first finger. All subjects were instructed to relax completely the muscles of the hand and arm. Audible feedback of the EMG signal was provided to assist them to meet this condition.

The brain was stimulated using a magnetic stimulator (Novametrix Magstim 200) with a 9cm circular coil centred over the vertex. The stimulation intensity was increased until it was just suprathreshold for a response in adductor pollicis and was then maintained at this level throughout the recording session.

Discrete cutaneous stimulation was employed by brushing the skin over the T1 dermatome, the muscle, the first carpo-metacarpal (C-MC) and the first metacarpo-phalangeal (MC-P) joints. In addition, the skin overlying the dorso-lateral aspect of the base of the thumb was stimulated at points on a 1.5cm grid using circular movements of a small stiff brush at each point. The EMG responses recorded from the surface electrodes were rectified and the voltage time integral calculated. Responses were averaged for each group of equivalent stimuli. A sequence of 16 brain shocks was administered as four sets of four stimuli consisting of one set without cutaneous stimulation, one set with cutaneous stimulation followed by a rest period (20s). The sequence was then repeated. The rest period was given to allow any persistent skin sensation to disappear before the next group of stimuli was given.

Results: Cutaneous stimulation produced facilitation of the adductor pollicis response to motor cortex stimulation at one or more of the sites tested in 8 of the 10 subjects. In subjects (n=7) showing facilitation at more than one site, the degree of facilitation was dependent upon the site of stimulation. Fig. 1 shows the distribution of responses for all ten subjects. Facilitation is clearly less evident on brushing the T1 dermatome.

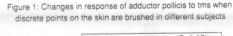

Figure 1: Changes in response of adductor pollicis to tms when discrete points on the skin are brushed in different subjects

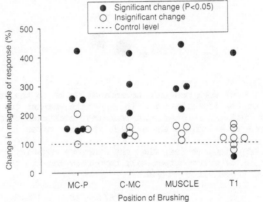

In the study shown in fig. 2 the size of the circle indicates the degree of facilitation of the adductor pollicis response to discrete cutaneous stimulation in one subject. The strongest facilitation occurs in response to stimulation of the skin over the joint lines.

Discussion: We have shown that contraction of the thumb adductor muscle elicited by transcranial stimulation of the motor cortex can be facilitated by cutaneous brushing. This contrasts with earlier findings (5) that revealed inhibition of cortically evoked contraction in response to electrical stimulation of a cutaneous nerve. A reason for this difference may be that facilitation in our experiments masks a weaker inhibition. Alternatively, electrical stimulation of the digital nerve may produe a discharge in afferents not excited by brushing the skin around the thenar eminence.

Figure 2: Changes in cortically evoked muscle responses
to discrete skin stimulation in a single subject

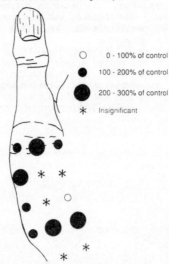

○   0 - 100% of control

●   100 - 200% of control

●   200 - 300% of control

∗   Insignificant

The present work provides no indication as to the central nervous location of the facilitation. To ascertain whether the facilitation is spinal or cortical further work is being undertaken using a mechanically drive probe to stimulate the skin at specific times in relation to cortical shocks.

In conclusion, we feel that the discrete organisation of cutaneous facilitation of motor output will have relevance to the therapeutic use of peripheral stimulation in man.

References

1. Goff B, (1969) Appropriate afferent stimulation.
    Physiotherapy 58, 13: 409-415
2. Barker AT, Jalinous R, Freeston IL (1985)   Non-invasive
    magnetic stimulation of the human motor cortex. Lancet 1, 1106-1107
3. Sherrington CS (1906) The integrative action of the nervous
    system. New York: Scribners
4. Hagbarth K-E (1952) Excitatory and inhibitory skin areas
    for flexor and extensor motoneurones. Acta. physiol.
    Scand 26 Suppl 94
5. Day BL, Dressler A, Maertens De Noorhout A, Marsden CD
    (1982) Differential effect of cutaneous stimuli on
    responses to electrical or magnetic stimulation of the
    human brain. J.Physiol 399 68P
6. Davey, NJ, Ellaway PH, Maskill DW, (1991) Facilitation
    by mechanical cutaneous stimulation of muscle responses
    to transcranial magnetic stimulation. J. Physiol. (in press)

EFFECTS OF FACILITATING POSITION ON H-REFLEX

K. Yanagisawa, R. Nakamura*, T. Fujiwara**, H. Saito
Tokyo Metropolitan College of Allied Medical Sciences, 7-2-10,
Higashioku, Arakawa-ku, Tokyo, JAPAN   *Touhoku Univ., **Shinshu Univ.

INTRODUCTION: Proprioceptive neuromuscular facilitation (PNF) (1)
utilizes specific starting position (PNF position) for each movement
pattern .   Kabat (2) assumed that PNF patterns are easy to be
executed and facilitate the alpha motoneurons of muscles related
to the movement. Our previous studies have indicated that simple
reaction time (RT) was fast at PNF positions of either the upper
or the lower extremities compared to neutral, i.e., kinesiological
reference, position (3). Also PNF position of the upper extremity
brought about the increase of peak force for fast knee extension
in isometric condition (4), and that of the upper extremity induced
cortical activation demonstrated by frequency analysis of EEG (5)
and/or by brain electrical activities map (BEAM)(6).   However,
PNF positions examined in our previous studies were not all of
them. According to Delwaide et al.(7) passive position changes
of the upper extremity in saggital plane induced the shift of
amplitude of H-reflex, which followed the pattern of hand-foot
reflex. Thus, there remain two questions: whether every PNF positions
could bring about the arousal response, and both non-specific arousal
response and the specific spinal reflex induced by the passive
postural changes of a limb are acting on motoneurons of the lower
extremity. In this study we analyzed H-response of normal subjects
at PNF and neutral positions of the shoulder or the hip, and
attempted to analyze the questions above mentioned.
METHODS: The experiment was performed on 24 male students of
a physical therapy school, aged 18 to 36 years. They were right-
handed by self report. The informed consent was obtained from all
subjects before participating the study.
      H-response of the left soleus muscle elicited by stimulation
of posterior tibial nerve was taken with surface electrodes at
neutral and PNF positions. The electric stimulation used during
experimental run was rectangular pulse with 1 msec duration in
1 Hz. The strength of stimulation before experimental run was 1.12
or 1.20 times of H-response threshold with double pulses with 1
msec, 6 msec interval, in 1 Hz. The H-responses were averaged 32
times in each trial.
      The subjects were randomly divided into two groups: the shoulder
(S) group, 10 males and the hip (H) group,14 males. The subjects
with closed eyes laid on a therapeutic bed. At neutral position,
both the shoulder and the hip were kept at 0 degree. In PNF positions
, the shoulder or the hip was passively kept at one of the following
positions: in S group, eight PNF positions of either left or right

shoulder and in H group, three PNF positions of the right hip. These
PNF positions are in the text book of PNF (1). It was impossible to
elicit H-response at Ext-Add-Ext/Rot position of the right hip.

Using H-response at neutral position as a control, the amplitude
of H-response at PNF positions were presented with percentage.

RESULTS: The stimulation current utilized range from 2.36 mA
to 6.38 mA (mean: 4.53 mA) in S group, and 2.70 mA to 7.50 mA
(mean:4.38 mA) in H group. The amplitude of H-response at neutral
position was from 0.50 mV to 1.84 mV in S group, and 0.26 mV to
3.93 mV in H group. M-wave was observed in two subjects in each
group.

Table 1 presents the percentages of the amplitude on PNF positions
to that on neutral position in S group. Compared to neutral position,
H-response was significantly greater at the extended abducted, and
internally rotated position of the left or right shoulder (p<0.05).
The amplitude of H-response between at other six PNF and neutral
positions were not different.

Table 2 shows the results of three PNF positions in H group.
The amplitude of H-response tended to be high at PNF positions with
flexion components (p<0.1), compared to neutral position.

Table 1. Means of H-response amplitude
in the shoulder PNF positions (%)

Position	Left Mean (SD)	Right Mean (SD)
Ext-Abd-I/R	122.5* (28.3)	127.2* (28.8)
Fl-Add-E/R	103.3 (17.1)	96.7 (20.0)
Ext-Add-I/R	95.4 (18.9)	89.0 (15.7)
Fl-Abd-E/R	95.7 (18.3)	110.7 (29.7)

Neutral Position: 100%, n=10, *:p<0.05

Table 2. Means of H-response
amplitude in the hip PNF
positions (%)

Position	Right Mean (SD)
Fl-Abd-I/R	111.1** (19.7)
Ext-Abd-I/R	95.4 (22.5)
Fl-ADD-E/R	114.9** (29.7)

Neutral Position: 100%,
n=14, **:p<0.1

DISCUSSION: Ext-Abd-Int/Rot positions of the shoulder that
facilitated H-response were kinesiologically extended position of
the shoulder. the other PNF positions of the shoulder that did not
facilitate H-response were flexed one. The results of this study
did not coincide with Delwaide's report, which indicated a reciprocal
effect of the both shoulder positions on the H-response of the soleus
muscle. It seems that the facilitation of the H-responses at two
PNF positions of the shoulder is due to cortical arousal rather
than the long spinal reflex such as hand-foot reflex. The certain
PNF position shortens not only the EMG-RT of the limb (3), also
vocal reaction time (8), and increases alpha band power revealed
by brain electrical map (6), compared to the neutral position.

Furthermore the certain PNF position of upper extremity induces the increase of the power of the quadriceps femoris (4). From these reports, it is considered that one of the PNF positions of the shoulder induce non specific arousal.

The amplitudes of H-responses tended to be high at the two flexed positions of the hip, compared to neutral position. Yanagisawa et al.(9) reported that the contralateral flexed position of the hip facilitated H-response of the soleus muscle and the extended position inhibited in saggital plane. It seems that the influence of crossed reflex brought about these results. The results of the PNF positions in complex plane were not clear-cut, compared to Yanagisawa's report that indicated the reciprocal effect of the contralateral hip position on the H-response. Therefore it is assumed that the results of the hip positions were due to the total effects of non specific arousal and specific spinal reflex such as crossed reflex.

CONCLUSIONS: The PNF positions with extension component in S group and with flexion component in H group facilitated H-response, but the other PNF positions did not induce such a phenomenon. The influence of the propriospinal reflex such as hand-foot reflex was not clear on H-response in S group. It seems that total effects of the arousal and the spinal reflex such as the crossed reflex reflected on H-response in H group.

REFERENCES

1. Knott M, Voss DD,(1968) Proprioceptive neuromuscular facilitation 2nd ed. New York, Harper and Row
2. Kabat H, (1965) Proprioceptive facilitation on therapeutic exercise.(edited by Licht,S 2nd ed,Elizabeth)New Haven,327-343
3. Nakamura R, Viel E (1974) The influence of position changes in the proximal joint on EMG-recording reaction time on key muscles in the human extremity. Proc. WCPT,7th Int. Congr.,119-123
4. Fujita M, Nakamura R (1986) The effects of PNF position of the upper extremity on rapid knee extension. Tohoku J Exp Med 150: 31-35
5. Chida T, Nakamura R, et al.(1983) EEG changes induced by passive postural changes. J Human Ergol 12:217-218
6. Hosokawa T, Nakamura R, et al.(1985) EEG activation induced by facilitating position. Tohoku J Exp Med 147:191-197
7. Delwaide PJ, Figiel C (1973) Influence de la position du membre superieur surl'excitabilite de l'arc soleair. Electromy Clin Neurophysiol 13:515-523
8. Nakamura R, (1983) Effect of facilitating positions on behavioral arousal. J J A Phys M Baln Clim 46:131-137
9. Yanagisawa K, Nakamura R,et al.(1989) Effect of the contralateral hip position in saggital plane on H-response of soleus muscle . Jap J Reh Med 26:244

FUNCTIONAL ARM MOVEMENT: THE RECOVERY OF MOTOR FUNCTION FOLLOWING STROKE

Catarina Broberg

Inst. Rehabilitation Medicine, Sahlgrenska Hospital, University of Gothenburg, Sweden

Introduction

Assessments of recovery of function following stroke has focused primarily on performance of activities of daily living and gross motor skill. Many studies indicate that a great proportion of hemiparetic patients make very limited recovery of motor ability, especially in the arm.(1) Studies on motor performance and effects of different therapies are usually made with patients in a cronic state of the disease. There are no studies on how the movement pattern develops during the recovery period, which is considered to occur during the first few months after stroke. Quantitative kinematic analysis provide a means for getting detailed information on motor behaviour. It also offers insight into the organization of movement and allows for developing new hypothesis on motor control and motor learning.(2)

The purpose of this study was to develop a means for systematic description of some of the qualitative aspects of movements seen during the revovery period after stroke and to identify measurement criteria that reflect the return of voluntary movements in the shoulder and elbow. The purpose was also to compare the results from the quantitative measurements with standard clinical assessments.

Methods

After giving their informed consent, four male and one female patients, 51 to 73 years old, suffering from subtotal hemiparesis due to cerebral infarction, were included. An opto-electronic camera system (IROS-3D, Remplir AB, Sweden) registered light pulses (0.5 ms) sequentially emitted (100 Hz) by infra red light-emitting diodes (LEDs) within a cube-shaped precalibrated measurement field. The LEDs were placed on the patients forehead, chest, shoulders, elbows and at the test object, a metal handle with a wooden knob fastened to a cylindrical horizontal plate (weight 550 grams). The LED position data were converted into cartesian room coordinates and stored. Analysis was made with the aid of a graphic work-station computer (Vax- station II, Digital Equipment Corp.) The displacement and tangential speed of the object, angular displacement and speed of the shoulder and elbow movements in the horizontal plane and associated movements of the body in the vertical plane were utilized for visualization and calculation. Parallel recordings were made with a video camera for subsequent visual control.

The patients, sitting in a chair without armrests, were instructed to perform two simple reaching movements "sagittally" (SAG) and "laterally" (LAT) as illustrated in Fig 1. The patient was

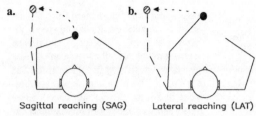

a. Sagittal reaching (SAG) **b.** Lateral reaching (LAT)

Figure 1. Test movements.

to place the object as fast as possible between two stands (height 54 cm) placed in front of him. Data were recorded during 10 secs. The affected arm was tested three times (and in one patient a fourth time) and the nonaffected arm was tested twice.

A neurological examination was performed by a physician and the following standard assessments were used to record clinical recovery at each test day: The Barthel ADL-index, The Fugl-Meyer motor assessment of upper extremity, the modified Ashworth scale of muscle spasticity and a self report on arm function.

Results

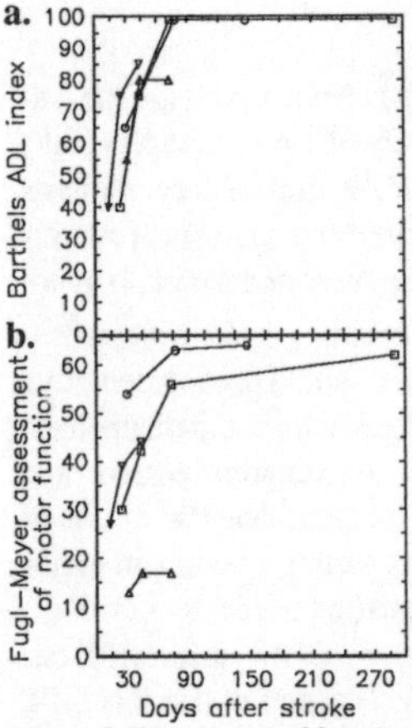

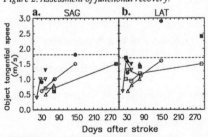

Figure 2. Assessment of functional recovery.

Figure 3. Tangential speed of object (see text for explanation).

Clinical recovery of ADL and motor function of the arm are shown in Fig 2 a and b. Patient 1 (P1, circles) and 2 (P2, squares) regained full ADL-capacity and 63 and 56 points respectively on the motor function test within 75 days after stroke. Patient 3 (P3, triangles up) and patient 4 (P4, triangles down) gained 80 and 85 points respectively on ADL capacity. Recovery of motor function was limited especially in P3. Muscular hypertonia was somewhat increased in all four patients at their first test (1 or 1+ in elbow flexors, but diminished in all but P3, who increased his score (3/2 in elbow flexors/extensors).

The tangential speed of the object is shown in Fig 3 a (SAG) and b. (LAT). Symbols see Fig 1. There was a decrease in speed of both the affected (open symbols) and the unaffected (solid symbols) arm at about 75 days after stroke especially in SAG as compared to one healthy middle-aged male (dotted line). P1 and P2 showed recovery of speed of both arms, but less in the affected one in LAT.

Analysis of the angular excursions of shoulder and elbow revealed that the coordination pattern was irregular and asynchronous in the affected as compared to the unaffected arm. Fig 4 a and b shows the raw tracings of the unaffected and affected arm of P2 in LAT. The different tracings are I: Movement excursion of object (cm), II and III: Shoulder

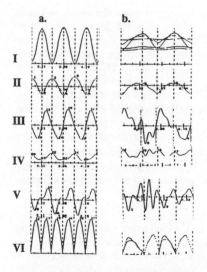

a. **b.**

I

II

III

IV

V

VI

Figure 4. Tracings of movement and speed obtained in one patient (details are given in text).

angle excursion (°) and speed (ms), IV and V: Elbow angular excursion and speed, VI: Tangential speed of object (meter/s). The asynchrony of the elbow movement was seen as an irregularity in angular speed See Fig 4 b, III. This phenomenon was interpreted to be due to "passive" associated movements and was true for all four patients but varied concerning joint and direction of movement. Full recovery of shoulder-elbow coordination and angular speed did nor occur, even in P1 and P2, who at 148 and 290 days after stroke respectivly reported "normal or almost normal use of the affected arm".

Discussion

Analysis of the data from kinematic measurements of recovery of motor function in the arm following stroke preliminary suggests that movement speed and analysis of coordination patterns can serve as a means to quantitate change over time in more detail than clinical tests. The measuring system described allows for testing of task-oriented movements, a prerequisite if the test should be representative for daily life activities. Though the test movements choosen were simple, the patients used different movement strategies. This indicates variability in the coordination pattern and suggests that the movements did not depend on spastic synergies, nor that the return of movements followed a certain order. These findings are in line with recent research on motor control theories, which has provided new paradigms on the understanding of motor control (2) and on coordination of arm movements.(3,4) The measurement system did not quite fulfill our demands in that i.e. reflexions of LEDs on the body sometimes spoiled the data collection. Still, kinematic measurement is considered a useful tool to study movement disorders.

References:

1. Parker VM, Wade DT, Langton Hewer R (1986) Loss of arm function after stroke: measurements, frequency and recovery. *Int Rehabil Med* 8:69-73

2. Scholtz JP (1990) Dynamic pattern theory - some implication for therapeutics. *Phys Ther* 70:827-842

3. Kaminski T, Gentile AM (1986) Joint control strategies and hand trajectories in multijoint pointing movements. *J Motor Behaviour* 18:262-278

4. Georgopoulos AP (1986) On reaching. *Ann Rev Neuroscience* 9: 147-170

5. Wing AM (1990) Recovery of elbow function in voluntary positioning of the hand following hemiplegia due to stroke. *J Neurol Neurosurg and Psychiatry* 53:126-134

THE EFFECT OF RESISTED EXERCISE ON ADULT NEUROMUSCULAR DISEASE

H.E. Lilley
University of Southampton, Hampshire, England
St. Vincent's Hospital, Melbourne, Victoria, Australia

Prescription of exercise for people with neuromuscular disease presents a dilemma for medical and physiotherapy staff. As a general rule, they are advised to be 'moderate' in their exercise whilst observing muscle wasting and progressive weakness.

The efficacy of therapeutic exercise in adult neuromuscular disease is relatively unresearched. There is a particular paucity in the literature on facioscapulohumeral dystrophy (FSHD) and limb girdle syndrome (LGS) (Vignos 1983; McCartney et al 1988; Milner-Brown & Miller 1988).

FSHD is an autosomal-dominant condition. The severity of muscle involvement varies from mild facial weakness to early severe disability involving upper and lower limbs and trunk. The reported incidence varies from 0.38:100,000 to 5.0:100,000. The pathological changes are not always distinctive. LGS describes a heterogeneous group comprising at least five subgroups. The pattern of inheritance is usually autosomal recessive. The pathological findings are indicative of myopathy.

In the medical literature there are clinical descriptions of people with FSHD who become weaker with 'excessive' exercise (Johnson & Braddom 1971). The resulting loss of muscle power appears to be permanent.

A study was undertaken to examine the effect of a six-week exercise programme for the quadriceps muscle.

Methodology

The study comprised five subjects (4 FSHD; 1 LGS). The following graduated, home-based, isotonic, resisted exercise programme was prescribed:

WEEK	EXERCISE
1	2 sets at 40% max.
2	2 sets at 50% max.
3	3 sets at 50% max.
4	1 set at 50% max.; 2 sets at 60% max.
5	1 set at 50% max.; 3 sets at 60% max.
6	1 set at 50% max.; 3 sets at 60% max.
7	1 set at 50% max.; 2 sets at 60% max.; 1 set at 70% max.
8	1 set at 50% max.; 1 set at 60% max.; 2 sets at 70% max.

TABLE 1: Graduated Exercise Programme

A set of exercises involved straightening and bending the knee six times.
The subjects exercised three times per week at the same time of day.
A standardised approach to seating for each subject was taken.

The two assessment tools used were the Musculoskeletal Evaluation,
Rehabilitation and Conditioning (MERAC) system and the maximum weight
lifted. The isotonic and isometric modes of the MERAC at 15°, 45° and
60° of knee extension (0° being full extension) were used.

An initial reliability study on equipment usage was undertaken. The
maximum weight lifted once was tested using either a DeLorme Boot (for
stronger subjects) or a specially-designed weight bag. The test position
for the maximum weight lifted and for exercising was standardised with
the hip maintained in 115° flexion.

The testing schedules were:

1. MERAC   - pre-exercise test weeks 1, 2 and 3
                      - exercise period test weeks 3, 6 and 8

2. Max. weight lifted - pre-exercise test weeks 1 and 2
                      - exercise period test weeks 2, 4, 6 and 8.

The withdrawal criterion was a loss of 20% of measured strength on any
exercise test. The weight to be lifted for exercise was recalculated
every two weeks at the time of the maximum weight lifted test.

An exercise demonstration session was undertaken. The subjects were
issued with standardised procedures, an exercise audiotape and written
instructions. Each subject completed an exercise diary.

<u>Results</u>

The MERAC reliability study was analysed using correlation coefficients.
The MERAC and maximum weight lifted during the study were analysed using
an ANOVA for repeated measures (p 0.05). Scheffe multiple range test
was done post hoc on significant F values from the ANOVA (p 0.05).

All subjects completed the exercise programme. Asymmetry in maximum
weight lifted was seen in the subject with LGS and in two of the
subjects with FSHD. Considerable intersubject variability was a
feature.

No loss of strength was seen on any measurement. There was a significant
increase in maximum weight lifted by the left leg and a trend toward an
increase on the right. No significant differences were seen at any angle
of the isometric testing. A significant difference was seen in range of
movement in the left leg on isotonic testing, but only between the first
and third pre-exercise tests.

Conclusion

It was evident that in the current study population, a closely-monitored, home-based, progressive, resisted, isotonic exercise programme did not lead to overwork weakness in the quadriceps. Indeed, all subjects showed an absolute increase in the maximum weight lifted. High technology muscle testing was not sensitive enough to detect the changes noted in maximum weight lifted. Despite the small number of subjects, which reflects the rarity of these conditions, the study demonstrated there is a potential for training in these people. It also highlights the need for further research in this area.

References

1. Vignos PJ (1983) Physical models of rehabilitation in neuromuscular disease. Muscle and Nerve 6:323-338

2. McCartney N, Moroz D, Garner SH, McComas AJ (1988) The effect of strength training in patients with selected neuromuscular disorders. Medicine and Science in Sport and Exercise 20:4:362-368

3. Milner-Brown HS, Miller RG (1988) Muscle strengthening through high-resistance weight training in patients with neuromuscular disorders. Archives of Physical Medicine and Rehabilitation 69:14-19

4. Johnson EW, Braddom R (1971) Overwork weakness in facioscapulohumeral muscular dystrophy. Archives of Physical Medicine and Rehabilitation 333-336.

EFFICACY OF FEEDBACK TRAINING IN LONG-STANDING FACIAL NERVE PARESIS
ROSS BR, NEDZELSKI JM, McLEAN JA

SUNNYBROOK HEALTH SCIENCE CENTRE
DEPARTMENTS OF PHYSIOTHERAPY AND OTOLARYNGOLOGY
2075 BAYVIEW AVE., TORONTO, ONTARIO, CANADA   M4N 3M5

Incomplete recovery of facial function following facial nerve injury as a result of Bell's palsy or post acoustic neuroma excision is seen in 25-30% of cases. Overall outcome is a result of aberrant reinnervation of the facial nerve and it is often stigmatized by synkinesis, mass movement and varying degrees of motor paresis. This prospective study examines the efficacy of EMG biofeedback versus mirror feedback as treatment strategies for long-standing facial nerve paresis.

None of the commonly applied physical therapy techniques used to treat facial palsy including electrical stimulation, routine exercise, and massage have successfully prevailed over the others and various controversial effects are found in the literature (1,2). Electromyographic (EMG) biofeedback for the re-education of facial muscles has been proposed to enhance facial function following facial paresis (3,4,5,). Existing case reports are retrospective in nature and furthermore they do not meet methodologic criteria for evaluating efficacy of intervention.

METHODS & MATERIALS

Thirty-one patients with a unilateral peripheral facial nerve injury of long standing duration (18 months minimum) consented to participate. The mean duration of facial nerve paresis was 46 months.

Prior to treatment allocation, patients were stratified according to the House Facial Nerve Grading System (6) and by the degree of synkinesis rated on a scale of zero to three (0 - normal; 1 - mild; 2 - moderate; 3 - severe). Twenty-four patients were randomly assigned to one of two training conditions: EMG biofeedback with mirror training (n=11) or mirror training alone (n=13). Seven rural patients who did not undergo treatment served as controls.

Treatment included specific retraining strategies using mirror exercises alone (mirror training group) or mirror exercises in combination with EMG biofeedback (EMG + mirror training group). The Hyperion Bioconditioner was the audiovisual feedback system used for monitoring and displaying two channels of muscle activity. The one year duration treatment protocol entailed thirty 60 minute sessions of structured therapy by a therapist skilled in the treatment of patients with facial nerve paresis. The selection of treatment strategies depended on clinical features of either hypertonus or hypotonus. Inhibition of undesired muscle activity on the involved side (i.e. synkinesis) or hyperactivity of the non-involved side was introduced early in training and reinforced throughout the course of treatment. All treatment subjects were instructed in a detailed individualized home program aided by the use of a mirror and consisting of specific action exercises that emphasized selective muscle control and symmetry of facial function (3,4).

Facial motor function was objectively quantified before, six and twelve months into treatment.

(i) Linear Measurement of Facial Movement.
Maximal facial expressions were quantified by linear measurement of surface anatomic landmarks (7) (Fig. 1). The distance between points at rest and during five standard facial expressions was measured using a hand caliper: Eyes closed tight and Forehead wrinkle (os-or); Nose wrinkle (ac-en); Broad smile (ch-sto) and Pout (sn-sl). The percent displacement (pD) was the change in distance (mm) divided by the resting distance (mm), then multiplied by 100. Intra-rater reliability of linear measurement of facial movement was previously evaluated with intraclass correlation co-efficients (ICC) in the range of 0.75 to 0.98.

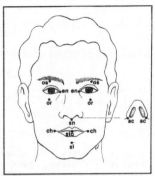

Figure 1

(ii) Visual assessment of voluntary movement.
Each subject was videotaped at rest and during eight standard facial expressions (forehead elevation, eye closure, even smile with mouth closed, broad smile with mouth open, bilateral snarl, unilateral smirk, pucker, lower lip out and down) using standardized photography. These tapes were randomized with respect to time and group before being sent to an independent experienced appraiser. A composite score was assigned to each facial expression using a voluntary score - 10 X (grade of synkinesis). Intra-rater reliability of voluntary movement scores was also evaluated with eight out of nine ICC reliability values being greater than 0.80.

RESULTS
Our results demonstrate the significant beneficial effect of feedback training with either mirror feedback alone or with the addition of EMG feedback. There was a clear noticeable increase in excursion of facial movement as demonstrated by the upwards slope in Fig. 2. The mean pD of groups over time zero to 12 months was statistically significant (p <.05). Similar improvements were demonstrated with respect to the visual assessment voluntary scores (p <.05). In contrast, patients in the 'no treatment' group demonstrated facial function measurements which indicated either deterioration or maintenance of the status quo (Fig. 2). There was no significant difference between EMG and mirror training alone. Patients exhibited less synkinesis with improved control of isolated voluntary facial movements (Fig. 3). Improvements were seen in resting symmetry, and in symmetry and excursion of expressions. (Fig. 4).

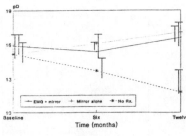

Figure 2

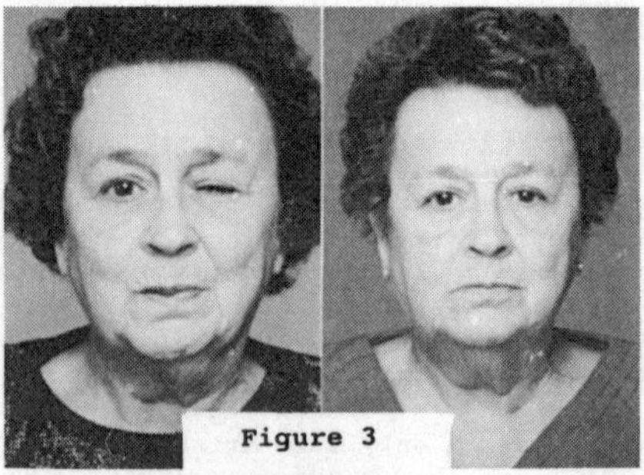

Figure 3

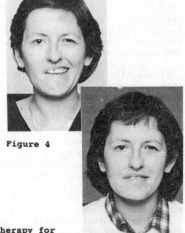

Fig. 3, 62 year old woman 2-1/2 years post Bell's palsy. Note reduced synkinesia with lip compression before and after mirror training.

Fig. 4, 30 year old woman 10 years post acoustic neuroma excision. Note improvement in symmetry for smile before and after mirror training.

Figure 4

CONCLUSION:

The positive results of this controlled study demonstrate that feedback training in combination with a structured home rehabilitation program is a clinically efficacious treatment for patients with facial nerve paresis.

REFERENCES

1. Mosforth J, Taverner D, (1958) Physiotherapy for Bell's Palsy. Brit Med J: 675-577.
2. Waxman B, (1984) Electrotherapy for treatment of facial paralysis (Bell's Palsy). Health Technology Assessment Reports, National Centre for Health Services Research 3: 27.
3. Balliet R, Shinn JB, Bach-y-Rita P, (1982) Facial paralysis rehabilitation: Re-training selective muscle control. Int Rehab Med 4:67-74.
4. Balliet R, (1987) Facial Paralysis. Manual of Physical Therapy Techniques, Payton (ed), Churchill Livingston Pub., N.Y., 41-76.
5. Brown DM, Nahai F, Wolf S, Basmajian JV, (1978) Electromyo-graphic biofeedback in the re-education of facial palsy. Am J Phys Med 4: 67-74.
6. House JW, (1983) Facial nerve grading systems. Laryngoscope 93: 1056-1069.
7. Burres SA, (1985) Facial Biomechanics: The standards of normal. Laryngoscope 95: 708-714.

TREATMENT IN SEVERE ADULT CEREBRAL PALSY WITH JAW DISLOCATION

M.Kazuki, K.Fukui, M.Satou
Department of Physical Therapy, Osaka Red Hospital for Pediatric
Orthopaedics(Otemaeseishigakuen), Osaka, Japan

Introduction:
   We report the case of severe adult cerebral palsy with jaw joint
dislocation. In a dental treatment, the left jaw joint of the patient
was dislocated by using a mouth gag. Soon after then, he suffered from
severe pain of the both jaw joints. The pain increased rigospasticity
of muscles in trunk and extremities. He was able to take neither a
resting supine nor a resting prone position, except a deleterious
opisthotonic posture. The pain and this posture prevented him from
eating, and he lost his weight from 35kg to 25kg for 70 days. Doctors
prescribed him a collar, jaw holder and muscle relaxants. But his pain
didn't subside. Finally he came to our hospital.

Case report:
   K. D.   male
(Perinatal condition)
   Birth weight was 3450g. Mature birth.
   He was taken into a couveuse because of febrile convulsion and
nuclear jaundice on seventh day after birth. It was not clear whether
he had exchange transfusion and photo therapy for nuclear jaundice.
(Present illness)
   At the age of 20 and a month the patient treated his teeth with a
mouth gag and then his left jaw joint was dislocated. He consulted
several hospitals, but his pain was not cured. At the age of 20 and
3 months he came to our hospital.
(Diagnosis)
   Cerebral palsy. Hypertonic athetosis. Left jaw joint dislocation
(Chief complaint)
   Severe pain of jaw joints

Treatment:
   He was treated by Vojta method four times per day for three months.

Hope of the patient and his family at the beginning of this treatment:
 I)Relieving his pain which was caused by left jaw joint dislocation.
 2)Decreasing rigospasticity of muscles in trunk and extremities.
 3)Improving his limited activity of daily living(ADL) which was caused
   by the pain and rigospasticity muscles.
   (About his ADL of before pain)
     He was not able to transfer himself to wheelchair, he could
   ambulate by himself. He was able to roll over and eat with his left
   hand without any help.
 4)His helper wanted to make it easier to take care of him.

Treatment process:
(At the beginning of the treatment) Fig.(I)(2)(3)
    The pain caused him to increase rigospasticity of muscles. He could
not take rest in neither the supine nor prone position. He could turn
his head only to the left. His cervical spine had a hyper lordotic
posture. His spine had rightside-curved scoliosis. The deformity of
ribs with sternum depression was presented. He held his jaw with his
left hand in order not to be dislocated. We asked the patient and his
mother to count how many times per day his jaw joint was dislocated.
But the dislocation happened too frequently to be counted. At the
biginning of treatment, Reflex turning was the only possibility.
After 3 weeks he took the sterting position of reflex creeping.
(One month after treatment)
    His jaw joint was almost stabilized one month after the beginning of
the treatment. He didn't have pain all day long. He was able to turn
his head to both sides. He didn't hold his jaw joint with his left
hand because of the disappearance of pain. He could use his left hand
freely again and sit on a wheelchair by himself. Though the pain was
relieved, he put a towel in his mouth in order to get the mental
stability.
(Two months after treatment)
    He didn't need a towel in his mouth. He was able to turn his head
from the left to right on his midline in supine position and supported
his body with his forearms steadily in prone and ambulate a wheelchair
by himself.
(Three months after treatment) Fig.(4)(5)(6)
    This thrapy improved his ribs deformity with sternum depression and
decreased hyper lordosis of cervical spine. He could support his body
firmly with his elbows in prone, but it was not perfect. He gained his
weight from 25kg to 30kg. The patient and his mother reported the
improvement of his autonomic nervous system as follows. He could
breathe easily. He had constipation for many years, but during the
treatment he had one defecation per day.

Results:
    The pain was relieved through the decrease of rigospasticity and the
improvement of posture. He could not only take a resting supine and
prone position but also ambulate by himself with wheelchair in sitting
position. He was able to eat by himself and gained his weight.

Discussion:
    The reflex locomotion of Vojta method consists of reflex creeping
and reflex turning. We treated a patient of severe adult cerebral palsy
y this fascillitation technicue. It is often said that Vojta method is
nly a baby treatment but this case gives us the following suggestion.
I)Vojta method can be applied to an adult cerebral palsy to decrease
   the rigospasticity of muscles and improve the asymmetrical deformed
   posture.
2)Patient can't take the position of sitting, on all fours and
   standing in treatment, we can treat him if he can have one of supine
   prone or side lying that basic postures in moter development.

3)In adult cerebral palsy, Vojta method is effective not only for the improvement of rigospasticity and posture but also autonomic nervous system.

Conclusion:
We described an adult cerebral palsy with severe deformity and jaw joint dislocation who was treated by Vojta method. This therapy relieved him from pain and improved his deformed posture.

Beginning of treatment   Three months after treatment

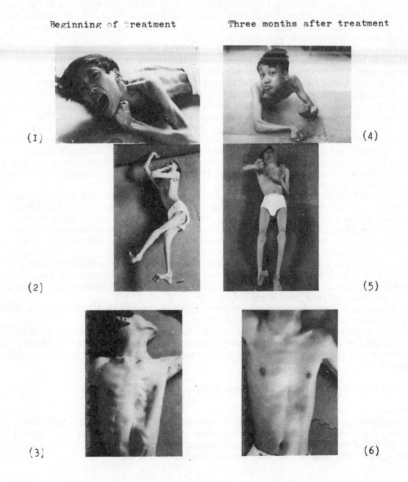

(1)

(4)

(2)

(5)

(3)

(6)

SELFTRAINING AD MODUM VOJTA, ADULT CEREBRAL PALSY - TWO CASESTUDIES.

B. Bäckström, K. Swanberg, H. Berglund, A-K Eriksson.
Kolbäckens habilitering S-90243 Umeå. Habiliteringscentralen Gammeläng S-961 37 Boden
Sweden.

The Vojta concept of treatment is based on provoking two inborn locomotor programmes, automatic creeping and turning. Locomotion always consist of the following distinct but inseparable elements: automatic control of the body position as a whole (postural control) ,the uprighting mechanisms necessary for the locomotion in question and the visible (phasic) movements of the particular type of locomotion (1).

The automatic movement patterns which in exact positions are provoked in treatment are global, the whole body including breathing, eye and mouth movements are included in coordinated muscle work. The locomotor programmes contain all necessary information to start different musclegroups in correct timing (2). The kinesiological content of reflex creeping and turning are well analysed and defined and contain, according to Vojta, building blocks on which the volitional movement of man is based (3). The inborn locomotion can be provoked in all humans, newborns as well as grownups, by means of proprioceptive stimulation. The stimulation is given on points of the body called triggerzones. Pressure is directed towards those points which alreadey in a newborn function as contact and support points to the surface. The automatic movement answers that appear during the treatment session will be more complete the longer the stimulation is given (timesummation) and the more triggerzones that are used in combination (spacesummation) (4,5). Thus inborn automatic locomotor programmes of man are used for treatment.

The idea of Vojta treatment is to strengthen the impact of the correct patterns, building blocks of developmental movement, by way of nonmotivated (automatic) movement answers. Wilful motivated movements are not wanted during treatment sessions since such movements in a person with a central nervous damage turn out on the terms of the lesion, pathologically. The influence on the pathological movement patterns will depend upon the extent of the lesion as well as the intensity and duration of treatment (6).

The treatment is used preventively for babies with a central coordination disturbance which might lead to cerebral palsy (7,8,9), for children with cerebral palsy in order to lessen pathology and promote function (10), as well as for children with congenital clubfoot (11), hip dislocation (12), torticollis (13) and spina bifida (14).

The locomotion is possible to provoke in grownup persons too in well defined positions. Wilful eyemovement may enhance the movement answer.

The aim of the following casestudies was to see if the creeping and turning as described by Vojta could be used as selftraining for adults with cerebral palsy. Would a training period aiming to affect developmental building blocks of movement improve motor function for daily living?

Case 1. Woman aged 21 years with spastic diplegia

Method:
Selftraining one hour twice daily leading to one session daily of approximately 11/2 hours during fifteen months. Positions used changed during the course of the study under supervision of the instructing physical theraput. Regular contact between trainee and PT was kept all through the study ranging from three times a week to once a month.

Evaluation was done by : 1) active and passive range of movement measurments of lower extremity joints. 2) videotape recordings of walking, climbing and descending stairs. 3) a videotaped statement by the trainee after completion of the training period.

Result:
1. active range of movement was increased in degrees as follows : hip abduction (10 bilaterally), hip extension (10 left, 12 right) and dorsal flektion of feet (15 left, 20 right)
2. walking pattern changed in flow and agility as seen on videotape.
3. The trainee stated several examples of improved motor function such as the ability to get in and out of a bathtub and in dancing. She experienced improved body appearance, agility, strength and endurance.

Case 2. Woman aged 28 years with spastic diplegia.

Method:
Selftraining 2x30 minutes daily for five months in prone and sidepositions. Contact with the instructing PT was to occur at the request of the trainee.
Evaluation was done by: 1) assessment of spacticity, passsive range of movement and muscle function to be administred by an unbiassed PT five times before, every six weeks during, and five times after conclusion of the study. 2) a weekly diary kept by the trainee.

Result:
1. The assessment showed lessened extensor spasticity of knees and hip and increased muscle strength in hip and kneeflektion and feet.
2. The diary expressed improvement regarding breathing posture, walking, climbing stairs and body appearance. The trainee stated contentment over the possibility to train "strength without increasing spacticity" and being able to do it at home "without correcting and evaluating PT hands".

Conclusion: It was possible to do selftraining based on the therapeutic concept of Vojta (regular provoking of inborn automatic locomotor patterns of creeping and turning in well defined positions) in two women with spastic diplegia.
The training aiming at affecting building blocks of developmental movement improved motor function for daily living in both cases registred objectively and subjectively .

References:
1. Vojta V (1984) The basic elements of treatment according to Vojta. Management of the motor disorders of children with cerebral palsy, Clinics in developmental medicine nr 90, Scrutton D (ed)
2. Brooks VB (1986) The neural basis of motor control. Oxford university press.
3. Vojta V (1988) Die cerebralen Bewegungsstörungen im Säuglingsalter, Früdiagnose und Frütherapie. Ferdinand Enke verlag, Stuttgart, 5th ed.
4. von Aufschneiter D (1989) Die Reflexlokomotion. Eine neuro-kinesiologische Behandlungsform nach Vaclav Vojta. Krankengymnasatische behandlung der infantile Zerebralparese. Feldkamp (ed) Pflaum verlag, München.
5. Wassermeyer D, Vojta V (1989) Aufgaben des Therapeuten bei der Krankengymnastik des symtomatischen Risikokindes nach Vojta. Krankengymnastik 41, 11:1120-1130.
6. Vojta V (1987) Zur Prognose der spät behandelten cerebralparetischen Kinder. Der Kinderarzt 18,9:1161-1166.
7. d´Avignon M, Noren L, Årman T (1981) Early physiotherapy ad modum Vojta or

Bobath in infants with suspected neuromotor disturbance. Neuropediatrics 12, 3: 232-241.

8. Brandt S, Lonstrup H, Marner T, Rump KJ, Selman P, Schack LK, d´Avignon M, Noren L, Árman T,(1980) Prevention of cerebral palsy in motor risk infants by treatment ad modum Vojta. Acta Pediatrica Scand 69:283-286.

9. Imamura ,Sakuma, Takahashi (1983) Followup study of children with cerebral coordination disturbance. Brain and development 5:311-314.

10. Kanda T, Ynge M, Yamori Y, Suzuki J, Sukase H (1984) Early physiotherapy in the treatment of spastic diplegia. Developmental medicine and child neurology 26:483-444.

11. Santori FS, Manili M, Havel J, Santori E, Martini G (1988) Possibilita di impiego della metodica Vojta nel trattamento del piede torto congenito. Europa Medicophysica 24, 2:103-110.

12. Niethard FU (1987) Die Vorbehandlung der kongenitalen Hüftgelenksluxation mit krankengymnastischer Therapie auf neurophysiologischer Basis. Z Orthop. 125 ,1: 28-34.

13. Vojta V, von Aufschneiter D , Wassermeyer D (1983) Der Geburtstraumatische Torticollis myogenes und seine krankengymnastische Behandlung nach Vojta. Krankengymnastik 4:191-197.

14. von Aufschneiter D (1981) Die krankengymnastische Behandlung des Spina bifida Kindes. Sozialpädiatrie in Praxis und Klinik 9:395-404.

Analysis of Component Times in the Stereotyped Movements of Upper Extremity in Patients with Parkinsonism

Iwatsuki,H., Muroga,T.(MD)
Dept.Phys.Ther. & Occup. Ther., Nagoya·Univ. Coll. of Tech.
1-1-20 Daikominami Higashiku Nagoya 461, Nagoya

The aim of this study is to evaluate clinical symptoms such as delay in motor initiation and clumsiness in movement of Parkinsonism (P) patients for certain tasks imposed on the upper extremity based on an analysis of reaction time, the time profile composing the reaction time, and the discharge pattern of active muscles. Further, we compared results on P patients with those from patients suffering cerebellar disorders that are known to slow similar symptoms, and investigated the functional difference between basal ganglia and cerebellum, or the two central control mechanisms underlying the voluntary movement.

Methods

Sixteen patients, ten males and six females, diagnosed as Parkisonism ranging in age from 47 to 77 years (mean 65.7), twelve patients, seven males and five females, diagnosed as Spinocerebellar degenerations (SCD) (mean 61.5) and fourteen control subjects, eight males and six females (mean 68.4). Patients with P and SCD could walk independently, although they had some difficulty in activities of daily living (ADL). All subjects were right-handed.

The subject was ordered to move the index finger as soon and correct as possible from the horizontal contact plate to the upper contact plate at 15 degrees, next to the other upper adductive contact plate and then return the horizontal plate by regular (0.2Hz) and random (less than 0.2Hz) signals of electrical stimulation (ES) to the opposite forearm. EMG activity of the deltoid was bipolarly recorded through surface electrodes attached 2-3 cm apart on the muscle belly at the same time. The motor components times were named as Fig.1.

Statistical methods; Values are presented as means ± SDs. Data were analyzed using the Student t-test, correlation coefficients and three-way analysis of variance (ANOVA). Differences were considered significant at $p < 0.05$.

Results

1. EMG activities and latent time

The latent time from the onset of ES to the appearance of grouping discharges was slightly longer in the P patients than in the control group, but it was significantly longer in the SCD patients than in the

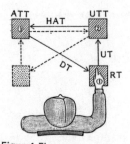

Figure1 Finger movements

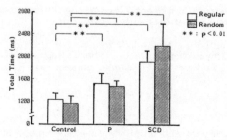

Figure2 Total time

control (p < 0.05).

2. Motor component times

Fig.2 shows the total time is longer in SCD patients than in P patients, but for both of these groups, it is significantly longer than in the control (p < 0.01), regardless of the stimulus condition. For both stimulus conditions, the total time in SCD patients was significantly longer than in P patients (p < 0.01). For normal subjects and P patients, the total time appeared to be reduced when irregular stimuli were given as opposed to regular stimuli. By contrast in SCD patients, the total time to irregular stimulation was more prolonged than for regular stimulation.

Table 1 represents the means and SDs of the times for a finger to reach the target (UT+HAT+ATT), from which it is apparent that for the control and P patients these values are lower when irregulaly stimulated than when regularly exicited, while for SCD patients the times for a finger to reach the target values tend to be higher when irregularly stimulated.

For the control, RT was about 273.6ms when regularly stimulated, and about 278.4ms when irregularly stimulated. For P, RT was about 290ms regardless of the stimulus condition. For SCD, RT was significantly greater than the corresponding values in the control (p < 0.01).

UT became greater in SCD than in P regardless stimulus condition, and the difference was significant (p < 0.05). The correlation between RT and UT was negative for the control under both stimulus conditions, but a positive correlation was observed under irregular stimulation in P and under two types of stimulation in SCD (Table 2).

Table1 Mean and SD of times for a finger to reach the target

	Regular	Random
Control	752.0±98.3	714.9±93.3
P	1006.9±103.7	926.5±104.8
SCD	1229.0±218.7	1330.7±286.2

** : p < 0.01

Table2 Correlation between reaction time (RT) and upward time (UT)

	Regular	Random
Control	-0.13	-0.19
P	-0.04	0.18
SCD	0.24	0.37

Discussion

The simple reaction time is delayed owing to changes in the brain substance, and the delay varies according to the side of the brain in which such abnormal changes are located, that is, whether they are in the left hemisphere or right hemiphere[1,2].

For P as well as the control, RT remained the same regardless of ES frequency, suggesting that in P there is no abnormality in ballistic movement initiated by the external stimulus. Goldberg[3] suggested that the roles of the individual parts of the central nervous system involved in voluntary movement vary according to the situation, and set forth a hypothesis that in voluntary movement, the basal ganglia-supplementary motor area link (of the medial system) plays a dominant role, while in movement initiated by external stimuli, the cerebellum-arcuate premotor area link (of the lateral system) becomes dominant.

According to this concept, P or a disease with disorders in the lateral systems more apt to create disturbances in movements triggered by external stimuli than in voluntary movements.

This is in according with the present results. By contrast, UT was significantly greater in P than in the control. This may be accounted for the existence of rigidity, tremor and disordered synchrony of the active muscles in P. The movement arrest characteristic to P impairs the rapid build-up of muscle contraction to effect movement, and this may be responsible for indistinctness of initial grouping discharge in P.

It was suggested that P patients meet the external task with self-paced and patterned motor performance.

References

1)Howes D, Boller F (1975) Evidence for forcal impairment from lesions of the right hemisphere. Brain 98:317-332

2)Yokochi F, Nakamura R, Nakabayashi H (1985) Reaction time of patients with Parkinson's disease, with reference to asymmetry of neurological signs. J Neur Neuros Psych 48:702-705

3)Goldberg, G (1985) Supplementary motor area structure and function review and hypotheses. Behav Brain Sci 8:567-615

4)Nakamura R, Mojica JAP, Yamada Y, Yokochi F (1989) Loss of reaction time specificity for movement direction in Parkinson's disease. Tohoku J exp Med 158: 9-16

5)Iwatsuki H, Muroga T, Kiyama T, Ida K et al.(1989) Analysis of component time in the stereotyped movements of upper extremities in patients with Parkinsonism. Rigaku ryohogaku 16:297-302

6)Evarts EV, Teravainen H, Calne DB (1981) Reaction time in Parkinson's disease. Brain 104: 167-186

PREVENTION OF SOLE WOUNDS IN INSENSITIVE FEET IN LEPROSY PATIENTS
UNDER THEIR NORMAL LIFE CONDITIONS

M. E. Mahato   M. N. Casablanca   P. Acharya
Leprosy Mission Hospital, Purulia, W.B., India

INTRODUCTION

Approximately 20% of present and former leprosy patients have posterior
tibial nerve damage at the level of the medial malleolus resulting in
sole sensory loss and intrinsic paralysis. Sole wounds, soft tissue damage
and bone loss often follow. These are among the major problems to be
contended with in leprosy work, because they lead to psycho-social
phenomena of stigma and job loss, and also to increased hospitalisation
and costs. The majority of leprosy patients have very low incomes. They
cannot afford to stop working or walking in order to heal sole wounds.
They are also unable to afford expensive special footwear to protect
their feet. Hence it became necessary to identify a way of reducing sole
wounds under local life conditions and using limited resources. With this
objective, a three year study project was initiated by ILEP/ with participants from different organisations and countries including The Leprosy
Mission Hospital, Purulia, India.

PATIENTS

In Purulia, initially a pilot group of 50 out-patients having tibial nerve
dysfunction with loss of protective sensation were chosen, 25 having sole
wounds, and 25 without sole wounds. During the 3 year study, 5 dropped out
for various reasons. The findings of the remaining 45 are considered in
this paper. They represent a cross section as regards age, sex, environment, leprosy and chemotherapy. There were 30 males and 15 females. Ages
ranged from 15 yrs to 68 yrs, the majority being in the 30-50 years age
group. Occupations include farmers, manual labourers, shop keepers,
musicians, students, housewives and unemployed. At the beginning of the
study 21 were on chemotherapy, but by the end of the 1st year, 33 had
finished treatment, 38 by the end of the 2nd year, and 42 by the end of
the 3rd year. The patients were out-patients taken from the Urban
Leprosy Control area of Purulia. Purulila is the district H.Q. town,
situated in the S.W. of West Bengal State (N.E.India) approximately
320 kms from Calcutta. It is predominantly an agricultural area. The
climate is sub-tropical, dry and drought prone in the summer months and
humid in the monsoon season. Temperatures range from 10°C to 45°C. The
area of Purulia town is 5.38 sq.km with a population of 100,000 and a
2-3 : 1,000 leprosy prevalence rate. The general socio-economic condition
is poor.

PROCEDURE

METHODS used to reduce sole wounds were as follows:-

1. Education and supervised practice of self-home care, including daily
   self examination of feet for signs of injury or pressure, daily water
   soaks, scraping and oiling (to prevent cracks and callous forming on

skin with no sweating) and early wound self care.

2. Raising of awareness of cause of wounds, and methods of injury
    avoidance and walking control in relation to their occupation and
    life style.

3. Provision of special minimum cost footwear, made using a micro-
    cellular rubber insole, a rubber tyre sole and leather straps,
    given to those who would wear them. Simple modifications to
    relieve pressure from scars and bony points were included when
    necessary.

At the beginning, all this was attempted in the clinics, but this proved
impossible in this situation because the patients were unwilling to be
observed in such open places among the general public. This also delayed
the whole team going on to the next clinic place. For these practical
reasons, the strategy was changed and the patients were called to the base
hospital. Some came but many did not, as they could not afford to lose a
day's wage. Finally the most suitable way found was to visit the patients
in their homes in the early morning before they left for work. This was
more advantageous as the education and practice could be done in the
privacy of the home; it could be adapted to the home situation; family members
could also be involved and it improved patient-therapist relationship.

PROGRESS of the study was monitored on a standard format giving details of
personal data; motor and sensory condition of the feet, tissue loss; history
and details of present sole wounds; type of footwear used; self care and
walking control attempted or planned. Details were recorded on the format
at the beginning of the study and thereafter at the end of each year for
3 years. At the beginning of the study many patients were on chemotherapy
and it was possible to see them monthly at the treatment clinics. However,
when the chemotherapy was completed the patients stopped coming to the
clinics and thereafter were seen approximately every 3 months in their homes.

TABLE I

Comparing the factors considered and their effect on the number of sole
wounds* and hospital usage in the two groups.

A   Those with sole wounds initially (21 patients),

and

B   Those without sole wounds initially (24 patients)

*   The term "Sole Wound" includes ulcers, open fissures and/or injuries.

TABLE I

No of Patients	Group	Baseline	1st Yr	2nd Yr	3rd Yr
Sole wound free through- out the year	A B	Nil 24	3 16	8 17	10 19
Wearing Special Footwear	A B	6 3	7 1	9 3	7 3
Wearing Other Footwear	A B	– –	14 22	12 21	14 16
Wearing No Footwear	A B	– –	Nil 1	Nil Nil	Nil 5
Doing self care regularly	A B	– –	12 13	12 16	16 18
Attempting walking control	A B	– –	4 6	5 7	4 6
No of days patients admitted to hospital for sole wounds	A B	– –	647 76	227 17	187 Nil

DISCUSSION

From the findings in Table I it can be observed that the number of patients remaining sole wound free increased (i.e. number of wounds decreased) through out the 3 years. The findings show clearly that those who had no initial sole wound sustained less wounds than those who had wounds initially. It was also noted that many patients treated their sole wounds at home in the early stages and they were quickly healed.

The number of patients wearing special footwear remained static and low. The special type of footwear is unacceptable to most patients for reasons discussed later. It was not given free or forced on the patients, because most of them would not have worn it. As this was a pilot group to minimise sole wounds under local conditions, it was given only to those who would genuinely utilise it.

The number of patients doing self-care regularly, increased over the 3 years. However, some patients for various reasons, could not or would not co-operate despite our efforts in this area. The number of patients attempting walking control remained low throughout the project.

The number of days that patients were admitted into hospital for sole wounds very noticeably decreased throughout the 3 years. In the 3rd year, one patient of the sole wound group insisted on a below-the-knee amputation for social reasons, although his foot condition did not warrant it. This increased the number of hospital days from 87 to 187.

PROBLEMS FACED

There is a good footwear department in Purulia and production and supply to patients proves no difficulty. However, this special footwear is unacceptable to the majority of patients for the following reasons :

a.   although at minimum cost it is still too expensive for many. It could have been given free of cost to the study group, but it is not possible to give free to all patients.

b.   it is recognisable as leprosy footwear and therefore carries stigma.

c.   it is not durable for some occupations (i.e. farming in wet paddy fields) and in the monsoon season.

It is difficult to get patients to come regularly to the clinics after they finish chemotherapy.

Visiting individual homes is very time consuming and expensive in terms of staff/work hours. Although done for this pilot group it would require changes in the present system and staff quota to do it for all who require it.

CONCLUSIONS

The study shows that :

1.   Sole wounds can be substantially reduced under local life conditions by teaching self care through supervised practice.

2.   This in turn reduces hospital usage and costs.

COMMENTS

1.   There is no doubt that the personal interest shown in the patients and the knowledge that they would be checked at any time increased compliance.

2.   As increasing numbers of leprosy patients are being cured and stopping chemotherapy, a new strategy must be devised to regularly monitor those with residual sensory deficiency and other deformities, encouraging and helping them to prevent further deformity.

3.   Even without protective footwear results show that sole wounds in insensitive feet can be reduced. The use of special footwear would reduce them even further. More research and effort must be given to provide acceptable durable, protective footwear at minimum cost.

4.   This is a joint study project of ILEP (International Federation of Anti-Leprosy Associations).

I gratefully acknowledge the help and co-operation of my colleagues at The Leprosy Mission Hospital, Purulia, also the advice and encouragement of Miss Jean Watson, Consultant Physiotherapist for The Leprosy Mission International and Mrs S Mondal for secretarial help.

CLINICAL ADVANCES IN THE USE OF THERAPEUTIC PRESSURE SPLINTS IN
NEUROLOGICALLY IMPAIRED ADULTS AND CHILDREN.

A.W.Thorp.

Work done at various locations.
Based at Deepsykehead,West Linton,Peeblesshire,EH46 7AY,Scotland.

During eight years of clinical work in a unit catering for the needs
of neurologically impaired adult patients with severe disability the
conditions found could be divided into two groups.
Group 1: Degenerating conditions with a slow onset over days,weeks
or months,in need of careful assessment and competent management to
maintain optimum ability for each patient.
Group 2: Conditions most serious at onset which was sudden, if the
medical condition of the patient could be stabilised then there was
a prospect of rehabilitation.
Stroke patients in the unit were being treated following the Concept
of Johnstone(1).Neurological impairment in other conditions sometimes presented with problems of tonal imbalance and sensory loss
similar to those found after stroke,so it seemed a reasonable assumption that use of the pressure splints would benefit patients with
other conditions.
Success with the arm splint when used to prevent or reverse flexion
contractures in the upper limb led to the development of two specific
types of leg splint which would allow a similar approach to the problem of flexor spasticity in the lower limbs.Both are single chamber
splints designed to inhibit increased flexor tone,one to support the
patient in standing,the other to be applied to the supine patient.
The splints are made of a specially developed clear pvc sheeting
forming a double sleeve which fits a limb and is then orally inflated.
Warm moist air from the lungs ensures that the inner layer moulds and
conforms exactly to the patient's limb giving pneumatic support with
all over even pressure.Lung pressure will not cause tissue damage to
the patient.A firm inflation pressure is seen to register at 40mm Hg
when tested with a manometer,pressures higher than this should not be
used.Always use a pressure that is comfortable for the patient and
always apply over a cotton sleeve or stocking to avoid sweat rash.
Splints are flexible but strong enough to support limbs placed in
desired inhibiting patterns. Comfortable because of the total skin
contact.With pneumatic pressure they give the stability of sustained
posture to a limb while at the same time they allow for muscle activity and controlled tonal flow within the splint.Where there is an
imbalance of muscle tone the splint may be used to help stabilise the
weight bearing limb in an inhibiting pattern,the therapist's hands
are now free to add weight to the limb or place a demand by increasing resistance.The tonal overflow arising from effort will be directed,by the correctly maintained pattern of inhibition,into the weak
synergy.When the inhibiting pattern has been firmly established then
further training can take place with a variety of planned activities,
for example in the Occupational therapy department or at home,thus

allowing for the constant repetition that is required for motor relearning.
Therapeutic splints may also be used passively to rest limbs in inhibiting patterns, best results are only obtained if the whole body be
correctly positioned. The prolonged stretch on muscles and tissues
during a resting period will maintain their length and pliability and
reduce spasticity.

RESTING SUPINE   WEIGHT BEARING

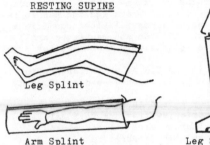
Leg Splint

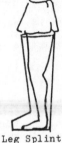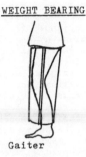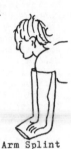

Arm Splint   Leg Splint   Gaiter   Arm Splint

Where appropriate,passive,assisted,or active range of movements may
be performed before removal of splints.
Splints applied to the ataxic patient have been found to give a welcome respite to patients agitated by the uncontrolled movement of
their limbs.
Loss of motor power becomes more disabling if associated with a loss
of tactile sensation, especially in the hand. The sensory input from
daily exercise sessions with the splints has been found to greatly
improve this lost sensation.
Intermittent pressure through the splints has brought good results
where proprioception is defective.
The splints already described are single chamber and used to combat
the problems of excesive flexor tone.If the problem is one of excesive extensor tone in the lower limbs and trunk,a different splint,the
leg gaiter should be used.
This splint has two chambers,each inflated separately.When correctly
applied it will support the standing patient in the pattern required
to inhibit excessive extensor tone.
Therapists need to recognise the different functions of these splints
and their methods of application in order to make the right choice
for each patient's therapy.
The therapist is constantly striving to achieve for the patient a
balance between inhibition and facilitation, normal movement depends
upon it.
Tonal flow is governed by posture and triggered by the weight bearing
responce.The position of the weight bearing base and the distribution
of weight through it determines the reflex activity required for altering tonal distribution through appropriate stabilising and moving
synergies. This is a constantly up-dating process responding to the
amount of movement of the centre of gravity in relation to the weight
bearing base.
Normal movement also depends upon normal sensation, so a disturbance

or defecit in the function of the modalities of sensation may result in faulty motor responses.

Treatment aims may vary from the achievement of normal movement to maintaining some sort of sitting balance.But, whatever the objective it must be realistic and will only be achieved if sound neurological principles are applied. These same principles must also apply to the manner in which the splints are used in treatment.

My involvement in a world wide teaching programme on the Johnstone Concept of stroke rehabilitation began eight years ago and has in recent years expanded to include MS and other neurological conditions. Some therapists attending worked with children and requested small splints for their patients.Prototype splints were then made for trial paediatric therapy.

Part of the original work was done in the U.S.A. on children with various conditions including cerebral palsy,closed head injury and brachial plexus injury(2).

Good initial results led to a further spread in the use of these splints in the U.K.,the Nordic Countries,Switzerland,Portugal and New Zealand.Children receiving the therapy were all neurologically impaired,the largest group were those with Cerebral palsy.

Splints for children are now being used in the following ways:
- to train standing balance in preparation for walking following derotational ostotomy of femur.
- to inhibit spasticity and maintain length and pliability of tissues.
- to facilitate passive/active movements.
- to give a sensory input and increase body awareness.
- to stabilise limbs for weight bearing using a correctly positioned base to influence tone, thus enabling the establishment of the central stability, balance and control that has to be achieved before normal movement can begin.

A programme of progression through neuro-developmental patterns has to be managed for the child where the disabilities are so great that instinctive progression has been lost.

Reports and observation during treatment sessions indicate that children welcome the splints in therapy. Carers and family members may be taught splint techniques so that treatment can continue during weekends and holidays.

Conclusion: when used competently,within the bounds of correctly applied neurology, therapeutic pressure splints offer a new dimension to therapists working with neurologically impaired patients,enabling the theories of management to become a practical reality.

References.
1 - Johnstone M (1991) Therapy for Stroke - Building on Experience. Churchill Livingstone, Medical Division,Longmann Group UK Ltd.
2 - Montgomery P (1989) Use of Air Splints in Brachial Plexus Injuries. APTA Pediatric Physical Therapy,Vol.1 No.2:85-86.

Footnote: The Urias Therapeutic Pressure Splints are manufactured by Svend Andersen Plastic Industri A/S, DK-4652, Haarlev, Denmark. A User's Guide is available with the splints.

EVALUATION OF REHABILITATION TREATMENT FOR PATIENTS WITH VESTIBULAR
DISORDERS.

M. Lessing-Turner, D. Ireland, T. Szturm[1]
[1]School of Medical Rehabilitation, University of Manitoba, Winnipeg,
Manitoba, Canada R3E OW3

INTRODUCTION
Disruption of the vestibular system is manifested in a number of disturbing signs and symptoms which may include all or a combination of the
following: postural imbalance, spontaneous nystagmus, blurred vision;
complaints of dizziness, nausea and disorientation. Recovery from vestibular
disorders involves both sensory substitution and adaptive CNS processes
(for review see 1-4). Goal directed activities under a variety of sensory
conditions must be encouraged even though it may initially aggravate
accompanying symptoms of motion stickness and vertigo. Rehabilitation has
been proposed for treatment of patients with certain vestibular deficits,
however, this treatment approach has only received sparse experimental
support[5-7]. The goal of this clinical trials study is to establish an
effective rehabilitation treatment program for patients with vestibular
disorders having a variety of clinical manifestations. The evaluation of
the rehabilitation program against traditional treatment is necessary to
lend support for such a program.

DESIGN
Patients diagnosed with peripheral vestibular loss or dysfunction as
assessed by history, measures of balance performance, caloric and head-shake
nystagmus tests, and no other observable neurological disorder were recruited.
Eighteen volunteers were randomly assigned to either:
(A) Home exercise group (n - 9, 4 females and 5 males): All subjects in
this group were instructed[8,9] to perform a modified version of the Cooksey-
Cawthorne head exercises[8,9,5] on a daily basis at home. These individuals
were given an education session, shown how to perform the exercises, and
contacted, by telephone, on a regular basis.
(B) Rehab Group (n = 9, 4 females and 5 males): These subjects received
predetermined rehabilitative therapy 3 times per week for 12 weeks. In
keeping with the present state of knowledge[1-9] the aim of treatment was to
mobilize sensory systems (including unaffected vestibular receptor
structures) involved in oculomotor and postural control. Training involved
standing activities, where appropriate, under a combination of the following
sensory conditions: varying support surface conditions such as compliant
or spongy surfaces of different qualities and degrees, and the use of a
narrow balance beam; various visual conditions such as eye closed, visual
stabilization, eye-head movements to stationary and moving visual targets,
optokinetic stimuli using an optokinetic drum, and dim light situations.
Biofeedback (auditory and visual) was provided using miniature force
sensing transducers (interlink Electronics, Santa Barbara CA., USA). A
Transducer was positioned under the balls and heels of the feet. The
conditioned transducer signals provided subjects with information regarding
position of the centre of foot pressure and relative amount of A-P body

sway during the different sensory conditions. For their home program they
were instructed to perform a modified version of the Cooksey-Cawthorne head
exercises.

PROCEDURES

A) Oculomotor Tests of Vestibular Function. Standard electronystagmyography
procedures[10] were followed to record eye movements using surface EOG
electrodes. The following tests were performed: (1) Chair rotations in the
dark to elicit pre-rotatory and post-rotatory vestibulo-ocular-reflex (VOR).
Two chair rotational velocities were used, 60_0/S. and 120_0/s, in clockwise
(cw) and counterclockwise (cc) direction. Time to reach target velocity was
4 seconds, and to decelerate to a stop was 2 seconds; (2) Optokinetic
stimulation. Sixty seconds into constant velocity chair rotation in the
dark the lights were turned on and the rotating subjects viewed a stationary
circular visual surround, consisting of a black and white striped pattern.
This elicited optokinetic nystagmus (OKN). The dependent parameters were
slow phase eye velocity (SPV) to determine the VOR gain, OKN gain, and VOR
time constant (TC). For both VOR gain and TC, the symmetry between left (L)
and right (R) responses were calculated as follows $(L - R) / (R + L) \times 100$.
B) Postural Related Tests of Vestibular Function: The Equitest apparatus
(NeuroCom Internatinal Inc.) was used to measure standing balance performance under a variety of altered visual and somatosensory conditions (for a
description of methods and data analysis see 11-13). In brief patients
were instructed to maintain standing balance for 20 seconds under the
following condition; (1) visual stabilization condition (SO#3); (2) support
surface stabilization (SO#4); (3) support surface stabilization with eyes
closed (SO#5); (4) a combination of visual stabilization and support surface
stabilization (SO#6). An equilibrium score was determined that quantifies
the extent to which the subject maintains the centre of mass within the
limits of stability. It is calculated as the difference in amplitude of
the maximal forward and backward A-P sway of the centre of foot pressure.
(see Table 1A). A strategy score was determined that indicates the extent
to which a subject uses ankle versus hip joint motion to correct body sway.
It is calculated as the difference in amplitude of the maximal to minimal
horizontal shear forces of the platform. (see Table 1B).

All tests were performed; 1 week prior to treatment (TEST 1), 6 weeks into
treatment (TEST 2), and at week 13 which was end of treatment (TEST 3).

RESULTS

For the Rehab group, the results presented in Table 1A and 1B demonstrate
a significant improvement in standing balance regulation under all demanding
sensory conditions. Some improvement occurred in the Home Exercise group, but
no statistical significance was evident.

OKN was within normal limits for all subjects. Based on a statistical
analysis (repeated measures ANOVA) of VOR gain, VOR TC and symmetry scores,
no significant effect of treatment could be demonstrated. In this regard,
it should be noted that; (a) the sample size was reduced because 2 subjects
had no VOR responses at either chair rotation velocity, and 4 subjects could
not tolerate the rotation test at 120_0/s; (b) for both groups the standard
error was large. Regardless, clear trends were observed. The Rehab group
exhibited improvement in L-R VOR gain symmetry, which was accompanied by
increases in L and R VOR gains. Similar findings were observed for VOR
time constants and respective symmetry scores. No consistent improvement
in symmetry scores were observed in the Home Exercise group. An increased
sample size will be required to substantiate the effects observed in the

Rehab group and not detectable in the Home Exercise group.

TABLE 1A and 1B – Group means and standard error of means (SEM) for the Equilibrium (1A) and Strategy (1B) scores. R = Rehab treatment group; HE = Home Exercise group. P values obtained from ANOVA (repeated measures model).

1A		TEST 1 MEAN (SEM)	TEST 2 MEAN (SEM)	TEST 3 MEAN (SEM)	P VALUE
SO #3	R	73.0 (4.9)	78.6 (3.7)	83.6 (3.2)	0.03
	HE	65.9 (10)	69.5 (7.6)	72.8 (8.2)	0.7
SO #4	R	65.6 (7.5)	75.2 (7.5)	78.3 (4.5)	0.04
	HE	67.3 (8.9)	65.1 (10.5)	67.7 (9.4)	0.8
SO #5	R	25.3 (6.7)	40.6 (9.3)	42.3 (8.5)	0.005
	HE	35.3 (8.3)	38.5 (8.3)	41.7 (8.5)	0.38
SO #6	R	30.3 (8.1)	44.3 (8.3)	48.3 (6.3)	0.002
	HE	35.1 (8.4)	39.7 (8.9)	42.3 (9.2)	0.26

1B		TEST 1 MEAN (SEM)	TEST 2 MEAN (SEM)	TEST 3 MEAN (SEM)	P VALUE
SO #3	R	86.3 (3.4)	94.1 (1.6)	94.8 (1.8)	0.03
	HE	83.8 (4.4)	82.8 (5.9)	82.9 (7.1)	0.8
SO #4	R	75.8 (4.4)	81.0 (3.2)	84.0 (2.2)	0.07
	HE	75.1 (4.4)	70.2 (7.7)	70.6 (7.8)	0.9
SO #5	R	50.7 (4.9)	57.8 (7.8)	58.9 (6.8)	0.3
	HE	45.2 (8.3)	50.1 (9.2)	55.2 (9.2)	0.4
SO #6	R	56.7 (5.3)	60.5 (7.2)	66.5 (4.2)	0.1
	HE	48.3 (7.6)	54.5 (10.2)	51.2 (10.1)	0.55

CONCLUSIONS

The main results show a significant effect of structured rehabilitative treatment on standing balance performance, and a positive effect on the magnitude and L-R symmetry of the vestibulo-ocular reflex response. By exposing vestibular patients to combinations of demanding somatosensory, visual and vestibular conditions and thus training the appropriate subsystem(s) involved in postural and oculomotor control (for review see 1-7), signs and symptoms of peripheral vestibular pathologies can be effectively managed.

REFERENCES

1. Igarashi M (1984). Acta Otolaryngol (Stockh); Suppl. 406:78-82.
2. Watt D, and Peterson B. (1988). IN: Vestibular Disorders. (eds)H. Barber and J. Sharpe. Year Book Medical Publishers Inc. Chicago. pp. 35-47.
3. Peppard, S., B, (1986). Laryngoscope 96:878-898.
4. Shumway-Cook A., and Horak F. (1990).Neurologic Clinics 8(2)441-457.
5. Norre, M.E. (1987). Am J Otolar 8:31-35. J. Laryngo & Otol 101:443-447.
6. Herdman, S. (1990). Physical Therapy 70(6)381-388.
7. Sheppard, N., Telian S., (1990). Neurologic Clinics 8(2)459-475.
8. Cawthorne, T. (1945). J. Chart Soc Physiother 106-107.
9. Cookery F., S. (1946). Proc. R. Soc. Med. 39:273-276.
10. Barber H O, Stockwell C W (1976). Manual of Electronystagmography. C.W. Mosby Co. St. Louis.
11. Black, F.O., et al (1988). Abnormal postural control associated with peripheral vestibular disorders. Progress in Brain Res. 76:263-275.
12. Vorhees R I (1989). Laryngoscope 99:995-1001.
13. Goebel J, Paige G (1989). Otolaryngo Head & Neck Syrgert. 100:553-558
*Supported by RHT Thorlakson Foundation Mb., Can., Mb. Med. Serv. Foundation

EVALUATION AND ANALYSIS OF STANDING BALANCE IN PATIENTS WITH CEREBELLAR ATAXIA AND CERVICAL MYELOPATHY.

YONEDA, Toshihiko, RPT,   KOBORI, Satoshi, M.Med.Sci.

Osaka University Hospital, Department of Physical Therapy, Osaka, Japan.

Kurume Institute of Technology, Department of Information Science and Electronics Engineering, Kurume, Japan.

[INTRODUCTION]

Stablizing upright posture (static standing balance) and weight-shifting in standing (dynamic standing balance) are fundamental and important functions for independent gait. Various disorders of the central nervous system and of the muscu-loskeltal system may interfere static and/or dynamic standing balance. Formerly these disturbances were evaluated by quali-tative tests such as one-leg standing test, Mann's test, tandem gait test and so on. These conventional methods, however, were not sufficient to assess disordered standing balance in physiotherapy.

The purpose of this study is to evaluate and analyse quantitatively the disordered standing balance resulting from neurological disorders such as cerebellar ataxia and cervical myelopathy.

[METHOD]

To evaluate static standing balance, we instructed patients to keep upright posture on a force platform(Kistler, 9281B11) for 30 seconds with minimum body sway. The body sway was measured as locus of the center of pressure in the following balancing activities: 1)standing with the eyes open and the feet 20 cm apart(EOFA), 2)standing with the eyes closed and the feet 20 cm apart(ECFA), 3)standing with the eyes open and the feet together(EOFT), and 4)standing with the eyes closed and the feet together(ECFT). In the eyes-open tests, the patients were instructed to watch a circle drawn on a wall(1.5 m ahead from the patients) at the height of the eyes, and the measurement was started about 10 seconds after they began to watch the circle. In the eyes-closed tests, the patients were instructed to close their eyes when they stood on the force platform, and the measurement was started about 10 seconds after marked body sway following eye-closing calmed down. The sam-pling frequency was set at 30 Hz.

Dynamic standing balance was evaluated by speed and accuracy in tracking of the center of pressure to a target which moves stepwise transversely on CRT. The subjects were instructed to keep upright posture on the force platform with the feet 20 cm apart and with equal loading of their weight on both legs. Then they were asked to watch their center of pressure and the target on CRT placed 1m ahead. Their center of pressure was displayed as a movable point on CRT in real time. Next, they were asked to trace the target moving randomly on CRT by moving their center of pressure. We measured the rise time(RT) of the tracking motion which was a duration needed to catch the target, and the mean of absolute error(ER) between the center of pressure and the actual target value during 1.5 seconds just after the rise time. RT is an index of speed, and ER is an index of accuracy. The time required for one trial was 60 seconds. The intervals of stepwise movements of target were from six to nine seconds, and one trial consisted of six to eight tracking motions. The amplitude of target movement, which was given randomly, was ranged from 6.2 to 10.0 cm. The sampling frequency was set at 33 Hz.

Values of the target and the center of pressure in each trial were analysed by the multiple regression method with a following formula;

$$\hat{C}(t)=b_0+b_1\Gamma(t-\tau)+b_2e(t)+b_3\dot{C}(t)$$

where, $\hat{C}$:estimated value of the center of pressure C, Γ: target value, e: error between the target and the center of pressure,

$\dot{C}$:velocity of the center of pressure C, τ :dead time, b_1,b_2,b_3:standard partial regression coefficients, b_0: constant term.

We examined fifty-two healthy persons in their 20's to 60's, twelve patients with cerebellar ataxia and twenty-seven patients with cervical myelopathy. Diseases of the patients in this study were shown in Table 1. Although the cerebellar and myelopathy patients in this study had impaired balance function in standing and walking, they could walk without support. All subjects in this study gave their informed consent.

The t-test was used to examine statistical difference between mean values of the subject groups.

[RESULTS]

1) Static Standing Balance (Table 2):

In every type of balancing activity, locus of the center of pressure was larger in the patients with cervical myelopathy than in the normal control, and it was largest in the patients with cerebellar ataxia. In order to elucidate the influence of closing the eyes on balance function, Romberg ratio(ECFT/EOFT) was calculated. This ratio was larger in the patients with cervical myelopathy than in the normal subjects, which means that the patients with cervical myelopathy showed larger body sway especially in the eyes-closed conditions. The ratio of the patients with cerebellar ataxia was not so large as that of the patients with cervical myelopathy and showed no statistical difference compared with the normal group.

2) Dynamic Standing Balance (Table 3):

The patients with cervical myelopathy showed longer Rise Time(RT) and almost same value of the error(ER) compared with the normal subjects. On the other hand, the patients with cerebellar ataxia showed longer RT and larger ER compared with the normal subjects. Regression line of ER onRT was similar between the normal group and the cervical myelopathy group, but quite different between the normal group and the cerebellar ataxia group. The multiple regression analysis revealed that the patients with cervical myelopathy showed smaller b_1 compared with the normal subjects, and that the patients with cerebellar ataxia showed the smallest b_1. Although the regression coefficients, b_2, b_3 of the three subject groups were small and almost negligible, the coefficient b_2 tended to be smaller in the cervical myelopathy group and larger in the cerebellar ataxia group compared with the normal group respectively. The dead time of the two patient groups was longer than that of the normal group. All subject groups showed very large multiple correlation coefficient that was similar to R=1.

[DISCUSSION]

1) Static Standing Balance:

The patients with cervical myelopathy showed larger body sway than the normal group, and the patients with cerebellar ataxia showed largest body sway in four types of balancing activities. There was statistical difference in locus of body sway between the cerebellar ataxia group and the cervical myelopathy group as well as between the cervical myelopathy group and the normal group. Besides, Romberg ratio was significantly larger in the cervical myelopathy group and not significantly larger in the cerebellar ataxia group compared with the normal group. Based on these data, we concluded that the patients with cervical myelopathy had instability in standing due to disturbances in proprioceptive and superficial sensation as well as spastic paresis, and that the patients with cerebellar ataxia showed more unstable standing even with visual feedback mainly because of disorders in postural control.

2) Dynamic Standing Balance:

The patients with cervical myelopathy showed longer RT and almost same value of ER compared with the normal subjects and the regression lines of ER on RT in both groups were almost equivalent. The patients with cervical myelopathy sacrificed speed for accuracy in the weight-shifting motion (speed-accuracy trade-off). This precedence of accuracy over speed is physiological principle of human performance. Therefore, normal postural control in dynamic standing balance is likely to be still working in the patients with cervical myelopathy in spite of significant sensory and motor disturbances. On the other hand, the patients with cerebellar ataxia showed inaccuracy even with slower speed, and the regression line of ER on RT in the patients with cerebellar ataxia was quite different from that in the normal subjects. From these data, we concluded that the patients with cerebellar ataxia had severely impaired balance function due to disturbed postural control mechanism.

The multiple correlation coefficient R was very large and substantially same as R=1(complete correlation) in any group, this multiple regression model was well fitted to this type of weight-shifting motion in both normal and neurologically disabled persons. The regression coefficient b_1 indicates contribution of a target value to movement of the center of pressure in the tracking motion. The mechanism of the contribution is explained by feedforward control triggered by visual input of a target. The regression coefficient b_2 expresses how visual feedback control contributes to movement of the center of pressure by correction of the error between the target and the center of pressure. Velocity of the center of pressure contributed little,if any, because the regression coefficient b_3 was negative and very small. The dead time τ means delay of motion. The regression coefficient b_1 was significantly larger in the patients with cerebellar ataxia and in the patients with cervical myelopathy compared with the normal subjects.

Summarizing these results, we supposed that the patients with cerebellar ataxia and cervical myelopathy had difficulty in controlling feedfowardly, and that they relied upon feedback control, which is more the case in the patients with cerebellar ataxia. This is supported by the data that the dead time was longer in both patient groups compared with the normal group, because feedback movement needs longer delay of motion than feedforward movement.

[CONCLUSION]

The disorders of static and dynamic standing balance in the patients with cerebellar ataxia and cervical myelopathy were evaluated and analysed quantitatively. The system of static and dynamic standing balance tests we developed should be applied to evaluation and treatment of physiotherapy for patients with neurological disorders.

Table 1. Diseases of the Patients in this study.

Cerebellar Ataxia:	Spinocerebellar Degeneration	10
	Cerebellar Tumor	1
	Cerebellar Atrophy	1
Cervical Myelopathy:	Cervical Spondylotic Myelopathy	16
	OPLL(Cervical Spine)	6
	Cervical Disc Herniation	3
	Cervical Cord Tumor	1
	Syringomyelia	1

Table 2. Results of the Static Standing Balance Test [Mean(SD)]

	EOFA	ECFA	EOFT	ECFT (cm)	Romberg ratio
					(ECFT/EOFT)
Normal younger	33.8(7.2)	41.7(7.9)	44.9(10.1)	66.2(15.8)	1.49(0.26)
elderly	37.4(8.3)	52.7(10.2)	50.2(8.2)	79.2(21.5)	1.56(0.25)
Myelopathy	43.4(11.6)	82.8(44.5)	69.6(23.4)	141.8(67.3)	2.02(0.56)
	NS	**N	**N	**N	**N
Cerebellar	107.3(63.5)	244.5(155.3)	172.4(69.5)	296.7(158.6)	1.87(0.52)
	**M	**M	**M	**N	NS

statistical difference   **N:p<.01 compared with normal subjects   **M:p<.01 compared with myelopathy patients   NS:not significant

Table 3. Results of the Dynamic Standing Balance Test [Mean(SD)]

	Normal	Myelopathy	Cerebellar
RT (sec)	1.41 (0.63)	1.74 (0.33) *N	1.90 (0.39) *N
ER (mm)	13.2 (2.8)	12.7 (3.6) NS	19.0 (5.2) **N
b1	0.964 (0.011)	0.958 (0.013) *N	0.941 (0.029) *N
b2	0.179 (0.021)	0.157 (0.032)	0.253 (0.107)
b3	-0.072 (0.013)	-0.049 (0.010)	-0.066 (0.017)
τ (sec)	0.83 (0.12)	1.11 (0.16) *N	1.01 (0.12) *N
R (median)	0.98	0.98	0.96

statistical significance   *N:p<.05, **N:p<.01 compared with normal subjects   NS: not significant

References:

1) Bohannon, R.W., et al.: Decrease in Timed Balance Test Scores with Aging. Phys. Ther. 64(7):1067-1070,1984.

2) Brooks, V.B.: The Neural Basis of Motor Control. Oxford University Press, New York, 1986.

3) Ikegami, A. et al.: Study on the Amplitude and Velocity of Movement of the Center of Gravity in Romberg's Posture. Vestibular and Visual Control on Posture and Locomotor Equilibrium. p331-334,1985.

4) Jansen, E.C., et al.: Quantitative Romberg's Test. Acta neurol. scandinav. 66:93-99,1982.

5) Kobori, S., et al.: The Evaluation and Analysis of Dynamic Balance by Means of Tracking Motion. Human Factors in Organizational Design and Management-III. p59-62,1990.

6) Murray, M.P., et al.: Normal postural stability and steadness:Quantitative assessment. J.Bone Joint surg.[Am]57:510-516,1975.

7) Schmidt, R.A.: Motor Control and Learning(second edition). Human Kinetics Publishers, Champaign, 1988.

8) Stribley, R.F., et al.: A Quantitative Study of Stance in Normal Subjects. Arch.Phys.Med.Rehabil.55:74-80,1974.

9) Thyssen,H.H., et al.: Normal ranges in reproducibility for quantitative Romberg's test. Acta neurol.scandinav.66:100-104,1982.

A STUDY TO DETERMINE POSSIBLE MILESTONES OF RECOVERY
IN GUILLAIN-BARRE SYNDROME

Jennifer Brackenreg and Yvonne Lewis
Physiotherapy Department The National Hospital for Neurology and
Neurosurgery, Queen Sq, London WC1N 3BG.

The National Hospital for Neurology and Neurosurgery (N.H.N.N.) receives
on average 27 patients per year with the diagnosis of Guillain-Barre
Syndrome (GBS). Physiotherapists are closely involved with these patients
from the moment of diagnosis in order to : -
1.) Establish a baseline assessment
2.) Maintain respiratory function throughout the acute stage
3.) Maintain optimal physical status throughout the course of the disease
4.) Assist recovery of function and ability once the acute stage of the
    disease has passed.
Consequently a large proportion of physiotherapy time is given over to the
management of patients with GBS.

This study was undertaken in conjunction with the Centre for Physiotherapy
Research, Strand, to determine whether patients with GBS follow a distinct
sequence of recovery. It is hoped to use such information to evaluate
methods of treatment and to accurately monitor individual patient progress.
It has previously been-demonstrated that predictable patterns of recovery
occur in patients following cerebral vascular accidents (ref. 1.). This
former work provided the background for this study.

A group of physiotherapists with experience of working with patients with
neurological disability, drew up an index of objectively recognisable
milestones. This was then piloted at the N.H.N.N. for one month. Ammend-
ments were then made based upon the comments received during this period.

A revised form was then sent to twenty teaching hospitals throughout
Britain. Reasons for the study and comprehensive instructions were given
in an accompanying letter. These letters were sent in June 1990 and
therapists were asked to return the forms by mid February 1991.

The participating therapists were requested to complete the form each week
from initial contact, through to cessation of physiotherapy intervention.
If a patient moved to another hospital, it was requested that the form was
sent with them. The form was specifically printed on A3 size paper,
folded to create 4 attached sides. This was to ensure that the instructions could not be detached from the table of milestones.

The form was sent to a named member of physiotherapy staff at each of the
hospitals (where possible). If additional forms were required, it was
suggested that the original form be photocopied. The teaching hospitals
were chosen at random - at this stage it was not taken into account whether
or not they were a receiving centre for GBS patients.

The form was also published in the September issue of the newsletter
belonging to the Association of Chartered Physiotherapists with an Interest

in Neurology (ACPIN). This publication included an explanation about the form and a request for assistance. The newsletter was distributed nationally.

In October 1990, a follow up letter, with further detail, was sent to the original group of hospitals and another copy of the form was enclosed.

In February 1991, 11 accurately completed forms were returned. The information is therefore considered limited, but the results have been analysed in the following manner :-
1.) The percentage of patients who achieved each milestone, week by week.
2.) Each patient's data was displayed in graph form, to assess pattern of recovery.
3.) Visual comparison of the graphs was made between each patient's results.

CONCLUSIONS

1.) A difference in pattern of recovery was noted between patients who had initially been diagnosed with GBS and then later revised to a diagnosis of chronic relapsing demyelinating disorder. This was evident in the graphical results, by the weekly fluctuation of milestones achieved and the period of time over which recovery occurred.

2.) A drop in the reported cases of patients with GBS occurred in the N.H.N.N. between the months of July and September.

3.) Patients with an accurate diagnosis of GBS achieved significant recovery by the 8th week (initial expectations had been that 14 weeks might be needed for patients to achieve the milestones tabled).

4.) A better response may have been achieved if a stamped addressed envelope had been sent with the forms.

5.) The number of responses are insufficient to draw any definitive conclusions from, but the information received so far is encouraging. A second stage to this study is therefore planned over a further 12 months, in order to increase the number of patients included in the study.

The second stage form will be modified in the following way : -

1.) The milestones will be arranged in a hierarchical form.

2.) Participating therapists will be requested to return the completed forms following the 8th assessment, or when the patient is discharged (whichever is sooner).

3.) The form will be sent to all the original participating hospitals with a letter thanking them for their earlier assistance, enclosing a summary of the results of stage one.

4.) Eight weeks after the distribution of this second stage form, a stamped addressed envelope will be sent for the return of any completed forms.

5.) Any patient sent from the N.H.N.N. with GBS, will be accompanied by a form and a stamped addressed envelope for return of the form after the 8th weekly assessment or when the patient is discharged from physiotherapy, whichever is sooner.

It is hoped that this study will identify whether milestones of recovery in GBS follow a predictable pattern. Such information may be used to compare different types of management; to evaluate the progress of individual patients and to help set realistic goals.

Reference

1. Partridge CJ; Johnstone M; Edwards S. "Recovery from Physical Disability after Stroke : Normal Patterns of Recovery". Lancet, Feb 14th 1987 : 373 375.

MS SCHOOL; A BIOPSYCHOSOCIAL INTERVENTION IN MULTIPLE SCLEROSIS.

Wikander B, Holmén A-M
Physiotherapy unit, Mölndal Hospital, S-431 80 Mölndal, Sweden.

INTRODUCTION

Recently a new concept of physiotherapy that broadens the therapeutic approach has been introduced (1). This concept is based on the fact that when a person is subjected to a life-long disease he needs a multifactorial intervention more than the conventional therapy offered to-day. This theory is built on the holistic perspective which means that the individual is recognized as a being where biological, psychological, and social factors meet and interact in a complex pattern. If anyone of these factors are under serious stress a chain reaction will be initiated and may end in a life crisis. It is obvious that a disease such as Multiple Sclerosis (MS) may bring about such a crisis. It is known that the ability to cope with a crisis differs between persons. One theory is that it is the individuals sense of coherence (SOC) that differs (2).

The multifactorial intervention of the present study consists of a series of physiotherapy sessions once a week during a four months' period with a constant group of patients with diagnosed and established Multiple Sclerosis. Every second time information is given about the disease, its symptoms and treatment, and its eventual consequences to the individuals personal life (3, 4, 5). A discussion follows and as it is the same people in the group every time, the physiotherapists and the patients get to know and trust each other well. This gives the physiotherapists a possibility to create an atmosphere of understanding, trust and openess that helps the individual to express his own worries, difficulties and experiences in a safe way (6). The hypothesis behind this work is that such a multifactorial intervention increases the individuals coping capacity through the support given by the physiotherapists and the fellow patients.

MATERIALS AND METHODS

PATIENTS
Twenty-three MS patients, registered at Mölndal Hospital, Physiotherapy unit, were chosen for this pilot study.

Nine patiens, 5 men and 4 women, aged 28-59 years (mean age 42) were consecutively chosen for the study. The following criteria were to be fulfilled:

- Diagnosed MS
- Referred to physiotherapy
- Living on their own outside institution

- Walking by themselves with or without cane/s
- No serious brain damage
- Holding a job

The remaining fourteen patients, 3 men and 11 women, aged 25-56 years (mean age 42) were included as a control group if fulfilling the criteria above listed.

THE MULTIFACTORIAL INTERVENTION, MS SCHOOL
The experimental group met once a week during a period of four months. The therapy consisted of:

- Pool exercises 20 minutes in colf water (8)
- Training session for 40 minutes
- Information for 40 minutes

INSTRUMENT

The level of coping capacity was established by using a modified version of the Sense of Coherence instrument (SOC) originally developed by Antonovsky, 1987. It consists of 29 items each with a maximum score of 100. The instrument has been found valid and reliable in measuring coping capacity after coronary artery by-pass grafting surgery (7).

RESULTS

The aim of this study was to measure if our multifactorial intervention, the MS school, increases the MS patients coping capacity. The impact of the disease on the patients well-being was seen from a biopsychosocial view. A modified version of SOC was used as an assessment instrument. Social and demographic data were taken from the patients medical records. The results indicate that our intervention at least in three cases increased the coping capacity from a low level to a normal level. Two patients decreased their level of coping capacity with ≥ 100 arb units and that corresponds well with their increasing symptoms during the period. Follow-ups will show if their coping capacity will increase when, or if, they get better.
The evaluation of the MS school shows that we succeeded in creating an atmosphere of trust and openess so that even embarrassing topics like incontinence were freely discussed. It also shows that it was, especially to the patients with a low coping capacity, a turning point to meet a person in the same situation getting on with life.
In the future the MS school will be offered to the patients at the same time as the doctor informs about the diagnosis (9).

IN CONCLUSION

The MS school and the self assessment instrument used may constitute useful tools for increasing and measuring the MS patients coping capacity and thereby Quality of Life.

1. Hansson M, Helgesson, Sonander G. Smärtskolan. Göteborg: Ciba-Geigy, 1986
2. Antonovsky A. Unraveling the Mystery of Health. San Francisco: Jossey-Bass, 1987
3. Chusid J G. Correlative Neuroanatomy and Functional Neurology. Lang, 1988
4. Hald T. The urinary bladder: neurology and dynamics. Baltimore: Williams and Wilkins, 1982
5. Olsson M. Multipel scleros, sjukdomsbild och behandling. Stockholm: 1983
6. Stewart D C, Sullivan T J. Illness behavior and sick role in chronic disease. The care of MS. Soc Sci Med 16:1397-404, 1982
7. Larsson P A, Karlsson I, Sundström C, Möller A, Sinderby C, Pettersson G. The impact of Biopsychosocial Factors on coping capacity after coronary by-pass surgery (in preparation)
8. Davis F A. Effects of Induced Hyperthermia in Multiple Sclerosis. Acta Neurol Scan 49:141-51, 1973
9. Fredriksson S. When and how should the patient be informed of the diagnosis of multiple sclerosis. Läkartidningen 86:3909-10, 1989

F-WAVES IN CEREBROVASCULAR DISEASE.

Toshiaki SUZUKI,   Isao TAKEDA, and   Tetsuji FUJIWARA
College of Medical Technology,   Kyoto University.
53 Kawahara-cho, Shogoin, Sakyo-ku Kyoto, Japan

Introduction

To clarify their neurophysiological application in the field of physical therapy, we investigated F-waves, which are presumed to reflect the 'backfiring' of motor neurons after antidromic activation induced by stimulation of the peripheral nerve. We reported that an increase in the strength of isometric contraction apparently led to enhanced excitability of anterior horn cells in the spinal cord, especially at maximum contraction, as the persistence of F-waves and amplitude ratio of F/M during isometric contraction were significantly greater than those in the relaxed state[1,2].

In the present study we focused on spinal motor neuron function in cerebrovascular disease (CVD) by analyzing the F-waves in bilateral upper extremities and the relationship of F-wave characteristics to neurological findings.

Materials and Method

Seventeen patients (10 males and 7 females),   mean age 61.1± 18.7 (range,49-79)years, were studied. Patients included 10 with cerebral infarction (3 with right and 7 with left hemiplegia) and 7 with cerebral hemorrhage (5 with right and 2 with left hemiplegia). Cortical location of lesion verified by computerized tomography scan of the brain was temporal in 14 patients,   frontal in 1,   temporo-occipital in 1, and temporo-parietal in 1. Patients with bilateral lesions of the brain or with severe agnosia, apraxia or aphasia were excluded from the present study.

After the patient rested for a while in a comfortable supine position, we measured the F-waves of the opponens pollicis muscle on the affected side in the relaxed state, and of that on the non-affected side in the relaxed state and 25%, 50%, 75% and 100% (maximum) isometric contraction.

A Viking (NICOLET) EMG machine was used to evoke F-waves. The intensity of constant current stimulation to the median nerve at the wrist was 20% supramaximal to evoke M response, and stimulus rate was 0.5Hz. The persistence, amplitude ratio of F/M, latency, duration and phase (number of peaks) of F-waves for 20 trials were analyzed. The amplitude ratio of F/M, latency, duration and phase were expressed as the mean value of 20 trials.

Neurological findings, including muscle tone, tendon reflex, Brunnstrom's motor function test, active movement, superficial sensation, deep sensation, agnosia, apraxia, aphasia and activities of daily living (ADL), were also evaluated. Findings for muscle tonus and tendon reflex were classified as increased, normal or decreased, those for active movement as normal or impaired, those for superficial sensation and deep sensation as normal or disturbed, those for agnosia, apraxia and aphasia as present or absent, those for ADL as independent or supported.

Results

1) Comparison of bilateral F-waves.

On the affected side, mean value for all subjects in the relaxed state was as follows: persistence, 86.0±20.9%; amplitude ratio of F/M, 4.25±2.31%; latency,27.6±3.23ms; duration,8.54±2.80ms and phase,2.95± 0.72. On the non-affected side,it was:persistence,70.7±26.0%; amplitude ratio of F/M,3.06±1.56%; latency,27.0±2.63ms; duration,8.39±1.21ms, and phase,2.91±0.50. Persistence and amplitude ratio of F/M were significantly higher on the affected side than on the non-affected side (p<0.05), but no significant difference between sides was found in latency, duration or phase.

On the non-affected side, no significant differences among the 4 contraction conditions for F-wave characteristics were found.

2) Relationship of F-wave characteristics to neurological findings.

Persistence and amplitude ratio of F/M on the affected side were correlated with muscle tonus and tendon reflex findings. Mean persistence and amplitude ratio of F/M on the affected side for 13 patients(76.5%) with increased muscle tonus and tendon reflex were 91.8± 18.6% and 4.92±2.23%, respectively, while for 4 patients(23.5%) with decreased muscle tonus and tendon reflex they were 67.2±18.0% and 2.10± 0.60%, respectively (p<0.05).

On the non-affected side, as on the affected side, F-wave characteristics were influenced by muscle tonus and tendon reflex findings.

Discussion

In the present study, we examined F-waves in patients with CVD and the relationship between F-wave characteristics and neurological findings.

According to Liberson et al[3], who was the first to study F-waves in patients with CVD, the amplitude ratio of F/M was significantly higher on the affected side than on the non-affected side because of the increased excitability of spinal motor neurons on the affected side. Fisher[4] also reported that the amplitude of F-waves was higher on the affected side than on the non-affected side, and that F-wave characteristics were closely associated with muscle tonus and tendon reflex findings. Our results for the affected side are compatible with those reported by Liberson et al. and Fisher, and indicate that findings for F-waves are an index of excitability at the spinal level in patients with CVD.

In the relaxed state, characteristics of F-waves on the non-affected side, like those on the affected side, were influenced by muscle tonus and tendon reflex. Durings isometric contraction, F-waves on the non-affected side showed no changes with varying strength of contraction. Although no previous reports describing F-waves on the non-affected side in the patients with CVD are available, it is well known that grasping strength, pinch strength and finger tapping scores for the non-affected side in CVD patients are significantly lower than scores for healthy subjects[5-8], and that there is positive correlation of scores on these tests for the non-affected side with those for the affected side[9].

Decreased function on the non-affected side is thought to be influenced by non-crossing anterior corticospinal and lateral corticospinal tracts on the affected side, as well as by the decreased nervous activity caused by disuse.

These findings suggest that F-waves can be used to investigate the hyperexcitability of spinal motor neurons resulting from lesion of upper motor neurons on the affected side, as well as to investigate the function of nervous on the non-affected side which are influenced by neurons on the affected side.

Conclusion

To investigate the characteristics of bilateral F-waves and their relationship to neurological findings in the patients with upper motor neuron lesion, we studied seventeen patients including 10 with unilateral cerebral infarction and 7 with unilateral cerebral hemorrhage.

In the relaxed state, persistence and amplitude ratio of F/M on the affected side were significantly higher($p<0.05$) than those on the non-affected side, these characteristics on both sides were influenced by muscle tonus and tendon reflex. No specific changes in F-wave characteristics during isometric contraction on the non-affected side were found.

We conclude that analysis of F-wave characteristics can be used to determine the excitability of spinal motor neurons not only on the affected side but also on the non-affected side in patients with cerebrovascular disease.

References

1. Suzuki T,Takeda I,Fujiwara T(1990) F wave in normal subject during isometric contraction and relaxation. Rigaku ryōhō jānaru 24;49-52.
2. Suzuki T,Takeda I,Fujiwara T(1991) F-wave response to changes in isometric contraction and to contralateral isometric contraction. Rigaku ryōhō jānaru 25 ; 125-128.
3. Liberson WT,Chen LY,Fok SK,Patel KK,Yu G,Fried P(1977) "H" reflexes and "F" waves in hemiplegics. Electromyogr clin Neurophysiol. 17;247 -264.
4. Fisher MA (1983) F response analysis of motor disorders of central origin. J Neurol Sci. 62; 13-22.
5. Jebsen RH (1971) Function of "normal" hand in stroke patients. Arch Phys Med Rehabil. 52; 170-174.
6. Wyke M (1972) The effects of brain lesions on the performance of bilateral arm movements. Neuropsychologia 9; 33-42.
7. Haaland KY,Delaney HD (1981) Motor deficits after left or right hemisphere damage due to stroke or tumor. Neuropsychologia 19;17-27.
8. Smutok MA,Grafman J,Salazar AM,Sweeney JK,Jonas BS,Dirocco PJ (1989) Effects of unilateral brain damage on contralateral and ipsilateral upper extremity function in hemiplegia. Phys Ther 69; 195-203.
9. Yagi M,So M,Kondo M,Hasue K,Kitamura M,Noguchi Y, Sugahara R,Sano S, Ariizumi M(1977) Function of the non-paretic limbs in hemiplegic patients (Part 4). Jap J Reh Med 14; 322-323.

HUNTINGTON'S DISEASE: DELIVERY OF PHYSICAL THERAPY SERVICES IN A GROUP SETTING.

I. W. Peacock
Huntington's Disease Project, 1631 North Vernon, Dearborn, Michigan 48128 U.S.A.

Huntington's Chorea or Huntington's Disease (HD) is a neurode-generative brain disorder which is transmitted by autosomal dominant inheritance. Major pathological changes in the brain are primarily in the basal ganglia althouth neurons may also be lost in the cortex, brain stem and cerebellum. Onset of mental, emotional and physical symptoms can vary from child-hood to advanced age but most often occurs between the ages of thirty-five and forty-five. Deterioration continues over a period of ten to twenty-five years to inevitable death.

Genetic counseling is the primary method for elimination of HD. Treatment in the USA is primarily in the area of drug therapy. Pharmacology has much to offer intreatment of depression or irrational behavior for HD patients and those at risk. However, the effects of drugs on uncontrolled movements may be only cosmetic and may sedate so that functional abilities are decreased. Informal observation seems to indicate (1) that some of the functional degeneration seen in HD may result from decreasing use of potential physical capacities, not necessa-rily in direct relationship to brain deterioration, and (2) therefore, maintenance of functional abilities within the limitations imposed by the CSN involvement should be possible. Meanwhile, most patients with HD have nophysical therapy service. Their need for assistance in maintaining function as long as possible is not being met. I propose a relatively simple exercise program to begin in early stages of HD and administered with minimum expense and professional time.

Consideration of the observed characteristics of HD is essen-tial in planning an exercise prlgram. Onset, rate of decline, sequence, severity, and the primary area of involvement may vary. Individualized home exercise programs should carry over the exercise program as based on the following characteristics:

The disease is known as Huntington's Chorea because patients first described had chorea or athetosis. Most HD patients do have involuntary movements at some time which may become completely debilitating in the cinal stages. Patients can maintain tonic contraction to prevent movement so efforts at control may further increase muscle tension. Some patients have rigidity rathan chorea or they may develop rigidity in later stages. RELAXATION TRAINING IS A PRIMARY NEED.

Lack of motor control may be apparent in varying degrees. In-coordination may involve small or large muscles. It may begin with very find coordination but ADL will be affected as the disease progresses. As large muscles are involved, ambulation will also be affected. COORDINATION TRAINING IS INDICATED.

Patients may lack freedom of movement, in varying degrees, which usually results in contractures. Often the cervical spine is affected early and lateral flexion may become impossible. ADL, ambulation, and other coordinations will be affected. EFFORTS TO INCREASE FLEXIBILITY ARE NEEDED.

Many patients exhibit a characteristic staggering gait which may be mistaken for drunkenness rather than a balance problem. Balance deficits and faulty directional control can result in falls and ADL problems. BALANCE TRAINING IS CLEARLY INDICATED.

Respiratory diseases affect most HD patients. Pneumonia is the most common cause of death. Breathing patterns often are uncontrolled, shallow, and erratic - evident inexhalation and coordinating breathing with swallowing. Patients may choke or aspirate food. Poor control of exhalation also affects speech. TRAINING IN BREATH CONTROL IS ESSENTIAL.

In my experience, loss of strength isnot a significant factor for relatively active patients in the earlier stages of HD. As involvement progresses, strength loss could be considerable. I do not routinely use resistance exercises or weights - which seemed to increase incoordination and tendion. Thatdoes not mean such an approach wouldnot be effective for some patients.

An active exercise program based on identified needs of the patients is the PT treatment of choice. Therefore, for most patients, exercises need to focus on relaxation, flexibility, coordination, balance, breath control and, to a lesser degree, strength. Any exercises that meet these criteria would be effective. They should be done regularly between PT visits.

The important factor in the effectiveness of the exercise program is the format for delivery of services. A small group of patients directed in exercises at regular intervals has many advantages over individual sessions. The most valuable result ofthe group therapy is the reinforcement and support which members give each other. None of my patients had ever met a person with HD except in their families. Acceptance by the group and individuals was apparent despite varied social competence, background, comprehension and physical ability.

Patients must follow instructions as precisely as possible in relation to direction, position, and speed. The cognitive aspect puts demands on the patient's ability to think, react, and cooperate. Observation, communication, and encouragement of peers helps to facilitate performance for most patients.

The supportive atmosphere may help "difficult" patients to participate in group activities. A small number, four to six patients, is potentially more effective than larger groups for more individualized supervision, peer relationships and use of space. A check-off exercise list is given to each patient for use at home. If it is to be continued indefinitely, there is need for supervision or at lease, encouragement of the patient in the home program. Exercising should not require hands-on therapy or add stress on the family. The specific exercises should be reviewed with each individual regularly. Audio tapes can also be helpful.

My therapy sessions end with a few recreational exercises. these may be loosely organized active games involving hitting, kicking, throwing, or catching. Music may be used for movement patterns, dancing or marching. Some activities may be more cognitive or involve fine coordination. Most of the patients enjoy such activities and join in freely. "Break times" as in any setting, are important for communication which may involve problem-solving or even peercounseling. The therapy group becomes a source of support in meaningful accomplishments both as reported in home and community activities as well as in the exercise program.

The group concept does involve some negative considerations. Patients need to be effective in most of the activities of the group. In my HD Project, only ambulatory patients were accepted. There is some dilution of individual attention. Being in a program also requires acceptance of the diagnosis, which some early patients tend to deny. They may not want to see the reality of other HD patients, especially if the involvement is marked. Out-patient individual therapy could be an effective entry route to a group. It should be noted that certain characteristics of some HD patients may impact on the effectiveness of PT services. The advantage of beginning a program early cannot be overemphasized. A pattern can then be established before the patient loses his self-esteem and motivation and gives up or the fears of the care givers have restricted his physical activities.

In conclusion, the delivery of PT in an exercise group proved to be effective because of the unique opporunity for patients to geve and receive support among their peers. Decrease in use of professional personnel and facilities is also cost-effective. Allowance of time and space for communication and recreational activities among group members is an important adjunct to the exercise program which maynot be feasible in all settings. The small group method has a potential for benefits beyond those possible in individual exercise situations for HD patients who can function in this setting.

References will be furnished upon request.

POSTER PRESENTATIONS

COGNITIVE PHYSIOTHERAPY FOR BRAIN-DAMAGED PATIENTS

Gitte Rasmussen

Center for Rehabilitation of Brain Damage, University of Copenhagen
Denmark.

The Center for Rehabilitation of Brain Damage was established in 1985
by Dr. Anne-Lise Christensen, a neuropsychologist. Over 100 patients
with post-acute brain-damage have been treated in a interdisciplinary
program. This program is inspired by the principles of the Russian
neuropsychologist A. R. Luria. His concept of higher cortical functions
as being social in origin, mediated by speech and conscious in their
performance has strongly influenced the physiotherapeutic training.

The physiotherapy program has evolved from a traditional Bobath oriented
concept to a more functional and cognitive approach, stressing memory,
concentration and learning. At the same time the patients are encouraged
to take responsibility for their own training with close guidance by the
therapists. New areas of physical training are being introduced, such as
learning to direct the morning gymnastic exercises for the whole group,
to manage to use the facilities in a fitness center and to sail a mini
12 Meter sailing boat - even with unilateral paralysis and cognitive
dysfunctioning.

The whole program is firmly structured and integrated in the "normal"
surroundings of the University, e.g. sharing the same transportation,
canteens and a nearby fitness center. New methods of evaluation have
been developed including the patients' own evaluation both physically
and psychologically.

Cognitive physiotherapy is not a name of a new system, but the label
which at present best covers the new functionally organized physiotherapy
for brain-damage in the post acute phase.

THE REHABILITATION OF BRAIN INJURED ADULTS WITH
AN ASSOCIATED BEHAVIOURAL DISTURBANCE THAT
PRECLUDES TREATMENT IN CONVENTIONAL SITUATIONS

J C Bentley, J A Shepherd, E V Thomson

Physiotherapy Department, Kemsley Unit
St.Andrew's Hospital, Northampton, U.K.

Introduction : The Kemsley Unit provides a structured and stimulating environment, conducive to the rehabilitation of patients with problem behaviours. It aims to modify behaviour in conjunction with maximising each individual's functional independence. The token economy system provides the framework for rehabilitation and the acquisition of functional skills provides the vehicle for learning control of unwanted behaviour. Emphasis is placed on the consistent and co-ordinated approach to behaviour and function by the interdisciplinary team.

Treatment : Patients follow a structured routine divided into : sessions, meal times and free time. Appropriate behaviour and effort are consistently rewarded to promote and subsequently reinforce acceptable behaviour and functional achievement. The functional skills which are taught in treatment sessions are incorporated into the daily activities to improve generalisation. As individuals learn to control behaviour and become more independent, ward based activities are generalised into community skills.

Results : Case notes are used to show how individuals learn to control unwanted behaviour and increase their functional independence as a preparation for integration into the wider community.

Conclusion : Successful rehabilitation of this difficult client group is achieved by a consistent and coordinated approach to both behaviour and acquisition of function.

CLINICAL CLASSIFICATION AND TENTATIVE PT PROGRAMME OF FRONTAL LOBE LESION

T Fukai[*] , H Hara[*] , T Fujiwara[**], M Inui[*] & T Mitsui[*],
*Dept. of Rehab. Matsumoto Kyoritu Hosp. Matsumoto,
390, JAPAN
**Sinshu Univ., School of Allied Med. Sciences,
Matsumoto, 390, JAPAN

Intoroduction:

The purpose of this study is to simplify the PT programm for the treatment of patients with lesions in the internal surface of the frontal lobe by classifying them into groups. But functional researches on the frontal lobe, especially the premotor cortex, started in the early part of the 20th century. And this field of study is today attracting great attention in the physical therapy of central nerves diseases[1]. As result, the frontal lobe assumes the role of initiating voluntary movements and coordinating the final reaction by integrating information from other cortical areas[2]. Therefore, the lesions in this area can often cause very complex clinical feature. To evaluate and analyze the lesions in the frontal lobe, it is nesessary to classify them into well-defined functional levels[3].

Subjects & Method

The paitients covered in this study were 35 cases aged 60 and above with lesions in their internal surface of the frontal lobe, who received hospital treatment in the Rehabilitation Department of the above-mentioned hospital during the period of April 1986 to December 1990. The average age of the patients (60 to 90 years of age) was 72.3. All the cases of 18 males and 17 females had been confirmed by the medical doctor with CT scan to have lesions in both sides of the frontal lobe.

Method

1. The patients were required to perform the following tasks and their movement patterns were analyzed:
(1)Ascent and descent of the stairs,(2)Walking with a gait assistive device, (3)walking with a wide-based cane, and (4)standing up.In the task of standing up, a handrail was prepaired before the patient so as to allow the shifting of the center of gravity forward.
2. Neurological signs of the lesion in the frontal lobe were investigated in regard to (1)forced grasp reaction, (2)abnormal muscule tone, (3)imitation behavior and (4)utilization behavior.
3. The Barthal's score at the plateau of function was determined.
4. The ADL independence and PT program were checked according to the hospital treatment records.

Results

Based on the finding in 1) to 4) above, the cases could be classified into the following five groups:(refarence rist 1)

(1)group 1: In 6 cases and capable of walking with a wide base cane, but in need of guidance as to optimal life environment and daily life program, (2)group 2: In 8 cases and capable of walking with a gait assistive device, (3) group 3: In 5 cases and capable of ascending and descending the stair and capable of assistive walk, (4) group 4: In 5 cases and capable of standing up, and (5) group 5: In 11 cases and bedrest completely. But in some paitients could flex and extend their knees in a play therapy using a ball and sit if so positioned.

As so the Barthal's score, five patients in group 1 showed high scores of 85 to 95 while others scored 65 below.

As for ADL independence, all the cases except those of group 1 required assistance or observation.

Discussion

The diseases in the frontal lobe, which cause disorder in programing, declease voluntary movements of the patients[4]. Thus the patients are in need of certain forms of assistance or observation in their daily living. These cases invariably show extremely low scores in the conventional Barthal's score or ADL independence classification, thus making it impossible to grasp the severity of the lesion. However, by paying attention to the ADL behavioral patterns or the neurological signs, it is possible to grade the cases into groups. Thus the author succeeded in grading them into five groups, using classification by ADL behavior as well as by capacity of executing assigned tasks. As a result, it was found that the most important point in PT evaluation and programming is whether the patient is able to stand up or not.For patients who can stand up, it is necessary to first assist them to go up and down the stairs and walk with a gait assistive device and then recomend to walk with a wide-based cane. For the patients who are unable to stand up, on the other hand, it is necessary to prevent the contracture of joints[5] such as the knee and induce the movements, such as flexion and extension, of the knee. Also, it was considered necessary to help the patient, who is lying in bed all day, to sit in a wheelchair. However, in any case, the patient requires certain assistance, so that the method and extent of assistance most appropriate for the patient's functional classification must be explained to the persons who give assistance to him or her.

Conclusion

1) Four tasks were assigned to the patients with complex symptoms resulting from lesions in the internal surface of the frontal lobe, and their behaviors were observed. Then a functional classification was attempted by compairing them with the neurological signs of the lesions in the frontal lobe.

2) The five classified groups represented and the PT program, which is based on whether the patient can stand up or not, must progress according to the stages of functional classification.

3) The programs for the patients who can not stand up require further investigation. It is deemed necessary to devise ways to effectively induce individual movements of the knees and other parts of the body as well as a therapy to combine individual movements into all integrated moovement.

	group 1 n=6	group 2 n=8	group 3 n=5	group 4 n=5	group 5 n=11
walking with wide-base cane	able	unable	←	←	←
walking with gait assistive device	able	←	unable	←	←
ascent and descent of the stairs	able	←	←	unable	←
standing up	able	←	←	←	unable
forced grasp reaction	release their hold voluntarily	evident			disappear
abnormal muscle tone		mild		moderate	severe
imitation behavior utilization behaivior	limited occation correctable	correctable	rare incorectable (case dependent)		disappear
excretion	under supervision		assistance encouragement		napkin

(Rist 1:Classification based on the finding in (1) to (4) method)

References

1)Steven P Wise, (1985) The Primate premotor cortex past, present and preparatory   Ann. Rev. Neurosci.
2)Bianchi,(1985) The function of the frontal lobe, Brain.
3)Henneman,(1980) Organization of the motor system, In Medical Physiology.
4)Roland PE,(1980) Forcal increase of cerebral blood flow during stereognotic testing in man . Arch Neurol, 33
5)HJ,Fruend (1984) The premotor syndrome in man : Evidence for innervation of proximal limb muscle. Exp Brain Res, 53

EFFECT OF THERAPEUTIC EXERCISE FOR THE VERTIGO WITH VESTIBULAR DISEQUILIBRIUM

○ Yasushi Uchiyama　　Department of Rehabilitation,
　 Koji Tokumasu　　　 Kitasato Institute Medical Center Hospital
　　　　　　　　　　　Arai 121-1 Kitamoto, Saitama, Japan 364

Introduction

The postural adjustments underlying good balance are the result of integration of afferent inputs, such as proprioceptive, visual, and vestibular inputs, into effective motor responses that minimize body sway[1,2]. Disorders involving any of these systems can cause disequilibrium. Peripheral vestibular disorders specially result in vertigo and frequently nausea and vomitting in addition to disequilibrium. Patients experience vertigo when moved rapidly with the head turned torsional nystagmus is induced.

A quantitative test relating to the functional performance of patients with vestibular disease is needed to evaluate improvement in vertigo and disequilibrium and to test the efficacy of training procedures. The authors have already focused on therapeutic exercise for vertigo, which led to the production of a scale of vertigo, and have described physical therapy management of vestibular disorders[3,4].

The purpose of this study was to analyze the relationship between the course of recovery from vertigo and therapeutic exercise for the disequilibrium.

Materials and Methods

Ten patients were referred to our hospital between August 1989 and March 1990 with peripheral vestibular disorder, including two with Meniere's disease, seven with benign paroxysmal positional vertigo, and one with delayed endolymphatic hydrops. They ranged in age from 39 to 75 (mean = 51.2). Five were male and five were female. Informed consent was obtained from all patients. To qualify for this study, subjects were required to have no history of central nervous system lesions.

Each patient was classified according to Tokumasu's scale for vertigo and body sway was measured when seated and standing. The vertigo scale was proposed by Tokumasu , a neuro-otologist, at the congress of the Japan Society for Equilibrium Research, the degree of impairment from the view point of nystagmus, vertigo, and symptoms of

Table : The scale of vertigo

V 8 : severe spontaneous vertigo, can not movement
V 6 : severe vertigo in provoking position
V 4 : vertigo at walking and/or standing, getting up
V 2 : vertigo when moved rapidly with the head turned
V 1 : vertigo feeling
V 0 : no symptom

N 2 : vomitting
N 1 : nausea and/or headache, neck pain
N 0 : no symptom

example; severe spontaneous vertigo and vomitting
V8 + N2 = 10
vertigo at walking and nausea
V4 + N1 = 5

the autonomic nervous system (Table) are taken into consideration.
Body sway is determined in the sitting position (sitting on a chair
without a back with the feet dangling without touching the floor), in
order to assess truncal equilibrium, and in the upright standing
position with feet kept 15 cm apart.   The measurement of sway was
performed with a system consisting of an Anima multicomponent force
measurement platform with a digital computer sampling at a rate of 20
Hz.   Center of pressure parameters, such as sway path, sway area,
mean displacement, and frequency analysis were measured over a 30
second period.
    Therapeutic exercise was performed combining visual, vestibular,
and proprioceptive stimuli administered by a physical therapist.
For the purpose of documentation of change of vertigo and equilibrium
function, the level of impairment was recorded at the onset of an
attack, at the start of physical therapy, and when the physical
therapy was finished.

Results
    All patients showed good recovery from vertigo after repeated
applications of the therapeutic exercise, and the scale of vertigo
also decreased (Fig. 1).   Subsequently, body equilibrium improved
significantly (Fig. 2).

Discussion
    The diagnosis of vestibular disease is usually made by a neuro-
otologist who would then refer the patient for physical therapy.   The
physical therapist should examine the patient to determine what
movement produce the vertigo and any balance problems associated with
activities of daily living[5].
    The results of this study indicate a recovery from vertigo, as

exemplified by the semicircular canals and ocular adapting, as a result of vestibular stimulation. Subsequently, body equilibrium also improves in term of proprioceptive and dynamic balance exercises.

The judgement as to the scale for vertigo is a simple, clinically applicable, semi-quantitative measure.

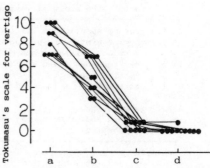

Figure 1 : Change of the scale of vertigo

a) at onset of an attack
b) at the start of physical therapy
c) at the finish of physical therapy
d) at follow up

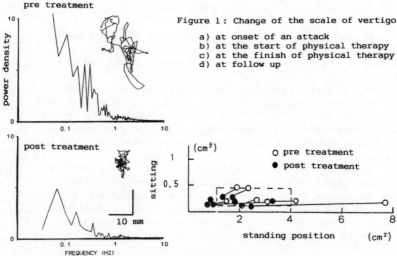

Figure 2 : Change of the sway area and frequency analysis

References

1) Chandler JM, Duncan PW, Studenski SA. Balance performance on the postural stress test:comparison of young adults, healthy elderly, and fallers. Phys Ther(70) 410-415, 1990.

2) Nashner LM, McCollum G. The organization of human postural movements: a formal basis and experimental synthesis. Behav Brain Sci(8) 135-172, 1985.

3) Tokumasu K. Rehabilitation for vertigo and disequilibrium. Jpn J. Otolaryng. Head and Neck Surgery (61) 257-264, 1989.

4) Uchiyama Y, Tokumasu K. Therapeutic Exercise for vertigo associated with vestibular disequilibrium. Equilibrium Res. (50), 1991.

5) Herdman SJ. Treatment of benign paroxymal positional vertigo. Phys Ther (70) 381-388, 1990.

LASER EVALUATION AND APPLICATION

LASER BIO-MODULATION IN PHYSIOTHERAPY

G. De Domenico
Electro-Physical Agents Laboratory, School of Physiotherapy,
Dalhousie University, Halifax, Nova Scotia, Canada.

Introduction In recent years, low-power laser energy has become widely used in Physiotherapy. In spite of its great popularity, it seems clear that there is great uncertainty with regard to the optimal use of the modality. The word **LASER** is an acronym for Light Amplification by Stimulated Emission of Radiation. But it is not 'Laser' that is given to the patient during these treatments. The term Laser describes a **process** used to produce light of a particular wavelength. Laser energy, is **light energy**.

Lasers are named after their **active medium**, this being the substance used to produce the lasing effect. This may be a gas such as Helium Neon (He Ne), a solid, for example a Ruby; or a semiconductor (Diode) such as Gallium Aluminium Arsenide (Ga Al As). In physiotherapy,the majority of lasers used are of the diode type, and most of these produce infrared energy. Laser energy is produced by electrical excitation of the atoms in the active medium to **emission levels**. This means that the atoms are excited to the point where electrons in their outer shells move to a higher orbit (atomic transitions). Energy is released whenever electrons fall back into a lower orbit. The 'packet' of energy released is known as a **photon**. The photons produced then collide with other electrons to continue the process. The world's first working laser (a Ruby laser) was reported by T.H. Maiman in 1960 [1].

In Physiotherapy, there are two main types of Laser device in common use. These are the gas and the diode Laser. In gas lasers, the beam may be directed directly onto the patients tissues, however in most cases, the beam of photons is directed using a fibre-optic cable. This type of cable produces a divergent beam at its end, due to the internal reflection that occurs along the cable. In the diode laser, the photons are given off in a divergent beam, directly from one end of the semiconductor material. The wavelength of most diode lasers is in the infrared range between about 770 and 1000 nm [1]. As with the gas laser, the divergent beam of the diode laser has important implications for dosage considerations when the probe is lifted off the skin surface.

Properties of Laser There are many properties of laser energy which are not relevant to their use in physiotherapy. In fact, it can be argued that the only property of lasers which is relevant to physiotherapy use, is the fact that the energy exists in a very narrow waveband of the electromagnetic spectrum. This is known as **monochromaticity** and is a function of the way in which the light energy is produced. The parallel property of the laser beam is a function of the **coherence** and **collimation** of the beam. These terms mean that the photons arrive at the target tissue in phase both temporally and spatially and that the beam is parallel. Those lasers in which the beam is parallel have implications for the industrial and medical (surgery) uses of laser energy. Once the laser beam has penetrated the skin surface the properties of collimation and coherence are lost because the tissues are not homogeneous.

Absorption and Penetration An area of concern with low-power laser use, is that of its absorption and penetration characteristics into human tissue. In general terms, the greater the absorption the less the penetration of an energy source; and vica versa. However, the most important criteria should be whether the energy is able to be absorbed in sufficient quantity, by the target tissues. Penetration is technically defined as the depth into the tissues at which 67% of the incident energy is absorbed by the tissues (or the depth at which 33% of the energy is left). Absorption on the other hand is dependant on the wavelength and frequency of the laser energy, and the absorption quality of the tissue i.e. certain tissues absorb laser energy more readily than others. In general, human skin absorbs more than 80% of laser energy within 3 to 4 mm.

Bio-Physical effects of Laser There are both **thermal** and **non-thermal** (**biological**) effects associated with laser produced energy. In order to produce significant thermal effects in human tissue, the average power of the laser must be greater than about 500 milliwatts. Since most physiotherapy lasers have an average power between 1 and 50 milliwatts, there are effectively no significant thermal effects. Of much greater interest to physiotherapists are the non-thermal (biological) effects. For the past fifteen years, there has been a great deal of interest in the biophysical effects of low-powered laser energy [2]. The physiological effects of laser energy have been extensively studied at cellular levels [2,3], however many of the mechanisms are not completely understood at the present time.

Although laser bio-modulation is surrounded by considerable controversy [4], it is not "magic". Even though many of the mechanisms are not fully understood, it seems reasonable to conclude that laser produced energy triggers cellular and possibly systemic effects, producing a facilitation of healing. Karu [2], suggests that the primary photoacceptor is the respiratory chain of the mitochondria. Energy absorbed here would increase cellular function This gives rise to the notion that laser energy can be used to both stimulate and inhibit cell function [2,4]. Indeed this is why the term 'laser bio-modulation' is preferable to the term 'laser bio-stimulation'. At the present time the clinical indications for laser treatment can be grouped into four main categories. These are: **Wound Healing, Recent Injuries, Pain Control and Arthritic Joints** [5,6,7,8]. These four categories of clinical applications of laser are not exhaustive, but they represent areas in which laser treatment has acquired some respectability.

Treatment Dosage The use of lasers in physiotherapy has been plagued by inconsistencies and controversy [9], particularly in regard to the the issue of dosage. The total energy delivered to the tissues is usually determined by controlling the exposure time. However, the average power and beam spot size are also important variables. Most diode lasers have an average power that varies widely, depending on the frequency of pulses. The formula required to determine the average power of a diode laser is as follows:
Average power (Watts)
  = **Frequency (Hz) x Pulse Width (sec) x Peak Power (W)**
For example, the average power of a laser with 1 watt of peak power and a 200 nanosecond pulse width, and frequency of 5000 Hz, is 1 milliwatt. Some diode lasers have a constant average power, regardless of frequency and do not require this formula.

Energy is quoted in Joules per sq. cm. (J/cm^2). Energy density, is the energy produced in a laser beam, per sec. The formula is given as:- **Energy Density** =

$$\frac{\textbf{Average Power (mW)}}{\textbf{Beam Spot Size (cm}^{-2}\textbf{)}} = mW / cm^2 / sec. = mJ / cm^2 = \textbf{J} / \textbf{cm}^2$$

In physiotherapy, doses of less than one Joule and up to 24 Joules per sq. cm. have been used. Unfortunately, at the present time there are no clear indications regarding the optimal dose required for specific clinical effects.

Energy Density at the Skin Surface   Since the tissues are not homogeneous, it is almost impossible to know with certainty, how much energy is being delivered to specific tissues under the skin. The exposure time required to deliver $1 \, J/cm^2$ is the main factor which needs to be known for any laser. The energy density of a laser with 2 mW of average power and beam spot size of $0.1 \, cm^{-2}$ is:-

$$= \frac{0.002}{0.1} = 20 \, mW / cm^2 / sec = 20 \, mJ / cm^2 = \mathbf{50 \ secs. \ to \ give} \ \mathbf{1 \, J / cm^2}$$

The energy density of a laser with a higher average power gives the same dose in a much shorter time. For example, the energy density at the skin surface, of a laser with 50 mW of average power, and beam spot size of $0.1 \, cm^{-2}$ is :-

$$= \frac{0.05}{0.1} = 0.5 \, W / cm^2 / sec = 0.5 \, J / cm^2 = \mathbf{2 \ secs. \ to \ give} \ \mathbf{1 \, J / cm^2}$$

Once the energy density of a laser probe is known, it is then possible to calculate how much energy is given to the patient during each treatment. In the future, research and clinical experience may indicate that a specific dose range is required to achieve certain clinical effects. If the exposure time for 1 Joule/cm^2 is known, then it is a simple matter to multiply or divide this figure to obtain the appropriate time. The most important information to give and locate in published reports, is the energy delivered to the tissues specified in J/cm^2. There is an urgent need for standardization of the way in which dosage is reported.

In Conclusion   Laser bio-modulation is rapidly expanding in physiotherapy. Whilst there is an ever increasing anecdotal clinical base for the use of lasers, there is still an urgent need for well controlled clinical studies. The most desirable features in a laser unit, are a high average power, large beam spot size, availability of probes with different wavelengths and high quality manufacture.

References
1. **Johnson J, Wojcikiewicz K** (1985) Laser Technology: An Individual Learning Course. Heathkit Educational Systems: Benton Harbour, Michigan.
2. **Karu T** (1989) Photobiology of low-power laser effects. Health Physics 56:691-704
3. **Young S, Bolton P, Dyson M, Harvey W, Diamantopoulos C** (1989) Macrophage responsiveness to light therapy. Lasers in Surgery and Medicine 9:497-505
4. **Basford JR** (1989) Low energy Laser therapy: Controversies and new research findings. Lasers in Surgery and Medicine 9:1-5
5. **Enwemeka CS** (1988) Laser biostimulation of healing wounds. Specific effects and mechanisms of action. Journal of Orthopaedic and Sports Physiotherapy 9:333-338
6. **Rochkind s, Rousso M, Nissan M, Villarreal M, Barr-Nea L, Rees D** (1989) Systemic effects of low-power laser irradiation on the peripheral and central nervous system , cutaneous wounds and burns. Lasers in Surgery and Medicine 9:174-182
7. **Harrison T** (1989) Laser acupuncture - A review. British Journal of Acupuncture 12,2:20-23
8. **Palmgren N, Jensen G, Kaae K, Windelin M, Colov H** (1989) Low-power laser therapy in rheumatoid arthritis. Lasers in Medical Science 4:193-196
9. **Enwemeka CS** (1990) Laser photostimulation. Clinical Management 10, 3::24-29

LASER-ACUPUNCTURE AND LASER-IRRADIATION IN PHYSICAL THERAPY

(Mrs.) W.E.Rodes-Bauer
Society for Soft Laser Research in Physical Therapy, Basel, Switzerland

Ladies and Gentlemen, dear Collegues,

My presentation will be structured as follows: First I'll give you a brief overview of the combination therapy I developed and practised now success-fully for 15 years in my institute. I will then deal briefly with the science of acupuncture. I will touch on different types of lasers and then give you a case history where laser-therapy was combined with physical therapy treatments and exercises.

The new combination therapy is based on some old precepts unfortunate-ly frequently neglected by current medical practitioners. They are: The concept of "total medicine" expressed in the old days as "body, mind, soul and will". -The need to treat the cause and not the symptom alone. - The recognition that the body of every living beeing has substantial innate recuperative capabili-ties, which can be stimulated by natural, non-chemical means. To this end Hypo-crates already built a natural solarium on the island of Kos, where length and strength of the exposure to sunlight could be controlled to some extent. From this follows, that a very thorough anamnesis, partially repeated at intervals throughout the treatment sessions, must preceed the diagnosis, which must be communicated to the patient in an understandable manner to strengthen his will to actively participate in his rehabilitation.

In combining acupuncture and Western school medicine we might be gui-ded by Julius Cesar's admonition: "Look into the past and you will gain much knowledge for the future".

Acupuncture is thousands of years old and usually defined as traditio-nal Chinese medicine. It is based both on a philosophy and on biological fac-tors, which have, in recent years been scientifically proven. The basic theory of the function of acupuncture is the so-called reestablishment of balance in the body and, to some extent, in the mind. The concept underlying traditional Chinese medicine is that of "total medicine" emphasizing prophylaxis. Under this concept the Chinese doctor was paid only as long as his charges were healthy, he received nothing when there were sick. A Chinese proverb says: A bad doctor heals an illness, a good doctor prevents it. It is wrong to believe that acu-puncture came to Europe fairly recently. We know that it was known and practised in Germany in the 13th century. A book showing Moxa type acupuncture, I'll ex-plain what this is in a moment, and explaining the indications treated, can be found in a museum in Munich. And, at the end of the 15th century Hyronimus Bosch, the Dutch painter, showed acupuncture with needles in his painting The Garden of Delights.

According to Chinese philosophy, energy, which is life, flows in and on the body along 12 imaginary axes called meridians. This flow passes numerous synapses called "points". These points are an accumulation of receptors and are connected to various organs and parts of the body. When these points are stimu-lated, a local reaction takes place and afferent reflexes are released to the spinal cord. They are then relayed to the thalamus from where they reach the telencephalon. From there they are influencing the organs or parts of the body connected to the points. Many points are connected to several parts of the body. This flowing energy is divided into a negative and a positive force called Yin and Yang. They correspond pretty much to our autonomic nervous system, to the parasympaticus and sympaticus. This energy flows in a certain rythm. When it is unimpeded, the sedative Yin and the tonic Yang are deemed in balance and the person is in a state of good health. When a trauma or illness occurs, the flow is impeded and the system is deemed to be unbalanced. Through stimulation of the acupuncture points the flow of energy is improved and the body balance reestablished. One of the most important effects of such stimulation is its impact on the spinal cord and the hypothalamus. In the dorsal horn system certain opioids are released and the hypothalamus causes an emission of endorphines. The production of endorphines interrupts the circulous vitiosus created by pain, muscle spasms, ischemia and irritation of nerves. It should be noted at this point, that Head's Zones, which lie along the bladder meridian, can be explained by this reaction. Similarly can be explained the reaction resulting from a stimulation of the connecting tissues. The interaction of the various acupuncture points is extremely complex and requires years of study and practice. The points can be stimulated by: the acupuncture needle of various lengths, the needle with an electrical charge, by neural therapy, by laser beam, by pressure resp. massage, by heat or cold application. In my opinion needle acupuncture and neural therapy should be practised by medical doctors only. The other means of stimulation should be employed by qualified physical therapists. A few minutes ago I mentioned stimulation of the acupuncture point by Moxa. The Chinese combine various herbs into a cigar-like bundle, which they light up and then hold the small fuming end over the point to be stimulated.

Before I turn to the laser, I would like briefly to mention auriculo-therapy. If you carefully look at a human ear, you can recognize the shape of a human embryo in the head-down position. All acupuncture points on the body are repeated in the ear. Ear acupuncture is effective more quickly than body acupuncture, because of the short distance from the ear to the brain. However, the effects of auriculo-therapy wear off quicker.

The word laser stands for Light Amplification by Stimulated Emission of Radiation. In popular terms: Laser light beams are parallel bundled light rays. More generally speaking, we can say that laser emission are coherent (i.e. uniformity of wave) monochromatic pure rays of light, in phase, with almost no divergence and very high brilliance at source. By brilliance is meant intensivity of energy at source. We differentiate between hard, mid, and soft lasers. Hard lasers, also called power lasers, use different means of bundling the rays. The results are light rays in different wave lengths of the spectrum. These lasers are used in surgery and, at very high frequences, in metallurgy. We use soft and mid-lasers, which are absolutely safe in use, except that they should not be directed into the eye for any length of time. For the stimulation of the acupuncture points and for irradiation we use soft lasers working with Helium-Neon gaz. They have a wave length of 632.8 nm. and, at the source, a diameter of 0.5 mm. The He-Ne lasers we use have a power output of 2mW and 6 mW. We use them with a continuous emission. Lower power output has a greater effect on chronic conditions. Higher output has a greater effect on acute conditions. The He-Ne laser beam has an average penetration of 1-2 cm. For deeper penetration in acupuncture of up to 5 cm as well as for irriadiation to improve circulation, especially locally and for quick relaxation of muscles we use a diode mid-laser.

It operates with GaAS   and emits at a wave length of 904 nm with a frequency of 200 nsec and an output 8W.

And now to the practical side: Some basic considerations of the combination therapy are: we know that swelling, tension, pain and spasms in the locomotorium and psychic conditions frequently hinder rehabilitation exercises. On the other hand we find among the effects of acupuncture: suppression of pain, improvement of the circulation, reduction of spasms and of inflammation and a balancing influence on the psychic condition. Irradiation furthers circulation locally and penetrates the bone. It reduces hematoma quickly, relaxes muscle tension and reduces inflammation locally.

The combination therapy usually consists of one or several of the following treatments: Laser-acupuncture and/or irradiation, application of heat or ice, massage, extension, PNF (Proprioceptive, Neuromuscular Facilitation technique) or Bobath or Vojta.

Among the indications treated successfully sofar, were: Cervical syndrome, brachialgia, migraine, torticollis, lumbago, siatic, PHS, tennis elbow, tendinitis, Cox-arthrosis, Gon-arthrosis, various types of fractures, asthma, bronchiectasis, emphysema, hemiplegia, and other cerebral insults.

Before giving you a case history, I'd like to tell you that some years ago, being fed up with hearing that the good results of our work were largely due to the placebo effect, I started to treat animals and experienced the same results. For instance, I treated horses for tendinitis, dogs for sciatic and cats for bronchial asthma.

Now I'd like to present a brief case history of a typical combination treatment. A 69 year old patient suffered a complicated fracture of the tibia and fibula in the lower right leg in an automobilie accident. The accident occurred on April 30th 1988, the osteotomy was performed on May 10th 1988. 16 screws were required and spongiosa from the spina iliaca was introduced into the f_acture. Immediately after the operation the following treatment was administered daily during 4 months: ice application, acupuncture, irradiation, massage, PNF. In view of the patients age and his condition resulting from an almost fatal accident 4 months prior to this one, the prediction after the successful operation was: healing of the fracture not before 10 months. In fact the fracture was closed 4 months after the operation. A year later the screws were removed and irradiation with the IR-diode laser was continued. Contrary to the expectations based on experience, the screw perforations of the bone began to fill slowly and close during the following one and a half years.

LASER-INDUCED CHANGES IN ARRHYTHMOGENESIS

V A Bobrov, V N Zalessky, E V Bobrova

Kavetsky Institute of Oncology Problems
Academy of Science Ukrainian SSR, Kiev,
*Strazhesko Research Institute of Cardiology, Kiev, USSR

The antitachiarrhythmic and autonomic nervous system stabilizating activities of laser-puncture (LP) were evaluated on the background of the basic (beta-blockers, etc) therapy in 98 patients with paroxysmal supraventricular tachycardia (PST). The monitoring used consisted of M-echocardiography, transesophageal ECG and Holter analysis (for hemodynamical and electro-physiological mechanisms of paroxysmal triggering), the LOBI-test (for psychological dysfunctions), the analysis of heart rate fluctuation (for autonomic nervous system dysfunctions). The alternating application of physical therapy - LP (He-Ne laser beam, 632.8 nm, c/w, multimode, $3-10 \times 10^{-3}$ W) and propranolol (Pr) (a half of the conventional dosage) resulted in reducing both PST events on set number and length ($P < 0.05$) so as in lowering of the rate of ventricular contractions frequency ($P < 0.002$).

Laserpuncture coupled with Pr was shown to provide control of tachiarrhythmia onset in patients with paroxysmal supraventricular tachycardia with concurrent LR produced a suppression of sympathetic effects of the mild beta-blocking type.

HELIUM-NEON LASER EFFECTS ON REGENERATION OF THE PERONEAL NERVE

G.F. Hamilton, T.K. Robinson, and R.H. Ray
Dept. of Physical Therapy, School of Allied Health Sciences, East
Carolina University, Greenville, NC, 27858, USA

Peripheral nerve injuries are prevalent problems in our society and frequently present a major challenge to health care providers. Nerve injury causes disruption of normal function, and when healing time is protracted, can result in major loss of extremity function and in some cases, gross deformity. If a physical therapeutic procedure was available which facilitated nerve healing and regenerative process, it would greatly enhance the contributions of physical therapists to the rehabilitation of the peripheral nerve injured patient.

Within the past decade, several studies have been conducted showing the efficacy of the Helium-Neon (HE-NE) laser on multiple areas of tissue function. Mester reported increased tensile strength, accelerated healing of burns, increased phagocytic activity of leukocytes, and increased collagen synthesis in animals.(1) Bostra, et al, demonstrated that a positive effect of the laser on wound healing existed by stimulating the secretion of fibroblasts in injured tissue.(2) Wolbarsht has shown that the morphophysiological state of nerve cells can be influenced by the radiation from a continuous HE-NE laser of low power. Experiments by Rakhishev and Tsoi, reported in Wobarsht demonstrated accelerated growth of somatic nerves with exposure to HE-NE laser radiation.(3) Walker and Akhanjee believe the peripheral nervous system possesses a previously unsuspected degree of photo sensitivity which may provide a rationale for the therapeutic applications of low power laser.(4) Although laser effects were not examined, Creager showed that regeneration of nerve axons occurred when the Nissel substance of the cell body synthesized protein for the repair of the damaged axons.(5) Rochkind, et al, conducted several studies examining the effect of low energy laser irradiation (LELI) on crush injuries of the sciatic nerve in rats. They reported significantly higher evoked action potentials in the treated limb, a contralateral limb effect, and that a 4-day delay in initiating laser treatment was less effective than if begun immediately following injury.(6-8) Additionally, in 1989 they reported a long term study of HE-NE irradiation applied 7 minutes daily for 20 days reduced the drop in nerve action potential, accelerated regeneration, increased vascularization of the nerve and that spinal cord irradiation diminished degeneration of the motor neuron.(9)

The purpose of this study was to examine the effect of clinical intensity low level laser irradiation upon healing in the crushed peroneal nerve of rabbits, as determined by alteration in amplitude of evoked action potentials across a surgically induced lesion.

METHOD

Following surgical preparation, peroneal nerves in both hind limbs

of 12 rabbits were crushed. The randomly assigned limb received 15 daily
laser treatments at 632.8 nM, applied at 1 mW to 6 points on a grid overlying the nerve for a dosage density of 3.82 J/sq.cm. per point and total
treatment to the area of 22.91 J/sq.cm. The other limb served as control.
Prior to nerve crush, and every third day thereafter, peroneal nerve conduction measurements were performed across the lesion in all limbs.

RESULTS

A split-plot ANOVA using the evoked compound action potentials
demonstrated a significant interaction ($p < .01$), indicating a different
pattern of recovery in treated compared to control limbs. Average
recovery 15 days following lesion was 67% for treated and 52% for control
limbs.

DISCUSSION

The results of this study demonstrated that treated and control limbs
of the rabbits responded differently over the 15 days of the experiment,
most probably due to a facilitative effect of Helium-Neon laser irradiation upon repair of the lesioned rabbit peroneal nerves.
    Critical review of the mean amplitude of evoked compound action
potentials from control and treated animals across the duration of the
study demonstrated an initial decline in amplitude, which reached its
lowest level on day three. This decline may have been attributed to edema
at the site of lesion or interruption of blood supply to fibers not
directly demaged by the nerve compression, resulting in the neuropraxic
response. From that point, the laser treated group had a more rapid
progression in recovery to day 15, at which time the amplitude of the
evoked electrical response between treated and control limbs was significant at the $p = .046$ level. Behavioral observations, such as reduction
in drop-foot, were consistent with the recovery in conduction amplitude.
    Various theories for the physiological effects of laser have been
advanced. Thermal effects were ruled out in this study since no rise in
temperature was found after 5 minutes of constant maximum radiation to
tissue directly overlying an implanted perineural thermal probe. No data
was produced to examine theories related to ATP or mitochondrial activity.
Taking into account the work of Creager, Mester and Rochkind, it is possible that greater increase in evoked potential amplitude of the laser
treated group was due to a facilitative effect on vascularization and
collagen synthesis. However, further studies are needed to critically
examine these theories.

CONCLUSION

The results of our study provide additional support for the utilization of low intensity laser irradiation to neural tissue in the presence
of neuropraxia. It was found the treated nerves showed an average
recovery of 67% of pre-lesion levels of conduction amplitude, whereas the
control group showed a 52% recovery 15 days post lesion. Although
theories exist to provide a rationale in support of its therapeutic
effect, the mechanism by which laser radiation influences tissue repair

is not well understood and deserves further research.

REFERENCES

1. Mester E, Spiry T, Szende B, Tota JG (1971) Effects of laser rays on
    wound healing. American Journal of Surgery, 122:532-535
2. Bostra K, Jucci A, Olliaro P, Quacci D, Sacchi S (1984) In Vitro
    fibroblast activation by laser irradiation at low energy: An
    electron microscopic study. Dermatologica 168:157-162
3. Wolbarsht ML, ed. (1983) Laser Applications in Medicine and Biology.
    New York, Plenum Press 3:76-126,234
4. Walker JB, Akhanjee LK (1985) Laser induced somatosensory evoked
    potentials: Evidence of photosensitivity in peripheral nerves.
    Brain Research 344:281-285
5. Creager J (1983) Human Anatomy and Physiology. Belmont, California:
    Wadsworth Publishing Co., 121
6. Rochkind S, Nissan M, Raxon N, Gartal A (1986) Electrophysiological
    effect of He-Ne laser on normal and injured sciatic nerve in the rat.
    ACTA Neurochirurgica 83:441-443
7. Rochkind S, Nissan M, Barrnea L, Raxon N, Schwartz M, Bartal A (1987)
    Response of peripheral nerve to HE-NE laser: Experimental studies.
    Lasers in Surgery and Medicine 7:441-443
8. Rochkind S, Barrnea L, Raxon N, Bartal A, Schwartz M (1987)
    Stimulatory effect of He-Ne low dose laser on injured sciatic nerves
    in rats. Neurosurgery 20:6, 843-847
9. Rochkind S, Russo M, Nissan M, Villarreal M, Barrnea L, Rees DG
    (1989) Systemic effects of low-power irradiation of the peripheral
    and central nervous system, cutaneous wounds and burns. Lasers in
    Surgery and Medicine 9:174-182

THE EFFECT OF PULSE REPETITION RATE IN LOW LEVEL LASER THERAPY
ON HUMAN PERIPHERAL BLOOD FLOW

D. Martin, J. Ravey, P McCoy, J Allen, & A. J. Bell.
Dept Occupational Therapy & Physiotherapy, Biomedical Sciences
Research Centre, University of Ulster, BT37 OQB, N Ireland

Introduction

Despite lack of clear information on the effects of Low Level
Laser Therapy (LLLT) physiotherapists are frequently using
this modality. This paper reports the findings of part of an
ongoing project which is investigating the effects of LLLT on
blood flow in humans.

Background

LLLT is widely used to promote tissue healing [1]. It has been
suggested that such effects may be mediated via the
circulatory system [2]. Blood flow in rat skin flaps was found
to increase following low intensity laser irradiation [3].
LLLT was also reported to increase blood flow in human cases
of vasomotor rhinitis [4] and mandibular fractures [5]. Other
studies using human subjects have suggested that LLLT causes
blood flow to increase in normal tissue [5,6]. These studies,
have suggested a laser induced increase in cutaneous blood
flow. This study proposes to investigate the effect of LLLT
on blood flow in normal deep skeletal muscle as a possible
explanation for the reduction of healing time in such a
tissue.

A secondary purpose of this study is to investigate if the
parameter of Pulse Repetition Rate (PRR) is important in
producing any changes in blood flow.

Methods

Subjects

24 healthy female volunteers, aged between 18-25 years were
recruited from within the University. All were informed of
the experimental procedure and signed a consent form. This
study was approved by the University Ethical Committee.

Procedure

A between groups experimental design was used with the
subjects randomly allocated into four groups, 6 per group.
The four groups were as follows - control (no laser); 20 mins

laser irradiation, PRR = 2.28Hz; 20 mins laser irradiation, PRR = 36.48Hz; 20 mins laser irradiation, PRR = 5000Hz.

The laser used was an Omega Technologies Biotherapy 3ML unit with a 31 diode cluster head (10 x 660nm + 10 x 950nm + 10 x 880 nm + 1 x 820 nm). This delivers a total incident power of 600 mW across a 12 sq.cm area. Laser was applied to the lateral aspect of the gastrocnemius bulk just distal to the knee joint. A non-contact technique of application was used to apply laser, as mechanical pressure on the muscle was found to interfere with blood flow. The distance between the laser and the leg was standardised at 1mm using a mechanical apparatus. The "beep" on the laser was turned off so that the subjects were unaware when laser was applied. Both subject and operator wore protective goggles.

Blood flow was measured using the technique of Strain Gauge Plethysmography. When used on the calf area this technique measures skeletal muscle blood flow [7] .

The subjects, having not exercised for at least 1 hour beforehand, lay in the supine position with the right leg bared. The leg was supported mechanically in a position of elevation just above the heart level with the knee in slight flexion. Throughout the procedure the subjects were told to maintain silence and remain still.

The subjects lay in this position for 10 minutes before measurements began. Five readings were used - 4 mins before laser (X); 2 mins before laser (A); after 10 mins irradiation (B); after 20 mins irradiation (C); 15 mins after the cessation of irradiation (D).

Results

The last four readings (A,B,C & D) were standardised as differences from the first reading (X). These difference scores (X-A; X-B; X-C; X-D) were analysed using a 2-way Analysis of Variance. The means, standard deviations (SD) and the standard errors of the means (SEM) are summarised in Table 1 and shown graphically in Fig. 1. The only statistically significant changes in blood flow were found in the 36.48 Hz group. Blood flow decreased after 10 mins irradiation ($p < 0.05$) and maintained at this level 15 mins after irradiation had ceased.

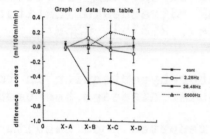

Summary Table of Means SDs & SEMs for difference scores

condition		difference scores (ml/100ml/min)			
		X-A	X-B	X-C	X-D
control	MEAN	0.00	0.02	0.00	0.02
	SD	0.06	0.04	0.00	0.04
	SEM	0.03	0.02	0.00	0.02
2.28Hz	MEAN	-0.02	0.12	-0.04	-0.08
	SD	0.08	0.38	0.30	0.30
	SEM	0.03	0.15	0.12	0.12
36.48Hz	MEAN	0.04	-0.48	-0.46	-0.56
	SD	0.09	0.55	0.30	0.64
	SEM	0.03	0.22	0.12	0.26
5000Hz	MEAN	0.00	0.00	0.21	0.14
	SD	0.00	0.23	0.36	0.24
	SEM	0.00	0.09	0.15	0.10

TABLE 1

Graph of data from table 1

Discussion

From these results it would appear that LLLT can influence skeletal muscle blood flow in humans. Why this is so is unclear and requires further investigation. From a therapeutic view, these changes in blood flow are small and their value questionable. However, more research is required to investigate any later effects. Most interestingly, this study suggests that PRR is an important parameter in LLLT. Again, more research is required into this aspect of LLLT.

References

1. BASFORD J R (1989). Lasers in Surgery and Medicine 9:1-5
2. GUBBIOTTI A (1984). Quadermia Dislaserterapia Notebook 1: 11-19
3. KAMI T, YOSHIMURA Y, NAKAJIMA T, et al (1985). Annals of Plastic Surgery 14:278-83
4. FILATOV V F & KALASHMIK M U (1986). Oto-Rino Laringologi Moskua 6:63-6
5. KATZ A (1987). Stomatologia Mosk 66:38-41.
6. DU RANN T, COETZEE S M, MOELICH M, et al (1988). South African Journal of Physiotherapy 44(3): 69-72
7. KEMPCZINSKI R F (1987) Practical non-invasive vascular diagnosis 2nd Ed. Tear Book Medical Publishers, Inc. Chicago, London.

ANTIHYPERTENSIVE ACTIVITY OF LASER BIOSTIMULATION THERAPY

V.N.Zalessky, V.I.Gordienko, V.A.Bobrov*

Kavetsky Institute of Oncology Problems, Kiev, 252127, USSR *Strazhesko Institute of Cardiology, Kiev, 252151, USSR

The role of risk factor-hypertension in the development of cardiovascular diseases has been emphasized in recent years.

Proceeding from the reported good results obtained in the course of treating early hypertension with physical therapy (traditional and laser acupuncture), the authors have subjected a group of 60 patients in the initial stage of the disease to laser biostimulation therapy (632.8 nm, 12 mW) in the following acupuncture points: H-7; Li-4; GV-6,7; S-36; SP-6 for 20 sec per point. The level of the patients' blood pressure was followed-up before and after the procedure (on the 10 and the 20 min). The course of treatment consisted of 12 procedures. All the patients were subjected to neurologic and somatic examinations prior to and after the treatment. The renal etiology of the disease was excluded. The changes in the prostaglandine levels (E-total, E_2)and thermographyc parameters of the patients induced by the treatment were recorded as well.

On the basis of the results obtained the authors recommend LBT as an effective part of hypertensive control programme.

SPINAL INJURIES

THE TEAM APPROACH FOR THE TREATMENT OF THE ACUTE SPINAL CORD INJURED
PATIENT IN THE INTENSIVE CARE UNIT

ME RINEHART, THOMAS JEFFERSON UNIVERSITY, DEPARTMENT OF PHYSICAL THERAPY,
130 SOUTH 9th STREET, SUITE 830 EDISON, PHILADELPHIA, PENNSYLVANIA, 19107

The individual who sustains a spinal cord injury (SCI) is
usually admitted to the intensive care unit (ICU) of an acute care
medical center. The ICU is the site of initial medical management
which typically is within the practice domain of the physician
and nurse. In the usual sense, routine rehabilitative management
is not initiated in the ICU. Guttman (1976) and Donovan (1984)
have stressed the importance of comprehensive care for the SCI
patient at the stage of initial ICU treatment.

Comprehensive rehabilitative care is essential for early
management of SCI. The rehabilitation team model (Rinehart, 1990)
is appropriate for use in the ICU. The team model supports the
concept of early management to optimize patient function. The
members of the rehabilitation team include: physicians (i.e.
neurosurgeons, orthopedic surgeon, physiatrists, internal medicine,
and etc.) nurses, physical therapists, occupational therapists,
social workers, psychologists, speech pathologists and respiratory
therapists.

TEAM DEVELOPMENT

The concepts of team development (Given, 1977) helps the
members to understand their role in patient management. Occasionally
traditional roles may overlap causing some minor irritation. The
concepts of team development and maintenance should be emphasized
at regular time intervals. The team should:
- Maintain effective communication systems
- Develop and maintain new approaches to problem-solving
- Accept differences of opinions
- Maintain tolerance of preconceived notions about
  emphasized roles
- Understand the perceived limitations of each professional
  and their discipline
- Maintain the goals of the patient's rehabilitation as
  the end-point and not a discipline specific ideology
- Establish and maintain weekly team care conferences

EVALUATION AND TREATMENT IN THE INTENSIVE CARE UNIT

Recognizing the important role of all team members in the rehabilitation effort, this presentation will focus on three health professions during the initial rehabilitation stage. The role of the nurse, physical therapist and occupational therapist in early rehabilitation will be discussed in detail. An evaluation of the patient is the first step in the rehabilitation process. The evaluation and assessment should include observation and testing of the neurological status, cardiopulmonary function, skin integrity and psychological status. If the team members coordinate their efforts, the tests will not have to be repeated as often and the expertise of each team member can be utilized. For instance, therapists have expertise in muscle testing and can help nurses become more proficient when performing the tests. Therapists participate in the nursing orientation course for the critical care unit at the Regional Spinal Cord Injury Center. They teach nurses how to perform more specific muscle tests and how to perform range of motion.

When establishing a treatment program in the ICU it is helpful to maintain open and on-going communication between the nurses, physical therapists and occupational therapists since the ICU is their domain. Some ways to maintain a good rapport with the nurses include:
° Review your goals so you both understand the outcomes you are working toward
° Establish a therapy schedule with the nurse, which is convenient for both team members
° Talk with the nurse on a daily basis about the care and progress of the patient
° Ask the nurse to demonstrate special treatments or procedures used in caring for the patient
° Establish approaches to treatment that facilitate the completion of each other's tasks (Rinehart, 1990)
° Assist with transfers or positioning of the patient
° Share the patient's reactions to treatment
° Be aware of the "atmosphere" in the ICU - is it short-staffed or is there a high census of complicated/time consuming patients
° Let the nurse know the therapist's limitations, both time and ability to proved equipment for the patient

When the daily schedule has been established treatment can be instituted. The treatment in the ICU consists of muscle strengthening, range of motion exercises, respiratory therapy and exercises, patient education and preparation for mobilization out of bed. If the patient is able, training for activities of daily living can be started.

SUMMARY

Comprehensive care of the spinal cord injured patient requires a team effort. The appreciation of each team member's contribution for the care and treatment of the spinal cord injured patient is enhanced using this model. Strategies to provide optimal patient care through the rehabilitation team model promotes the process of team development.

References

1. Donovan WH, Carter RE, Bedbrook GM, et al (1984) Incidence of medical complications in spinal cord injury: patients in specialized compared with non-specialized centers. Paraplegia 22:282-290

2. Given B, Simmons S, (1971) The interdisciplinary health-care team. Nur For 16:165-184

3. Guttman L, (1976) Spinal Cord Injuries - Comprehensive management and research. Oxford, Blackwell Scientific Publications, 22-47

4. Rinehart ME, (1990) Early mobilization in acute spinal cord injury: a collaborative approach. Critical Care Nursing Clinics of North America 2:399-405

This paper was supported in part by The National Institute on Disability and Rehabilitation Research, Department of Education, Washington, D.C. through the Regional Spinal Cord Injury Center of Delaware Valley, Philadelphia, PA. Grant #H133N0027

ENERGY CONSUPTION IN PARAPLEGICS WALKING

R. Puricelli*, S. Miglierina*, M. Lusvardi°
                                    M. Divani°
* Varese Hospital - Varese - Italy
° Officine Ortopediche Rizzoli S.p.A. - Bologna
  Italy

Energy consumption in 17 paraplegics with lesion level between T3 and L2 has been studied using a new measuring device. The instruments is named "COSMED K2" and measures, besides the oxigen consumption, other interesting parameters. The patients wore the Vannini-Rizzoli Stabilizing Lower Limb Orthoses, an orthosis shaped as a boot, that allow them to stand without any support and to walk using a walking frame. The patients have been evaluated in three different conditions: resting, standing and walking and the results have been compared to an healthy group. In every condition only the data related to the steady state have been considered. During walking the energy consumption for paraplegics has been 53.5 cal/min/kg verse 82.9 in the healthy group. The cost is obviously bigger. This is due to the slowness of walking in paraplegics, performed with swinging movements of the lower limbs. Other patients, using different orthoses, have been tested with the same methodology. The res' its seem to indicate that walking with the V-R.S.L.L.O. is a good energy saving rehabilitative therapy.

VENTILATORY DYSFUNCTION AND RESPIRATORY REHABILITATION IN POST TRAUMATIC
TETRAPLEGIA

Dr P Gounden
Department of Physiotherapy, University of Durban-Westville and King Edward VIII
Hospital.

INTRODUCTION

The neuromuscular respiratory insufficiency in tetraplegia is secondary to paralysis of the
intercostal and abdominal muscles [1,2,3,4].

The expiratory muscle force is reduced to less than 40 per cent of its normal values causing
a serious impairment in the patient's ability to cough [4,5,6]. Vital capacity has been shown
to drop to levels less than 50 per cent of its normal values [7,8,9]. These factors are
closely associated with the incidence of hypostatic pneumonia which has been shown to be one
of the leading causes of death in tetraplegia [10,11,12].

The existing protocol for pulmonary care in tetraplegia is one of carer and therapist
orientation with very little patient involvement. In order to allow the tetraplegic the
opportunity to develop his respiratory capacity to optimal levels there must be a shift of
responsibility from carer to patient. This could be accomplished with the aid of a specific
training programme involving progressive resistive loading on accessory expiratory muscles
in tetraplegics with low cervical cord lesions.

PRELIMINARY STUDY

Electromyographic (EMG) examination of the clavicular part of pectoralis major during active
expiration in ten patients showed increased phasic activity while the patient was tested in
supine. The increase in phasic EMG activity occurred simultaneously with resisted expiration as shown in Fig (1). This showed that the expiratory function of the clavicular part
of the pectoralis major to be posture dependent Fig. (1).

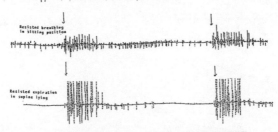

FIGURE 1 : PHASIC MOTOR UNIT ACTIVITY IN THE CLAVICULAR PART OF THE PECTORALIS MAJOR
MUSCLE DURING REST AND DURING FORCED RESISTED EXPIRATION WITH THE SUBJECT
IN SITTING AND IN THE LYING POSITION

PROGRESSIVE RESISTIVE LOADING ON ACCESSORY EXPIRATORY MUSCLES IN TETRAPLEGIA

METHOD:

To investigate the effects of progressive resistive loading on accessory expiratory muscles
in tetraplegia, 40 such patients undergoing standard pulmonary rehabilitation were randomly
assigned to control (n = 20) and experimental (n =20) groups. The latter consisted of eight

females and 32 males with an average age of 31 years. Their lesions were between the fifth and eight cervical segments. The majority of the patients sustained their injury during motor vehicle accidents.

Prior to training, measurements of maximum expiratory mouth pressure and vital capacity were obtained from each group. The experimental group underwent eight weeks of training. The training involved the use of the PFLEX muscle trainer which allowed the patient to expire against a predetermined resistance. The initial resistive load was set at a level equivalent to 60 per cent of the patient's maximum expiratory mouth pressure. Each subject was required to train for half an hour each day for six days a week. The resistive load was increased at two weekly intervals to ensure optimal loading throughout the training period.

The control group was excluded from any form of strenuous training, but continued with the standard pulmonary care which involved conventional breathing exercises and assistance in coughing.

RESULTS: (Fig. 2 and 3).

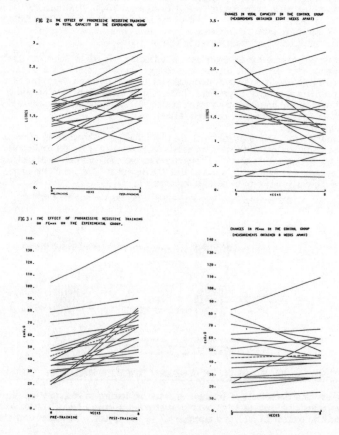

FIG 2: THE EFFECT OF PROGRESSIVE RESISTIVE TRAINING ON VITAL CAPACITY IN THE EXPERIMENTAL GROUP

CHANGES IN VITAL CAPACITY IN THE CONTROL GROUP (MEASUREMENTS OBTAINED EIGHT WEEKS APART)

FIG 3: THE EFFECT OF PROGRESSIVE RESISTIVE TRAINING ON PEmax ON THE EXPERIMENTAL GROUP.

CHANGES IN PEmax IN THE CONTROL GROUP (MEASUREMENTS OBTAINED 8 WEEKS APART)

The eight weeks course of progressive resistive loading on accessory expiratory muscles showed a significant improvement in vital capacity (p = 0,0001; pre-mean 1.48; post-mean 1.98) and a dramatic improvement in expiratory muscle strength (p = 0,001; pre-mean 43.76, post-mean 68) Fig. (2,3). Comparison of the values in the control group which were obtained eight weeks apart, showed no significant changes.

DISCUSSION:

The significant improvement in accessory expiratory muscle strength as represented by the increase in maximum expiratory mouth pressures could be attributed to several factors:

(i) An improvement which could be due to muscle fibre hypertrophy.

(ii) The threshold of training stimulus might have initiated the recruitment of a larger portion of the partially innervated muscles.

(iii) Beside the known accessory expiratory muscles, the serratus anterior muscle as well as other upper thoracic muscle (spared by the lesion) may also have a role in the mechanism of active expiration in tetraplegia. The training stimulus might have recruited active contraction in these muscles.

The study also showed that effective strength training should involve the use of near maximal resistances throughout the allotted training period. Clinical evidence showed enhancement in the patient's ability to cough.

REFERENCES:

1. McCagg C. Post-operative management and acute rehabilitation of patients with spinal cord injuries. Orthop Clin Norm Am (1986); 17(1):171-182.

2. Massery M. An innovative approach to assistive cough techniques. Top Acute Care Trauma Rehabil. 1987; 1(3):73-85.

3. Carter RE. Respiratory aspects of spinal cord injury management. Paraplegia (1987); 25:262-266.

4. Fugl-Meyer AR. Effects of respiratory muscle paralysis in tetraplegic and paraplegic patients. Scand J Rehab Med 1971; 3:141-150.

5. Axen K, Pineda H, Shunfenthal H, Haas F. Diaphragmatic function following cervical cord injury. Arch Phys Med Rehabilitation (1985); 66:219-222.

6. Momichan JC, Mitchel L, Westbrook PR. Pulmonary dysfunction following traumatic quadriplegia, recognition, prevention and treatment. JAMA (1980); 243:528-531.

7. Haas F, Axen K, Pineda H, Gandino D, Haas A. Temporal pulmonary function changes in cervical cord injury. Arch Phys Med Rehabil (1985); 66:139-144.

8. Guttman L, Silver J. Electromyographic studies on reflex activity of the intercostal and abdominal muscles in cervical cord lesion. Paraplegia (1965); 3:1.

9. Estenne M, De Troyer A. Relationship between respiratory muscle electromyogram and rib cage motion in tetraplegia. Am Rev Respir Dis (1985); 134:53-59.

10. De Troyer A, Estenne M, Heilporn A. Mechanism of an active expiration in tetraplegic subjects. N Engl J Med (1986); 314(12):740-744.

11. McMichan JC, Michel L, Westbrook PR. Pulmonary dysfunction following traumatic quadriplegia: recognition, prevention and treatment, JAMA (1980); 243:528-531.

12. Ledsome JR,, Sharp JM. Pulmonary function in acute cervical cord injury. Am Rev Respir Dis (1981); 124:41-44.

THE USE OF THE FLEXION WITHDRAWAL REFLEX IN SPINAL CORD INJURED PATIENTS

A. C. B Smith, M. H. Granat, B. J. Andrews.
Bioengineering Unit, University of Strathclyde, Glasgow, Scotland.

INTRODUCTION

The flexion withdrawal reflex (FWR) is a polysynaptic spinal reflex evoked by nociceptive stimuli. It may be elicited by mechanical or electrical stimulation at various sites on the lower limb. The reflex is a primitive protective mechanism enabling a rapid withdrawal from danger by producing flexion of the hip and knee, and dorsiflexion of the ankle. Functional movements can be produced by means of this reflex, and have been utilised for gait in lower limb Functional Electrical Stimulation (FES) systems. The use of FES for gait was first proposed by Liberson in 1961 [1] for hemiplegic subjects, and later applied to paraplegic subjects by Krajl [2]. In these applications the swing phase of gait was produced by eliciting the FWR at the site of the common peroneal nerve. FES has been shown to have a greater potential in incomplete spinal cord injury (ISCI) subjects than complete spinal cord injury subjects [3]. Previous studies in the value of FES for ISCI subjects have demonstrated the use of the FWR in gait [4] but have not evaluated any therapeutic effects, or reported any additional increase in mobility as a result of using FES. As the proportion of ISCI patients presenting to spinal injury units is steadily increasing [5] it is important to identify rehabilitation techniques which will be of value to this group of patients.

The aim of this paper is to demonstrate the therapeutic and functional value of the FWR elicited by FES during gait in a group of ISCI subjects.

MATERIALS AND METHODS

Six patients who had sustained an incomplete lesion of the spinal cord were selected. Patient details are given in table 1. All had completed a standard post-injury rehabilitation programme and were capable of varying degrees of ambulation in orthoses. An individualised FES gait system was devised for each patient in which the FWR was elicited bilaterally in subjects C, E and F, on the right leg for subjects A, B and D. A stimulator was used daily at home by each subject for approximately six months.

Table 1. PATIENT DETAILS.

PATIENT	AGE	YEARS POST INJURY	LESION OF SPINAL CORD	MOBILITY AIDS % time using wheelchair
A	20	2	C4 incomplete	R. AFO No wheelchair
B	31	10	L1 incomplete	R. AFO No wheelchair
C	35	4	T12 incomplete	2 AFO's Wheelchair 90%
D	35	18	C3/4 incomplete	R. AFO Wheelchair 10%
E	40	5	T6 incomplete	2 KAFO's Wheelchair 100%
F	27	5	T12 motor complete	2 KAFO's Wheelchair 100%

Tests to evaluate the outcome of the FES gait programme were carried out at the commencement of the programme and at the end of the FES gait phase. These were:

a) **Muscle strength tests (MST):-** All lower limb muscle groups were evaluated by the same physiotherapist using the Oxford Scale of muscle strength.

b) **Performance of gait:-** At the end of the FES gait programme temporal and spacial gait parameters and heart rate were measured during gait using either the subjects' normal orthoses or using FES. The gait test were performed on five separate occasions with each form of orthoses. The physiological cost of gait was quantified using the Physiological Cost Index (PCI) [7]. This is the ratio of the increase in heart rate at the end of walking to walking speed.

c) **Activities of Daily Living (ADL):-** The modified Barthel Index [8] was used to evaluate the degree of independence in areas of mobility and self care.

d) **Subjective assessment:-** A history was taken of each individual's degree of mobility. This comprised their maximum walking distance, ability to negotiate kerbs and stairs, and problems of access, with their consequent restrictions to daily life.

RESULTS

Measured parameters:- The MST results were analysed using the Wilcoxon matched-pairs sign ranks test; each muscle group was evaluated separately. Results of the hip flexors are shown in Figure 1. There was a significant increase in the strength of the hip flexors (p < 0.05) for the group as a whole. Individually, bilateral increase in hip flexor strength was seen in subjects A, B, C and E. A two-tailed independent t-test was used for the gait parameters with a significance level of 0.05. There was no significant change in the PCI for the group as a whole. Subject B had an increase in stride length using the FWR, but there was no change in stride length for the group as a whole. Subject E scored an increase in the category of mobility in The Barthel Index.

Fig (i). OXFORD SCALE GRADINGS OF HIP FLEXORS PRE AND POST USE OF FWR

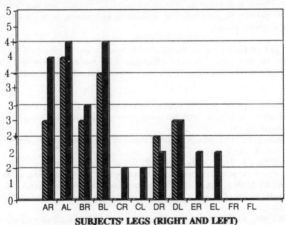

SUBJECTS' LEGS (RIGHT AND LEFT)

Mobility: In all except subject B, some value in walking using the FWR was derived, however, there were varying degrees of functional benefit. For subjects C and D the benefits were not sufficient to outweigh some of the technical disadvantages of the system. Subject A was able, using the FWR, to use both legs to initiate a step when negotiating stairs, where previously he could only do so with his left leg. He reported that his maximum walking distance increased when using FES and that gait was less tiring. Subject C had a more normal gait pattern using FES. The FWR produced sufficient flexion to enable him to negotiate kerbs and small steps without having to lift his body by means of his upper limbs. Subject D had a more natural gait pattern using FES, however functional use was restricted by habituation of the reflex, resulting in deterioration of hip flexion. Subject E was able using the FWR to walk without orthoses or help, and as a result of this walked daily within the house. This compared favourably with her conventional orthosis where she was dependent on her husband for don/doffing of the orthoses and to stand and walk. At the end of the programme her voluntary strength had increased sufficiently for her to walk independently without using FES or orthoses. As a result of this she was not dependent on the use of disabled toilets when out in the community, enabling her to travel more widely. Subject F walked for exercise only, but used FES in preference to her bilateral KAFO's. She reported that FES was less cumbersome, easier to don/doff, and cosmetically more acceptable.

DISCUSSION

The results of the MST suggest that the use of the FWR can produce strengthening of the hip flexors in ISCI subjects where there is some preserved motor control. However, it was not possible to predict from the initial strength what improvement can be achieved. As there was no increase in the PCI, and therefore no increase in effort using the FWR, this technique may be a preferential hip flexor strengthening method, enabling full activation of the muscle. In this way patients who are unable to initiate hip flexion with voluntary effort may use the FWR to re-educate the muscle group. It may be that a mechanism of facilitation occurs when using the FWR, as there is reinforcement of the muscle fibres under voluntary control by those contracting as a result of the stimulation only.

Our results show that in addition to hip flexor strengthening, the use of FES in preference to conventional orthoses may be indicated in some ISCI patients for the following reasons:

1) Improvement in the gait pattern as demonstrated in 5 of the subjects may be useful for re-education of gait in early rehabilitation; 2) Improvement in ability to negotiate steps and kerbs; 3) The FES system is easier to apply, and more cosmetically acceptable; consequently subjects who walked for exercise only tend to walk more frequently using FES.

The use of FES as an orthosis is therefore of value in selected ISCI subjects and has the advantage of being reusable by other patients if discarded. The limitations were shown to be in the problems of habituation and in the hardware design.

CONCLUSIONS

The use of the FWR in gait for the ISCI produces therapeutic benefits, and in some subjects produces an improvement in mobility. We believe the FWR has a role to play in the rehabilitation of ISCI patients. The findings of this study suggest that further research into these problems of habituation and hardware design would be worthwhile.

REFERENCES

1. Liberson WT, Holmquest HJ, Scott D, Dow A (1961) Functional Electrical Therapy: stimulation of the peroneal nerve synchronised with the swing phase of the gait in hemiplegic patients. Arch. Phys. Med. Rehabil., 42:101
2. Kralj A, Grobelnik S (1973) Functional electrical stimulation - A new hope for paraplegic patients? Bulletin Prosthetic Research, 10-20:75-102
3. Bajd T, Kralj A, Turk R, Benko H, Sega J (1989) Use of functional electrical stimulation in the rehabilitation of patients with incomplete spinal cord injuries. J. Biomed. Eng. 11:96-102.
4. Bajd T, Andrews BJ, Kralj A, Katakis J (1986) Restoration of walking in patients with incomplete spinal cord injuries by use of electrical stimulation - preliminary results. Clinical Prosthetics and Orthotics, 10:111-114.
5. Bedbrook GM (1985) A balanced viewpoint in the early management of patients with spinal injuries who have neurological damage. Paraplegia, 23:8-15.
6. Steven MM, Capell HA, Sturrock RD, MacGregor J (1983) The physiological cost of gait (PCG) : A new technique for evaluating nonsteroidal anti-inflammatory drugs in rheumatoid arthritis. British J. Rheumatology, 22:141-145.
7. Granger CV, Albrecht GL, Hamilton BB (1979) Outcome of comprehensive medical rehabilitation: Measurement by PULSES profile and the Barthel Index. Arch. Phys. Med. Rehab., 60:145-154.

ACKNOWLEDGEMENTS This study was supported by the Scottish Home and Health Department. The authors like to thank the staff and patients of Philipshill hospital, Glasgow, Scotland.

DIAPHRAGMATIC FORCE AND FATIGUE DURING TRUNK FLEXION IN THE TETRAPLEGIC PATIENT

Christer Sinderby, Lars Sullivan and Lars Lindström.
Spinal Injuries Unit Inst. of Neurosurgery and Dept. of Clinical Data Processing, Sahlgrenska Hospital, S-413 45 Gothenburg, Sweden.

The interaction between the abdominal and the paravertebral muscles, with respect to trunk extension, has been scrutinized by several authors (1, 2, 3). Few studies have been designed to investigate the ability of the diaphragm as a sufficient trunk extensor. Recently, Hemborg et al (4) described that during heavy lifting in normals the paravertebral EMG signal strenght was inversly related to the EMG signal strenght obtained in the eight intercostal space, the latter assumed to represent diaphragmatic EMG activity.

In a series of studies we found that both voluntary and involuntary trunk flexions in cervical cord injuries (CCI) patients were accompanied by increase in gastric pressure and continuous diaphragmatic EMG activity with markedly increased amplitude (5). Similar tracings were also shown during the first revolutions of arm cranking in CCI patients with poor triceps. These findings were regarded to reflect a compensatory diaphragmatic contraction in order to increase abdominal pressure and thereby prevent a narrowing between the lower thorax aperture and the symphysis.

To study how this mechanism affects the diaphragm with respect to force and ischaemic fatigue, we measured the ventilation, the intraabdominal and intrathoracic pressures and the diaphragmatic EMG response to sustained trunk flexion in a group of six patients with complete motor paralysis from level C5 to C8.

MATERIAL AND METHODS

All patients were studied sitting in their own wheelchairs. Respiratory flow was measured at the mouth and volume was obtained by integration of flow. A quadruple-lumen balloon catheter was introduced to the stomach via the nose and anchored against the cardia, to measure gastric and esophageal pressures (Pga and Pes) as well as the transdiapragmatic pressure difference (Pdi). The latter represents force developed by the diaphragm. Normalisation of the transdiaphragmatic pressure was obtained by calculating the change in Pdi during trunk flexion, (Pdi_{flex}) as a fraction of the maximal transdiaphragmatic pressure (Pdi_{max}). The latter obtained during maximal inspiratory efforts against closed airways. The catheter was counterbalanced by a small weight which was attached proximal to the nostrils.

Two cobalt EMG electrodes on the catheter registered the crural diaphragmatic EMG signals. The EMG signal strength (EMGdi) were normalized according to the formula:

$$\Delta EMGdi = (EMGdi_{flex} - EMGdi_{rest})/EMGdi_{rest}.$$

To quantify diaphragmatic EMG fatigue, we used power spectrum analysis of the EMG (6). Decreases in the diaphragmatic EMG center frequency CFdi were verified by linear regression analysis. Further details of the method are presented in another paper in this proceeding (7).

To achieve a trunk flexion, the patients were instructed to lift their arms and cross them on the chest and then bend forward to the outermost position that could be maintained without falling. They were urged to remain in this position as long as possible. The maximal trunk angle during trunk flexion was measured with a goniometer, with the vertical plane as reference. The exercise was performed on an arm ergometer. To establish the influence of the passive increase in Pga during trunk flexion, two patients were examined in supported trunk flexion at 45°.

RESULTS

Clear drops in CFdi were observed in all patients but one during the period of sustained trunk flexion. The average time of sustained trunk flexion in all patients was 38.5 seconds (range 11-60 seconds), at a mean trunk flexion angle of 15° (range 0-30°). Uninterrupted EMGdi activity throughout the period was found in all patients. The mean increase in ΔEMGdi was 1.2 times the resting level (SD 0.44). Mean $\Delta Pdi_{flex}/Pdi_{max}$ was 0.33 (SD 0.05), where Pdi was dominated by Pga, with a Pga/Pdi ratio of 0.81 (SD 0.07).

In one patient there was a marked rise in the Pga/Pdi ratio, from 0.42 at rest to 0.91 during sustained trunk flexion, possibly indicating a passive increase in Pga. In the remaining patients there was a less than 10 per cent change in the Pga/Pdi ratio. In the two patients who performed supported trunk flexion to 45°, the end-expiratory Pga was 0.2 and 0.5 kPa, respectively.

The median Ti/Ttot for all patients ranged from 0.28 to 1.0 with a large intra-individual fluctuation. Due to the variation in Ti/Ttot and the possibilities of a passive increase in ΔPdi_{flex}, we did not calculate the product of Ti/Ttot and $\Delta Pdi_{flex}/Pdi_{max}$.

In periods when all ΔEMGdi observations exceeded the baseline (EMG signal strength at rest) by 50 per cent or more, there was frequently a clear decrease in CFdi. This is illustrated in Figure 1, showing one patient (panel a), who held his breath throughout trunk flexion, with an ΔEMGdi range of 0.6 - 3.3 and a progressive decline in CFdi, and one patient (panel b), who had the least irregular Ti/Ttot, with an increase in CFdi, and an ΔEMGdi ranging from -0.1 to 2.8.

All patients perceived the trunk flexion as increasingly strenuous and accompanied by breathing difficulties. The sensation of loading was located to the chest and/or upper abdomen. During trunk flexion, heart rate (HR) increased by a median of 8.0 beats/minute (range 0-37 beats/minute).

This study shows that patients with cervical cord lesions develop clear EMG signs of diaphragmatic fatigue when they bend forward. We emphasize the need for differing strategies in the short and long-term treatment of CCI patients and suggest that longitudinal evaluation of their diaphragmatic function may be useful for the dosage of training.

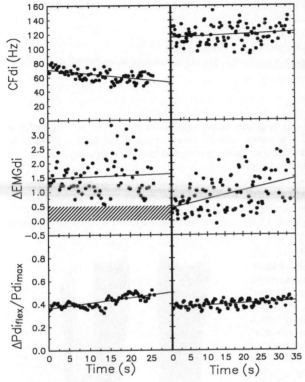

Figure 1. The time plots of the EMGdi centre frequency (CFdi) (upper panels), the ΔEMGdi (middle panels) and the $\Delta Pdi_{flex}/Pdi_{max}$ ratio (lower panels) in one patient who holds his breath and show decreasing CFdi (left panel) and one patient who have a median Ti/ Ttot of 0.5 (right panel) during the sustained trunk flexion and show a stable CFdi. Decrease in CFdi was frequently associated with a gap between the baseline EMGdi signal strength (EMGdi at rest) and the observed ΔEMGdi values at trunk flexion (shaded area, left middle panel). In the right panel, the rythmic variation in $\Delta Pdi_{flex}/Pdi_{max}$ tracings and frequent returns of ΔEMGdi to its baseline level indicate that duty cycle governs diaphragmatic fatigue also when the breathing pattern consists of a continuous postural EMGdi-activity with a superimposed phasic respiratory activity.

REFERENCES

1. Andersson G. B. J., R. Örtengren and A. Nachemson. Intradiskal pressure, intra-abdominal pressure and myoelectric activity related to posture and loading. *Clin. Orthop. 129: 156-164, 1977.*

2. Örtengren R., G. B. J. Andersson and A. Nachemson. Studies of relationships between lumbar disc pressure, myoelectric back muscle activity, and intra-abdominal (intragastric) pressure. *Spine.* 6: 98-108, 1981.

3. Hemborg B. Intraabdominal pressure and trunk muscle activity during lifting. Thesis. Lund University. 1983.

4. Wedin S., R. Leanderson and E. Knutsson. The effect of voluntary diaphragmatic activation on back lifting. *Scand. J. Rehab. Med.* 20: 129-132, 1988.

5. Sinderby C., P. Ingvarsson, L. Sullivan, I. Wickström and L. Lindström. The role of the diaphragm in trunk extension in tetraplegia. *Paraplegia.* in press.

6. Lindström L., R. Kadefors and I. Petersén. An electromyographic index for localized muscle fatigue. *J. Appl. Physiol.* 43: 750-754, 1977.

7. Sinderby C., L. Sullivan and L. Lindström. Evaluation of diaphragmatic force and fatigue in practical situations. In *Proceeding WCPT 11th International Congress,* London 1991.

THE VANNINI-RIZZOLI STABILIZING LOWER LIMB ORTHOSES

M. Lusvardi
Officine Ortopediche Rizzoli S.p.A. - Bologna Italy

The Bologna Boots were originally developped during the first 80's by Officine Ortopediche Rizzoli in cooperation with the Montecatone Rehabilitation Hospital to allow paraplegics to stand, with no hand support, and to walk reciprocally, with the aid of a reciprocal walker or quad-canes.

At that time we were well aware of the design compromise that this new orthosis, as any other walking system, had to satisfy. We wanted to emphasize the independence that a paraplegic could achieve, giving him an orthosis lightweight and easy to don and doff, and to supply a device cosmetically acceptable, since we found it to be an important factor to our patients.

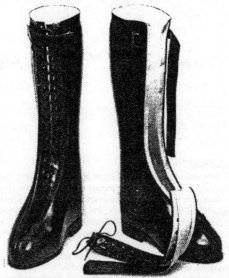

Fig.1 The Vannini-Rizzoli stabilizing lower limb orthoses

The Bologna Boot (Fig. 1) is a custom made ankle-foot orthosis, shaped as a boot. It's characterized by a rigid structure, an half shell made in composite material (fiberglasses and resins) which blocks the patient's ankle at approximately 10 degrees of plantarflexion, thus shifting his center of gravity forward on the metatarsal heads. The rigid sole, made in polyurethane foam, should be modified, during the standing test, putting wedges or soles below it, thus permitting the patient to stand hand-free in a good alignment.

The skeletal structure of the boots is internally padded with pe- lite to prevent the possibility of pressure sores. The cosmetic appeareance of the V-RSLLO is a high leather boot extending to a level just below the tibial tuberosity. It's fastened by a central lace and two zippers located on either side of the boots.

In order to be fitted with the Bologna Boots a patient must present full range of motion to all the joints of the lower limbs and no muscle contractures. The upper extremities must be functional with good grasp, being able to support the patient's body weight.

We have fitted up to now hundreds of paraplegics with different level of lesions among thoracics and lumbars, either complete or incomplete. The energy consumption analysis has shown us that, due to the differences in speed, a good degre of functional independence can be reached with low lesion or incomplete subjects, while for high lesions the boots can be considered an exercise orthosis.

As per other orthosis also the Bologna Boots are part of a complete rehabilitative treatment. The pre-orthosis training program consists of 3-5 hours daily for 4 weeks; stratching of the joints, standing balance, trunk stabilization are some of the activities. There are also mat exercise geared to reciprocating movements of the sholder, hips and knee. The patient must learn how to shift his body weight from one leg to the other and to perform swinging movements of the lower limbs..

Donning and doffing is very easy and can be performed while sitting in a wheelchair. The anterior part of the boot is unfasten and the foot correctly positioned inside the orthosis. The laces are adjusted the first time, then the patient has only to fasten the two zippers.

Standing is achieved by the patient pushing on his upper extremity to lift all his body weight. Once standing this posture is maintained without any hand support because the angle at which the foot is positioned in the orthosis stabilizes the knee. By controlling the balance of the upper body, the pelvis, hips and knee are held in a slightly extended position. Although this position, up to now we have not received any report of knee legament damage.

Walking is achieved by shifting the body weight on one leg. Pushing on the upper extremities and tilting the pelvis one foot is cleared off the ground. A step is then completed by moving the unweighted foot forward in a pendulum fashion toghether with the progression of the pelvis.

As a consequence of static equilibrium our patients can perform manual activities. They can work at a counter or in a small workshop. They can use the toilet or talk at the telephone while standing, walk around the house..

Using the Hoffer scale we can refer to our patients as to household ambulators or to community ambulators depending on their level of injury.

During the presentation we will also show a short video regarding the gait analysis conducted in our laboratory.

Effects of Sport Activity on Physical Fitness of Paraplegic
Patients.

Ronikier A. Magiera A., Milewski P.
Faculty of Rehabilitation, Academy of Physical Education,
ul. Marymoncka 34, 04-811 Warsaw, Poland.

The range of metabolic changes in the organism during
physical exercises are a sensitive physiological criterion for
the evaluation of individual physical efficiency. The study of
the physiological responses and energy expenditure during
exercise is of particular importance in the rehabilitation
treatment of patients with various groups of diseases since
this treatment is a therapeutic factor which must be used
particularly rationally.

Determination of the optimal value of the exercise to be
applied in individual cases of disability is connected with
considerable difficulties, since in the pertinent literature
no normal values and indices can be found which would
determine the degree of exercise tolerance in various groups
of diseases. It is not known either what degree of fitness
should be achieved by a given patient at a given stage of
rehabilitation treatment. The normal and standard values
determined for the population of healthy subjects cannot be
applied in the physiology of exercise in the disabled persons.

However, it is known without doubt that the consequences
of diseases or injuries with reduction of motor activity of
the organism decrease the Physical Fitness (PF) of the patient
measured with such physiological parameters as the PWC test,
efficiency of mechanical work, oxygen consumption, energy cost
of the exercise or responses of the cardiovascular and
respiratory systems.

Only little attention has been given to the evaluation of
physiological parameters of the physical activity of the
Spinal Cord Injury (SCI) patients during rehabilitation
process. This may mean also, that in many cases rehabilitation
treatment is conducted irrationally due to incorrect dosage of
workload during exercises.

Method and material.

The physiological observations were carried out in a group
of 16 paraplegics (age 25-44 years old); 5 of them
participated in basketball games on wheelchairs and 11
participated in a three-week fitness course of exercises in
the Metropolitan Rehabilitation Center, Konstancin – Warsaw.
The energy expenditure was measured during basketball game and
exercises preceding the game and another group underwent the
PWC 170 test before and after a course of training. The energy

hypokinesia of paraplegic patients the value of PWC 170 test was decreased by 20–45%. Our results show that three-week intensive training significantly improves patients' PF but this improvement (9–65% of PWC 170 test value) was strongly correlated with SCI level.

The oxygen consumption of paraplegics during basketball game on wheelchairs was in the studied group about 1200 ml O2/min, which may be regarded as a very exhausting workload, exceeding by 200 ml O2/min the oxygen cost during upright body position locomotion, which is treated by many authors as a very heavy effort in SCI patients (Merkel [5], Glaser [1], Mattsson [4], Nene [6]).

In the studies of Zwiren [8] the paraplegics not engaged in exercises program could achieve VO2max value of 1380 ml O2/min but could not exceed the consumption of oxygen over 1800 ml O2/min.

However, it may be assumed that basketball playing on wheelchairs is for a disabled person a very attractive form of rehabilitation treatment which in view of of the intensity of the physical effort improves significantly his PF.

The paraplegics should be told that exercises increasing endurance, improving physical efficiency and increasing muscle strength are indispensable for them since the remaining active muscle must take over all motor functions lost due to the trauma. These are often everyday functions of the disabled person such as locomotion, self care etc. Improved PF will facilitate the life of the paraplegics and will accelerate the progress of rehabilitation.

References.
1. Glaser R. (1985): Exercise and locomotion for the spinal cord injured. Exercise and Sport Scien. Rev., vol.13.
2. Gordon E, Van der Walde H (1956): Energy requirements in paraplegic ambulation. Arch. Phys. Med. Rehab. 37:256.
3. Kofsky R, Davis G, Shepard R., Jackson R (1983): Assessment of physical fitness of disabled adults. Eur. J. Appl. Phys. 51:109.
4. Mattsson E (1989): Energy cost of level walking. Scand. J. Reh. Med. Supp. 23.
5. Merkel K, Miller N, Westbrook P, Mervitt J. (1984): Energy expenditure of paraplegic patients standing and walking with two knee – ankle – foot orthoses. Arch. Phys. Med. Rehab. 65:3.
6. Nene A, Orth D, Orth M (1989): Energy cost of paraplegic locomotion with ORLAU Para Walker. Paraplegia 27:1.
7. Odden J (1979): Early mobilization of paraplegic patients after traumatic spinal cord injuries. J. Appl. Physiology 15:1159.
8. Zwiren L, Bar-or O (1975): Responses to exercises of paraplegics who differ in conditioning level. Med. Scien. in Sports 7:2:94–98.

expenditure was determined by the open indirect calorymetry method using a Kafrani-Michailis gasometer and Scholander oxygen gasanalyser (the obtained gasometric data were calculated for standard conditions STPD). The PWC 170 test was carried out in morning hours using manually driven TUNTURI cycloergometer, heart rate HR was measured using physiograph with standard electrodes.

Results.

Table 1.
Mean physiological parameters of paraplegics (n=5)

TEST DATA	VE BTPS (1/min)	VO2 STPD (ml/min)	VO2 STPD (ml/min/ kg b.w.)	ENERGY EXPEND. (kc/min)	HR (b./ min)
REST 10 min	11.70	338	4.69	1.70	80
TACTIC EXERCISES	18.20	898	12.40	4.49	118
GAME 15 min	31.40	1200	16.60	5.99	124

Table 2.
Physical Work Capacity (PWC) and Heart Rate Restitution Time (HR-RT) of paraplegics (SCI levels: D3-D5 n=4, D8-L2 n=7)

TEST DATA	PWC 170 (Watt)	HR-RT (min)
PRE-COURSE	126.7	15.8
POST-COURSE	160.8	12.2

Discussion.
    The number of patients was to small for drawing of any too far reaching conclusions, but it may be supposed that all studied patients had before the training course a very low fitness level. It may suggest that outside the rehabilitation center they performed exercises rarely and lost early physical efficiency which is so necessary for everyday life.
    Gordon [2] stated that in paraplegia only 30-40% of the total muscle mass participates in the energy metabolism, and that this value depends on the level of SCI. Kofsky and Davis [3] studied the PF of paraplegics in relation to the level of SCI and physical activity. Results of these investigations indicate that the level of SCI as well as the range of physical activity have an important effect of PF of paraplegics. Odeen [7] demonstrated that during 20 days of

CLINICAL PROBLEMS WITH LOWER LIMB PROGRAMMES OF FUNCTIONAL ELECTRICAL STIMULATION FOR SPINAL CORD INJURY PATIENTS

FMD Barr
F.E.S Research Unit. Royal National Orthopaedic Hospital
Stanmore, England.

INTRODUCTION

Functional Electrical Stimulation (FES), the activation of paretic muscle by electrical stimulation of motor nerves, has been used in the rehabilitation spinal cord injury patients for 30 years (Cybulski 1984, Peckham 1987). Programmes of electrical stimulation to the lower limb have been developed at the Spinal Injuries Unit at the Royal National Orthopaedic Hospital over the past five years, with the aim of restoring standing and walking in paraplegic patients in order to provide physiological, physical and psychological gains for that individual (Barr 1987, 1989). Despite the explicit patient selection criteria devised through experience during these programmes, physiological and practical problems were still experienced by patients at the outset and throughout the course of a stimulation programme, resulting in patients' withdrawal.

The aim of this paper is to identify the broad spectrum of problems incurred by patients following a lower limb programme of FES and to discuss their management and subsequent outcome with a view to facilitating prophylactic measures for future programmes.

METHODS

Patients were selected to undergo a 12 week lower limb exercise programme of FES using the criteria shown:-

1. To have sustained a spinal cord injury between the levels T1 - 12, resulting in a clinically complete upper motor neurone paralysis.
2. Absence of contractures and pressure sores of the lower limb.
3. Absence of excess spasticity.
4. To have completed a full rehabilitation programme and to be following a regular standing programme.

The stimulation programme comprised two components, dynamic and static muscle contraction of the quadriceps and glutei and common peroneal nerve stimulation producing a flexor withdrawal response (Barr 1987, 1989). The exercise programme was progressed by increasing the duration of the stimulation period and by addition of weights during the dynamic phase of the exercise.

Assessments were conducted to examine physiological change; muscle power and spasticity were measured using a robotic dynamometer - the Kinetic Communicator (KIN COM) (Barr 1989), muscle bulk using CT scanning and circulatory responses using contact thermography (Barr 1987). Questionnaires and patient interviews were conducted to discuss the social and psychological implications of the programme.

RESULTS

Lower Motor Neurone Dysfunction

Lower motor neurone dysfunction presented in five patients, manifested as diffuse EMG abnormality and isolated peripheral nerve damage. Muscle strengthening was not achieved in those with diffuse EMG abnormality and therefore the patients were unable to progress to standing. Patients exhibiting isolated peripheral damage to the common peroneal nerve achieved standing but were unable to progress to a walking programme.

Spasticity

An increase in muscle spasticity was recorded in 85% of the patient population. The use of medication (Baclofen) in two subjects with a severe increase in spasticity following stimulation, caused a minimal reduction in the level of spasticity and a decrease in muscle force of the quadriceps muscle such that the patients were unable to achieve standing.

Cessation of stimulation in these cases restored the degree of spasticity to its pre-stimulation level.

Soft Tissue Damage & Articular Changes

Many of the patients involved in the lower limb programmes experienced a decrease in joint range of movement, particularly in the ankle and foot. Inaccurate placement of electrodes led to a lack of strengthening in the anterior tibial muscles and an increase in plantar spasticity with resultant shortening of the gastrocnemius muscle. In standing, the loss of plantargrade position of the foot caused flexion at the hips and a subsequent increase in lumbar lordosis, resulting in poor standing posture.

These subjects were retaught correct passive stretching, encouraged to rest in prone lying and instructed to stand daily for a minimum period of thirty minutes. All patients regained hip extension and ankle range of movement to plantar grade.

Osteophyte formation in the cruciate ligaments was seen in one patient. Radiographic examination had not been made prior to commencing stimulation and therefore no comparison could be made. Routine Xray examination of knee joint was subsequently introduced into the preliminary assessment protocol.

Postural Deformity

When quadriceps were stimulated in isolation, patients stood with some hip flexion and an increased lumbar lordosis. This posture was corrected to the midline with the application of gluteal stimulation and voluntary contraction of latissimus dorsi to stabilise the upper trunk.

Spinal deformity was seen in three patients with complete lesions at the level of T10, T6 and T7: postural scoliosis in the first two, as a result of surgery for implantation of a bladder controller in one individual and in the second patient as a result of poor sitting posture. The third patient presented with a marked lumbar lordosis in the standing position which was uncorrectable with gluteal and paraspinal stimulation and required a spinal fusion using Harrington rods. The patient was able to resume his standing programme after six months with corrected posture.

Patient Perceptions

The nature and number of assessment procedures in general did not disturb the patients although several patients were unwilling to undergo repeat muscle biopsy on completion of the programme.

The practical application of the stimulation was not perceived by the patients to be problem although weekly reassessment showed errors in some patients' method of stimulation i.e. starting position for exercise and electrode application. The time taken to perform the stimulation caused problems related to restriction of activities and boredom but all patients felt that they had made a commitment to the programme and therefore had to prioritise their leisure time accordingly.

Despite clear explanation at the outset, of the limited objectives and goals of the programme, patients felt hurt, disappointed, and saddened, by the outcome, particularly those who did not achieve standing due to poor muscle strengthening. Regardless of the outcome of the stimulation, patients commented that during the course of the programme they had reflected upon their injury, their capabilities in the wheelchair and some felt that they had finally come to realise that they would never be able to walk again. These findings highlight the need for further counselling and psychological support throughout the course of the programme.

CONCLUSION

From the study, it is evident that a broad spectrum of problems of a physiological, physical, social and psychological nature may present in paraplegic individuals participating in a lower limb programme of Functional Electrical Stimulation. The author stresses the need for systematic study of patients by a multidisciplinary team in order to minimise these incidences. Sensitive and objective assessment and measurement must be continued throughout the course of a stimulation programme as well as at the time of entry, with a full awareness of the potential problems which may develop.

Acknowledgements

The author wishes to thank ASPIRE, the Milly Apthorpe Charitable Trust and Opportunities for the Disabled for their support in this work.

REFERENCES

1. Cybulski G, Penn R, Jaeger R (1984) Lower extremity Functional Neuromuscular Stimulation in cases of spinal cord injury. Neurosurg. 15(1) 132 - 146.

2. Peckham PH. (1987) Functional Electrical Stimulation: Current status and future prospects of applications to the neuromuscular system in spinal cord injury. Paraplegia 25:279 - 288.

3. Barr FMD, Bayley JIL, Middleton FRI, Moffat B. (1987) Functional Electrical Stimulation: Practical Experience in the clinical setting. Proc. IX International Symposium of External Control of Human Extremities. Belgrade.

4. Barr FMD, Moffat B. (1989) Practical considerations in gait restoration by means of FES. Proc. Biological Engineering Society meeting. Electrical Stimulation of Muscle. Hexham.

5. Barr FMD, Moffat B, Bayley JIL, Middleton FRI (1989) Evaluation of the effects of Functional Electrical Stimulation on muscle power and spasticity in spinal cord injury patients. Clin. Rehab. 3:17 - 22.

FUNCTIONAL ELECTRICAL STIMULATION (FES) IN THE GAIT TRAINING OF THE TETRAPARETIC PATIENT

M.M.Primožič, T.Krizmanič, P.Obreza
University Rehabilitation Institute, Linhartova 51
61000 Ljubljana, Slovenia, Yugoslavia

INTRODUCTION

Functional electrical stimulation (FES) is a modern method in the field of rehabilitation medicine (1). It's aim is to restore the function of paralysed or paretic muscles. By applying FES we elicite muscle contraction to achieve useful functional movement. The method came into everyday practice at our institution after an extensive research has been done in collaboration with the group of scientists at the Institute Joseph Stephan in Ljubljana (2,3). The analogies of FES widely applied in medicine are cardiac pacemakers, electrical stimulation of the urinary bladder and the pain relieving transcutaneous electrical nerve stimulation (4).

DESCRIPTION OF THE METHOD

FES is applied predominantly to the patients with lesion in the upper motor neurone. The main candidates are:

- patients with hemiplegia or hemiparesis due to cerebral lesion (injury, stroke)
- children with cerebral palsy
- patients with lesion of the spinal cord.

It is important to emphasize that in the case of the lesion of the upper motor neurons the reflex arc is maintained. This fact enables FES to be applied. Without a functioning reflex arc FES is useless. The basic premis for FES is a viable muscle which can still be indirectly or directly contracted by the electrical currents (5).

By applying FES a motor or mixed nerve is stimulated above the threshold of the motor fibres. The mechanical response is an ordinary muscle twitch. By applying above 20 impulses per second a tetanic contraction of the muscle appears. In this way we are able to carry out the desired movements of various muscles and muscle groups.

Parameters of stimulation in FES are the following:

- duration of impulses about 0,5 msec.
- frequency from 20 - 50 Hz
- intensity usually to 60 V, rarely up to 100 V
- use of the mono or biphasic impulses.

The most widely used functional electrical stimulation device at our institution is the so called functional electrical peroneal stimulator for correction of dorsiflexion and eversion of the spastic equinovarus in the swing phase of gait in patients with this problem (6).

CASE PRESENTATION

On videotape (15 min) the authors present a successfull 6 month recovery of gait in a 37 year old patient with the luxation of vertebrae C IV and C V resulting in tetraplegia immediately after the car accident, and slowly evolving into the spastic tetraparesis. Due to the instability of the vertebrae a surgical spondylodesis was done.

The gait training started 4 months after injury. FES was applied on regular basis to stimulate the right peroneal nerve facilitating the flexor response of the paretic lower extremity which enabled the patient to make an efficient step forward. The clinical stimulator AM 5 developed and produced at the University Rehabilitation Institute Ljubljana was applied. The amplitude of current was 70 V, impulse duration was 0,5 msec and frequency 40 Hz. Besides FES the patient was given all the neccessary conventional physiotherapy for spinal cord injuries.

RESULTS

After 6 months of gait training the patient was able to walk independently with crutches and returned to work.

CONCLUSION

The authors consider FES an important physiotherapeutic method for the restoration of gait in patients with incomplete spinal cord injury.

REFERENCES

1. Štefančič M (ed.). Seminar on functional electrical stimulation. University Rehabilitation Institute, Ljubljana, 1986: 1-104.
2. Vodovnik L, Bajd T, Kralj A. The impact of biomechanics on the neuromuscular rehabilitation. In: Raul H, Ghista DN, Rau G (eds.): Perspectives in biomechanics, Vol.1, part B. Commemorating the First international conference on mechanics in medicine and biology, Aachen, 1978: 26-29.
3. Vodovnik L. Influence of electrical stimulation on some abnormal motor function in man. World congress on medical physics and biomedical engineering, Hamburg, 1982: 84.
4. Štefančič M, Jelnikar T. Evalvacija protibolečinskega aparata PEBA. University Rehabilitation Institute, Ljubljana, 1980.
5. Kralj A, Bajd T, Turk R. Electrical stimulation providing functional use of paraplegic patient muscles. Med Prog Technol 1980; 7: 3-9.
6. Liberson WT, Holmquest HJ, Scott D, Dow M. Functional electrotherapy: stimulation of the peroneal nerve synchronized with the swing phase of gait of hemiplegic patients. Arch Phys Med 1961; 42: 24-36.

POSTER PRESENTATIONS

AN ISOTONIC STRENGTH TRAINING PROGRAM FOR TRUNK EXTENSION IN PARAPLEGIC INDIVIDUALS USING THE MEDX[TM]. *

N P Fisher, H A Schulte
University of Florida, College of Health Related Professions,
Department of Physical Therapy, Gainesville, Florida 32610-0154 USA

Traditionally, strengthening of the upper extremity and shoulder girdle musculature with arm ergometry or weight lifting has been a major focus for those with paralyzed lower limbs. The use of variable resistance or isokinetic equipment can augment the traditional means by which therapists document objective information about muscle strength and endurance with the neurologically impaired population. In spite of voluminous reports of studies with able-bodied subjects utilizing various kinds of variable resistance equipment, limited experimental work has been published in the area of the neurologically impaired population; in particular spinal cord injury (SCI).

Recently, the development of a lumbar extension machine has provided the means for isometric and isotonic testing and training of trunk extensors in a seated position. This allows for the potential utilization of this equipment by paraplegics. This machine is designed to restrict the role in which the pelvic muscles influence the force production of the lumbar extensors[1] thus giving therapists a means to obtain objective measurements. Therefore, the purpose of this study was to investigate the efficacy of testing and strengthening spared trunk extension musculature using the MedX[TM] with a sample of healthy paraplegic individuals.

Twenty five volunteers were initially interviewed for potential participation in the training program. Selection criteria included documented medical evidence of spinal stability, wheelchair utilization for at least 75% of their locomotion, independence in functional transfers, activities of daily living and bladder management. An initial screening or review of current x-rays was performed by an orthopedic surgeon on all subjects prior to participation.

* MedX Corporation, Ocala, Fl. 32670

Ultimately, five healthy volunteers with SCI (4 male paraplegics and 1 female paraplegic with lesions ranging from T5 to T12 participated in a 12 session training program (2 days per week for 6 weeks). The mean age of the subjects was 26.4 ± 6.3 years.

Subjects transferred to the MedX[TM] and were seated with the top of their thighs approximately horizontal with the seat. The footplate provided counter pressure bilaterally through the tibia and femur so that the femurs were positioned into the posterior aspect of the acetabulum[1]. The top of the thighs were prevented from moving by a wide belt secured snugly across the lap, and this in turn prevented the femurs from moving upwards. Arm, head and trunk weight were counterbalanced for gravitational forces. The position of the head and arms was also standardized so that reproducible positioning could occur. To monitor the pressure on the femurs, a sphygmomanometer cuff was placed across the thighs underneath the wide lap belt, and maintained at a pressure of 60 to 70 mmHG throughout the sessions. This precaution was taken because it was felt that appropriate feedback was unable to be communicated regarding belt tightness, since the SCI subjects had impaired or absent position, pressure and pain sensation.

Each subject performed isometric strength test-retest sessions on the MedX[TM] extension machine prior to and after an isotonic training phase. Testing consisted of maximum voluntary trunk extension at seven standard positions on the MedX[TM] through a 72° ($72,^{\circ} 60,^{\circ} 48,^{\circ} 36',^{\circ} 24,^{\circ} 12,^{\circ} 0^{\circ}$) arc of trunk flexion. Training consisted of concentric and eccentric trunk extension, through the same 72° arc of trunk movement against a variable resistance for 3 minutes in duration. Torque production during isometric testing and the amount of resistance during dynamic extension exercises were recorded and analyzed. Sessions were separated by a minimum of two days. Dynamic strength testing consisted of subjects performing an isotonic trunk extension exercise using the MedX[TM] until volitional fatigue. The testing on the first day, during the pre-training test-retest session, was considered a practice day to familiarize the subjects with the testing equipment and the protocols.

Most subjects were able to produce force at all seven positions (except two subjects with high level thoracic lesions, who could not obtain force production at 0°) during the isometric strength tests. These subjects also demonstrated an increase in their isometric torque production when measured pre- and post training. Torque production in the forward flexed position (72°) was higher than values at the extended position (0°). The average amount of torque production (9 to 60 Nm) was markedly reduced for this population when compared to healthy subjects[2,3] (236 to 465 Nm) and chronic low back pain[3] (150 to 372 Nm).

During the course of the study, no session had to be discontinued because of adverse effects. No modifications were made to enable this group to utilize the MedX[TM].

It was felt that torque production was generated from spared neck, shoulder-girdle (latissimus dorsi) and upper thoracic musculature. The ability to recruit these muscles as a collective group, rather than focusing on isolated muscles, is more representative of how these muscles work in performing every day functional activities.

This study demonstrates the feasibility of using an isotonic trunk extension machine with a group of SCI individuals. All subjects completed the study without any adverse effects. This study showed that repeated measurements of isometric trunk extension strength at multiple angles were highly reproducible (r^2 = .91 to .99). Although not statistically significant, all subjects increased the amount of torque produced at multiple positions throughout a full ROM, pre- and post-training.

These subjects demonstrated high levels of motivation and functional independence, which may be reflective of the low magnitude of the gains in isometric torque production. It was felt that strict inclusion criteria were necessary because of the lack of any previous documentation in the literature using this type of equipment with SCI individuals. Isotonic exercise training for 2x/week for 6 weeks was effective at improving dynamic strength of the trunk extensors, which was demonstrated by an increase in dynamic weight load (p < .002) and duration of time the initial weight load was moved (p < .003). Future directions should include longitudinal studies which utilize a random sampling of a larger number of SCI subjects and matched control group. Various combinations of intensity, duration and frequency should be explored in exercise studies, and the specific effectiveness upon the quadriplegic and paraplegic populations. Future applications of this type of training program with a SCI population who are still in an inpatient rehabilitation setting, should be examined to evaluate the relationship between strength gains and the attainment of functional goals for discharge.

REFERENCES
1 Jones A, Pollock M, Graves J, Fulton M, et al. The Lumbar Spine. Santa Barbara, Sequoia Communications, 1988

2 Pollock ML, Leggett SH, Graves JE, Jones A, et al. Effect of resistance training on lumbar strength. Amer J Sports Med, 1989 (in press)

3 Robinson, ME, Greene AF, Graves JE, O'Connor P, et al. Isometric strength differences between chronic low back pain patients and normal controls. (in review)

This study was supported by a grant from the Paralyzed veterans of America.

CARDIOPULMONARY RESPONSES TO ARM-CRANKING,
WHEELCHAIR-PROPELLING, AND CRUTCH-WALKING
IN SPINAL CORD INJURIES

KWAN-HWA LIN, MU-JUNG KAO, I-NAN LIEN,
JIN-SHIN LAI

DEPT OF PHYSICAL THERAPY
SCHOOL OF REHABILITATION MEDICINE
NATIONAL TAIWAN UNIVERSITY
TAIPEI, TAIWAN, REPUBLIC OF CHINA

<u>Introduction:</u> The endurance training for paraplegics is very
important. The cardiopulmonary responses during maximal arm
exercise and at anaerobic threshold between paraplegics and
the able-bodied were studied in order to provide informations
for effective exercise program.

<u>Trearment:</u> Study was performed in 35 male paraplegics and
35 matched able-bodied. The seated subject was asked to
crank the Monark arm ergometer with resistance increasing
progressively until exhausted. The expired gas was collected
and analyzed by MGC 2000. Heart rate was also measured during
wheelchair-propelling and crutch-walking.

<u>Results:</u> During maximal arm exercise, the oxygen consumption
and O_2 pulse in T1-L2 paraplegics were significantly ($p < 0.01$)
lower than that of the able-bodied. However, the ventilatory
equivalent was not significantly different. At anaerobic
threshold, the oxygen consumption and O_2 pulse was lower than
the able-bodied only in T1-T5 paraplegics. The heart rate
during wheelchair-propelling was significantly less than
that at anaerobic threshold, but the heart rate during
crutch-walking was significantly higher.

<u>Conclusions:</u> The low oxygen consumption in paraplegics ,
especially in high thoracic lesions, might be primarily
due to the reduced cardiac function which could be resulted
from the inadequate daily activities. To exercise near the
anaerobic threshold is suggested.

TYPES OF INDEPENDENT LIVING WITH CERVICAL CORD INJURY

K.Hiruma,   H.Kawai

Physical Rehabilitation Section,Tokyo Metropolitan
Rehabilitation Center, Tokyo,   Japan

Introduction : About 20 years before, in Japan the cervical cord injured had been forced to be in hospital because of their medical care and management.In these days, leaving hospital and living in home together with familiese or in single is taken as a matter of course.Considering their rehabilitation programme, if they want to live in home independently we have to have skills to help their lives.In the captioned Tokyo Metropolitan Rehabilitation Center, the physical therapists have been making their enthusiastic effors to aid those cervical cord injured for their various living skills necessary for their daily life in their home in order that they can have more fulfilled and better life in their living area while they have a handicap there.The purpose of this presentation is to illustrate and discuss about two clients with cervical cord injury who have been in community independently after the training of our Center.

Treatment : 6~9 months rehabilitation programme is described, including self-control for health,for instance, urinary tract control and decubitus control, adaptation to housing and etc.

Conclusion : A cervical cord injured who is male,33 years old, his former job was a teacher,gets the pension of Workmen's Accident Compensation Insurance,lives in home by himself hiring a private home-helper as he needs.Another is female,33 years old,and a recipient of public assistance, lives in a public housing for the disabled getting a public home-helper 2 hours a day,twice a week.

TEMPERO MANDIBULAR JOINT DYSFUNCTION

Dentistry and Physical Therapy- A TMJ Approach
F. Fischer D.D.S., R. Mele R.P.T.

Dental, Head and Neck Trauma,
Teporomandibular Joint Disorders
26381 Southfield Rd.; Southfield, Michigan   48076   USA

The unique relationship between dentistry and physical therapy which prevails in our facility is designed to provide maximal care under one roof primarily for victims of traumatically-induced tempromandibular joint dysfunction and dental trauma.

What causes TMJ dysfunction? The symptoms of TMJ dysfunction are frequently manifested following a traumatic injury to the head, face, jaw, or indirect injury such as cervical trauma-hyperextension/flexion injury, and are frequently more severe on one particular side. This may occur abruptly or even months after the injury.

The balance of the temporomandibular joint, along with the head and neck, is maintained by a precise and complex balance of craniofacial and cervical musculatures. Discriminatory contraction of the various head and neck muscles is necessary to move the mandible precisely and allow effective functioning. A sound understanding of orthopedic principles is necessary for evaluation and treatment of the various disorders of the temporomandibular joint.

The articular surface of the TMJ must be maintained in constant contact. This contact is produced by the muscles that pull across the joint. (The elevators . . the temporalis, masseter and medial pterygoid). Temporomandibular joint dysfunction results when there is dysharmony in the components of the joint system.

The temporomandibular joint is designed to function in a friction free manner. On occasion, clicking, popping, or grinding sounds may be heard from the joint. Such sounds are abnormal, and can occur when the disc in the joint is pushed forward; the back ligament of the disc becomes stretched and inflamed, and the condyles in the joint make the displaced disc pop when the jaw is opened and closed. After many years of this, there may be arthritic changes in the joint, a one-way degenerative process. This damage to the TMJ and the associated muscle spasm causes pain, not only in the joints themselves, but through muscle spasm to other parts of the body, resulting in many of the symptoms that are associated with TMJ.

Diagnosis is made upon determining history and onset of symptoms, and prescribing tomograms or TMJ transcranial xrays showing bone anatomy of the joint. The articular disc, being of cartilage material, soft tissue density, does not show up on xrays. We, therefore, refer patients for CAT-scan (Computerized Axial Tomography) or MRI (Magnetic Resonance Imaging) in order to view the position or displacement of the articular disc. Doppler auscultation studies are also utilized for diagnostic purposes to determine dysfunctional condylar movement along the articular surface.

Diagnostically, incisal jaw opening 42 to 52 mm is considered within normal limits. Lateral movements should be 10 to 12 mm to the right and to the left. If one demonstrates a restricted lateral movement, it would be the opposite joint that is causing the restriction. For example, if right lateral movement is 8 mm, it would be the left joint that is causing the dysfunction.

Most temporomandibular joint dysfunctions can be managed with a combined treatment plan of medications, orthotic appliances, physical therapy and home exercises, and dietary restrictions such as soft foods. The function of the temporomandibular joint orthotic appliance is to break the cycle of pain and to improve the musculoskeletal balance, thereby inhibiting pain. Another function of the appliance is to reduce the displaced articular disc. The use of the appliance will allow the spastic jaw/craniofacial musculatures to relax and allow the mandible to be repositioned in a harmonious, stable, stress-free position. The appliance must be worn initially 24 hours a day, and then an attempt to wean the patient off the appliance is recommended.

In the physical therapy aspect of care of temporomandibular joint dysfunction, the physical therapist is involved in two primary areas: identification of goals and objectives for each individual patient, and implementation of a comprehensive treatment program for that individual patient.

Physical therapy goals for this malady are often dictated by the post-traumatic-stress nature of the injuries. This can be complex, involving not only identification of orthognathic problems associated with the TMJ dysfunction, but factors such as posture, the body's upper quarter musculature imbalances, and various degrees of harmful psychosomatic behaviors. Overall, TMJ symptomatic problems could be identified as simply a limitation in mandibular dynamics, frequently masked by other symptomatic pains such as chronic headaches, teeth clenching or grinding, ringing, throbbing or swishing in the ears or earaches, constant stress, face and neck pain, sensitive hearing or hearing loss, difficulty swallowing, dizziness, shoulder pain, and stiffness associated with cervical-neck movement patterns.

Physical therapy goals may include: 1. Increase/decrease mandibular dynamics to be within normal limits; 2. Correction of mandibular and/or maxillofacial muscle imbalances; 3. Correction of cervical muscle imbalances; 4. Correction of postural abnormalities as related to TMJ and cervical spine disorders; and 5. Identification and retraining of stress lifestyle changes and overall behavorial changes.

Physical therapy patients generally have a series of five to six sessions with the physical therapist immediately followed by a treatment session with the attending dentist. This unique relationship between the dental therapeutics and physical therapy sessions is designed to enhance the ability to detect subtle gains made through physical therapy which can immediately be capitalized upon by the dentist.

Our comprehensive physical therapy program incorporates mobilization and disc recapturing techniques, postural and strengthening exercises, complemented by basic physical therapy modalities to insure long-lasting carryover of positive behavior patterns.

In conclusion, interdisciplinary work of physical therapy and dentistry enhances both professions' ability to successfully treat patients with temporomandibular joint dysfunction.

An investigation into the inter-relationship between clinical measurement of cervical posture, and X-ray measurement of cervical lordosis and Hyoid bone position.

Bryden, L., Power, A.,
The Royal Free Hospital, Hampstead, London.

ABSTRACT
The link between temperomandibular joint (TMJ) dysfunction, cervical spine dysfunction and hyoid bone position is unclear to date. This study looks at measuring static cervical posture both clinically and on X-ray and compares these measurements to the Hyoid bone position on X-ray. It has been suggested that abnormal hyoid bone position can affect mandibular and consequently TMJ mechanics,which in turn may lead to TMJ pathomechanics and dysfunction.
Five female subjects aged between 18 and 37, all of which were attending an orthodontic clinic at the time of data collection were analysed. The authors conclude that due to a limited sample size the results were not statistically significant. However trends in data would tend to indicate that a relationship does exist between clinical and x-ray measured cervical posture and that the degree of elevation or depression of the hyoid bone tends to reflect cervical posture.
If these trends are accurate, then clinicians who deal with both TMJ and cervical dysfunction must be aware of the inter-relationship these structures have and the ramifications of cervical dysfunction possibly leading to TMJ problems.

INTRODUCTION
TMJ dysfunction is a syndrome which has attracted increasing attention by dentists and physiotherapists over the past ten years.
Several authors claim that the head, neck, hyoid, mandible and shoulder girdle form an interdependent biomechanical unit. Therefore dysfunction in one area may lead to dysfunction in another area by altering the position and thereby the function of structures in relation to one another.
Various studies (1.,2.,3.) using cephalometric x-rays have investigated the inter-relationship between TMJ biomechanics, head and neck posture, hyoid position, tongue position and occlusal patterns. Only a few authors have studied hyoid position on x-ray in relation to the mandible, cervical posture on x-ray and clinical cervical posture. All of these authors recognise the unique anatomy of the hyoid which provides attachment for the muscles, ligaments and fascia of pharynx, mandible, cranium and cervical spine.
In reviewing the literature on measurement of hyoid bone position authors vary greatly in their methods of measurement(1.,4.). Literature is also lacking in the measurement of cervical spine posture on x-ray in relation to hyoid and mandibular position.
Few of the postural studies compare the changes of clinical cervical posture to cervical posture on x-ray, even though many authors (5.,6.,7.) state that a forward head posture is commonly observed on patients with TMJ dysfunction and cervical spine dysfunction. This raises the question of whether patients are asymptomatic and who have forward head postures are at risk of developing TMJ dysfunction.
The hypotheses under investigation are:
1. that there is a relationship between hyoid position on x-ray and cervical posture measured clinically.
2. that there is a relationship between hyoid position on x-ray and cervical curvature on x-ray.

METHOD
Five subjects between the age of 18 and 37 years underwent on x-ray examination followed by a clinical postural assessment. Apparatus reliability,

inter and intra-operator reliability were calculated prior to the investigation and showed high reproducibility.
Measurement of clinical cervical posture was determined by using a posture profile apparatus. X-ray measurements of cervical posture and hyoid position were calculated from lateral cephalometric x-rays. (1.)(Figs. 1.and 2.)

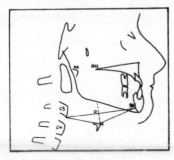

Figure 1. THE HYOID TRIANGLE
Reproduced from Bibby et al.(1.)

Figure 2. Clinical Measurement of Posture.

RESULTS
The data was analysed using Spearman's correlation test. The results showed:
1. a strong correlation($p < .0001$) between hyoid position on x-ray and cervical curvature on x-ray.
2. a strong positive correlation ($p<.0001$) between hyoid position on x-ray and clinical cervical posture.
3. a positive correlation($p<.01$) between clinical cervical posture and cervical curvature on x-ray.

Table 1. Summary of Results

Patient	Degree of Cervical Lordosis (high figure indicates greater degree of lordosis)	Degree of Cervical Lordosis on X-ray + = Lordosis − = Kyphosis	Position of Hyoid Bone in relation to C3-RGN on X-ray. + = below line − = above line
1	44	+4.0	+2.0
2	56	+1.0	−1.0
3	56	−2.0	−1.5
4	38	+6.0	+8.0
5	57	−4.0	−3.0

DISCUSSION
The sample size needs to be increased to validate the trend shown by the first five subjects.
The results support Rocabado (2.,7.) who states that a normal cervical posture on x-ray will give a hyoid position below a line drawn between C3 and the mandibular symphysis (C3-RGN),(Fig.1.).When there is a straightening or kyphosis of the cervical curvature he states that the hyoid bone will be on or above the line C3 -RGN. Rocabado also related these three positions of the hyoid bone to the craniovertebral angle but states that the position of the hyoid bone is more related to the curvature of the cervical spine than to the craniovertebral relationship.
The results of this study showed that the relationship between clinical measurement of the cervical spine and the hyoid bone position was different to the relationship demonstrated between x-ray measurement of cervical posture and hyoid position, although in both cases a relationship existed. On clinical measurement a greater degree of cervical lordosis correlated to a hyoid position on or above the line C3-RGN. When measured on x-ray a tendency towards straightness or kyphosis of the cervical spine correlated with a hyoid

position above this line. It is therefore interesting to examine a third relationship, that between the clinical and x-ray measurement of cervical posture. Here the results show that an increased clinical measurement of lordosis correlates with an x-ray measurement of reduced lordosis.
The results are also in agreement with authors who have linked changes in the position of the mandible to changes in cervical spine posture (8.,6.).
In this study the craniovertebral relationship has not been investigated and it's effect on the measurements we have taken are unknown. A previous study (9.) found that there was no significant correlation between hyoid bone position and the magnitude of change in head position and this is supported by Rocabado(2.).

SUMMARY AND CONCLUSIONS
Due to the small sample size this study can only be considered to be a pilot study. However if the trends are accurate then cervical spine posture and hyoid bone position are related and thus cervical posture may have an effect on TMJ mechanics and visa-versa.
This raises the question of whether or not subjects with a forward head posture are at risk of developing TMJ dysfunction and indicates that clinicians dealing with problems of both the cervical spine and TMJ need to be aware of the relationship between these two areas.
Also of importance is that clinical observation of cervical spine posture may be misleading in that apparent lordotic postures in the clinical situation may actually be kyphotic in the mid and lower cervical spine when viewed on x-ray.

REFERENCES
1.Bibby, R.E. & Preston, C.B.,(1981) The Hyoid Triangle. American Journal of orthodontics. 80, (1). 92-97.
2.Rocabado, M.,(1983) Biomechanical Relationship of the Cranial, Cervical, and Hyoid Regions. Physical Therapy. 1:3, 62-66.
3.Tallgren, A. & Solow, B.,(1984) Long-term changes in hyoid bone position and craniocervical posture in complete denture wearers. ACTA Odontol.Scand.42:257-267.
4.Stepovich, M.L.,(1965) A Cephalometric Positional Study of the Hyoid Bone. American Journal of Orthodontics.882-900:Dec.
5.Friedman, M.H. & Weisberg, J.,(1982) Application of Orthopaedic Principles in Evaluation of the Temporomandibular Joint. Physical Therapy. 62:5, 597-602.
6.Passero, P.L., Wyman, B.S., Bell, J.W., Hirschey, S.A. & Schlosser, W.S.,(1985) Temporomandibular Joint Dysfunction Syndrome: A Clinical Report. Physical Therapy. 65:8, 1203-1207.
7.Rocabado, M.,(1981) Diagnosis and Treatment of Abnormal Craniocervical and Craniomandibular Mechanics. Rocabado Institute.1-21.
8.Mohl, N.,(1976) Head Posture and its Role in Occlusion. N. Y. Dental Journal.42:January, 17-23.
9.Gustavsson, U., Hansson, G., Holmqvist, A. & Lundberg, M.,(1972)Hyoid Bone Position in Relation to Posture. Swedish Dental Journal. 65, 411-421.

MANUAL THERAPY IN POST-INJECTION TRISMUS - TWO CASE REPORTS

YADAVA N.S.   SUPDT. PHYSIOTHERAPIST
RATTAN P.   SENIOR PHYSIOTHERAPIST
UTREJA A.   ASSOC.PROF.DENTAL SURG.

POSTGRADUATE INSTITUTE OF MEDICAL EDUCATION AND RESEARCH
                CHANDIGARH (INDIA)

INTRODUCTION : Trismus is the inability to open the mouth partially or completely. It can be due to various reasons like tetanus, inflammation or spasm of masticatory muscles as a result of infection or trauma, T.M.joint arthritis, T.M. joint sublaxation or fracture dislocation of the condyloid process of mandible.

Rarely it may be due to an injection in the medial pterygoid muscle. Medial pterogoid muscle is a thick quardriangular muscle, main fibres arising from medial surface of lateral pterygoid plate of sphenoid bone and from the grooved surface of pyramidal process of palatine bone. It passes downward slightly laterally and posteriorly attaching to the inner surface of the mandibular angle. It is supplied by trigeminal nerve.

When an injection is given in the muscle, the trauma may lead to moderate degree of temporary trismus which recovers with assisted mouth exercises. However, at times it may persist for considerable time which is due to the formation of a band of fibrous scar tissue present in the vicinity of pterygoid muscle which restricts normal opening of the mouth.

'Seward' in hospital practice estimates this occurance as only two to three times in 100,000 cases.

CASE NO. 1

I.J. 41 years old male reported to the department with inability to open the mouth for the past 10 days. 12 days earlier he visited a dentist for the treatment of his left lower second molar. An inferior alveolar block of 'Xylocaine and Adrenalin' was given and temporary filling done. Within 2 days patient complained of pain and developed complete trismus for which he consulted the dentist again. He was advised to do hot fomentation and active mouth opening exercise which did not improve his condition at all. History of injection 2-3 days prior to inability to open the mouth in absence of any other trauma clearly indicated that it was a case of 'Post-injection trismus'.

CASE NO. II

S.L.52 M, inability to open mouth 15 days. History of left 2nd mollar extraction. Patient received 2-3 pricks of anaesthetic injection and stiches were done after extraction which were removed after 5 days. In the evening patient complained of inability to open mouth and mild pain radiating up and down the jaw. Pain killers gave no relief. From history and absence of any other disease, diagnosis of trismus was confirmed.

INVESTIGATIONS/EXAMINATION

1. Pain and tenderness over(left) T.M.joint area, probably due to spasm of medial pterygoid muscle.

2. Opening of mouth not more than 1 Cm.

3. Painful clenching of teeth and difficulty in mastication.

4. Some spasm over cervical and trapizius region.

5. No fever, swelling or sensory loss, ruling out infection or nerve involvement.

6. Deviation of mandible on opening of mouth.

7. CAT Scan of T.M. joint revealed normal study.

CASE I- TREATMENT

Physiotherapy treatment was instituted on the same day which consisted of ultra-sonics, heat and manual therapy,

-   10 sittings of ultra-sonic 1 watt/Cm for 3 mts over the pterygoid muscle were given.

-   5 Sittings of hot packs covering neck and (left) side of the face were given. It was discontinued once tenderness and pain disappeared.

-   For its deeper heating effects diathermy was started after 5 sittings and 10 sittings were given in all.

-   Since the patient was unable to open the mouth, manual therapy in the form of external friction massage over pterygoid muscle and lateral mobilisation of jaw within the limits of pain was given. 3 cervical manipulations relieved cervical and trepizius muscle spasm. Manual assisted and resisted mouth opening exercises were also given.

On 5th days, when opening of mouth increased to more than one finger, per oral manipulation of T.M.joint as per 'Cyriax' technique was started. Pain and tenderness subsided after 7 sittings and mastication became normal. After 10 sittings, mouth opening increased to 2 fingers, but deviation of mouth persisted. In all it took 15 sittings for the patient to be fully asymptomatic.

CASE II TREATMENT

For 2-3 days patient had dental gauge and exercises
at home only with no relief. Physiotherapy started on 15th
day in form of U.S. and external manipulation. After 4 days
one finger opening of mouth was possible. Now per-oral manipulation and US were carried on for one week. Patient made
near normal recovery before stopping the treatment.

TECHNIQUE OF MANIPULATION

If the trismus is on left side the therapist
stabilises the(left) Frontotemporal area with his left hand.
Fingers of right hand grip the mandible and by putting the
right thumb on the left molars medially, the mandible is
distracted downwards and outwards from temporal bone. When
adequate separation is achieved after few seconds of triction
this movement is repeated slowly and rythmically,5-7 times.

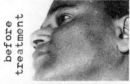

before treatment   during treatment   after treatment

CONCLUSION : Both the patients were treated with special
manual therapy technique alongwith palliative physiotherapy
for relief of pain and spasm. They responded very well leading
to full recovery. Therefore, this non-invasive method is
strongly recommended in comparison to treatment like manipulation under general anesthesia or surgery etc. which has its
own inherent problems. It is also evident that this method
will prove useful in other non-infective condition like T.M.
arthritis muscle spasm etc. which restricts mouth opening.

REFERENCES

1.   H.C.Killey/L.W,Kay; (1969) Prevention of complica-
      tions in dental surgery, E & S livingstone Ltd
      Edinburg and London P 69, 70

2.   John Warfel(1974) The head, neck and Trunk; lea and
      febriger, Philadelphia, P.32.

3.   James Cyriax(1971) Text book of orthopaedic medicine
      Vol.2.

4.   Joyce Sheriff; Temporo-mandibular joint pain-I and
      K.Smith, temporo mandibular joint pain-2(1989);
      Physiotherapy, Vol. 75, No.9, P.502-3-4.

5.   Tipton Paul A.: (1990) Temporomandibular Joint
      Dysfunction – A Restorative Dentist's View.
      Physiotherapy, Vol. 10,P.608-610.

AUTHORS INDEX

AUTHORS INDEX

L Dawson	O-289	183
G De Domenico	O-314	606
G De Domenico	O-139	1083
L de Groot	O-275	1199
J Dekker	P-046	1679
J Dekker	O-262	99
W H M den Hartog	O-471	1584
A Devreese	O-108	872
W de Weerdt	O-123	510
K J Dick	O-356	1230
E Domholdt	O-096	1664
M Donaghy	O-131	975
A Dossa	O-491	937
A Dossa	P-084	50
A Dossa	O-361	1763
B R Durward	P-035	857
B R Durward	O-191	1292
B R Durward	O-181	447
E L Eddy	O-351	207
J E Edelstein	O-380	414
S K Effgen	O-428	1233
D J El-Din	O-454	1716
F Endo	O-312	600
M Engardt	O-220	1298
M Engardt	O-022	472
C S Enwemeka	O-215	812
C S Enwemeka	O-061	673
A Eriksson	O-070	734
A Eriksson	O-216	815
N T Farina	O-346	192
A J Fernando	O-193	228
N P Fisher	O-011	403
N P Fisher	P-051	1125
T Fujiwara	O-317	614
T Fukai	P-065	1075
M C Fyfe	O-375	1385
R Gailey	O-185	655
R Gailey	O-058	647
R Gailey	O-054	635
R Gailey	O-056	641
R Gailey	O-183	650
R Gant	O-484	1473
J M Gardner	P-011	623
B A Garrett	P-076	1555
L Gatsi	O-221	1301
C G Gaughwin	O-472	1587
C Gauthier-Gagnon	O-187	661
M R Gersh	O-062	676
L S Gifford	1FOMT-005	1785
D G Gilbert	O-008	395
M E Glendinning	O-218	1732
L Golin	O-057	644
M Goodman	O-414	1754
M Goodman	O-279	1211
H Gosselink	P-056	953

S A Hyde	O-271	1190
U Ingwersen	P-059	1545
B Ireland	O-152	15
S H Irwin-Carruthers	P-075	1552
S H Irwin-Carruthers	O-473	1590
H Ito	O-229	1006
N Ito	O-331	1367
T Iwasaki	O-188	1283
H Iwatsuki	O-419	1043
J A Jackson	O-352	210
J M Jackson	O-446	514
J E Jackson	O-234	1741
R Jackson	O-389	1401
S E Jackson	O-292	1741
J A Jameson	O-098	1670
J A Jameson	O-474	1593
M-H Jan	P-024	1492
G-B Jarnlo	O-382	420
M L Jayne	P-050	125
W J Jefferson	P-016	632
S Jensen	P-071	89
A Y M Jones	O-080	763
A Y M Jones	O-295	270
C B Jones	O-326	716
M C Jones	O-028	548
G A Jull	P-032	850
Y P Kane	O-387	1395
S-L Karppi	O-304	1343
T L Kauffman	P-013	625
S P Kaye	O-235	1744
M Kazuki	O-417	1037
K M Kerr	P-030	844
R Keskinen-Rosenqvist	O-065	687
G L Key	O-311c	1638
E M L Kinnear	O-089	1643
J A Klaber Moffett	O-079	760
L C Kloth	O-084	788
B W Koes	O-002	374
J M Kottoor	O-475	1596
A Koube	O-178	438
M W Krause	P-019	779
S Kukkonen	O-155	22
A Kumai	P-039	1511
H Kuroki	P-062	539
A Kusoffsky	O-448	520
A Kvaale	O-260	93
A Kvaale	O-284	116
J L Lacey	O-274	1196
R K Ladyshewsky	O-460	308
R K Ladyshewsky	O-348	198
L C W Laidler	O-090	1646
L C W Laidler	O-476	1599
L Lannefors	O-242	912
J Latimer	O-001	371
H T Law	O-431	1243

J Laycock	O-109	875
L Lee	O-374	286
C I Leiper	O-383	423
M Lessing-Turner	O-422	1053
D Lester	O-114	894
S Levitt	O-373	283
S Levitt	O-429	1236
J Y Li	O-212	804
C A Liggins	O-308	699
H E Lilley	O-370	1031
K-H Lin	P-052	1128
I Lindstrom	O-439	138
C B Liston	O-004	153
C B Liston	O-201	242
D Littler	P-029	841
A E Ljunggren	O-302	1337
R B Lode	O-151	10
T M Long	O-282	1220
T M Long	O-280	1214
T M Long	O-277	1205
R B Lopopolo	O-099	1673
O M Lundby	O-425	561
M Lusvardi	O-244	1112
M E Lynch	O-228	1005
M MacKay-Lyons	O-132	978
M MacKay-Lyons	O-172	1274
F Macchiavello	P-026	1494
S F H Mackintosh	O-392	1408
M E Mahato	O-420	1046
M J Majsak	O-231	1012
E Mälkiä	O-306	1349
E Mälkiä	O-162	1160
P Mancilla	O-293	266
K J Manella	O-390	1404
C J Manheim	P-018	778
C J Manheim	O-309	702
J Mantle	O-434	884
T Marovino	O-073	746
E Marshall	O-467	220
D Martin	O-324	1093
S C Martin	O-355	1227
K Maruta	O-334	1377
D W Maskill	O-367	1022
M R Mason	O-330	1366
S Matsumura	O-381	417
H J Matthews	O-395	1416
E Mattsson	O-485	1476
E Mattsson	O-180	444
M J Mayston	O-391	1405
H McBurney	O-489	931
A McCoy	O-163	1161
M P McCoy	O-192	225
M P McCoy	O-462	312
M P McCoy	O-005	156
C L McGarvey	O-052	594

C L McGarvey	O-055	638
T C McGarvey	O-033	1575
C C McGinley	O-290	257
J M McIntosh	O-087	795
J M McIntosh	O-034	1577
J M McIntosh	P-044	1526
J M McMeeken	O-322	1358
A McMillan	O-362	1766
C A Meaden	O-043	1622
R Mele	O-146	1133
A Middleditch	1FOMT-002	1779
E C Minnigh	O-372	282
S Miyashita	P-036	858
S Moe	O-437	135
B Mokhtar	O-077	756
G Möller	O-236	1747
K Monsen	O-066	690
M Moon	O-285	119
M Moon	P-021	781
M Moon	P-045	1531
G Mooney	K-004	1567
E T Morris	O-173	1277
M E Morris	O-021	469
M E Morris	O-119	496
S C Morrison	O-316	611
J R Morton	O-401	1427
A M Moseley	O-177	998
R M B Mpofu	O-349	201
A A Mugglestone	P-043	1523
A A Mugglestone	O-081	766
S Mungovan	O-025	478
S F Mungovan	O-222	1304
I M Musa	O-256	168
R H Mushet	O-442	1456
R S Myers	O-200	241
R S Myers	O-088	798
U Myhr	O-332	1373
I Nara	O-450	526
O N Narbekov	O-320	715
R A Newton	O-176	995
R A Newton	O-013	406
V M Nieland	O-345	189
A M Nieuwboer	O-210	1710
E Nikola	P-023	1489
L Nilsson-Wikmar	O-006	389
L Nilsson	O-026	481
N Nirsimloo	O-086	794
N Nirsimloo	O-083	787
J E Nitschke	O-126	960
L A Nordholm	O-465	214
A S Norlen	O-490	934
L L K Noronen	P-073	323
J C Nosworthy	O-340	925
R L Nutt	O-335	1380
S H Nyyssonen	P-069	84

C M O'Hagan	O-014	409
B Oberg	O-404	1434
B Oberg	O-443	1459
U Oberg	O-100	823
G I Odia	O-113	891
S Ogiwara	O-441	1453
H Okeke	O-101	826
L Olséni	O-336	915
E Olsson	O-384	453
E Olsson	O-182	450
E Olsson	O-015	429
R A B Oostendorp	O-048	584
Z Z Osmonbekova	P-025	1493
A Overmire	O-457	1725
B Pangrsic	O-124	511
A Parry	O-313	603
C J Partridge	O-379	412
C J Partridge	O-118	493
J Paul	O-160	37
I W Peacock	O-481	1068
G Peninou	O-191a	1295
J Perks	O-156	25
S Petersen-Testrup	O-091	1647
P Petriccione de Vadi	O-082	769
L A Pfalzer	O-436	132
G Pierron	O-127	963
J J M Pool	O-129	967
A Poulis	O-249	1312
S Poulis	O-482	1467
T Poyhonen	P-038	1508
T Poyhonen	P-037	1505
E Price	O-270	1187
M M Primozic	O-247	1120
R Puricelli	O-143	1102
P Rafferty	O-007	392
M R Raji	O-469	819
E L Ramsden	O-198	237
E L Ramsden	O-136	164
E L Ramsden	O-194	236
G Rasmussen	P-063	1073
M J Reid Campion	O-174	988
C A Richardson	O-102	829
M Rigo	O-252	1319
A Riising	O-196	233
M E Rinehart	O-142	1099
M E Rinehart	P-072	251
M B Rinne	O-153	18
P A Roche	O-286	122
P A Roche	P-027	1497
W E Rodes-Bauer	O-140	1086
D Rodriguez	O-203	1689
A Ronikier	O-245	1114
B Rosblad	O-170	1180
B R Ross	O-416	1034
G Rossi	P-042	1520

P J Rowe	O-027	545
P J Rowe	O-385	456
P J Rowe	O-388	1398
G Roxendal	O-063	681
A Ryhanen	P-040	1514
M Sabbahi	O-044	1625
N Sabiel	P-006	1259
C Sackley	O-023	475
G Saeboe	O-265	106
M Sakamoto	O-305	1346
T Sakamoto	O-059	667
S Sakoh	O-329	1363
P M Salter	O-208	1704
M K Sanford	P-078	1557
S Sastre	O-250	1315
S Saunders	O-319	714
M N Sauriol	O-458	304
R J Savage	O-338	921
E Schell	O-032	560
G Schmuck	O-426	564
E Schweizer	P-003	1254
S M Scott	O-072	743
D R Scrutton	L-004	367
I Searles	P-002	1253
D M Selkowitz	O-227	1001
K Shepard	O-363	1769
K F Shepard	O-343	301
R B Shepherd	O-190	1289
T D Shields	O-085	791
L Silverstolpe	O-069	731
J Sim	O-207	1701
J D Simpson	O-333	1376
C Sinderby	O-239	903
C Sinderby	O-243	1109
M A Skinner	O-291	260
E M Sluijs	O-154	21
E M Sluijs	P-083	49
A C B Smith	P-028	1498
A C B Smith	O-145	1106
E Smith	O-092	1650
K M Sodring	O-116	487
P Solomon	P-048	1681
P Solomon	O-258	173
Zh B Soodonbekova	O-451	529
F K St George	O-300	1331
K H Stappaerts	O-350	204
B Steinrud	O-195	230
C H Stenstrom	O-031	557
A T Sterle	O-053	597
C Stevens	O-164	1164
S J Stikeleather	O-400	384
K Stiller	O-240	906
L I Strand	O-261	96
R Strom	P-085	53
M J Sullivan	O-276	1202

N T Watts	O-219	1735
B Webber	L-002	351
L Weidenhielm	O-030	552
A Weiner	O-051	591
H R Weiss	O-339	922
G Wennerberg	O-067	693
H Wennergren	O-010	400
E Wersall-Robertson	O-029	549
M G Westmorland	O-410	332
P C Westwood	P-015	631
J R Wheeler	P-082	48
B Wikander	O-479	1062
K E Wilk	O-403	1433
K E Wilk	O-049	585
C Willèn	O-042	1619
J E Williams	O-050	586
R Williams	O-259	176
M A Willson	O-046	1631
A Winberg	O-133	981
L Wingate	O-110	878
E Wolgast	O-357	66
P G Wood	O-464	318
P G Wood	O-297	276
N S Yadava	O-148	1139
M Yamada	P-061	536
M Yamaguchi	O-394	1413
C Yamamoto	O-241	909
K Yanagisawa	O-368	1025
A Ye Asheraliyeva	O-078	759
M Yekutiel	O-449	523
T Yoneda	O-423	1056
J E Zachazewski	O-179	441
V N Zalessky	O-141	1089
V N Zalessky	O-325	1096